Immunotherapy Against Lung Cancer

Shvetank Bhatt • Rajaraman Eri Eri •
Bey-Hing Goh • Keshav Raj Paudel •
Terezinha de Jesus Andreoli Pinto •
Kamal Dua
Editors

Immunotherapy Against Lung Cancer

Emerging Opportunities and Challenges

Springer

Editors
Shvetank Bhatt
School of Health Sciences and Technology
Dr. Vishwanath Karad MIT World Peace University
Pune, Maharashtra, India

Bey-Hing Goh
Sunway Biofunctional Molecules Discovery Centre (SBMDC), School of Medical and Life Sciences
Sunway University
Bandar Sunway, Selangor, Malaysia

Terezinha de Jesus Andreoli Pinto
School of Pharmaceutical Sciences
University of Sao Paulo
Sao Paulo, São Paulo, Brazil

Rajaraman Eri Eri
STEM College
RMIT University
Melbourne, VIC, Australia

Keshav Raj Paudel
Faculty of Science
University of Technology Sydney
Camperdown, NSW, Australia

Kamal Dua
Discipline of Pharmacy, Graduate School of Health, Faculty of Health
University of Technology Sydney
Schofields, NSW, Australia

ISBN 978-981-99-7140-4 ISBN 978-981-99-7141-1 (eBook)
https://doi.org/10.1007/978-981-99-7141-1

This Springer imprint is published by the registered company Springer Nature Singapore Pte Ltd.
The registered company address is: 152 Beach Road, #21-01/04 Gateway East, Singapore 189721, Singapore

Paper in this product is recyclable.

*"In memory of my beloved sister, Shipra,
who lost her life in the battle against cancer"*

Dr. Shvetank Bhatt

Preface

Cancer is a leading cause of death worldwide, accounting for nearly ten million deaths in 2020, or nearly one in six deaths. Head and Neck, breast, liver, pancreatic, gastro-esophageal, bladder, lung, colorectal, blood, and prostate cancers are the most common cancers. Cancer occurs when cells in the body start multiplying in an uncontrollable manner. This is due to modifications in apoptotic pathways and related mechanisms. The diseases normally start with a small area and become localized, and in the later stages cells become metastasized in different locations in the body.

Immunotherapy is a newer and potential treatment approach that has emerged for the treatment of various types of cancers and works through the stimulation of the immunity of the patient. The goal of cancer immunotherapy is to boost or restore the ability of the immune system to detect and destroy cancer cells by overcoming the mechanisms by which tumors evade and suppress the immune response in essence to shift the equilibrium back in favor of immune protection. The hallmark of the adaptive immune response is specificity and long-term memory, which, when present, can result in durable responses. These therapies are more active against cancer cells which have tumor microenvironment around them. Some tumors like lung cancer, bladder cancer, and renal cell carcinoma have a rich immune microenvironment and respond well to immunotherapy.

The treatment of lung cancer includes surgery, radiotherapy, chemotherapy, targeted therapy, and the most advanced immunotherapy. These therapies are specifically targeted and having less side effects as compared to conventional chemotherapy. Immunotherapies such as PD-1/PD-L1 inhibitors, CTLA-4 inhibitors, IDO inhibitors, LAG-3 inhibitors, and TGF-β inhibitors are in clinical trials and are receiving approval for the treatment of lung cancer. These therapies are also evaluated as monotherapy or in combination with other chemotherapy or targeted therapy for their anticancer activity. In addition to above treatments, various vaccines and oncolytic viruses also have significant potential for the treatment of lung cancer. These drugs increase the overall survival and progression-free survival of lung cancer patients. The chapters in this book cover all the major immunotherapeutic approaches used for the treatment of lung cancer.

We hope the book shall be a useful compilation for undergraduate, postgraduate, doctoral students, and researchers working in cancer and drug delivery research,

research and development, and national research institutes. We hope to receive feedback, suggestions, and inputs from researchers and students that will help improve the next edition of the book.

Pune, Maharashtra, India — Shvetank Bhatt
Melbourne, VIC, Australia — Rajaraman Eri Eri
Bandar Sunway, Selangor, Malaysia — Bey-Hing Goh
Camperdown, NSW, Australia — Keshav Raj Paudel
Sao Paulo, São Paulo, Brazil — Terezinha de Jesus Andreoli Pinto
Schofields, NSW, Australia — Kamal Dua

Acknowledgments

I would like to express my sincere gratitude to the Honorable Founder-President, Dr. Vishwanath Karad, and Executive President, Mr. Rahul V. Karad, of Dr. Vishwanath Karad MIT World Peace University, Pune, India, for their motivation. My heartfelt thanks go to Dr. Neeraj Mahindroo, Professor and Dean of the School of Health Sciences and Technology at Dr. Vishwanath Karad MIT World Peace University, Pune, India, for his continuous support during the writing of this book. Finally, I would like to extend my gratitude to the faculty members of the School of Health Sciences and Technology at Dr. Vishwanath Karad MIT World Peace University, Pune, India.

Dr. Shvetank Bhatt

Contents

About the Editors

Shvetank Bhatt is currently working as an Associate Professor in the School of Health Sciences and Technology, Dr. Vishwanath Karad MIT World Peace University, Pune, Maharashtra, India. He has done M.Pharm in Pharmacology from Manipal College of Pharmaceutical Sciences, MAHE, Manipal, Karnataka, and Ph.D. in Neuropharmacology from Birla Institute of Technology & Science (BITS) Pilani, Pilani Campus, Rajasthan. He has a total 16 years of industrial and academic research experience. His area of specialization is CNS disorders, pain, inflammation, and immuno-oncology. He is a recipient of Prof. Duggirala Visweswaram & Prof. Sreemantalu Satyanarayana Award (Best Paper in Pharmacology-IJPER) in 2012 and 2014. He has published more than 90 papers in various journals of national and international repute. He has also published two books with Springer. He is a life member of Association of Pharmaceutical Teachers of India (APTI) and Indian Pharmacological Society (IPS).

Rajaraman Eri is the Associate Dean at the School of Science at RMIT University in Melbourne. Prof. Eri is a veterinarian turned biomedical scientist who specializes in research investigations into colorectal cancer, functional foods (dietary fiber),clinical nutrition, and gut health. Raj was awarded a master's degree in Veterinary Medicine (TN Veterinary and Animal Sciences University, India) followed by his Ph.D. from the University of Queensland in molecular and cell biology in 2001. His subsequent postdoctoral training in the USA included research work mainly investigating both innate and adaptive immune responses and associated aspects of clinical translation. Between 2006 and 2010, Dr. Raj joined UQ-Mater Medical Research Institute, Brisbane, as a senior research officer where he was involved in groundbreaking work illustrating the role of endoplasmic reticulum stress in the pathogenesis of bowel diseases. In late 2010, he joined UTAS as an independent investigator developing a research laboratory dedicated to gut health, establishing an international reputation in this area over a decade. On the teaching side, he coordinates and teaches in the fields of biosciences, immunology, nutrition, and biochemistry. Dr. Raj has won multiple teaching awards including the Australian national citation for excellence in teaching in 2017.

Bey Hing Goh is a full-time professor of biochemistry at Sunway University (Malaysia) and leads the Sunway Biofunctional Molecules Discovery Centre (SBMD). His research focuses on the functionality of natural products from herbs, microbes, and algae. With over 200 scientific articles, books, and patents, he has over 8000 citations and an H-index of 51. Goh provides professional advice to biotech, aquaculture, and wellness companies and excels in education—receiving awards for teaching innovation. Goh's contributions to research, education, and community, together with his dedication to biology, earned him recognition as a Top 10 Outstanding Young Malaysian in 2020 and placed him as the first Malaysian on the Advisory Board of the International Natural Product Sciences Taskforce.

Keshav Raj Paudel is a recipient of IASLC fellowship (currently at mid-career researcher stage) at the Centre for Inflammation, Centenary Institute/UTS. He completed his Ph.D. (2017) from Mokpo National University, South Korea, and started his first postdoctoral research at the University of Texas Health Science Center at Houston Texas, USA-2018, on a NIH-funded project.

He is an emerging scientist with good scientific track records demonstrated through his publications and successful grants. After joining UTS in 2019 for a second postdoctoral position, his research trajectory is continuously upraising in the field of translational research with a major focus on r^ $690K), including IASLC ECR fellowship-2019 (lead CI) and TSANZ grant-in-aid-2021 (lead CI). He has published more than 130 peer-reviewed scientific articles in leading journals such as the *European Respiratory Journal, Trends in Food Science and Technology, Medical Journal of Australia, Medicinal Research Review, Cell reports, Cell death and disease,* and *Journal of Controlled Release, Critical Reviews in Food Science and Nutrition.* He has also published six book chapters and one book as an editor. His scientific publications have been cited more than 2900 times, with an h-index of 30 and an i-10 index of 60 (google scholar). He is also a reviewer of more than 50 journals reviewing 145 papers so far and editor of more than 10 journals handling 115 papers so far.

Terezinha de Jesus Andreoli Pinto is a full Professor at the School of Pharmaceutical Sciences, University of Sao Paulo. Professor Terezinha holds more than 40 years of sound experience in academia and researches on parenteral (formulation, analytical, microbiological, and performance methods) and medical devices. Professor Terezinha authored 180 articles in scientific journals, more than 12 book chapters, and also holds two patents. Alongside her career, Professor Terezinha took on management roles in the University, such as being dean of School of Pharmacy for two mandates (2004–2008 and 2012–2016) and also being chair of Deliberative Board of FURP—a pharmaceutical firm that manufactures products from the WHO Essential Medicines list, run by Sao Paulo State Government. Strong scientific skills coupled with leadership and management abilities enabled her to establish agreements with internationally prestigious institutions, including the University of Alberta, Lisbon, and Bath. Under her supervision, the CONFAR Laboratory was set up, the only Brazilian state university laboratory accredited by the National Institute of Metrology, Quality and Technology (INMETRO) (ISO/IEC 17025) and authorized by the National Agency of Sanitary Surveillance (ANVISA) and the Ministry of Agriculture, Livestock, and Supplies (MAPA), and is considered a reference both in Brazil and overseas, in the analytical area. Professor Terezinha is also involved with standard-setting activities in agencies such as Brazilian Pharmacopeia (as coordinator of the Brazilian Pharmacopeia Drug Product and Medical Devices technical committee, and currently member of Biological and Biotechnological Products Committee), International Standard Organization (ISO) as Brazilian Association of Technical Norms (ABNT) representative, and also the United States Pharmacopeia stakeholder with participation in convention current cycle.

Kamal Dua is a Senior Lecturer in the Discipline of Pharmacy at the Graduate School of Health, University of Technology Sydney (UTS), Australia. He has research experience of over 13 years in the field of drug delivery systems targeting inflammatory diseases. Dr. Dua is also a Node Leader of Drug Delivery Research in the Centre for Inflammation at Centenary Institute/UTS, where the targets identified from the research projects are pursued to develop novel formulations as the first step towards translation into clinics. Dr. Dua conducts research in two complementary areas: drug delivery and immunology, specifically addressing how these disciplines can advance one another, helping the community to live longer and healthier. This is evidenced by his extensive publication record in reputed journals. Dr. Dua's research interests focus on harnessing the pharmaceutical potential of modulating critical regulators such as Interleukins and microRNAs and developing new and effective drug delivery formulations for the management of chronic airway diseases. He has published more than 100 research articles in peer-reviewed international journals and authored or coauthored four books. He is an active member of many national and international professional societies.

Introduction to Lung Cancer

1

Rohini Pujari, Sujit Kumar Sah, and Shvetank Bhatt

1.1 Introduction

Worldwide, there are many different cancers that affect people, most of which are characterised by uncontrolled cell growth and the spread of cancerous cells into neighbouring local tissues. Lung cancer has been one of the most frequently diagnosed cancer types in the globe for many years. Lung cancer accounts for 11.6% of all cancer diagnoses globally, and both cancer incidence and mortality rates are growing (Sung et al. 2021).

With 18.4% of all cancer fatalities still attributable to lung cancer, this disease continues to be the biggest financial and social burden on society. The unchecked division of aberrant cells in one or both lungs is known as lung cancer. According to incidence and death rates, it is the most frequent cancer in males, and it is the second most common illness in women after breast cancer (Carbone et al. 2015).

1.2 Etiology of Lung Cancer

Only 10–15% of lung cancer diagnoses occur in people who have never smoked, with long-term smoking accounting for the vast majority (90%) of instances (Huang et al. 2022). The risk of developing lung cancer is highest among smokers over 50 who have a history of smoking, and moreover, the male smokers are at the highest risk. Lung cancer risk factors include smoking, radon gas exposure, asbestos exposure, air pollution, and genetic predisposition. According to Neal et al. (2019), smoking is responsible for about three-fourths of lung cancer diagnoses, with the

R. Pujari · S. K. Sah · S. Bhatt (✉)
School of Health Sciences and Technology, Dr. Vishwanath Karad MIT World Peace University, Pune, Maharashtra, India

S. Bhatt et al. (eds.), *Immunotherapy Against Lung Cancer*,
https://doi.org/10.1007/978-981-99-7141-1_1

remaining instances being caused by radon exposure, environmental pollution, and occupation-specific variables.

The danger rises when additional chemicals, including asbestos, are exposed. The risk of lung cancer is increased by 20–30% by passive smoking. Radiation for the treatment of cancers other than lung cancer, particularly non-Hodgkin's lymphoma and breast cancer, is another issue (Lorigan et al. 2005). Exposure to metals including chromium, nickel, arsenic, and polycyclic aromatic hydrocarbons is also connected to lung cancer. Independent of smoking, lung conditions such idiopathic pulmonary fibrosis raise the risk of lung cancer (Burns 2000).

Exposure to asbestos, particularly occupational exposure, increases the chance of developing lung cancer in a dose-dependent manner that varies depending on the kind of asbestos fibre. The risk of asbestos exposure outside of the workplace is less clear (Wagner 1997). Lung cancer risk among uranium workers exposed to radon was minimal but considerable (Grosche et al. 2006). Radon has also been shown to accumulate in homes as a consequence of uranium and radium decay. Residential radon poses significant risks, especially for smokers, and is thought to be responsible for 2% of lung cancer deaths in Europe, according to a meta-analysis of research conducted on that continent (Darby et al. 2005).

Epigenetic changes and genetic damage to DNA are additional causes of cancer. The routine functions of the cell, such as cell division, DNA repair, and apoptosis are affected by these alterations. These aberrant cells fail to carry out typical lung cell functions and do not grow into sound lung tissue. As more damage builds up, the likelihood of developing cancer increases (Cagle et al. 2013) (Fig. 1.1).

1.3 Epidemiology of Lung Cancer

Lung cancer cases make up the majority of cancer diagnoses worldwide (12.4% of all cancer diagnoses), as well as the majority of cancer-related deaths. According to the American Cancer Society's estimations, over 234,000 new instances of lung cancer are diagnosed each year, and over 154,000 people die as a result of lung cancer in the United States (Siegel et al. 2017). With an expected 1.8 million fatalities, lung cancer continued to be the most common kind of cancer mortality globally, according to the Global Cancer Statistics report from 2020 (Sung et al. 2021).

History suggests that the industrialised world is the only place where the lung cancer pandemic exists. Recent data indicate a sharp increase in the prevalence of lung cancer, with 49.9% of newly diagnosed cases occurring in developing nations (Barta et al. 2019). Men in the United States experience higher death rates than women do. Overall lung cancer incidence is not associated with racial difference; however, African American males have a greater age-dependant death rate than their Caucasian counterparts. Women are not treated differently in this regard (Alberg and Samet 2003).

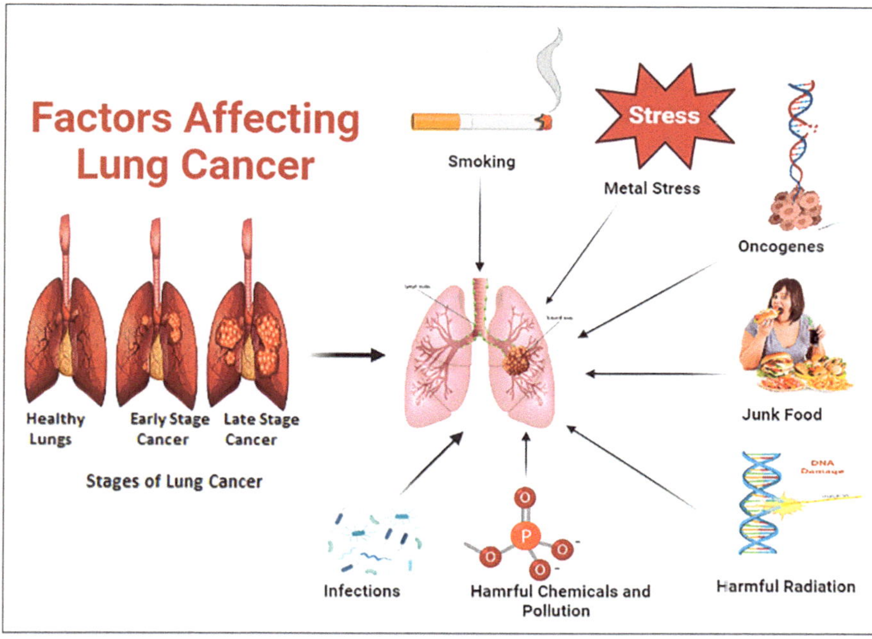

Fig. 1.1 Risk factors causing lung cancer

1.4 Classification of Lung Cancer

Non-small-cell lung cancer (NSCLC), which makes up 80–85% of all lung cancer cases, and small-cell lung cancer (SCLC), which makes up the remaining 15–20% of cases, are the two broad groups into which lung cancers are divided by the World Health Organisation (WHO). It turns out that both NSCLC and SCLC kinds of metastatic lung cancer have low survival rates, with a 5-year survival rate of only 4% (Nicholson et al. 2022).

(a) **Small-cell lung cancer (SCLC):** Heavy smokers are almost usually diagnosed with this kind of cancer. Small-cell lung cancer (SCLC), which accounts for around 15% of all lung tumours, is distinguished by an exceedingly rapid rate of proliferation, a considerable tendency for early metastasis, and a grim prognosis. With exposure to cigarette carcinogens, risk of SCLC increases. When they are diagnosed, the majority of patients have metastatic disease; just one-third have earlier-stage illness that can be treated with potentially curative multimodality therapy. According to the extent of the illness, SCLC is divided into two categories: LD-SCLC (limited disease SCLC) and ED-SCLC (extensive disease SCLC) (Aisner et al. 1990; Nicholson et al. 2022).

(b) **Non-small-cell lung cancer (NSCLC):** The term "non-small-cell lung cancer" refers to a group of lung tumours that exhibit comparable characteristics.

NSCLC include large cell carcinoma (LCC), adenocarcinoma (LUAD), and squamous cell carcinoma (LUSC). Several categories can be subcategorised within each subclass based on the molecular targetable genetic profile (Nicholson et al. 2022).

1.5 Pathophysiology of Lung Cancer

The pathophysiology of lung cancer is incredibly intricate and yet not fully understood. Lung epithelial dysplasia is thought to be brought on by repeated exposure to pollutants like cigarette smoke. Oncogenes or tumour suppressor genes become active or become inactive throughout the aetiology of lung cancer. These genes become mutated as a result of carcinogens, which results in genetic changes that have an impact on protein synthesis (Cagle et al. 2013). In turn, this disrupts the cell cycle and promotes the cancer development. MYC, BCL2, and p53 for SCLC and EGFR, KRAS, and p16 for NSCLC are the most frequent genetic alterations linked to the development of lung cancer (Lindeman et al. 2013, 2018).

In 10–30% of lung adenocarcinomas, mutations in the K-ras proto-oncogene are to blame. About 4% of non-small-cell lung cancers include an EML4-ALK tyrosine kinase fusion gene. Cancer suppressor genes may become inactive as a result of epigenetic modifications, such as variations in DNA methylation, histone tail modification, or microRNA control. The epidermal growth factor receptor (EGFR) controls several cellular processes, including cell division, apoptosis, angiogenesis, and tumour invasion. NSCLC frequently harbours EGFR mutations and amplifications, which provide the basis for EGFR inhibitor treatment (Lindeman et al. 2018).

1.6 Diagnosis

Tumours develop over time as a result of the aberrant cells, impairing lung function. This is mostly due to the absence of recognisable symptoms in the early stages of the illness, which causes a delayed diagnosis. Patients with lung cancer may either have no symptoms at all or experience a wide range of symptoms, including tiredness, unexplained weight loss, anorexia, coughing, dyspnoea, haemoptysis, and chest discomfort (Balata et al. 2022). Therefore, early lung cancer detection has shown to be rather difficult for medical experts due to the presence of non-specific symptoms. A Swedish research found that patients with lung cancer must wait 6 months between the start of symptoms and the start of treatment (Ellis and Vandermeer 2011). Lung cancer can be pathologically diagnosed via cytological or histological techniques. Clinical classification of lung cancer divides it into two categories. Both SCLC and NSCLC fall under this category. Adenocarcinomas, big cell cancers, and squamous cell cancers are the three other histological forms of NSCLC that are often detected (Bradley et al. 2019). Several techniques are employed as histological methods of analysis for identifying lung cancer, including light microscopy, bronchoscopic biopsies, needle biopsies, coupled with surgical biopsy procedures such pneumonectomy, lobectomy, excisional wedge biopsy, or thoracoscopy (Travis 2002).

1.7 Treatment Strategies

There is a crucial necessity for effective techniques to treat lung cancer, especially late-stage malignancies, despite the fact that numerous anti-cancer treatments, such as surgery, irradiation and chemotherapy, are utilised to treat NSCLC and SCLC. The lack of a platform for early-stage diagnosis and the late onset of symptoms in the course of the illness limit treatment options and survival in NSCLC, making the prognosis difficult (Zappa and Mousa 2016).

The most effective screening method now available for lung cancer patients is low-dose computed tomography (LDCT). Only 5% of the 15 million high-risk people in the USA who have been urged to get screened have so far used LDCT. Low early detection efficiency, false-positive detection, radiation risk, and a lack of resources for a CT-based screening programme are all problems with LDCT (Ramalingam and Belani 2008).

Although tumour resection, treatment, and a successful outcome are more likely with early detection, lung cancer is fatal at later stages due to the lack of an appropriate screening platform, the disease's metastatic nature, genetic heterogeneity, and a minimal response to chemotherapy (Howington et al. 2013). Although they have proved to have a limited overall survival (OS) and hazardous side effects, still recommended treatments for locally progressed and metastatic cancers include chemotherapy and radiation.

Targeted medications have become standard therapies for NSCLC patients with actionable oncogenic alterations. In certain instances, this has boosted progression-free survival (PFS) and overall survival (OS). Targeted treatments differ from chemotherapy in their adverse effect profiles and may not always provide long-lasting therapeutic effects (Masters et al. 2015).

Based on how far the disease has spread, SCLC is divided into two categories: limited disease SCLC (LD-SCLC) and extended disease SCLC (ED-SCLC). The prognosis is still poor due to aggressive progression, a lack of early diagnosis methods, a lack of effective treatment alternatives, and the constant development of new chemotherapeutic medicines (Hiddinga et al. 2021). Chemotherapy (cisplatin or carboplatin with etoposide) coupled with thoracic radiation is a common treatment plan for LD-SCLC (Früh et al. 2013). SCLC reacts initially favourably to chemotherapy and radiation, but frequently relapses, which negatively impacts survival. Due to a lack of early detection methods, a scarcity of tissue available for clinical research, tumour genetic heterogeneity, and a lack of knowledge of molecular mechanisms causing rapid progression and therapeutic resistance, the median survival (MS) rate for this group of patients is roughly 7–12 months (van Meerbeeck et al. 2011). Limited, positive outcomes have been observed in clinical trials of novel medicines and targeted molecular therapies for SCLC (De Ruysscher et al.

2016). A novel therapeutic method with a durable response is thus urgently needed. Figure 1.2 shows various treatment modalities of lung cancer.

Recent studies have improved our knowledge of how the immune system responds to cancer and how to strengthen it, which has significantly improved cancer immunotherapy (Chen and Mellman 2013). Regardless of the histology or driver mutational status, immunotherapy has the potential to be effective and result in durable remission, particularly in patients who show a response (Kawakami 2016). Cancer immunotherapy seeks to instigate (or re-instigate) a cellular immune response, particularly the T-cell-mediated tumour-specific antigen (TSA) and tumour-associated antigens (TAA)-directed cytotoxicity that can target and eradicate a tumour (McGranahan et al. 2016). By boosting the number of tumour-specific antibodies, natural killer (NK) cells, dendritic cells (DCs), macrophages (M), and cytokines in the blood plasma, immune-modulatory medications can also combat cancer cells (Xin Yu et al. 2019). However, due to insufficient immune responses, immunotherapy has recently been deemed inappropriate for treating lung cancer (Vinay et al. 2015). Lung cancer immunotherapy is difficult because the cells modulate immune-suppressive cytokines secretion, T-cell-mediated cytotoxicity, and loss of major histocompatibility complex (MHC) expression, which reduce the overall immunological response (Osmani et al. 2018). Since it was recently discovered how immunogenic lung cancer is at the molecular level, many immunotherapies have been created to treat lung cancer. Examples of immunotherapy treatment techniques include therapeutic vaccines, immune modulators, autologous cellular therapies,

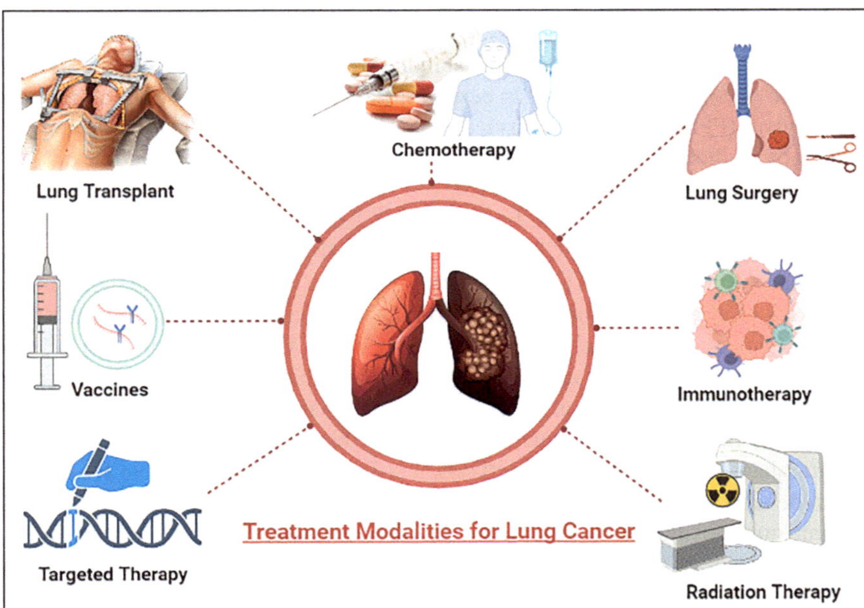

Fig. 1.2 Treatment approaches for lung cancer

and monoclonal antibodies (mAbs) targeted against checkpoint inhibitor signals linked to activated T cells and/or cancer cells. It is desirable to combine different medicines or therapeutic techniques with immunotherapy, nevertheless, as each therapeutic strategy has unique benefits and drawbacks (Vétizou et al. 2015).

1.8 Conclusion

Lung cancer is a significant issue for world health. Several methods are required to eradicate this malignancy. More stringent enforcement of tobacco control regulations is essential. Early detection initiatives should be put in place to lower lung cancer mortality. Adjuvant and induction therapies are expected to benefit from targeted medicines and immune checkpoint inhibitors, which have improved the treatment of metastatic cancers, even though chemotherapy remains the mainstay of care. Novel immunotherapeutic approach have a lot of potential. The molecular biology of lung cancer should be better understood to enable rational medication design.

References

Aisner SC, Finkelstein DM, Ettinger DS, Abeloff MD, Ruckdeschel JC, Eggleston JC (1990) The clinical significance of variant-morphology small-cell carcinoma of the lung. J Clin Oncol 8(3):402–408

Alberg AJ, Samet JM (2003) Epidemiology of lung cancer. Chest 123(1 Suppl):21s–49s

Balata H, Quaife SL, Craig C, Ryan DJ, Bradley P, Crosbie PAJ, Murray RL, Evison M (2022) Early diagnosis and lung cancer screening. Clin Oncol (R Coll Radiol) 34(11):708–715

Barta JA, Powell CA, Wisnivesky JP (2019) Global epidemiology of lung cancer. Ann Glob Health 85(1):8

Bradley SH, Kennedy MPT, Neal RD (2019) Recognising lung cancer in primary care. Adv Ther 36(1):19–30

Burns DM (2000) Primary prevention, smoking, and smoking cessation: implications for future trends in lung cancer prevention. Cancer 89(11 Suppl):2506–2509

Cagle PT, Allen TC, Olsen RJ (2013) Lung cancer biomarkers: present status and future developments. Arch Pathol Lab Med 137(9):1191–1198

Carbone DP, Gandara DR, Antonia SJ, Zielinski C, Paz-Ares L (2015) Non-small-cell lung cancer: role of the immune system and potential for immunotherapy. J Thorac Oncol 10(7):974–984

Chen DS, Mellman I (2013) Oncology meets immunology: the cancer-immunity cycle. Immunity 39(1):1–10

Darby S, Hill D, Auvinen A, Barros-Dios JM, Baysson H, Bochicchio F, Deo H, Falk R, Forastiere F, Hakama M, Heid I, Kreienbrock L, Kreuzer M, Lagarde F, Mäkeläinen I, Muirhead C, Oberaigner W, Pershagen G, Ruano-Ravina A, Ruosteenoja E, Rosario AS, Tirmarche M, Tomásek L, Whitley E, Wichmann HE, Doll R (2005) Radon in homes and risk of lung cancer: collaborative analysis of individual data from 13 European case-control studies. BMJ 330(7485):223

De Ruysscher D, Lueza B, Le Péchoux C, Johnson DH, O'Brien M, Murray N, Spiro S, Wang X, Takada M, Lebeau B, Blackstock W, Skarlos D, Baas P, Choy H, Price A, Seymour L, Arriagada R, Pignon JP (2016) Impact of thoracic radiotherapy timing in limited-stage small-cell lung cancer: usefulness of the individual patient data meta-analysis. Ann Oncol 27(10):1818–1828

Ellis PM, Vandermeer R (2011) Delays in the diagnosis of lung cancer. J Thorac Dis 3(3):183–188
Früh M, De Ruysscher D, Popat S, Crinò L, Peters S, Felip E (2013) Small-cell lung cancer (SCLC): ESMO clinical practice guidelines for diagnosis, treatment and follow-up. Ann Oncol 24 Suppl 6:vi99–v105
Grosche B, Kreuzer M, Kreisheimer M, Schnelzer M, Tschense A (2006) Lung cancer risk among German male uranium miners: a cohort study, 1946-1998. Br J Cancer 95(9):1280–1287
Hiddinga BI, Raskin J, Janssens A, Pauwels P, Meerbeeck JPV (2021) Recent developments in the treatment of small cell lung cancer. Eur Respir Rev 30(161):210079
Howington JA, Blum MG, Chang AC, Balekian AA, Murthy SC (2013) Treatment of stage I and II non-small cell lung cancer: diagnosis and management of lung cancer, 3rd ed: American College of Chest Physicians evidence-based clinical practice guidelines. Chest 143(5 Suppl):e278S–e313S
Huang J, Deng Y, Tin MS, Lok V, Ngai CH, Zhang L, Lucero-Prisno DE 3rd, Xu W, Zheng ZJ, Elcarte E, Withers M, Wong MCS (2022) Distribution, risk factors, and temporal trends for lung cancer incidence and mortality: a global analysis. Chest 161(4):1101–1111
Kawakami Y (2016) Introduction: cancer immunology special issue-immunotherapy. Int Immunol 28(7):317
Lindeman NI, Cagle PT, Beasley MB, Chitale DA, Dacic S, Giaccone G, Jenkins RB, Kwiatkowski DJ, Saldivar JS, Squire J, Thunnissen E, Ladanyi M, College of American Pathologists International Association for the Study of Lung and P. Association for Molecular (2013) Molecular testing guideline for selection of lung cancer patients for EGFR and ALK tyrosine kinase inhibitors: guideline from the College of American Pathologists, International Association for the Study of Lung Cancer, and Association for Molecular Pathology. J Mol Diagn 15(4):415–453
Lindeman NI, Cagle PT, Aisner DL, Arcila ME, Beasley MB, Bernicker EH, Colasacco C, Dacic S, Hirsch FR, Kerr K, Kwiatkowski DJ, Ladanyi M, Nowak JA, Sholl L, Temple-Smolkin R, Solomon B, Souter LH, Thunnissen E, Tsao MS, Ventura CB, Wynes MW, Yatabe Y (2018) Updated molecular testing guideline for the selection of lung cancer patients for treatment with targeted tyrosine kinase inhibitors: guideline from the College of American Pathologists, the International Association for the Study of Lung Cancer, and the Association for Molecular Pathology. J Mol Diagn 20(2):129–159
Lorigan P, Radford J, Howell A, Thatcher N (2005) Lung cancer after treatment for Hodgkin's lymphoma: a systematic review. Lancet Oncol 6(10):773–779
Masters GA, Temin S, Azzoli CG, Giaccone G, Baker S Jr, Brahmer JR, Ellis PM, Gajra A, Rackear N, Schiller JH, Smith TJ, Strawn JR, Trent D, Johnson DH (2015) Systemic therapy for stage IV non-small-cell lung cancer: American Society of Clinical Oncology clinical practice guideline update. J Clin Oncol 33(30):3488–3515
McGranahan N, Furness AJ, Rosenthal R, Ramskov S, Lyngaa R, Saini SK, Jamal-Hanjani M, Wilson GA, Birkbak NJ, Hiley CT, Watkins TB, Shafi S, Murugaesu N, Mitter R, Akarca AU, Linares J, Marafioti T, Henry JY, Van Allen EM, Miao D, Schilling B, Schadendorf D, Garraway LA, Makarov V, Rizvi NA, Snyder A, Hellmann MD, Merghoub T, Wolchok JD, Shukla SA, Wu CJ, Peggs KS, Chan TA, Hadrup SR, Quezada SA, Swanton C (2016) Clonal neoantigens elicit T cell immunoreactivity and sensitivity to immune checkpoint blockade. Science 351(6280):1463–1469
Neal RD, Sun F, Emery JD, Callister ME (2019) Lung cancer. BMJ 365:l1725
Nicholson AG, Tsao MS, Beasley MB, Borczuk AC, Brambilla E, Cooper WA, Dacic S, Jain D, Kerr KM, Lantuejoul S, Noguchi M, Papotti M, Rekhtman N, Scagliotti G, van Schil P, Sholl L, Yatabe Y, Yoshida A, Travis WD (2022) The 2021 WHO classification of lung tumors: impact of advances since 2015. J Thorac Oncol 17(3):362–387
Osmani L, Askin F, Gabrielson E, Li QK (2018) Current WHO guidelines and the critical role of immunohistochemical markers in the subclassification of non-small cell lung carcinoma (NSCLC): moving from targeted therapy to immunotherapy. Semin Cancer Biol 52(Pt 1):103–109

Ramalingam S, Belani C (2008) Systemic chemotherapy for advanced non-small cell lung cancer: recent advances and future directions. Oncologist 13(Suppl 1):5–13

Siegel RL, Miller KD, Jemal A (2017) Cancer statistics, 2017. CA Cancer J Clin 67(1):7–30

Sung H, Ferlay J, Siegel RL, Laversanne M, Soerjomataram I, Jemal A, Bray F (2021) Global cancer statistics 2020: GLOBOCAN estimates of incidence and mortality worldwide for 36 cancers in 185 countries. CA Cancer J Clin 71(3):209–249

Travis WD (2002) Pathology of lung cancer. Clin Chest Med 23(1):65–81, viii

van Meerbeeck JP, Fennell DA, De Ruysscher DK (2011) Small-cell lung cancer. Lancet 378(9804):1741–1755

Vétizou M, Pitt JM, Daillère R, Lepage P, Waldschmitt N, Flament C, Rusakiewicz S, Routy B, Roberti MP, Duong CP, Poirier-Colame V, Roux A, Becharef S, Formenti S, Golden E, Cording S, Eberl G, Schlitzer A, Ginhoux F, Mani S, Yamazaki T, Jacquelot N, Enot DP, Bérard M, Nigou J, Opolon P, Eggermont A, Woerther PL, Chachaty E, Chaput N, Robert C, Mateus C, Kroemer G, Raoult D, Boneca IG, Carbonnel F, Chamaillard M, Zitvogel L (2015) Anticancer immunotherapy by CTLA-4 blockade relies on the gut microbiota. Science 350(6264):1079–1084

Vinay DS, Ryan EP, Pawelec G, Talib WH, Stagg J, Elkord E, Lichtor T, Decker WK, Whelan RL, Kumara H, Signori E, Honoki K, Georgakilas AG, Amin A, Helferich WG, Boosani CS, Guha G, Ciriolo MR, Chen S, Mohammed SI, Azmi AS, Keith WN, Bilsland A, Bhakta D, Halicka D, Fujii H, Aquilano K, Ashraf SS, Nowsheen S, Yang X, Choi BK, Kwon BS (2015) Immune evasion in cancer: mechanistic basis and therapeutic strategies. Semin Cancer Biol 35(Suppl):S185–s198

Wagner GR (1997) Asbestosis and silicosis. Lancet 349(9061):1311–1315

Xin Yu J, Hubbard-Lucey VM, Tang J (2019) Immuno-oncology drug development goes global. Nat Rev Drug Discov 18(12):899–900

Zappa C, Mousa SA (2016) Non-small cell lung cancer: current treatment and future advances. Transl Lung Cancer Res 5(3):288–300

Immunobiology of Lung Cancer

2

Priyanka, Shireen Sheikh Nishad, and Pratima Tripathi

2.1 Introduction

Cancer results due to suppression of host immune system. Due to uncontrolled cell division, immune system fails to recognise these abnormal cells which results in cancers. Leukaemia is most common type of cancer seen in subjects associated with weak immunity. Therefore, cancer can be simply defined as an abnormal immune system tolerance to uncontrolled dividing cells. These cells that divide in uncontrolled manner will escape the cell checkpoint control due to several reasons such as self-antigens, self-tolerance (de la Cruz-Merino et al. 2008). This tumour-induced immune tolerance is the main aspect of cancer immunotherapy. The hypothesis that host's immune system can control the extravasation of cancer was first proposed by "Paul Ehrlich" in 1909, and further, Thomas and Burnet termed it as immune surveillance in mid-twentieth century. Immune cells such as regulatory T cells (Tregs), NK cells, macrophages play a major role in tumour growth suppression. Apart from these CD4+ and CD8+ T cell activity also contributes in suppressing the tumour growth. From these various studies, it is clear that both innate immunity and adaptive immunity have a role in immune response. Cancer immune-based therapy is further classified into both active immunotherapy and passive immunotherapy (de la Cruz-Merino et al. 2008). Passive immunotherapy mainly includes monoclonal antibodies, which acts against similarly exposed antigens in a tumour cell linage. Example includes adoptive immunotherapy, in which the lymphocytes are isolated immunogenically, in vitro, and then they are infused passively. This is a promising approach in melanoma. Active immunotherapy includes stimulation of immune system through subject's own immune mechanism (Lake and Van der Most 2006). It involves tumour vaccination or specific immunogenic therapy. Various number of

Priyanka · S. S. Nishad · P. Tripathi (✉)
Department of Biotechnology, National Institute of Pharmaceutical Education and Research, Raebareli, Uttar Pradesh, India

S. Bhatt et al. (eds.), *Immunotherapy Against Lung Cancer*,
https://doi.org/10.1007/978-981-99-7141-1_2

therapeutic vaccines are available which include purified tumour antigens or antigen-presenting cell-based vaccines, DNA vaccines, viral vectors, and killed tumour-based vaccines. Some of specific immune responses based on tumour infiltration are sort of interest but due to lack of real clinical efficacy is the rule.

From various studies, it is clear that due to improper functioning or inability of immune cells, to infiltrate, they become more active and prone to cause cancer when encountered with tumour-inducing antigen in vivo. Development of some methods such as stimulating antigen presenting cells (APCs) can activate immune system against tumour and helps in tumour surveillance. When compared to chemotherapy or radiotherapy, the immunotherapy has more advantage, such as it is site or target-specific and less likely to cause adverse effects, and it has less interference with other types of therapies, which makes immunotherapy as the best approach in cancer treatment. From this discussion, we have an idea about how the immune system is a active and effective "gate-keeper" of cancer. Innate immunity also plays a role in cancer regulation. Anti-cancer activity is primarily mediated by natural killer (NK) cells, macrophages, T and B lymphocytes, neutrophils, which further are capable of generation of memory and cytotoxic cells, which control the extrusion of tumour both systemically and locally. Some cytokines like IL-10 and transforming growth factors (TGF-B) are associated with suppression of immune mechanism. Tregs are actively associated in regulation or inhibition of anti-tumour functions of tumour-specific T cells. These Tregs get deposited at the tumour site, and they directly suppress cytotoxic T-cell response against the growing tumours (Lake and Van der Most 2006). The overall role of Tregs in tumours is not totally clear yet, and further investigations are going on.

Tumour P^{53} is a tumour-suppressing factor involved in controlling the overgrowth of cancer. Any mutation or loss of function in wild-type P^{53} may lead to cancer. It is clear that P^{53} status is profound to have immunological response in cancer regulation. P^{53} also induces cell arrest once the cells have been stressed or damage is resolved. It also enhances the oncogenic signalling pathways and considered as the hallmark of malignant transformations. It also has the ability to induce other biological pathways (Casares et al. 2005). Thus, P^{53} plays a role in tumour-induced immune system cross walk. P^{53} is activated by various signals, including cell damage, genotoxicity, starvation, and oncogene activation. Type 1 interferons and CCL-5 can promote the tumour-suppressing function of P^{53} via destruction or arresting of cell cycle and leads to apoptosis. Some of the cytokines can also both inhibit and induce the functions of P^{53}.

2.2 Innate and Adaptive Immune System Regulation of Cancer

Innate and adaptive immune system cells play an important role in cancer growth regulation. Although it is often assumed that a tumour-specific immune response will restrict cancer growth, it is apparent that various kinds of inflammation induced in a tumour can also lead to cancer proliferation, invasion, and dissemination

(Gajewski et al. 2013). The immune system cells that are seen invading human cancer are diverse and include both innate immune system cells (e.g., macrophage, neutrophils) and cells associated with an adaptive immune response (e.g., T and B cells). However, mounting data suggest that certain cancer patients establish an adaptive immune response particularly directed against antigenic proteins produced in their tumours. Various adaptive and innate immune cells are involved in cancer proliferation or regulation.

NK, natural killer T (NKT), and Gamma delta (γδ) T cells, among other innate immune cells, are essential for defending the host against cancer as shown in Fig. 2.1. Gamma delta (γδ) T cells are the prototype of 'unconventional' T cells and represent a relatively small subset of T cells in peripheral blood. They are defined by expression of heterodimeric T- cell receptors (TCRs) composed of γ and δ chains. Through a small number of germ line–encoded pattern recognition receptors, such as TLRs, macrophages, and dendritic cells (DCs) in particular serve as important sensors of encroaching pathogens and cancer cells. Nuclear factor (NF)-jB and type-1 interferon pathways are activated upon recognition of pathogen-derived ligands by TLRs, a variety of cells, including dendritic cells and T cells. This results in the production of proinflammatory cytokines, which are crucial for inducing CD4 T cells to differentiate into T helper (Th) 1, Th2 Th17, and regulatory T (Treg) cells. According to recent research, Treg cells are essential for suppressing immunological reactions and promoting immune tolerance to cancer and infectious illnesses (Vesely et al. 2011). A specialised subgroup of T cells called Tregs function to inhibit immunological response, preserving homeostasis and self-tolerance. Tregs have been demonstrated to have the ability to suppress T-cell growth and cytokine production, and they are essential for avoiding autoimmunity. Of special note, Treg cell suppression can be reversed only with the help of the human TLR8 signalling pathway. TLRs control innate immune responses, which are mediated by Treg, dendritic, and other immune cells, to control cancer immunity and tolerance (Fig. 2.2).

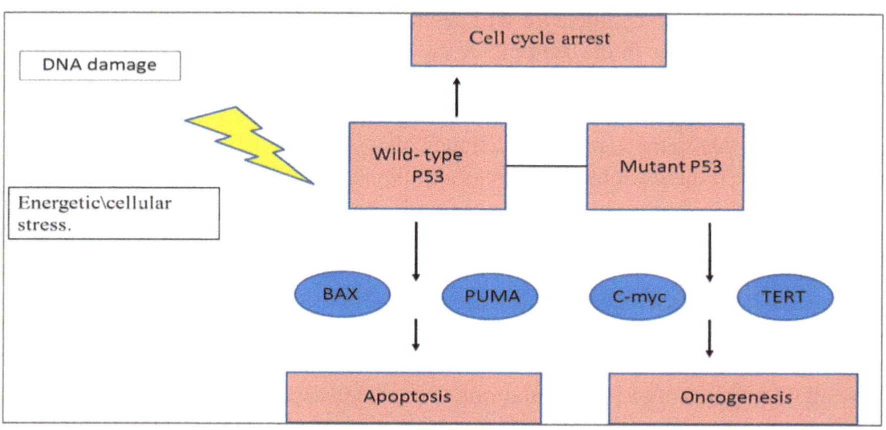

Fig. 2.1 Superior-negative effect of mutant P^{53} on wild-type P^{53} induces malignant transformation due to upregulation or expression of C-myc and TERT (telomerase reverse transcriptase)

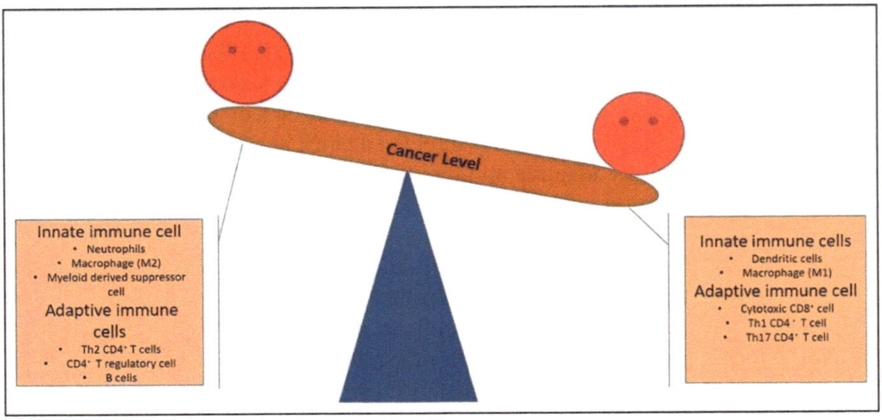

Fig. 2.2 Innate and adaptive immune regulation of cancer

2.3 Molecular Mechanism of Cancer

The normal cells and nuclear material get injured due to various external factors such as chemicals, radiation, and viruses. But in many conditions, we can detect the DNA damage and successfully repair the DNA. But in some conditions due to inherited mutations in genes affecting DNA repair and genes affecting cell growth or apoptosis are responsible for the failure of DNA repair and the BRCA1 gene, has most mutations, and if it is inherited, then the DNA repair diminishes. Those patients have higher risk of breast cancer and GU malignancies. In abnormal cells, if the DNA damages, the cell will undergo apoptotic pathway, but if the apoptotic pathway is disturbed, then those cells won't kill themselves appropriately. So those are inherited mutations that can impact the DNA damage (Weinberg 1983). If the DNA repair doesn't take place, then we will accumulate mutations in either somatic cell or genome. Mutations in the genome of the somatic cell can potentially cause activation of growth-promoting oncogenes. Oncogenes are those genes that normally regulate cell proliferation, but if they turned on, they may become cancerous cells. Alternatively due to these mutations, it may also lead to inactivation of tumour suppressor genes. If either of these happens simultaneously, then it leads to unregulated cell proliferation. Normal cells are constantly turning over, and at the same time, they normally die due to natural apoptosis. But due to these mutations in the genome of somatic cells, it leads to alternations in genes that regulate apoptosis which further results in decrease in apoptosis (Murphy 2001). Both unregulated cell proliferation (uncontrolled growth) and failure of apoptosis result in clonal expansion of normal cell. With the clonal expansion when the genetic instability that doesn't kill the cell, it acquires additional mutations. Due to cell expansion, it leads to outgrowing its vascular supply (i.e., angiogenesis) and due to escape from immune surveillance mechanism (Wolf 2006). All these parameters lead to tumour progression and lead to malignant neoplasm (Martin and Gutkind 2008). Now the cell has acquired

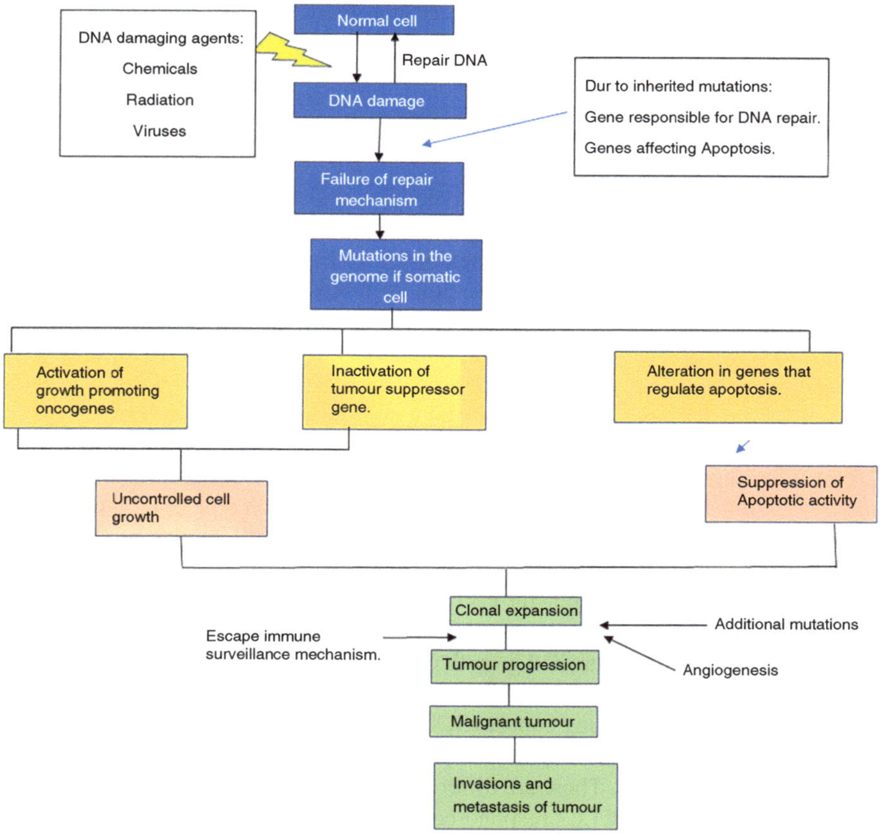

Fig. 2.3 Molecular mechanism of cancer

all other mutations and continues to grow without any exogenous stimulus. It further acquires the malignant potential by invading or by breaking off into blood stream or lymphatic system results into invasions and metastasis of tumour (Lin et al. 1997) (Fig. 2.3).

2.4 Lung Cancer

Lung cancer is one the most common cancers seen worldwide. In the USA, it is the second most common type of cancer diagnosed. Tobacco smoking is considered as one of the most important causes of lung cancer. When compared to non-cigarette smokers, cigarette smokers have 80–90% increased risk of lung cancer. Women are more prone to cause lung cancer compared to men (Minna et al. 2002). In the USA, it is the second most common cancer in men after prostate cancer as well as in women after breast cancer, while it is seen that there is a decreased risk with the cessation of smoking after a lag period of ~7 years.

2.5 Genetic Epidemiology

In cigarette smokers, due to addiction of nicotine, it leads to increase in the carcinogens like poly aromatic hydrocarbons (PAH) and nicotine-derived nitrosamine ketone (NNK). They are generally metabolically inactive, but once they become metabolically active, it leads to formation of DNA adducts (Schabath and Cote 2019). These DNA adducts can either repair the normal cell or may lead to cell death due to apoptosis or sometimes may modify into mutations like k-ras and p^{53}. These mutations are the main cause of lung cancer (Fig. 2.4).

Activated carcinogens lead to DNA adducts formation and may further lead to mutations. Mutations mainly include conversion of G to T (Wistuba and Gazdar 2006). This mutation may be sometimes forming silent type of mutations, but sometimes they may become too wild and due to increase in such type of mutations leads to defective gene coding and further leads to formation of defective protein which leads to cancers (Spiro and Silvestri 2005).

When we inhale, lungs transfer O_2 from the atmosphere to the tissues and also remove CO_2 from the tissues and get rid of it when we expel the air outside. Lung cancer is caused by uncontrolled growth of cells and spread of some cells from the lungs. Lung cancer is further classified into two types. Non-small-cell lung cancer (NSCLC) and small-cell lung cancer (SCLC). NSCLC is the most common type of cancer seen in most of the lung cancer patients. NSCLC makes up about 80–90% among most of the cases. There are different types of NSCLCs (Alberg et al. 2005). Most of the types of NSCLCs respond best to the treatment in their early stages of the disease malignancies. There are of two common types: (1) squamous cell lung carcinoma and (2) adenocarcinomas.

In squamous cell lung carcinoma, there is about ~30% malignant prevalence. It starts from the cells that line the tracts of the respiratory system. Adenocarcinomas typically include three different subtypes. It usually starts from the outer part of the lungs. The three subtypes are adenocarcinoma in situ (AIS), adeno squamous carcinoma, large cell carcinoma. Adenocarcinoma in situ (AIS) is a rarest subtype that

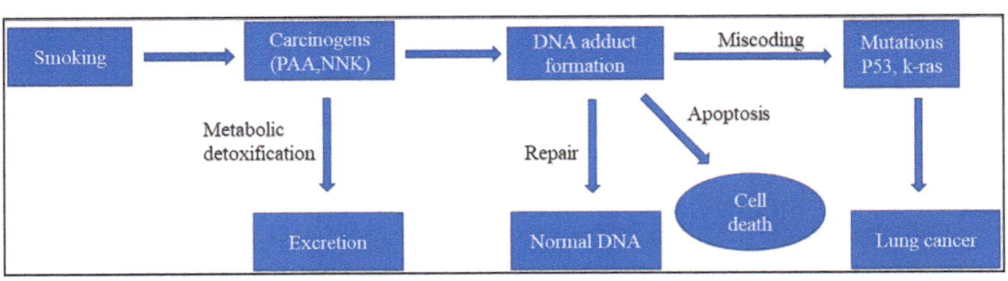

Fig. 2.4 Genetic epidemiology of lung cancer

usually starts from the smaller air sacs of the lungs, i.e., alveoli. Compared to other subtypes, this is not that aggressive and can be easily cured with treatment. Adeno squamous carcinoma is a mixture of both squamous and cells that produce the mucus. Large cell carcinoma is the major and fastest growing type of NSCLC, and it cannot be further classified into any type of cancer. Small-cell lung cancer has about ~15–20% malignant prevalence (Risch 2001). Compared to NSCLC, SCLC is more aggressive and death-causing. Sometimes SCLC responds best for chemotherapies but only in initial stages. However, it doesn't respond that much when compared to NSCLC. Mesothelioma is a type of cancer caused due to overexposure to asbestos. It generally starts with neuroendocrine cells (the cells that produce hormones). This type of cancer is wilder and more aggressive, and it does not respond well to any such treatment such as NSCLC and SCLC.

Cigarette is the main cause of lung cancer. Signs and symptoms include tiredness, facial/neck swelling, fatigue, sudden weight loss, dyspnoea, chest pain, cough, haemoptysis, loss of appetite, trouble swallowing, lumps in collar bone, yellowing of the skin, shoulder pain, swelling of the face and upper body parts, lack of perspiration on one side of the face, balancing issues, dizziness, etc. All include the symptoms of NSCLC. Risk factors of LC include cigarette smoking, nickel, arsenic (air pollution), radon, tar, family history, personal history, previous radiation therapy to chest, second-hand smoking, etc. All of these factors include the risk factors of lung cancers (Hemminki et al. 2004).

Diagnosis of lung cancer includes imaging tests, sputum cytology, and bronchoscopy. Imaging tests include CT scan, MRI, X-ray, and PET scan. They produce detailed and much smaller lesions through which it will be easier to identify the invasion or progress of the cancer. Sputum cytology includes cough from the subject, which is examined in the microscope to determine the presence of cancer cells. Bronchoscopy involves the passage of narrow tube down into the throat to closely examine the invasion of cancer present in the lungs. Lung biopsy can also be performed in the diagnosis of lung cancer. In this, a piece of tissue is taken to examine the tumour cells present in the lung. Sometimes it may be painful, but it gives the exact results in the case of any type of tumours (Fong et al. 2002). Generally, biopsy is performed under the sedation of the subject. Biopsy is performed using different methods such as mediastinoscopy and lung needle biopsy. Mediastinoscopy includes incision at the base of the neck, and a light pipe-like instrument is inserted into the neck along with some surgical devices. It is generally done in the presence of anaesthesia. Lung needle biopsy is performed by inserting a needle through the chest wall into the infected lung. Needle biopsy is also performed for testing of lymph nodes. It is generally performed in the presence of sedative action by giving anaesthesia to the patient. If biopsy gives positive results, it confirms the presence of cancers. Additional tests such as bone scan are also required further to understand the level of cancer invasion or spread.

Sometimes lung cancer also causes neuroendocrine cell cancer. Neuroendocrinal cell cancer produces parathyroid-like substance, ACTH-like substance, and ADH (Anti Diuretic Hormone)-like substances. These cells mimic other hormonal cells that produce in our body. Parathyroid hormone targets the bone and leads to breakdown of the bone which results in release of minerals such as calcium from the bone into the blood (Fong et al. 2017). Increase in the calcium levels leads to accumulation of calcium in the blood and results in a condition called hypercalcemia. ACTH-like substances stimulate the adrenal glands to produce more cortisol.

This leads to increase in the stress and increase in sympathetic activity. ADH-like substances target the kidneys to stimulate neurons to reuptake the water and thus, increase in water retention.

Lung cancer is further divided into several stages based on their level of invasion or spread. These stages give a clear idea during the time of treatment and also help in selection of best possible treatment method based on different stages in the different individuals. Non-small-cell lung cancer includes stage 1, stage 2, stage 3, stage 3A, stage 3B, and stage 4. Stage 1 includes cancer that starts from the inner lining of the lung pipe. It is usually present within the lung instead of outside the lung. Stage 2 includes the cancer that generally starts in the lymph nodes of the lungs and presents within the lungs. Stage 3 includes the cancer that is present within the lungs and lymph node, and sometimes it is present in the middle of the chest. Stage 3A includes cancer that is present in the lymph nodes and only on one side of the lung, usually where the cancer first begins to start (Rom et al. 1991). It is a type of benign tumour. In stage 3B, the cancer starts from one lung and passes to the opposite side of the lung or to lymph nodes over the collar bone. Stage 4 includes cancer that is spread overall in both the lungs and extends outside the lungs. Small-cell lung cancer involves two stages, limited and extensive stage. In limited stage, it involves the spread of cancer within the lung or to the opposite lung. But in extensive stage, it generally includes the spread of cancer to one lung or opposite lung, or to one lymph node or opposite node, or fluid around the lung, bone marrow, and distant organs.

2.6 Tobacco as a Prominent Cause of Lung Cancer

When you smoke, harmful gases enter your lungs, travel through your bloodstream, and then reach every organ in your body. Tobacco leaf, which has nicotine and a number of other chemicals, is used to make cigarettes. Numerous harmful substances, including PAA and NKK48, are released while the tobacco and compounds burn. Smoking produces carcinogenic chemicals like carbon monoxide and nitrogen oxide, as well as minute amounts of radioactive particles. All tobacco products, including cigarettes, pipes, and smokeless varieties like chewing tobacco and snuff, are harmful. The addictive substance in cigarettes is nicotine. Nicotine enters the bloodstream after being inhaled and travels to the brain (Gomperts et al. 2011). When the brain is continually exposed to nicotine, it causes a pleasurable feeling and desensitises the brain.

2.7 Major Health Effects of Smoking

People who smoke often pass away at a younger age than non-smokers, as smoking causes death. In fact, smoking is a contributing factor in one in five deaths in the United States. In addition to raising the chance of death from COPD, smoking raises the risk of heart disease, heart attacks, strokes, lung cancer in both men and women. Smoking also increases the risk of cardiovascular disease because nicotine enhances the release of epinephrine as it passes through the adrenal gland, a blood pressure–raising hormone. In addition, the lining of the arteries' inner walls can be harmed by carbon monoxide and nicotine46. Atherosclerosis is a disorder where fatty deposits called plaques build up at the sites of injuries and grow large enough to constrict the arteries and significantly limit blood flow.

In coronary artery disease, atherosclerosis causes the blood vessels that carry oxygen-rich blood to the heart to constrict, increasing the risk of a heart attack. Smoking increases the chance of blood clots by making platelets in the blood clump together. Peripheral vascular disease—in which atherosclerotic plaques obstruct the major arteries in your arms and legs—is caused more likely by smoking. Smoking can also result in an abdominal aortic aneurysm, which runs across the abdomen and includes aorta enlargement or weakening (Fong et al. 2017).

Two significant lung organs are also harmed by smoking. Airways are also referred to as bronchial tubes and alveoli are tiny air sacs. Air enters the lungs through the trachea, also known as the windpipe, with each breath. Afterward, air enters countless tiny alveoli where oxygen from the air enters your bloodstream and waste products, such as carbon dioxide, exit the bloodstream (Rom et al. 1991). Cilia, which resemble tiny hairs, border the bronchial passages and remove toxic particles from the lungs. The lining of the bronchial tubes becomes irritated by cigarette smoke, swelling and secreting more mucus as a result. Additionally, cigarette smoke slows down the cilia's mobility, causing some smoke and mucus to stay in the lungs. Some of the cilia recover while you sleep and start expelling more mucus and contaminants from your lungs. The body coughs repeatedly in an effort to eliminate the mucus (Gomperts et al. 2011), a disease referred to as smoker's cough.

Chronic bronchitis develops over time as cilia quit functioning. Breathing becomes challenging as airways get congested with scarring. Lung disease susceptibility has increased. Additionally, harming alveoli and hindering the exchange of oxygen and carbon dioxide is cigarette smoke. Emphysema (a condition in which one must gasp for every breath and wear an oxygen tube under the nose in order to breathe) is also caused by a lack of oxygen reaching the blood over time. Chronic obstructive pulmonary disease (COPD) is the collective term for chronic bronchitis and emphysema. COPD is a condition that slowly impairs breathing and has no known cure (Anichini et al. 2020).

At least 40 chemicals that cause cancer are present in cigarette smoke (Lavin et al. 2017). Carcinogens include substances like cyanide, formaldehyde, benzene, and ammonia. Healthy cells in the body divide, expand, and then die. DNA, the genetic material found inside each cell, controls this process. Toxic substances can harm the DNA of healthy cells if you smoke. Damaged cells consequently divide uncontrollably and produce new, unhealthy cells, which can then spread to other areas of your body. With more than a million new cases diagnosed each year, lung cancer is the most prevalent cancer in the world. Other organs of the body, including the blood and bone marrow, mouth, larynx, throat, oesophagus, stomach, pancreas, kidney, bladder, uterus, and cervix, might develop cancer as a result of harmful compounds in cigarettes.

Men and women who smoke can become infertile. Smoking while pregnant exposes the unborn child to the toxic compounds included in cigarettes, increasing the risk of low birth weight, miscarriage, preterm delivery, stillbirth, infant mortality, and sudden infant death syndrome (Kitajima et al. 2019). Smoking is harmful at any stage of breast-feeding. Through breast milk, nicotine enters the baby and can result in agitation, a rapid heartbeat, nausea, disturbed sleep, or diarrhoea. Other negative health impacts include low bone density in women, an increased risk of hip fracture in women, gum disease, which frequently necessitates tooth removal surgery, a malfunctioning immune system, and sluggish wound healing in men.

2.8 Immune Escape Mechanism in Lung Cancer

Immune escape mechanisms are seen at every phase of lung cancer development. The progression of precursor lesions into the invasive phase is conquered by a diverse range of immune evasion strategies (Anichini et al. 2020). Tumour cells survive and become aggressive to initial phase because of this immune escape. At the beginning, anti-tumour activity and immune response are in equilibrium (Lavin et al. 2017). But when the tumour starts to invade, then the immune escape becomes dependent and further leads to increase in the tumour cells population. Immune escape pathways help to explain innate and acquired resistance of NSCLC to immunotherapy (immune checkpoint blockade, ICB) targeting immunological checkpoints (Gomperts et al. 2011). Immunoediting selects neoplastic cells with subclonal loss of heterozygosity at the HLA loci in tumours with significant tumour mutational burden (TMB) (Kitajima et al. 2019), neoantigen loss, in intra-tumour heterogeneity for neoantigens, and also the development of an immune suppressive microenvironment. All of these reduce the effectiveness of cancer immunotherapy in NSCLC. Due to the function of the genetic modifications, they carry some type of molecular subgroups of NSCLC that exhibit distinct mechanisms that may influence the resistance to immunotherapy. Genetic mutations include increase of EGFR, STK11, which is associated with STING silencing. In total, 3.1% of AIS/MIA have HLA loss of heterozygosity (LOH) in contrast to 16.7% of LUAD samples. LOH is observed in all subtypes of lung cancer except in AAH lesions. Changes in the genomic expression, DNA methylation associated with the loss of heterozygosity and further lesions of AAH (Teixeira et al. 2019). In conclusion, advanced invasive LUSC and pre-invasive bronchial lesions at the CIS stage share a common number of genomic changes, while the benign and cancerous lesions differ in terms of transcriptome and also in some of the epigenetic modifications (Mascaux et al. 2019).

2.9 Immune Response to Lung Cancer

Immune system helps in protection the body against invading bacteria and other foreign microorganisms and helps in maintenance of good health of individuals (Domagala-Kulawik et al. 2014). In cancer patients, immune system plays a significant role as cancer weakens the immune system and due to chemotherapy, targeted anti-cancer drugs, radiotherapy, and usage of high dose of steroids suppress the body's natural immune response (Alberg et al. 2013). Due to suppression of immune regulation, it leads to a number of diseases. As immune system also helps in fighting back against the cancer, some cells of immune system can recognise the cancerous cells and attack them and kill them (Dail et al. 1995). Certain cells involved in the tumour suppression are neutrophils, B cells and T cells, Natural killer cells, dendritic cells, and macrophages (Raire and Dail 2008).

Neutrophils help in fighting the infection (Kryczek et al. 2011). They move to the infected areas and stick over the area where these infectious agents are present and release chemicals that are useful for killing the infectious agents such as viruses or bacteria. Low neutrophil count in the blood leads to increase in the infection (Franceschi et al. 2000). B cells and T cells get activated in the presence of any infectious antigens or tumour antigens (Skotarenko et al. 2014). T cells release certain interleukins such as IL-4, IL-7, IL-38, and other cytokines that help in detection of these antigens and help to get rid of them from the body (Vermaelen and Pauwels 2005). B cells due to activation of dendritic cells get activated and help in production of antibodies against the respective antigens, when they are exposed to certain type of antigenic response. These antibodies bind to the epitope of the infectious antigen and form antigen–antibody complex which is further engulfed by macrophages or either directly killed by the natural killer cells present in the body (Nielsen et al. 2004) (Fig. 2.5).

Recent studies have found that in the case of long metastasis, when the Th17(T helper 17) cells are transferred (Orentas et al. 2006), these Th17 cells enter into the lung cell surface where the tumour antigens are present and recognise these tumour antigens (D'Ambrosio 2006). These T cells secrete IL-17 (Viehl et al. 2006). Once

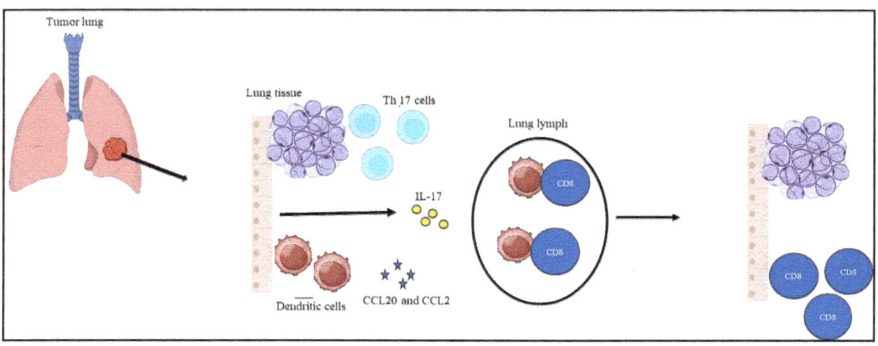

Fig. 2.5 Immune regulation against lung cancer

they recognise this antigen, they get activated and attack the lung cells and tumour cells to produce chemokines like CCL-20 and CCL-2, these chemokine agents provoke the inflammation and lead to migration of dendritic cells from the circulation to the lung tissue (Erfani et al. 2014). As a consequence, these dendritic cells uptake tumour antigens that are present in the lining of lung tissue and then migrate to the lung lymph node to process and present the antigen to CD8 cells (Sánchez-Margalet et al. 2019). These cells are also called as antigen-presenting cells. The anti-tumour CD8 cells come back into the lining of the lung and kill the tumour antigens and thus help in elimination of the tumour cells from the body (Schneider et al. 2011).

2.10 Future Perspectives

NSCLC can be efficiently detected, treated, and prevented with a combination of chemotherapeutics, gene therapy, immunotherapy, artificial intelligence, and computational techniques. Although chemotherapy is a better alternative for treating NSCLC, but it causes side effects that attribute the lives of patients to a higher risk. Chemotherapeutics' clinical trials and their potential impacts should be carried out in a way that prevents possible future adverse effects. A common treatment that blocks the pan kinase enzyme is gene therapy. REQORSA is one of the main types of gene therapy for treatment of lung cancer. These medicines still have a few adverse reactions that must be treated immediately. The primary kind of lung cancer treatment that can be added in future perspectives is immunotherapy using antigen-specific vaccinations that will be the most prominent treatment for lung cancer.

2.11 Conclusion

The global burden of morbidity and mortality from lung cancer is enormous, and it also places a heavy financial strain on the world's health systems. The main lung cancer screening trials' findings may suggest a chance to combat this problem at the secondary level, even if quitting smoking should be the foundation for minimising the severe effects of this public health hazard. To end this serious condition, additional efforts from a variety of actors—including politicians, stakeholders, healthcare workers, and researchers—will be required.

References

Alberg AJ, Brock MV, Samet JM (2005) Epidemiology of lung cancer: looking to the future. J Clin Oncol 23(14):3175–3185

Alberg AJ, Brock MV, Ford JG, Samet JM, Spivack SD (2013) Epidemiology of lung cancer: diagnosis and management of lung cancer: American College of Chest Physicians evidence- based clinical practice guidelines. Chest 143(5):e1S–e29S

Anichini A, Perotti VE, Sgambelluri F, Mortarini R (2020) Immune escape mechanisms in non-small cell lung cancer. Cancers 12(12):3605

Casares N, Pequignot MO, Tesniere A (2005) Caspase-dependent immunogenicity of doxorubicin-induced tumor cell death. J Exp Med 202:1691–1701
D'Ambrosio D (2006) Regulatory T cells: how do they find their space in the immunological arena. Semin Cancer Biol 16(2):91–97
Dail DH, Hammar SP, Colby TV, Dail DH (1995) Uncommon tumors. In: Pulmonary pathology—tumors, pp 157–341
de la Cruz-Merino L, Grande-Pulido E, Albero-Tamarit A (2008) Cancer and immune response: old and new evidence for future challenges. Oncogene 13:1245–1256
Domagala-Kulawik J, Osinska I, Hoser G (2014) Mechanisms of immune response regulation in lung cancer. Transl Lung Cancer Res 3(1):15
Erfani N, Hamedi-Shahraki M, Rezaeifard S, Haghshenas M, Rasouli M, Samsami DA (2014) FoxP3+ regulatory T cells in peripheral blood of patients with epithelialovarian cancer. Iran J Immunol 11(2):105–112
Fong KM, Sekido Y, Minna JD (2002) The molecular basis of lung carcinogenesis. In: The molecular basis of human cancer. Humana Press, Totowa, NJ, pp 379–405
Fong KM, Larsen JE, Wright C, Sriram K, Davidson M, Daniels M, Sekido Y, Bowman RV, Yang IA, Minna JD (2017) Molecular basis of lung carcinogenesis. In: The molecular basis of human cancer, pp 447–496
Franceschi C, Bonafè M, Valensin S, Olivieri F, De Luca M, Ottaviani E, De Benedictus G (2000) Inflamm aging: an evolutionary perspective on immunosenescence. Ann N Y Acad Sci 908(1):244–254
Gajewski TF, Schreiber H, Yang-xin F (2013) Innate and adaptive immune cells in the tumor microenvironment. Nat Immunol 14(10):1014–1022
Gomperts BN, Spira A, Massion PP, Walser TC, Wistuba II, Minna JD, Dubinett SM (2011) Evolving concepts in lung carcinogenesis. Semin Respir Crit Care Med 32(01):032–043
Hemminki K, Rawal R, Chen B, Bermejo JL (2004) Genetic epidemiology of cancer: from families to heritable genes. Int J Cancer 111(6):944–950
Kitajima S, Ivanova E, Guo S, Yoshida R, Campisi M, Sundararaman SK, Tange S, Mitsuishi Y, Thai TC, Masuda S, Piel BP (2019) Suppression of STING associated with LKB1 loss in KRAS-driven lung cancer silencing of STING in KRAS-LKB1–mutant lung cancer. Cancer Discov 9(1):34–45
Kryczek I, Wu K, Zhao E, Wei S, Vatan L, Szeliga W, Huang E, Greenson J, Chang A, Roliński J, Radwan P (2011) IL-17+ regulatory T cells in the microenvironments of chronic inflammation and cancer. J Immunol 186(7):4388–4395
Lake RA, Van der Most RG (2006) A better way for a cancer cell to die. N Engl J Med 354:2503–2504
Lavin Y, Kobayashi S, Leader A, Amir EA, Elefant N, Bigenwald C, Remark R, Sweeney R, Becker CD, Levine JH, Meinhof K (2017) Innate immune landscape in early lung adenocarcinoma by paired single-cell analyses. Cell 169(4):750–765
Lin JK, Chen YC, Huang YT, Lin Shiau SY (1997) Suppression of protein kinase C and nuclear oncogene expression as possible molecular mechanisms of cancer chemoprevention by apigenin and curcumin. J Cell Biochem 67(S28–29):39–48
Martin D, Gutkind JS (2008) Human tumor-associated viruses and new insights into the molecular mechanisms of cancer. Oncogene 27(2):S31–S42
Mascaux C, Angelova M, Vasaturo A, Beane J, Hijazi K, Anthoine G, Buttard B, Rothe F, Willard-Gallo K, Haller A, Ninane V (2019) Immune evasion before tumour invasion in early lung squamous carcinogenesis. Nature 571(7766):570–575
Minna JD, Roth JA, Gazdar AF (2002) Focus on lung cancer. Cancer Cell 1(1):49–52
Murphy PM (2001) Chemokines and the molecular basis of cancer metastasis. N Engl J Med 345(11):833–835
Nielsen J, Holm TL, Claesson MH (2004) CD4+ CD25+ regulatory T cells: II. Origin, disease models and clinical aspects. APMIS 112(10):642–650
Orentas RJ, Kohler ME, Johnson BD (2006) Suppression of anti-cancer immunity by regulatory T cells: back to the future. Semin Cancer Biol 16(2):137–149

Raire AE, Dail DH (2008) Miscellaneous tumors and tumor-like proliferations of the lung. In: Dail and Hammar's pulmonary pathology: volume II: neoplastic lung disease, pp 500–541
Risch N (2001) The genetic epidemiology of cancer: interpreting family and twin studies and their implications for molecular genetic approaches. Cancer Epidemiol Biomark Prev 10(7):733–741
Rom WN, Travis WD, Brody AR (1991) Cellular and molecular basis of the Asbestos-related diseases. Am Rev Respir Dis 143:408–422
Sánchez-Margalet V, Barco-Sánchez A, Vilariño-García T, Jiménez-Cortegana C, Pérez- Pérez A, Henao-Carrasco F, Virizuela-Echaburu JA, Nogales-Fernández E, Álamo-de la Gala MC, Lobo-Acosta MA, Palazón-Carrión N (2019) Circulating regulatory T cells from breast cancer patients in response to neoadjuvant chemotherapy. Transl Cancer Res 8(1):59
Schabath MB, Cote ML (2019) Cancer progress and priorities: lung cancer. Cancer Epidemiol Biomark Prev 10:1563–1579
Schneider T, Kimpfler S, Warth A, Schnabel PA, Dienemann H, Schadendorf D, Hoffmann H, Umansky V (2011) Foxp3+ regulatory T cells and natural killer cells distinctlyinfiltrate primary tumors and draining lymph nodes in pulmonary adenocarcinoma. J Thorac Oncol 6(3):432–438
Skotarenko LV, Vorotnikov IK, Kadagidze ZG, Shamilov FA (2014) The specific features of T cell immunity in breast cancer. Tumors Female Reprod Syst 4:24–27
Spiro SG, Silvestri GA (2005) One hundred years of lung cancer. Am J Respir Crit Care Med 172(5):523–529
Teixeira VH, Pipinikas CP, Pennycuick A, Lee-Six H, Chandrasekharan D, Beane J, Morris TJ, Karpathakis A, Feber A, Breeze CE, Ntolios P (2019) Deciphering the genomic, epigenomic, and transcriptomic landscapes of pre-invasive lung cancer lesions. Nat Med 25(3):517–525
Vermaelen K, Pauwels R (2005) Pulmonary dendritic cells. Am J Respir Crit Care Med 172(5):530–551
Vesely MD, Kershaw MH, Schreiber RD, Smyth MJ (2011) Natural innate and adaptive immunity to cancer. Annu Rev Immunol 29:235–271
Viehl CT, Moore TT, Liyanage UK, Frey DM, Ehlers JP, Eberlein TJ, Goedegebuure PS, Linehan DC (2006) Depletion of CD4+ CD25+ regulatory T cells promotes a tumor-specific immune response in pancreas cancer–bearing mice. Ann Surg Oncol 13:1252–1258
Weinberg RA (1983) A molecular basis of cancer. Sci Am 249(5):126–143
Wistuba II, Gazdar AF (2006) Lung cancer preneoplasia. Annu Rev Pathol 1:331–348
Wolf K, Fried P (2006) Molecular mechanisms of cancer cell invasion and plasticity. Br J Dermatol 154(s1):11–15

3 Evolution of Lung Cancer Treatment from Classical Chemotherapy to Advanced Immunotherapy

Subiksha Maheshkumar, Diwahar Prakash, Ashwin Subramanian, Gayathri Devi Muthukumarasamy, Rishmitha Duraisamy, Gayathri Gopal, Shibi Muralidar, and Senthil Visaga Ambi

3.1 Introduction

Cancer is a genetic disorder that is characterized by genomic instability, in which a great number of point mutations build up and structural changes take place as the tumour progresses. These genetic changes may result in tumour antigens, which the immune system may identify as non-self and which may cause cellular immunological responses. Because immune cells infiltrate the tumour microenvironment (TME) and influence the control of cancer progression, the immune system is crucial to immunosurveillance. The 5-year overall survival rate for non-small-cell lung cancer (NSCLC) in the United States is still only 18.1%, despite improvements in surgery, chemoradiotherapy, and targeted molecular therapy for patients with lung cancer (Chen et al. 2022). Accelerated technical advancement has allowed for

Subiksha Maheshkumar and Diwahar Prakash contributed equally with all other contributors.

S. Maheshkumar · D. Prakash · A. Subramanian · G. D. Muthukumarasamy · R. Duraisamy · S. Muralidar
Biopharmaceutical Research Lab, Anusandhan Kendra-1, School of Chemical and Biotechnology, SASTRA Deemed-to-be-University, Thanjavur, Tamil Nadu, India

G. Gopal · S. V. Ambi (✉)
Biopharmaceutical Research Lab, Anusandhan Kendra-1, School of Chemical and Biotechnology, SASTRA Deemed-to-be-University, Thanjavur, Tamil Nadu, India

Department of Bioengineering, School of Chemical and Biotechnology, SASTRA Deemed-to-be-University, Thanjavur, Tamil Nadu, India
e-mail: senthilvisagaambi@scbt.sastra.edu

S. Bhatt et al. (eds.), *Immunotherapy Against Lung Cancer*,
https://doi.org/10.1007/978-981-99-7141-1_3

extensive research of tumour genomes and increased understanding of the intricacy of cancer cytogenetics and evolution. Immunotherapy has emerged as a breakthrough in the treatment of tumours in recent years. It is frequently utilized in the clinic and is anticipated to introduce a novel approach to the cancer therapeutics due to its long-lasting effects and low incidence of side effects. Most of the initially susceptible individuals, meanwhile, eventually develop immunological drug resistance. Drug resistance is currently the biggest issue in the treatment of tumours; hence, this should be a focus. Immunotherapy, which tries to enhance innate defences to eliminate malignant cells, is a significant advancement in the treatment of cancer. It completely altered the oncology field (Yu et al. 2020). Although the concept of using the host immune system to fight cancer dates back to the early twentieth century, significant progress was achieved in the recent clinical investigations. It completely altered the oncology field (Yu et al. 2020).

Although the concept of using the host immune system to fight cancer dates back to the early twentieth century, significant progress has been made in recent basic and clinical studies. Immunotherapy has shown substantial responses in a clinical setting at the range of cancer types while having modest response rates and uncertain underlying mechanisms. Because immune cells are the biological foundation of immunotherapy-based cancer treatment, it is essential to comprehend the immunological infiltrates in the TME in order to improve response rates and develop novel therapeutic strategies. The suggested course of treatment may vary depending on the type and stage of the cancer, probable adverse effects, the patient's choices, and general health. During surgery, the entire lung tumour as well as any nearby lymph nodes in the chest may be removed. A border or margin of healthy lung tissue must be present around the tumour when it is removed. A "negative margin" indicates that no tumour cell was discovered in the healthy tissue around the tumour when the pathologist examined the lung or a portion of the lung that was surgically removed. In order to reduce the risk of recurrence, additional therapies can be given both before and after the surgery. Before the procedure, cancer patients may get neoadjuvant therapy, sometimes referred to as induction therapy (Toschi et al. 2017). This kind of therapy is utilized to lessen the scope of surgery in addition to treating the original tumour and reducing your chance of recurrence. Treatment that is given following surgery is called adjuvant therapy. It aims to eradicate any lung cancer cells that could still be present in the body following surgery. Although there is always a chance that the cancer will return, this reduces that risk (Chen et al. 2022).

Radiation therapy and systemic ailments including chemotherapy, targeted therapy, and immunotherapy are some of the adjuvant therapies utilized for NSCLC. Radiation therapy eliminates the tumour cells that are exposed to the radiation beam, and the non-cancerous cells that are also in its path are susceptible to damage. Chemotherapy is being prevalently used to suppress the tumour growth, proliferation, and production of new cancer cells. It has been showed to prolong and improve the quality of life in individuals with lung cancer. Concurrent chemoradiotherapy refers to the administration of chemotherapy and radiation therapy at the same time. Also known as sequential chemoradiotherapy, they can be administered one after the other (Boolell et al. 2015). Immunotherapy has emerged as a breakthrough in the treatment of tumours in recent years. It is frequently utilized in the clinic due to its long-lasting effects and lack of side effects and is anticipated to introduce a novel approach to the treatment of tumours (Chaft et al. 2021; Toschi et al. 2017).

This chapter discusses the conventional cancer treatment options and the significance of therapeutic options available for lung cancer. The chapter will introduce the evolution of lung carcinoma treatment in the context of surgery, chemotherapy, radiation therapy, and immunotherapy. The mechanistic concepts of the treatment strategies in handling individuals with lung cancer are focused in this chapter, with the outline on the recent advances in the combination therapy and how the therapeutic strategies have progressed according to the evolution of cancer gene make-up.

3.2 Conventional Lung Cancer Treatments

3.2.1 Chemotherapy

There are various treatment strategies used to treat lung cancer. They include surgery, radiotherapy, and chemotherapy. Among these, chemotherapy plays a vital role in treating malignant tumours by using anti-cancer drugs to kill cancer cells. The common side effects of chemotherapy are cardiac toxicity, hair loss, nausea, vomiting, neuropathy, gastrointestinal disorders, and vascular toxicity. Despite all these side effects, chemotherapy has been an effective cancer treatment for decades since it can be combined with radiation or surgical therapy. The mainstream chemotherapeutic drugs approved by NCCN guidelines include cisplatin, methotrexate, doxorubicin, and ifosfamide for the first line of chemotherapy treatment (Biermann et al. 2017). Chemotherapy can be administered through intravenous injection, pills, or fluids. The chemotherapy can be classified as single-agent chemotherapy or combinational chemotherapy. The different ways of using chemotherapy are adjuvant therapy, curative therapy, and neoadjuvant therapy.

3.2.1.1 Chemotherapy in Lung Cancer

The small-cell lung cancer (SCLC) occurs in the tissues of the lungs, and they are considered as the rare and aggressive type of lung cancer. Overall diagnosis of SCLC patients is 15% when compared to other lung cancer types. Non-small-cell lung cancer (NSCLC) is most common type of cancer especially in women. NSCLC grows and spreads slower than small-cell lung cancer. For early stages of NSCLC (stage I, II, IIIA) surgical resection is recommended, and for II–IIIA stages adjuvant platinum-based chemotherapy is recommended (Alexander et al. 2020). Single-agent chemotherapy is a rarely used treatment strategy except in early phase of drug development. During the 1980s, the response rate of combinational chemotherapy in lung cancer treatment was 20–50%, and few complete responses in NSCLC when compared to the single-agent chemotherapy. Most used combinations are etoposide and cisplatin, cyclophosphamide + doxorubicin and etoposide, cyclophosphamide + doxorubicin + etoposide. The effect of combinational chemotherapy has caused minimal differences in patients with squamous cell cancer (SCC), adenocarcinoma, or large cell cancer (IJsselmuiden and Faden 1992).

3.2.2 Radiation Therapy

Radiation therapy (RT) is one among the three therapies to treat cancer. RT is mainly used therapy in most types of solid tumours, selected hematologic malignancies. RT minimally inhibits the proliferation of selected benign tumours. The ultimate aim of RT is to cure cancer locally without the excess side effects. The factors that affect the results of radiation therapy are type of tumour, area of location of tumour, regional extent, and the accuracy in calculated radiation dose. In association with surgery or chemotherapy, RT is used in most of the cancer patients as neoadjuvant treatment. Early effects of radiations are skin erythema, mucositis, and late effects include carcinogenesis and fibrosis. Approximately 65% of all cancer patients require radiotherapy alone or with the combination of chemotherapeutic drugs or surgery (Mehta et al. 2012). Radiation damages the genetic material (DNA) present inside the cancer cells. If the cancer cells are not able to repair it, the cell will not be able to produce the new cells, and it may die. The major side effects of radiation therapy are loss of appetite, skin irritation in the treated area, and extreme fatigue.

3.2.2.1 Radiation Therapy in Lung Cancer

RT technologies evolve rapidly with more accuracy, and the accuracy of RT depends on imaging. The four-dimensional computed tomography (4DCT) is routinely used RT which measures the specific motion of the patients, which ensures prescribed dose delivery in patients regardless of their position (Vinod and Hau 2020). The respiratory gating (RG) is an alternative technique that is used to measure tumour motion. RG is applied to the metastatic tumours. This system uses chest/abdomen markers and infrared camera to find the normal respiratory cycle of patients. Respiratory gating delivers the radiation, only when the tumour is in the treatment field. This respiratory gating can be achieved by breath hold techniques, at the particular point in respiratory cycle the patient holds their breath, and the treatment is given in increments only during the breath hold. This can be much more challenging for patients with lung disease. Respiratory-gated radiation therapy seems to be necessary to reduce the acute toxicity, pulmonary, cardiac, and during the chest irradiation, oesophageal late toxicities (Giraud et al. 2011).

Radiation therapy for NSCLC: For the peripherally located stage I-IIA (NSCLC), stereotactic ablative body radiotherapy (SABR) is the standard of care for the patients who do not adopt the surgery. For the third stage of NSCLC, concurrent chemo-radiation is usually preferable (Bradley et al. 2020). Adjuvant immunotherapy is recommended as a benefit for the patients who do not progress after the concurrent chemotherapy and the fourth stage of NSCLC cannot be cured (Antonia et al. 2017, 2018).

Radiation therapy for SCLC: Thoracic radiotherapy is recommended for SCLC patients in stage I–III (limited stage), and the two meta-analyses showed survival rate of 5.4%. For extensive stage, palliative platinum-based chemotherapy is highly recommended (Murray and Turrisi 2006).

3.2.3 Surgery

Surgery plays a vital role in diagnosing cancer and determining the staging. Special surgery techniques employed for cancer are cryosurgery, laser surgery, Mohs surgery, laparoscopic surgery, and robotic surgery (Wright et al. 2002). Cancer cells enter circulation, tackle immune cell, reach a distant site, invade, and proliferate there. This process is known as metastasis. The immune cells present in blood such as macrophages and natural killer cells are involved in eliminating cancer cells (Natural et al. 1999). Development of new metastatic disease can be inhibited by neutrophil extracellular trap (NET) inhibition after the surgery (Tohme et al. 2016).

3.2.3.1 Role of Surgery in Lung Cancer Treatment

Surgery is preferred for early-stage NSCLC patients, but not suitable for patients with metastatic disease. The NSCLC has its own types: lobectomy, segmentectomy, and pneumonectomy (Frank and Detterbeck 2018). For SCLC, surgery is not practised widely because SCLC spreads rapidly throughout the body, removing it all by this treatment is not possible. So, treatments like chemotherapy, radiotherapy, and immunotherapy are preferred.

3.3 Chemotherapy

3.3.1 Origin

Dr. Paul Ehrlich, a famous German Scientist, started producing medications to cure infectious disorders in the 1900s. The concept of "chemotherapy," was first established by him, which he categorized as the employment of chemicals to treat disease. At a point, they realized that the cure rates were promisingly increasing than the local cancer treatments by 33%. Then surgery and radiation therapy were most commonly used by clinicians to treat cancer in the 1960s. Further studies have shown that chemotherapy and other treatments may treat patients with chronic malignancies (DeVita and Chu 2008). Before the introduction of chemotherapy, probative treatment impacted a halfway survival of 2–4 months for metastatic lung cancer. The clinical benefits of early chemotherapy medicines like methotrexate and doxorubicin were not much efficient. The survivors of lung cancer have not improved until platinum and new-generation chemotherapeutic medications were used in the late 1900s. Pemetrexed, a chemotherapeutic medication with documented efficacy in treating lung cancer, reached the market in the early 2000s. Pemetrexed revealed substantial remedial advantage in non-squamous versus scaled histology in the Phase 3 JMDB research, validating that histology is crucial in treating lung cancer. In the mid-2000s and early 2010s, anti-angiogenic medications like bevacizumab and novel medicine delivery methods similar to albumin-bound nanoparticle paclitaxel (nab-paclitaxel) have exhibited therapeutic improvements in terms of efficiency and safety (Lee 2019).

3.3.2 Mechanism of Action

The primary mechanism of action of chemotherapeutic drug is to stop abnormal cell division. Many drugs act on the cells in the gap phases, especially between the G1 and S phases, to inhibit the process of DNA synthesis. By making the drugs act during the gap phases, we can stop the cells from synthesizing the DNA (G1 Phase) or inhibit them from cell division (G2 Phase). Cancer therapeutic drugs affect both the normal cells and the malignant cells. It is the biggest challenge in the field of cancer. However, there is an increased chance of recovery for the normal cells from minor damage during chemotherapy, and malignant cells have increased chances for cell death. The increased chance of death for malignant cells is the critical factor that chemotherapy exploits to increase the success rate of the treatment (Thirumaran et al. 2007).

3.3.2.1 Alkylating Agents

Covalent bonds are created when alkylating chemicals interact with electron-rich atoms. Classical alkylating chemicals typically transfer a methyl group containing single carbon, which may contain long hydrocarbons, known as an alkane. The interactions with DNA bases are the most significant regarding the anticancer activity of the drug candidate. Alkylating agents include the medications such as Melphalan, Busulfan, Chlorambucil, Mechlorethamine, Temozolomide, Cyclophosphamide, Ifosfamide, Carmustine, Dacarbazine, and Procarbazin (Ralhan and Kaur 2007).

3.3.2.2 DNA Topoisomerase Inhibitors

DNA transcription and replication cause twists in DNA, in which DNA topoisomerases may unwind. DNA topoisomerases I and II, found in cells, work by severing the DNA backbone on both strands, depending on the situation, relieving torsional stress, and finally relegating the fragmented DNA backbone. These enzymes regulate transcription and replication and are found in huge structure in the cell nucleus. The following compounds block the topoisomerase enzyme in cancer cells, thereby inhibiting its proliferation: plant alkaloids like camptothecin and its semi-synthetic derivatives like irinotecan and topotecan, anti-tumour antibiotic doxorubicin derived from *Streptomyces peucetius var. caesius* that inhibits topoisomerase II enzyme, platinum compounds like cisplatin, carboplatin, and oxaliplatin, and antimetabolites inhibiting the nucleoside synthesis pathways (Thirumaran et al. 2007).

Stage III B and stage IV NSCLC patients cannot be cured by surgery; hence, painless chemotherapy was chosen as the choice of treatment. On that note, topoisomerase I inhibitors like camptothecin and its derivative, topoisomerase II inhibitors like etoposide, ifosfamide, and platinum derivatives are commonly used to reduce cancer. Usage of topotecan in combination with carboplatin reduces toxicity in the kidney, nerve cells, and bones in comparison to other platinum combinations. SCLC patients are treated with topoisomerase I inhibitors like camptothecin and its derivative, topoisomerase II inhibitors like etoposide, doxorubicin, vincristine, and cyclophosphoamide. Resistance to topoisomerase inhibitors arises when there is insufficiency in drug accumulation at enzyme-binding site, response of the cells to topoisomerase inhibitors, chromosomal alterations, and alterations in topoisomerase enzymes (Chhatriwala et al. 2006).

3.3.3 Resistance to Chemotherapy

3.3.3.1 Small-Cell Lung Cancer

The process is complicated as many factors, such as mutations at the genetic or epigenetic levels of the critical genes, could result in drug resistance. Some of SCLC's recognized drug resistance mechanisms are the overexpression of MDR-related proteins, aberrant intracellular enzyme expression, cellular death escape, abnormalities in cellular repair systems, cancer stem cell lines, and other factors. However, these are not the only reason for drug resistance, there may be other unidentified processes also. Several innovative methods have been created to treat NSCLC, most notably molecular targeted therapy, improving the prognosis of patients (Zhou et al. 2019).

Tumour cells may develop cross-resistance, or MDR, after repeated exposure to a particular chemotherapeutic agent. MDR refers to drug resistance to a wide variety of structurally and functionally distinct substances. It has to do with the increased expression of ATP-binding cassette (ABC) transmembrane transport protein drug pumps, such as P-glycoprotein (P-gp), which is encoded by the MDR1 gene, multidrug resistance-associated protein (MRP, including MRP1 and MRP2), lung resistance protein (LRP), which mediates transport processes within the cell, and RLIP76, a non-ABC transport protein, among others. The MDR is manifested by blocking DNA-targeted chemotherapeutic drugs. In chemo-naive SCLC cells, there was a substantial negative connection with P-gp and MRP1 expression and insignificant correlation with LRP expression for more excellent chemotherapy responsiveness (Zhou et al. 2019).

In individuals with relapsed disease, Pgp and MRP1 expression was noticeably elevated in cells that are in metastatic state. These findings imply that P-gp and MRP1 may be more closely related to chemotherapy resistance in SCLC than LRP. Because of enhanced efflux due to RLIP76 overexpression, cancer cells acquire more resistance towards chemotherapeutic drugs resulting in a drop in intracellular concentration of the medications. Sal-like protein 4 (Sall4) is a transcription factor with a zinc finger. Human foetal livers express SALL4, while adult livers in good condition do not. There was a considerable rise in SALL4 expression in the chemotherapy-resistant SCLC cell line. SALL4 was downregulated, which made chemotherapy-resistant SCLC cell lines more drug-sensitive. Key enzymes that transform sphingosine into sphingosine-1phosphate (S1P), a bioactive lipid known to control inflammation, are sphingosine kinase (SphK) types 1 and 2. According to a study, SPHK1 is crucial for controlling SCLC multidrug resistance (Zhou et al. 2019).

3.3.3.2 Non-Small-Cell Lung Cancer (NSCLC)

Drug resistance is a serious hurdle to invariable chemotherapeutic usage. This phenomenon, which comes from the natural ability of cancer cells to create variant cells in response to an unfavourable selection of any form, is generally a problematic component of cancer therapy. The heterogeneity of tumours are due to numerous chromosomal abnormalities in different types of cells comprising tumour. Due to the genetic flexibility of cancer, the unfavourable selection imposed by utilizing cytotoxic treatments can readily result in the formation of mutant cells. Consequently, the similar strategy that destroys cancer cells may also enforce a selection for treatment resistance. Treatment resistance is a critical challenge in clinical oncology, which often results in patient's mortality (Min and Lee 2021).

DNA structure changes because of DNA adducts formed by platinum compounds leading to the DNA repair machinery that guards against apoptosis. Therefore, resistance to platinum-based chemotherapeutic drugs is mediated by the activation of the DNA repair mechanism. Due to the polar nature of platinum compounds, a variety of parameters, including pH and the quantities of sodium and potassium ions, can influence how well platinum derivatives are absorbed. The resistance to platinum compounds was created by the decontamination and silencing of platinum compounds, such as the attachment of a platinum compound to metallothionein or the binding of glutathione (GSH) to cisplatin by glutathione S-transferase (GST) and excretion through MRP2/ABCC2. The DNA adduct formation due to platinum derivatives stimulates response due to DNA, culminating in cell cycle arrest and death. The genes expression is adjusted in a stable and heritable way by epigenetic modulation, which includes modifications in DNA and histones instead of mutations in DNA. The result of platinum drug treatment has been regulated by changes in epigenetic modifications and the expression of epigenetic modifiers. Epithelial–mesenchymal transition (EMT), changing epithelial cells into mesenchymal states, is critical in providing cancer cells cellular flexibility and creating tumour heterogeneity. Researchers suggested that the EMT programme activation contributes significantly to drug resistance by accelerating the transition of non-cancer stem cells to cancer stem cells (Min and Lee 2021).

3.3.4 Side Effects

There has been a cohort investigation of lung cancer patients taking chemotherapy in Australia. Patients self-reported the adverse effects that they encountered. By cancer sort and grade, the prevalence, incident rates, and frequency of side effects were assessed, and cumulative incidence curves for each side effect were generated (Pearce et al. 2017).

Despite more treatment, top three adverse effects of the patients, dyspnoea, haemorrhage, and tiredness, remain unchanged from beginning to end. On the other hand, dyspnoea and profuse bleeding were moved to positions two and three owing to exhaustion, which was increased in importance. Only 50% of cancer patients receiving radiation or chemotherapy believe that they have various treatment options. The results presented here demonstrate the viability, efficacy, and significance of using a patient-focused strategy to involve individuals by enlisting them in research that impacts them and involves them in the execution, translation, and dissemination of the results (Islam et al. 2019).

3.4 Immunotherapy

The survival rate of lung cancer is very less when compared to other types. Earlier immunotherapy failed in curing the disease, but now it's emerging as one of the leading treatments which comparatively increases the overall survival rate and has fewer side effects that are not so serious. Immunotherapy targets specific parts of the immune system to detect and kill cancer cells. Immunotherapy can be done in two ways: either by body's own immune system which can fight against the cancer cells or by preparing a substance in the lab and introducing it into the body to fight against the cancer cells. Among all the treatments, immunotherapy is the best because it has less survival rate and fewer side effects. Some of these are fatigue, diarrhoea, dizziness, fever, and cold. Some of that can also be life-threatening like autoimmune reactions and infusion reactions (Bar et al. 2019).

3.4.1 Origin

Immunotherapy has become one of the most leading treatments for cancer and cancer-related diseases, but the concept of immunotherapy has been discussed for past two decades. The objective of immunotherapy is to balance the human defence system to destroy tumour cells and at the same time side effects should also be less. In the history of immunotherapy, there are many rises and falls in search of treatment to cure cancer-like diseases using body's own immune system. The first regression was noticed in mid-eighteenth century when erysipelas was accidentally infected to patients with cancer. Coly, father of immunotherapy, purposely infected a person with erysipelas to cure and noticed a shrinkage in malignancy; later the causative agent of erysipelas was noticed but was disapproved by Mr. Burnet, who developed "acquired immunological tolerance" theory which claims that the immunotherapy would be much more complicated for body's defence system to differentiate among normal and tumour cells. This contradictory thought increased the complexity level of immunotherapy in oncogene. After several arguments, Mr. Burnet developed another thesis "immunosurveillance theory" which promotes the idea of immunotherapy. Later this was proved by stating that T cells can kill cancer cell by mutation and provide responses against tumour cells. Soon immunotherapy entered oncology. There are several types of immunotherapies used in cancer treatments. They include oncolytic virus-mediated therapies, cytokine-targeted therapy, adaptive cell transfer, immune checkpoint inhibitor, targeting B cells and NK cells (Wang et al. 2020).

3.4.2 Mechanism of Action

T cells can distinguish normal cells and cancer cells by recognizing the receptors present on its surface. Cancer cells are normal cells that are mutated, more the mutations, more easily it recognizes, but T cells only recognize the cancer cell but does not destroy it; this is because the PDL-1 molecule present in the tumour cell when binds with the PD-1 proteins of T cells prevents the elimination of cancerous cells. Here immune checkpoint inhibitor comes into play which protects binding of PDL-1 and PD-1 which leads to destroying of cancer cells. These inhibitory signals being targeted come from a number of sources (Calles and Álvarez 2019).

Our body's immune system has a significant role in controlling the proliferation of tumours or neoplasm. Certain types of inflammatory response may lead to promotion of neoplasm, whereas the tumour-specific adaptive immune response can regulate the tumour growth. It is a process in which each step requires regulation of different kinds of factors to manage great balance between immune activity and autoimmunity. In order to avoid autoimmunity activation and proliferation of T lymphocytes, they are regulated by immune checkpoints. The most preferable checkpoint pathways are cytotoxic T-lymphocyte-associated antigen 4 and PD-1. Treatment of lung cancer using monoclonal antibodies prevents side effects. Programmed cell death domain (PD-1) is an immunotherapeutic target, whose inhibition enhances anti-cancer immune response and tumour apoptosis. Pre-treatment of advance NSCLC patients with monoclonal antibody shows higher PD-1 blockage when compared to chemotherapy. Monoclonal antibodies are available to block EGFR (Epidermal Growth Factor Receptor) and immune checkpoints. Some commonly used monoclonal antibodies to treat lung cancer include Pembrolizumab (PD-L1 blocker), Durvalumab (bind to PD-1 and CD80), Necitumumab (EGFR inhibitor), Nivolumab (disrupt signal for T cell activation and proliferation). Other monoclonal antibodies include Sinitilimab, Gemiplimab, Atezolizumab, and Ipilimumab. The main immune checkpoint pathways are CTLA-4, PDL-1, and PD-1. The healthy cell of the body is protected by activating and suppressing T cells. Vaccines improves the activation of tumour-specific T cells and B cells. It also harnesses the immune recognition of specific antigens. There are different types of vaccines used for treating cell-based, protein, and genetic vaccines (Naddafi 2019).

3.4.3 Clinical Trials

Lung cancer is one of the common life-threatening diseases which consumes three-fourths of the lung cancer is non-small-cell lung cancer. Clinical trials were conducted for the patients with non-small-cell lung cancer (NSCLC). FDA approved two immune checkpoints for treatment of advanced NSCLC. Primary-care treatment for lung cancer is divided into three different phases (1) Radical therapy is provided to patients with early-stage of non-specific cell lung cancer. (2) Cancer vaccination is antigen-specific immunotherapy which is also one of the clinical trials practised which produces antigen-specific antibodies (Declerck and Vansteenkiste

2014). For patients with advanced non-small-cell lung cancer, platinum doublet chemotherapy is used which extends the survival period up to 10 months. Whereas the usage of checkpoint inhibitors PDL-1 for the treatment of advanced NSCLC is said to be best as it has fewer side effects and the overall survival rate is also high (Calles and Álvarez 2019).

3.4.4 Efficacy of Immunotherapy for Lung Cancer

Immunotherapy is a kind of treatment where our immune system is boosted up to fight against cancer. The eradication of healthy cells is prevented by the action of tumour-specific T cells, which binds specifically to receptors on cancer cell. Generally, the tumour neoantigen is recognized by antigen-presenting cells (dendritic cell), which carries them to the primary lymphoid organ (lymph node), where T cells gets matured upon recognition and attachment of T cell receptor (TCR), major histocompatibility complex I (MHC-I), and CD 40 ligation. The activated T cells enter circulation, interact with tumour, survive immune suppression in tumour microenvironment, and attack them (Steven et al. 2016). Antigen-specific vaccines that are specific to tumour antigens, cancer vaccines, monoclonal antibodies, immune checkpoint inhibitors which negatively regulate immune system activation, CTLA-4 and PD-1 blockers are widely used strategies in immunotherapy. Immunotherapy initially didn't work for lung cancer because of primary and acquired resistance. These resistances were due to inadequate accumulation of mutated tumour antigens, reduced cross-presentation that suppress dendritic cell migration, lack of necessary signals from CD-40, and ineffective lysed tumour cell presentation in cancer vaccines. Some of the promising immunotherapies include chimeric antigen receptor (CAR) and CD3-based dual specific receptors (Kinoshita et al. 2021).

3.5 Road Map from Chemotherapy to Immunotherapy

The unavoidable side effects of chemotherapy and the development of mutations and drug resistance paved way to the discovery of anti-angiogenic and targeted therapies. Anti-angiogenic drugs inhibit the blood vessel formation in cancer cells and thereby hinder the supply of nutrients to them. Researchers and doctors have discovered that the chemotherapeutic drugs act variably among patients in cohorts. This led to the discovery of targeted therapies where specific cancer genes, and cancer proteins like EGFR, ALK, HER2, KRAS, ROS, NTRK fusion genes, RET fusion genes are targeted to reduce cancer progression. The chance of normal cells getting destroyed in targeted therapy is very less, since it is more specific. Though the drugs work specifically to cancer genes or proteins with lesser side effects, they are highly expensive and take longer time to recover. Similarly personalized or precision medicines designed based on genetic makeup of an individual also face the same drawbacks. Hence, researchers have aimed to boost the immune response of the host to tackle cancer progression. This idea has led to the invention of immunotherapy. Some of the treatment strategies followed after understanding the drawbacks of chemotherapy, treatments that show better results in combination with chemotherapy, and the treatments that were into practice before the emergence of immunotherapy have been discussed below.

3.5.1 Anti-Angiogenic Therapy

Vascular Endothelial Growth Factor (VEGF) is responsible for angiogenesis in normal and cancer cells to supply nutrients through the blood. Of all four VEGF families, VEGF A is closely associated with NSCLC. It has two receptors, and the treatment strategies aim to target these receptors of VEGF that could control cancer progression. AVAiL and AVAPERL studies showed varied Progression Free Survival (PFS) and Overall Survival (OS) rates when Bevacizumab (a monoclonal VEGFA Inhibitor) along with chemotherapy is tested for its action in non-squamous NSCLC patients. Its usage showed adverse effects like pulmonary haemorrhage, haemoptysis, and pulmonary embolism. A recombinant human fusion protein called Aflibercept (an isoform of anti-VEGF A and anti-VEGF B), when administered in tumour-progressing NSCLC patients who had already undergone platinum-based doublet therapy, showed reduced thromboembolic effect and progression. Administration of Nintedanib (a tyrosine kinase inhibitor for VEGF receptor) and Ramucirumab reduced haemorrhagic side effects in adenocarcinoma and squamous cell carcinoma patients, respectively (Tian and Cao 2020).

3.5.2 Targeted Therapy

3.5.2.1 Target as Epidermal Growth Factor Receptor (EGFR)/ ERBB/HER

EGFR, upon activation by its ligand EGF, regulates effector signalling pathways like RAS, AKT, and STAT. Nearly 20% of adenocarcinoma occurs due to EGFR overexpression and mutations. Deletion of exon 19, or point mutation in exon 21 (L858R), is common among them. The first-generation Tyrosine Kinase inhibitors (TKI) like Gefitinib and Erlotinib target the intracellular domain of EGFR and exhibit competitive, reversible binding. This process inhibits cell proliferation and induces apoptosis. Though it has side effects like diarrhoea, nausea, and acneiform rashes, it is considered a superior strategy to chemotherapy for EGFR-mutated NSCLC. A missense mutation in T790M resists first-generation EGFR TKI and paves the way for second-generation EGFR TKI's like Afatinib, Dacomitinib, and Neratinib. They are pan-ErbB inhibitors that bind irreversibly to EGFR carrying T790M mutation, Her2 and Her4 mutation. They considerably respond to other uncommon EGFR mutations. Third-generation EGFR TKIs like Rociletinib and AZD9291 inhibit T790M mutation and exhibit a minimal effect on other members of the ErbB family. Anti-EGFR monoclonal antibodies like Cetuximab and

Necitumumab are prescribed to squamous cell cancer patients with EGFR mutations since they actively block the ligand-binding site of EGFR-1. An EGFR mutant NSCLC patient, when treated with Cetuximab and Afatinib, showed a 29% of response rate. Grade 3 toxicity patients undergoing this combination of treatments showed 99% side effects. Patients with cancer progression after EGFR TKI treatment are advised to temporarily cease the treatment and continue with Gefitinib instead of platinum-based doublet chemotherapy (Metro and Crinò 2012).

3.5.2.2 Target as Anaplastic Lymphoma Kinase (ALK)

ALK gene mutations like EML4-ALK fusion, L1196M, and G1269A lead to lung cancer. A first-generation ALK TKI known as Crizotinib (a small molecule inhibitor) blocks cell cycle at the G1-S phase and kills them. Its usage leads to visual disturbances, diarrhoea, vomiting, and benign cyst formation in the kidney. The emergence of resistance for Crizotinib occurs because of the substitution of C1156Y, G1202R mutation, and gatekeeper mutation (L1196M), thereby bringing Ceritinib (a second-generation ALK TKI) into existence. Ceritinib showed a response rate of 58% in ALK-positive NSCLC patients who were newly exposed to ALK TKI therapy and had already undergone Crizotinib therapy. Alextinib, a more potent second-generation ALK TKI, showed a 93.5% response rate in NSCLC patients with ALK mutations. Alextinib replaces first-generation ALK TKI since it has greater CNS penetration capacity, thereby preventing brain metastasis. A new approach targeting heat shock protein 90 (Hsp90) using Crizotinib showed positive activity in tumour regression (Boolell et al. 2015).

3.5.2.3 Other Common Drug Targets

When Hepatocyte Growth Factor (HGF) ligand binds to MET (Proto-oncogene) receptor, it activates AKT, RAS, MAPK, and PLC signalling pathways involved in invasion and metastasis. Approximately 40–50% of MET Receptor is expressed in NSCLC. MET TKI like Tivantinib, Cabozantinib, Crizotinib, Foretinib and MET monoclonal antibodies like Ficlatuzumab, AMG 102, and Onartuzumab are used as treatment strategies to minimize them. Nearly 4% of lung adenocarcinoma due to C-MET gene amplification is treated using Crizotinib and Cabozantinib (Korpanty et al. 2014). Proto-oncogene (ROS 1 gene) fusion, or rearrangement with CD74, SLC24A2, EZR, and FIG genes, leads to 1.5% of adenocarcinoma having similar clinical presentation like ALK mutations; hence, Crizotinib was administered to treat this type of NSCLC. It showed a 72% response rate with 19.2 months of PFS (Boolell et al. 2015). Nearly 1.7% of lung adenocarcinoma occurs due to RET fusion genes harbouring. They include CCDC6, NCOA4, KIF5B, and TRIM33. Among them, KIF5B fusion is the most resistant. They are treated using multi-kinase inhibitors like Sunitinib, Vandetanib, Sorafenib, Lenvatinib, and Cabozantinib (Bronte et al. 2019). BRAF is a part of the MAPK signalling pathway that is involved in cell regulation and cell growth. BRAF (V600 E) mutation leads to 2% of adenocarcinoma and SCC and is treated using Dabrafenib. On the other hand, some treatments do not work efficiently. KRAS mutations lead to 30% of lung adenocarcinoma, which was aimed to treat with Selumitinib and Docetaxel but failed to stop cancer progression. Similarly, IGFR (Insulin Growth Factor Receptor) and FGFR (Fibroblast Growth Factor Receptor) amplifications were aimed at reducing cancer progression using Figitumumab and AZD4547 but failed. Discoidin Domain Receptor (DRR) mutation leads to 4% of SCC. Treating this type of mutation using an oral TKI (Dasatinib) does not stop cancer progression (Boolell et al. 2015).

3.6 Combination Therapy

3.6.1 Chemotherapy with Immunotherapy

Chemotherapy is a widely used approach to treat cancer by administering medications that destroy cancer cells. Yet, emerging research suggests that chemotherapy could also boost the response to immunotherapy for cancer. This is accomplished by several mechanisms, including the release of tumour-specific antigens, upregulation of MHC expression, elevation of cytotoxic lymphocytes to regulatory T cells ratio, and reduction of myeloid-derived suppressor cells. The phase 2 KEYNOTE-021G trial determined the predominance of combining immunotherapy and chemotherapy in advanced NSCLC (Salas-Benito et al. 2021). The KEYNOTE-189 trial showed substantial improvement for Progression-Free Survival and Overall Survival rate, no matter the PD-L1 category (Lee 2019). A phase 1/2 study evaluated the combination of pembrolizumab with pemetrexed and carboplatin (CIT) as an alternative first-line therapeutic approach for NSCLC patients with 50% tumour PD-L1 expression. There was a higher response rate in the CIT combination group (55%) when compared to the group that received chemotherapy alone (29%) (Lee 2019; Salas-Benito et al. 2021). PD-1/PD-L1–blocking-based combinations, such as ipilimumab + nivolumab and atezolizumab + bevacizumab + chemotherapy, have recently been validated for NSCLC patient as first-line treatment. Additionally beneficial was nivolumab used in conjunction with chemotherapy and bevacizumab. In SCLC, addition of PD-L1 blockade with atezolizumab or durvalumab to standard platinum + etoposide yields better results than chemotherapy alone. Pembrolizumab with etoposide + carboplatin has been reported in a phase III trial (Salas-Benito et al. 2021). In KEYNOTE-021, the response rate to pembrolizumab/carboplatin plus paclitaxel was 52%; however, this increased up to 70% when patients were treated with pembrolizumab/carboplatin plus pemetrexed. In a different study using atezolizumab in combination with various chemotherapies, response rates ranged from 60% to 75% (Hellmann et al. 2016). Through the activation of NF-B, CD8+ T-cells, PD-L1, APC maturation, MHC class I presentation, and the downregulation of immunosuppressive cells, chemotherapy affects the immune system. To assess the security and effectiveness of immune checkpoint inhibitors in combination with platinum-based chemotherapy, various clinical trials are being developed (Lazzari et al. 2018). The KEYNOTE-021 research revealed that the most effective combination of treatments was pembrolizumab with carboplatin and paclitaxel, carboplatin, paclitaxel, and bevacizumab, or carboplatin and pemetrexed, yielding an overall response rate (ORR) of 52%. These results imply that chemotherapy may alter immune function (Hellmann et al. 2016; Lazzari et al. 2018).

3.6.2 Immunotherapy with Radiation Therapy

The RT for NSCLC has been established to improve median OS and PFS when administered prior to pembrolizumab treatment. Generally, RT is used for palliative care; however, this research indicates that there may be an additional benefit to using it beforehand (Heinzerling et al. 2021). Individuals who had radiation prior to beginning nivolumab experienced a higher overall response rate compared to those who had not. Further research has been conducted to explore the potential synergistic effect of combining this treatment with fractionated radiation or SBRT (Heinzerling et al. 2021). At one metastatic site prior to treatment, 76 patients were randomly assigned to receive pembrolizumab with or without SBRT. Although the overall response rate increased by 50% from 18% to 36%, the predetermined endpoint was not reached. The outcomes of radiation therapy and immunotherapy have been studied in a number of prospective trials in patients with more regionally advanced or oligometastatic NSCLC. In a single-arm phase II trial with recently published results, pembrolizumab was administered 4–12 weeks after local therapy. Patients with three or fewer locations of oligometastatic illness are being randomly assigned in the ongoing phase III trial to receive continuing maintenance therapy as opposed to local radiation therapy or surgery (Heinzerling et al. 2021; Miller et al. 2018).

3.6.3 Chemotherapy with Radiation Therapy

Cancer cells can avoid growth inhibition and immunosurveillance. CAR T-cell therapy is based on T cells that have undergone genetic modification to incorporate a CAR that allows them to recognize cancer cells without the aid of MHC proteins. These transformed T cells require both extracellular, tumour recognition and intracellular transmembrane components for growth. The use of CAR T-cells in solid tumours exhibits a peculiar challenge to successfully deliver the genetically modified T cells to the target and spread this response in a hostile TME (Miller et al. 2018). When combined with immunotherapy, radiotherapy has immunomodulatory effects that can be used. Carcinoembryonic antigen (CEA) and mesothelin-expressing tumours are two instances of radiotherapy-inducing tumour-associated antigens. By increasing the expression of the Fas gene in cancer cells that also express CEA, radiotherapy can more effectively treat these cancer cells. However, it can also present a challenge to T-cell therapy due to issues related to trafficking and chemotaxis. This means that while radiotherapy can have benefits for treating cancer, it may also affect the ability of T-cell therapies to reach and target cancer cells. CAR T-cell therapy is being investigated for metastatic NSCLC at the National Institutes of Health in a phase II clinical trial.

However, using CAR T cells in solid tumours presents a unique challenge (Miller et al. 2018; Lazzari et al. 2018).

3.7 Conclusion

Over the past few years, lung cancer medications have rapidly advanced beyond chemotherapy. The identification of oncogenic driver mutations has provided fresh therapeutic options for cancer treatment as well as new methods for categorizing NSCLC. TKIs that are appropriate have been employed to successfully target EGFR mutations and ALK gene rearrangements. Targeted medicines have also been employed in early clinical studies to investigate other driver mutations such ROS, MET, RET, and BRAF. New methods in the research of immuno-oncology have extended the scope for the use of inhibitors that are key for the immune system routes for recognizing cancer cells. Compelling evidences suggest that cancers are reducing post immune and targeted therapies which has given rise to investment of fund from pharmaceutical firms, philanthropists, and the government. The effectiveness of lung cancer treatments has augmented over the past 15 decades, moving from general surgery to molecule-specific targeted therapy and immunotherapy. More cutting-edge and extraordinary medicines are anticipated to enter the field as our understanding of the immune-cancer connection expands. After the development of complicated sub-clonal lesions, cancer can be challenging to treat with chemotherapy and targeted molecular therapies since it is a developing genetic disease. Future immunotherapies will focus on the mutant proteins that are created as neoantigens as a result of the slow accumulation of genetic alterations. Current developments include the discovery of new pharmaceuticals and the blending of various medications. Combining multiple forms of treatment with immunotherapy is a viable treatment approach if the adverse effects of the medications can be managed.

Author Contributions Subiksha Maheshkumar, Diwahar Prakash & Ashwin Subramanian: Writing - Original Draft, Writing - Review & Editing, Collection of data; Gayathri Devi Muthukumarasamy & Rishmitha Duraisamy: Writing - Original Draft, Collection of data; Gayathri Gopal & Shibi Muralidar: Writing - Review & Editing; Senthil Visaga Ambi: Conceptualization, Visualization, Supervision, and Writing - Review & Editing.

Conflict of Interest The authors declare no conflict of interest.

Acknowledgments The authors express their gratitude to SASTRA-Deemed-to-be-University, Tamil Nadu, India, for infrastructure and financial support. The authors also extend their appreciation for the contribution of Biopharmaceutical research lab members, SASTRA-Deemed-to-be-University.

References

Alexander M, Kim SY, Cheng H (2020) Update 2020: management of non-small cell lung cancer. Lung 198(6):897–907. https://doi.org/10.1007/s00408-020-00407-5

Antonia SJ, Villegas A, Daniel D, Vicente D, Murakami S, Hui R, Yokoi T, Chiappori A, Lee KH, de Wit M, Cho BC, Bourhaba M, Quantin X, Tokito T, Mekhail T, Planchard D, Kim Y-C, Karapetis CS, Hiret S, Özgüroğlu M (2017) Durvalumab after chemoradiotherapy in stage III non–small-cell lung cancer. N Engl J Med 377(20):1919–1929. https://doi.org/10.1056/nejmoa1709937

Antonia SJ, Villegas A, Daniel D, Vicente D, Murakami S, Hui R, Kurata T, Chiappori A, Lee KH, de Wit M, Cho BC, Bourhaba M, Quantin X, Tokito T, Mekhail T, Planchard D, Kim Y-C, Karapetis CS, Hiret S, Özgüroğlu M (2018) Overall survival with durvalumab after chemoradiotherapy in stage III NSCLC. N Engl J Med 379(24):2342–2350. https://doi.org/10.1056/nejmoa1809697

Bar J, Ofek E, Barshack I, Gottfried T, Zadok O, Kamer I, Urban D, Perelman M, Onn A (2019) Lung cancer transformation to small cell lung cancer as a mechanism of resistance to immunotherapy in non-small cell lung cancer. Lung Cancer 138:109–115. https://doi.org/10.1016/j.lungcan.2019.09.025

Biermann JS, Chow W, Reed DR, Lucas D, Adkins DR, Agulnik M, Benjamin RS, Brigman B, Budd GT, Curry WT, Didwania A, Fabbri N, Hornicek FJ, Kuechle JB, Lindskog D, Mayerson J, McGarry SV, Million L, Morris CD, Scavone JL (2017) NCCN guidelines insights: bone cancer, version 2.2017. J Natl Compr Cancer Netw 15(2):155–167. https://doi.org/10.6004/jnccn.2017.0017

Boolell V, Alamgeer M, Watkins DN, Ganju V (2015) The evolution of therapies in non-small cell lung cancer. Cancers 7(3):1815–1846. https://doi.org/10.3390/cancers7030864

Bradley JD, Hu C, Komaki RR, Masters GA, Blumenschein GR, Schild SE, Bogart JA, Forster KM, Magliocco AM, Kavadi VS, Narayan S, Iyengar P, Robinson CG, Wynn RB, Koprowski CD, Olson MR, Meng J, Paulus R, Curran WJ, Choy H (2020) Long-term results of NRG oncology RTOG 0617: standard-versus high-dose chemoradiotherapy with or without cetuximab for unresectable stage III non-small-cell lung cancer. J Clin Oncol 38(7):706–714. https://doi.org/10.1200/JCO.19.01162

Bronte G, Ulivi P, Verlicchi A, Cravero P, Delmonte A, Crinò L (2019) Targeting RET-rearranged non-small-cell lung cancer: future prospects. Lung Cancer (Auckl) 10:27–36. https://doi.org/10.2147/LCTT.S192830

Calles A, Álvarez GACSR (2019) The role of immunotherapy in small cell lung cancer. Clin Transl Oncol 961:0123456789. https://doi.org/10.1007/s12094-018-02011-9

Chaft JE, Rimner A, Weder W, Azzoli CG, Kris MG, Cascone T (2021) Evolution of systemic therapy for stages I–III non-metastatic non-small-cell lung cancer. Nat Rev Clin Oncol 18:547–557. https://doi.org/10.1038/s41571-021-00501-4

Chen S, Qiao Y, Chen J, Li Y, Xie J, Cui P, Huang Z, Huang D (2022) Evolutions in the management of non-small cell lung cancer: a bibliometric study from the 100 most impactful articles in the field. Front Oncol 12:1–15. https://doi.org/10.3389/fonc.2022.939838

Chhatriwala H, Jafri N, Salgia R (2006) A review of topoisomerase inhibition in lung cancer. Cancer Biol Ther 5(12):1600–1607. https://doi.org/10.4161/cbt.5.12.3546

Declerck S, Vansteenkiste J (2014) Immunotherapy for lung cancer: ongoing clinical trials. Future Oncol 10:91–105

DeVita VT, Chu E (2008) A history of cancer chemotherapy. Cancer Res 68(21):8643–8653. https://doi.org/10.1158/0008-5472.CAN-07-6611

Frank C, Detterbeck (2018) The eighth edition TNM stage classification for lung cancer: What does it mean on main street? The Journal of Thoracic and Cardiovascular Surgery, 155(1): 356–359. https://doi.org/10.1016/j.jtcvs.2017.08.138.

Giraud P, Morvan E, Claude L, Mornex F, Le Pechoux C, Bachaud JM, Boisselier P, Beckendorf V, Morelle M, Carrère MO (2011) Respiratory gating techniques for optimization of lung cancer radiotherapy. J Thorac Oncol 6(12):2058–2068. https://doi.org/10.1097/JTO.0b013e3182307ec2

Heinzerling JH, Mileham KF, Simone CB (2021) The utilization of immunotherapy with radiation therapy in lung cancer: a narrative review. Transl Cancer Res 10(5):2596–2608. https://doi.org/10.21037/tcr-20-2241

Hellmann MD, Li BT, Chaft JE, Kris MG (2016) Chemotherapy remains an essential element of personalized care for persons with lung cancers. Ann Oncol 27(10):1829–1835. https://doi.org/10.1093/ANNONC/MDW271

IJsselmuiden CB, Faden RR (1992) The New England Journal of Medicine Downloaded from nejm.org on January 31, 2011. For personal use only. No other uses without permission. Copyright © 1992 Massachusetts medical society. All rights reserved 326

Islam KM, Anggondowati T, Deviany PE, Ryan JE, Fetrick A, Bagenda D, Copur MS, Tolentino A, Vaziri I, McKean HA, Dunder S, Gray JE, Huang C, Ganti AK (2019) Patient preferences of chemotherapy treatment options and tolerance of chemotherapy side effects in advanced stage lung cancer. BMC Cancer 19(1):1–9. https://doi.org/10.1186/s12885-019-6054-x

Kinoshita T, Terai H, Yaguchi T (2021) Clinical efficacy and future prospects of immunotherapy in lung cancer. Life 11(10):1–16. https://doi.org/10.3390/life11101029

Korpanty GJ, Graham DM, Vincent MD, Leighl NB (2014) Biomarkers that currently effect clinical practice in lung cancer: EGFR, ALK, MET, ROS-1 and KRAS. Front Oncol 4:1–26. https://doi.org/10.3389/fonc.2014.00204

Lazzari C, Karachaliou N, Bulotta A, Viganó M, Mirabile A, Brioschi E, Santarpia M, Gianni L, Rosell R, Gregorc V (2018) Combination of immunotherapy with chemotherapy and radiotherapy in lung cancer: is this the beginning of the end for cancer? Ther Adv Med Oncol 10:1–12. https://doi.org/10.1177/1758835918762094

Lee SH (2019) Chemotherapy for lung cancer in the era of personalized medicine. Tuberc Respir Dis 82(3):179–189. https://doi.org/10.4046/trd.2018.0068

Mehta N, King CR, Agazaryan N, Steinberg M, Hua A, Lee P (2012) Stereotactic body radiation therapy and 3-dimensional conformal radiotherapy for stage I non-small cell lung cancer: a pooled analysis of biological equivalent dose and local control. Pract Radiat Oncol 2(4):288–295. https://doi.org/10.1016/j.prro.2011.10.004

Metro G, Crinò L (2012) Advances on EGFR mutation for lung cancer. Transl Lung Cancer Res 1(1):5–13. https://doi.org/10.3978/j.issn.2218-6751.2011.12.01

Miller ED, Fisher JL, Haglund KE, Grecula JC, Xu-Welliver M, Bertino EM, He K, Shields PG, Carbone DP, Williams TM, Otterson GA, Bazan JG (2018) The addition of chemotherapy to radiation therapy improves survival in elderly patients with stage III non–small cell lung cancer. J Thorac Oncol 13(3):426–435. https://doi.org/10.1016/j.jtho.2017.11.135

Min HY, Lee HY (2021) Mechanisms of resistance to chemotherapy in non-small cell lung cancer. Arch Pharm Res 44(2):146–164. https://doi.org/10.1007/s12272-021-01312-y

Murray N, Turrisi AT (2006) A review of first-line treatment for small-cell lung cancer. J Thorac Oncol 1(3):270–278. https://doi.org/10.1016/S1556-0864(15)31579-3

Naddafi F (2019) Monoclonal antibodies in non-small-cell lung cancer: light at the end of the tunnel. Trends Med 19(3):1–5. https://doi.org/10.15761/tim.1000190

Natural N, Defense I, Rushfeldt C, Sveinbjørnsson B, Seljelid R (1999) Early events of hepatic metastasis formation in mice: role of Kupffer early events of hepatic metastasis formation in mice: role of Kupffer and NK-cells in Natural and interferon-γ-stimulated defense. J Surgl Res *82*(2):209–215. https://doi.org/10.1006/jsre.1998.5532

Pearce A, Haas M, Viney R, Pearson S, Haywood P, Brown C, Ward R (2017) Mức Độ Nghiêm Trọng Của Tác Dụng Phụ.Pdf. 1–12

Ralhan R, Kaur J (2007) Alkylating agents and cancer therapy. Expert Opin Ther Pat 17(9):1061–1075. https://doi.org/10.1517/13543776.17.9.1061

Salas-Benito D, Pérez-Gracia JL, Ponz-Sarvisé M, Rodriguez-Ruiz ME, Martínez-Forero I, Castañón E, López-Picazo JM, Sanmamed MF, Melero I (2021) Paradigms on immunotherapy combinations with chemotherapy. Cancer Discov 11(6):1353–1367. https://doi.org/10.1158/2159-8290.CD-20-1312

Steven A, Fisher SA, Robinson BW (2016) Immunotherapy for lung cancer. Respirology 21(5):821–833. https://doi.org/10.1111/resp.12789

Thirumaran R, Prendergast GC, Gilman PB (2007) Cytotoxic chemotherapy in clinical treatment of cancer. In: Cancer immunotherapy: immune suppression and tumor growth. Elsevier Inc. https://doi.org/10.1016/B978-012372551-6/50071-7

Tian W, Cao C (2020) Anti-angiogenic therapy in the treatment of non-small cell. Lung Cancer 13:12113–12129
Tohme S, Yazdani HO, Al-Khafaji AB, Chidi AP, Loughran P, Mowen K, Wang Y, Simmons RL, Huang H, Tsung A (2016) Neutrophil extracellular traps promote the development and progression of liver metastases after surgical stress. Cancer Res 76(6):1367–1380. https://doi.org/10.1158/0008-5472.CAN-15-1591
Toschi L, Rossi S, Finocchiaro G, Santoro A (2017) Non-small cell lung cancer treatment (r)evolution: ten years of advances and more to come. Nat Rev Clin Oncol 11:1–14
Vinod SK, Hau E (2020) Radiotherapy treatment for lung cancer: current status and future directions. Respirology 25(S2):61–71. https://doi.org/10.1111/resp.13870
Wang F, Wang S, Zhou Q (2020) The resistance mechanisms of lung cancer immunotherapy. Front Oncol 10:1–22. https://doi.org/10.3389/fonc.2020.568059
Wright CJ, Chambers GK, Robens-paradise Y (2002) Evaluation of indications for and outcomes of elective surgery. CMAJ 167:461
Yu S, Wang R, Tang H, Wang L, Zhang Z, Yang S, Jiao S, Wu X, Wang S, Wang M, Xu C, Wang Q, Wu Y (2020) Evolution of lung cancer in the context of immunotherapy. Clin Med Insights Oncol 14:1179554920979697. https://doi.org/10.1177/1179554920979697
Zhou J, Li Z, Li J, Gao B, Song W (2019) Chemotherapy resistance molecular mechanism in small cell lung cancer. Curr Mol Med 19(3):157–163. https://doi.org/10.2174/1566524019666190226104909

Revolutionizing Lung Cancer Treatment: Recent Breakthroughs in Immunotherapy

4

Kuttiappan Anitha, Santenna Chenchula, Parameshwar Ravula, Chikatipalli Radhika, and Shvetank Bhatt

4.1 Introduction to Lung Cancer

Lung cancer, the third most prevalent disease, is the leading cause of cancer-related death worldwide (Naumov et al. 2009). In 2020 alone, it resulted in approximately 1.8 million deaths globally (Naumov et al. 2009). Within the United States, there are over 230,000 new cases of lung cancer and 130,000 deaths reported each year (Naumov et al. 2009). Based on the histological appearance, lung cancer is classified into small-cell lung cancer (SCLC), a neuroendocrine tumour, and non-small-cell lung cancer (NSCLC) (Naumov et al. 2009). Overall, NSCLCs account for approximately 80–85% of all lung malignancies in humans, while SCLC constitutes the remaining 15–20% of lung cancer cases (Naumov et al. 2009; Hottel et al. 2018). The non-small-cell lung cancer, which is further classified into two primary subgroups, including squamous cell carcinoma (SCC), adenocarcinoma (ADC), and

P. Ravula
Department of Pharmacology, SPTM, SVKM's Narsee Monjee Institute of Management Studies (NMIMS) Deemed-to-University, Shirpur, Maharashtra, India
e-mail: kuttiappan.anitha@nmims.edu

S. Chenchula
Clinical Pharmacology, All India Institute of Medical Sciences (AIIMS), Bhopal, Madhya Pradesh, India

P. Ravula
Amity Institute of Pharmacy, Amity University Madhya Pradesh (AUMP), Gwalior, India

C. Radhika
Department of pharmacology, Sri Venkateshwara College of Pharmacy, Chittoor, Andhra Pradesh, India

S. Bhatt
School of Health Sciences and Technology, Dr. Vishwanath Karad MIT World Peace University, Pune, Maharashtra, India

S. Bhatt et al. (eds.), *Immunotherapy Against Lung Cancer*,
https://doi.org/10.1007/978-981-99-7141-1_4

large-cell carcinoma (LCC), each with distinct characteristics and varied responses to treatments (Naumov et al. 2009). Although SCLC is less common, it is known to be more aggressive, by its rapid doubling time, high growth fraction, and the early development of metastases (Naumov et al. 2009). Early identification plays a crucial role in determining the survival rates of lung cancer patients, and surgical removal of tumour tissue is generally the recommended treatment (Hottel et al. 2018).

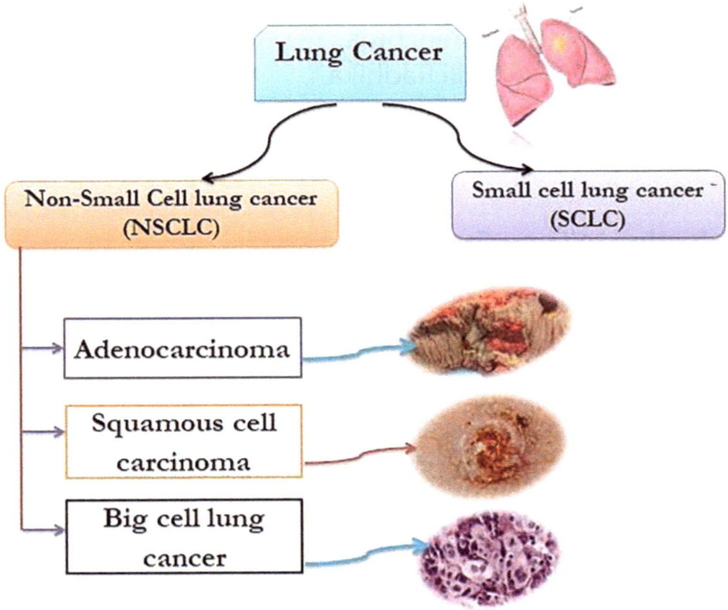

In the early stages of NSCLC, surgical resection offers the best opportunity for long-term survival and cure in patients with resectable NSCLC or stage I or II NSCLC, while patients with stage I or II disease who are not candidates for surgical resection or who refuse surgery may be candidates for nonsurgical local therapy with radiation, and both chemotherapy and radiation are suggested for stage III disease or locally advanced cancer (Rosell et al. 2017). While researchers continue to explore new therapeutic alternatives for all stages of the disease, there have been some positive developments in the treatment of advanced-stage lung cancer. One notable advancement is the use of epidermal growth factor receptor tyrosine kinase inhibitors (EGFR-TKIs) as the primary first-line choice for treating EGFR-mutant NSCLC, which has significantly advanced targeted therapy for malignant lung cancers. Additionally, the introduction of immunotherapies to EGFR-TKI therapies, aiming to dual-block the VEGF/EGFR pathways in preclinical models of EGFR-mutant NSCLC, has shown promising results in reversing primary or acquired resistance to EGFR-TKIs (Saito et al. 2019). Hence, there is an urgent need for novel therapeutic techniques to achieve more effective lung cancer treatment.

4.2 Recent Breakthroughs in Immunotherapy for NSCLC

Preliminary studies have demonstrated that the significance of downregulating lung cancer cells includes TAP1 and/or TAP2, which makes them resistant to TCR-dependent lysis. It is worth noting that TAP deficit has been observed in various human malignancies, such as cervical carcinoma, head and neck carcinoma, melanoma, gastric cancer, and lung cancer, and is associated with the evasion of immune system surveillance (Marincola et al. 2000). In fact, approximately 70% of non-small-cell lung cancer (NSCLC) cases exhibit low levels of TAP1 and/or TAP2 expression.

4.2.1 Developments in Perioperative Immunotherapy

Immunotherapy has gone from the advanced to the early phases, increasing the likelihood that patients with early-stage NSCLC would survive. There has been a substantial change in how things are done recently that NSCLC patients are treated. Many clinical trials, including those on postoperative immune adjuvant therapy and immune neoadjuvant therapy, are now in progress. The results of several ongoing clinical trials will determine the direction of future treatment. We believe that these discoveries may benefit lung cancer perioperative care (Abele and Tampe 2006).

4.2.2 Research on Circulating Tumour DNA (ctDNA) as Effective Biomarkers

The 2021 European Society of Medical Oncology (ESMO) Congress published the results of ctDNA as a potential biomarker, showing that ctDNA positivity is associated with poor prognosis in DFS. However, interestingly, atezolizumab showed improved DFS outcomes for patients with Stage II-IIIA cancers, irrespective of ctDNA status. Further analysis demonstrated that the level of PD-L1 expression, rather than ctDNA, was the biomarker influencing patient prognosis (Setiadi et al. 2007). Therefore, ctDNA cannot be solely used for screening potential candidates for adjuvant immunotherapy, as both ctDNA-positive and ctDNA-negative individuals can benefit from immunotherapy.

Immunotherapy has evolved from being primarily used in advanced stages to being employed in early stages, with the aim of improving cure rates for patients with early-stage NSCLC. Adjuvant and neoadjuvant perioperative treatments have the potential to enhance disease outcomes in NSCLC. The treatment landscape for NSCLC patients has witnessed significant changes in recent years, with ongoing clinical trials exploring immune neoadjuvant therapy and postoperative immune adjuvant therapy. The findings from these trials will shape future treatment approaches. Consequently, it is anticipated that these discoveries will provide valuable insights for perioperative lung cancer treatment (Einstein et al. 2009).

4.2.3 Approaches in Adjuvant Immunotherapy

Adjuvant therapy is widely utilized for the treatment of early and locally advanced cancers that respond to local therapy. The objective of adjuvant systemic chemotherapy in cancer treatment is to improve local control by eradicating micrometastatic disease that may have developed after surgery. Adjuvant chemotherapy has become the standard of care for patients with resected stage II-III NSCLC and is now being considered for stage IB disease, offering a 5-year overall survival (OS) benefit of approximately 5%. Notably, previous studies have indicated a significant advantage in disease-free survival, leading to FDA approval of targeted EGFR treatment for 3 years in the adjuvant setting (Leibowitz et al. 2011). In a clinical trial evaluating the efficacy of ICI in patients with early-stage lung cancer who had completed radical therapy, including surgery and postoperative adjuvant chemotherapy, atezolizumab adjuvant immunotherapy significantly improved disease-free survival (DFS) compared to Best Supportive Care (BSC) in Stage II-IIIA NSCLC patients (Borghaei et al. 2021).

4.2.4 The Concept of Neoadjuvant Immunotherapy

In a previous study investigating immunotherapy as postoperative neoadjuvant therapy for NSCLC, 21 patients who received two cycles of nivolumab before surgery were enrolled. The results demonstrated a 45% major pathologic response rate (MPR) for nivolumab neoadjuvant therapy, a 70% 24-month recurrence-free survival (RFS), and a 10% pathologic complete response (pCR). This groundbreaking experiment ushered in a new era of perioperative immunotherapy and confirmed the clinical efficacy and safety of neoadjuvant ICI monotherapy (Anagnostou et al. 2018).

4.2.5 Immunotherapy for Advanced NSCLC

Immunotherapy has revolutionized the treatment of advanced NSCLC, transforming the way lung cancer is managed. Following initial evidence that immunotherapy could improve overall survival (OS) in advanced NSCLC patients, it became the standard second-line treatment for patients without driver gene mutations (Chen et al. 2021). Immunotherapy in combination with chemotherapy has successfully treated the entire group of patients with advanced NSCLC and negative driver genes. Additionally, novel techniques such as dual immunotherapy and combined immunological and antivascular therapy continue to expand the scope of immunotherapy.

4.2.6 Combined Immunotherapy and Chemotherapy

Chemotherapy and immunotherapy are now considered to be the mainstay of care for people with non-small-cell lung cancer. According to preclinical research, combination therapy that includes synergistic immunomodulation may enhance immune-mediated cancer death and disrupt the immunosuppressive tumour microenvironment, which hinders immune detection. Clinical trials of chemo-immunotherapy, which demonstrated improved and long-term benefits, have demonstrated this potential synergy or complementary activity. The CameL study was the first Phase III clinical trial to include participants without systemic therapy who had Stage IIIB or IV EGFR/ALK wild-type non-squamous NSCLC. The most recent data showed that chemotherapy and immunotherapy together significantly improved objective response rate to a significant level (Ren et al. 2022).

The data from CameL-sq study reported that camrelizumab was used as the first-line treatment for EGFR/ALK-negative unresectable locally advanced or metastatic squamous NSCLC. It was also combined with paclitaxel and carboplatin. Chemotherapy alone was found to be less effective than chemotherapy with immunotherapy, with a much better ORR (64.8% vs. 36.7%) and longer PFS (8.5 vs. 4.9 months). The 2- and 3-year survival rates were about 20% higher in the camrelizumab plus chemotherapy group than in the chemotherapy alone group (53.4% vs. 35.0%, 42.8% vs. 23.7%, HR = 0.57, 95% CI: 0.44–0.74, p 0.0001) and significantly reduced death risk by 43% (Sahin et al. 2017).

Novel Immunotherapy is the mainstay treatment for advanced NSCLC, and medicines like PD-1/PD-L1 have been licenced as first-line monotherapy or in conjunction with chemotherapy. However, in clinical trials, the median PFS (mPFS) was less than 1 year, indicating that a new treatment strategy is required to enhance the outcome.

4.2.6.1 Combined Immunization with JAK Inhibitors

Despite tremendous breakthroughs in the treatment of NSCLC with surgery, radiation, and chemotherapy, patients with advanced cancer continue to have a poor prognosis and significantly varying clinical outcomes because of tumour recurrence, and metastasis needs developing vaccination in conjunction with JAK inhibitors. In the first-line treatment of metastatic NSCLC with PD-L1 50%, a Phase II clinical study's results, which were showed that pembrolizumab combined with itacitinib (INCB039110, a JAK inhibitor), had a 12-week ORR of 62% and an mPFS of 23.4 months, achieving a significant and sustained ORR that is anticipated to become a treatment trend (Ubenik 2003).

4.2.6.2 Immunization Combined with Poly ADP-Ribose Polymerase (PARP) Inhibitors

The first clinically approved drugs that use synthetic lethality were PARP inhibitors, which were first introduced in 2005 as a cancer-targeting strategy. They have changed the natural history of a disease with high genetic complexity and defective DNA repair via the homologous recombination pathway, and they have significantly improved the therapy of advanced NSCLS. PARP inhibitor-induced DNA damage may modify tumour immunogenicity and sensitize tumours to PD-1/PD-L1 blockade, potentially resulting in more persistent PD-1/PD-L1 blockade than a single-drug anti-tumour response (Ishii et al. 2015). Patients with EGFR/ALK wild-type metastatic NSCLC and no disease progression (PD) in the initial treatment were randomly assigned to durvalumab plus olaparib or durvalumab monotherapy as first-line therapy for advancement of therapy (Wang et al. 2023).

4.2.7 Immune Combination Antibody–Drug Conjugate (ADC)

TROPION-Lung02's Phase Ib study employed a two-drug or three-drug combination therapy strategy that included Dato-DXd and pembrolizumab chemotherapy, the dual regimen was more secure than the triple regimen (Domvri et al. 2020). Findings of the study have shown that Datopotamabderuxtecan (DS-1062a, ADC), a TROP-2-targeting ADC, showing efficacy and tolerability as monotherapy in patients with relapsed/refractory advanced/metastatic NSCLC. The triple regimen exhibited significant chemotherapy-related side effects, but there was no significant difference between the two regimens in immune-related side effects. ADC immuno-combination appears to be successful. The dual regimen's first-line treatment had an overall remission rate of 62%, whereas the triple regimen achieved an ORR of 80%.

4.2.8 Anti PD-1 and PD-L1 Inhibitors in NSCLC

The immunological checkpoint receptor programmed cell death protein-1 (PD-1) induces and maintains tolerance in lymphocytes such as T cells, invariant natural killer T (iNKT) cells, and natural killer (NK) cells. Immune checkpoint inhibition with PD-1 inhibition restores the lymphocytic immunostimulatory phenotype and has been utilized to treat several malignancies. While immune checkpoint inhibition has been shown to provide good anticancer therapy outcomes, its overall response rate remains low in a significant proportion of cancer patients (Reck et al. 2019).

While immune checkpoint inhibition has been shown to provide good anti-cancer therapy outcomes, its overall response rate remains low in a significant proportion of cancer patients. A key unmet need in cancer therapy is the development of novel pharmacologic approaches to minimize resistance rates associated with immune checkpoint suppression. Furthermore, resistance to anti-PD-1/PD-L1 immunotherapy correlates to failure and poor prognosis in patients with advanced NSCLC receiving anti-PD-1/PD-L1 therapy. An immune checkpoint inhibitor (ICI) is a medication that targets an inhibitory immune checkpoint molecule, such as programmed death-ligand 1 (PD-L1) and its receptor, programmed death-1 (PD-1) or cytotoxic T-lymphocyte-associated antigen 4 (CTLA-4). In the treatment of NSCLC, agents that suppress PD-1/PD-L1 signalling have shown encouraging outcomes (Felip et al. 2021). In the PEARLS/KEYNOTE-091 trial, among almost 1200 patients with completely resected stage IB ($T \geq 4$ cm) to IIIA NSCLC, adjuvant pembrolizumab improved DFS relative to placebo in the overall group (54 vs. 42 months; HR 0.76), with a non-significant trend toward improvement in those with tumour PD-L1 ≥ 50%. Two PD-1 antibodies (nivolumab and pembrolizumab) and two PD-L1 antibodies (atezolizumab and durvalumab) have been approved for the treatment of NSCLC by the US Food and Drug Administration (FDA) and/or the European Medicines Agency (EMA) (Table 4.1).

4.2.9 Novel Immune Checkpoint Inhibitor Under Investigation in In Advanced Non-Small-Cell Lung Cancer (NSCLC) Treatment

Several new combinations are currently being investigated in advanced non-small-cell lung cancer (NSCLC). In the preliminary results of Study 16,113, a total of 466 patients were randomly assigned to receive chemotherapy with or without cemiplimab. The group receiving cemiplimab demonstrated an improvement in median overall survival, with rates of 22 months compared to 13 months in the

Table 4.1 The PD-1/PD-L1 inhibitors licenced for clinical use or under clinical trials for 1062 NSCLC treatment

Checkpoint	Blocking agent	IgG isotype and characteristics	Clinical stage
PD-1	Pembrolizumab (MK3475, Keytruda, lambrolizumab)	Humanized IgG4 mAb	EMA, FDA approved for second-line NSCLC treatment
	Nivolumab (BMS936558, OPDIVO, MDX-1106, ONO-4538)	Fully human IgG4 mAb	FDA approved for first-line and second-line NSCLC
	REGN2810	Humanized IgG4 mAb	Phase I
	MEDI0680 (AMP-514)	Humanized IgG4 mAb	Phase I
	PDR001	Humanized IgG4 mAb	Phase I
PD-L1	Avelumab (Bavencio, MSB0010718C)	Fully human IgG1 mAb	FDA-approved treatment for metastatic MCC
	BMS-936559 (MDX1105)	Fully high-affinity human IgG4	Phase I
	Durvalumab (MEDI4736, Infinzi)	Human IgG1-κ mAb	FDA approved for treatment of unresectable stage III NSCLC without relapse after platinum-based chemoradiation
	Atezolizumab (Tecentriq, MPDL3280A, RG7446)	High-affinity human IgG1	FDA approved for second-line NSCLC

FDA Food and Drug Administration, *Ig* immunoglobulin, *mAb* monoclonal antibody, *NSCLC* non-small-cell lung cancer, *PD-1* programmed death-1, *PD-L1* programmed death-ligand 1, *PD-L2* programmed death-ligand 2

chemotherapy-only group. Furthermore, the cemiplimab group experienced low rates of serious adverse events. Similarly, the POSEIDON trial revealed that the addition of tremelimumab plus durvalumab to chemotherapy led to an improvement in median survival, with rates of 15 months compared to 11 months in the chemotherapy-only group. Additionally, acceptable rates of grade ≥ 3 toxicity were observed. These compelling results have resulted in the approval of combinations of cemiplimab, as well as tremelimumab/durvalumab, by the US Food and Drug Administration for the treatment of advanced NSCLC cases that lack certain driver mutations.

4.3 Recent Breakthroughs in Immunotherapy for SCLC

The SCLCs make up roughly 10%–15% of all lung cancers, which were most lethal malignancies and a major health riddle, which are poorly differentiated, high-grade neuroendocrine tumours. Small-cell lung cancer (SCLC) is a particularly lethal illness that is distinguished by early metastasis, rapid progression, and the absence of a feasible solution after recurrence. Etoposide-platinum (EP) therapy has been the standard of care for SCLC for the past 30 years. Finding new treatments for SCLC is essential and required. Immunotherapy, including immuno-checkpoint blockers such as PD-1, CTLA-4, and other proteins linked with cytotoxic T lymphocytes, has made significant strides in the treatment of SCLC patients over the past 5 years, and for some patients, it has even replaced first-line therapy (Ott et al. 2017). Traditional chemotherapy procedures or specific drugs, such the transcription inhibitor lurbinectedin and the alkylating agent temozolomide, are expected to develop into innovative immunotherapeutic drugs because they have been found to have immunomodulatory properties.

Although it is generally established that these molecules are not yet targetable, the two most frequent genetic alterations found in SCLC are TP53 and RB1 mutations. The immune system may be exposed to new antigens because of radiation treatment, and the presence of mesenchymal-derived suppressor cells may be reduced, partially altering the tumour microenvironment and inducing an anti-tumour immune response locally (Martoglio and Dobberstein 1998). Radiation treatment can cause tumour cells to undergo apoptosis. As a result, combining radiation and immunotherapy for cancer treatment makes sense.

According to recent studies, a mechanism known as cancer immune surveillance, to control the emergence and expansion of tumours, the immune system is essential. T cell and natural killer cell dysfunction is promoted by the addition of regulatory T cells (Tregs), tumours can avoid immune monitoring. Patients with SCLC are known to be in an immunosuppressive condition, which may have an impact on their prognosis. For instance, compared to non-SCLC (NSCLC), SCLC more frequently results in the decrease of inflammation in pre-existing T cells (Traxler 2003). Although they have a limited effectiveness, small-molecule antiangiogenic medications (anlotinib) have made some headway in the treatment of SCLC. Immunotherapy using checkpoint inhibitors has not kept pace with that for

SCLC patients with non-small-cell lung cancer, and the role of immunotherapy in the treatment of SCLC is now well clearly known.

4.4 Lung Cancer Targeted Therapy and Traditional Chemotherapy

Regarding treating advanced NSCLC, treatment for lung cancer has undergone a dramatic transformation because of immunotherapy. Immunotherapy is the second-line treatment for people without driver gene changes, this was first demonstrated to increase overall survival (OS) in individuals with advanced NSCLC (Segovia-Mendoza et al. 2015). First-line monotherapy of immunotherapy for NSCLC patients with high PD-L1 expression improved survival, paving the way for the first-line chemotherapy-free approach. Immunotherapy combined with chemotherapy is currently the standard of care for all patients with advanced NSCLC and negative driver genes, and strategies like dual immunotherapy, combined immunological and antivascular therapy further improve the therapeutic options (Reguart and Remon 2015).

4.5 Combined Immunotherapy and Chemotherapy

By increasing the mutational load of cancer cells and the level of human leukocyte antigen (HLA) expression, these chemotherapeutic agents have been shown in preclinical models to potentiate immune responses against cancer cells. This enhances the ability of cytotoxic T lymphocytes (CTL) to recognize cancer cells. Moreover, following neoadjuvant chemotherapy treatments in SCC patients, myeloid-derived suppressor cells activity reduced and cancer cells expression of PD-L1r. These results could be in favour of chemotherapy and immunotherapy regimens for lung cancer (Garon et al. 2014). In patients with EGFR mutations and ALK rearrangements, tyrosine kinase inhibitors are frequently utilized as the first-line therapy. TKIs are non-peptide substances that resemble adenosine triphosphate (ATP). This makes it possible for them to engage in ATP-binding area competition with protein kinases, blocking phosphorylation and activation of the intracellular signaling cascades, and so reducing the development and death of cancer cells (Rudin et al. 2016). According to the findings of multiple phase III clinical studies, these tailored treatments enhance rate of response, progression-free their survival, as well as quality of life when compared to traditional first-line platinum-based chemotherapy.

4.6 Theranostic in Lung Cancer

Nanoparticles have recently been effectively shaped, created, and used for cancer theranostic in lung cancer. Chemotherapy is the most often employed lung cancer treatment approach. One of the biggest hurdles to the clinical efficacy of lung cancer treatment is inadequate drug concentration in tumour tissue (Jett et al. 2013). To successfully treat those who have advanced stage or metastasis lung cancer, it is increasingly necessary to detect a number of theranostic indications. The development of theranostic stools over ultrasensitive along with precise evaluation of theranostic indicators, competence to detect and determine tumours at its infancy of rapid resolution, and early adaptation forecast to cancer therapy will also be determined by new assisting tools like AI. Even though combining therapy and diagnostic into a single theranostic platform should have many benefits (Kroemer et al. 2013), the pharmacokinetics and dynamics of the imaging and tumour targeting components can differ, which could cause serious manufacturing issues and depicted in (Fig. 4.1). Minimum biomarkers are necessary to assess the status of PD-L1, ROS1, ALK, BRAF, and EGFR in individuals with metastatic lung adenocarcinoma (Deng et al. 2014). Cancer therapy using theranostic is based on evidence and precise prescriptions, ensuring the proper medication at the right time, enlightening the quality of health, and to provide cost effective medications and facilities.

Recent advancement in therapy of lung cancer includes imaging and treatment using nanotheranostics. Due to their advantageous photophysical characteristics, porphyrins have proven particularly effective for photodynamic treatment (PDT) and cancer imaging. More countries have approved the use of hematoporphyrin derivative (HpD), porfimer sodium, for the identification and photodynamic therapy of endobronchial, esophageal, lung, proximal bladder, stomach, and cervical cancers (VanderLaan et al. 2018a). Laserphyrin 664 has been given PDT approval in Japan to treat centrally confined, early-stage lung carcinoma. Fluorine-18 coupled with deoxy glucose (FDG), a nuclear medicine imaging technique, is usually paired with PET (positron emission tomography) (Ilie and Hofman 2012). Theranostic is most repeatedly used to treat lung cancer bone metastases that have disseminated to the bones fastly.

4.7 Neoepitopes as Therapeutic Targets for Lung Cancer

It has been recognized for decades that somatic or passenger mutations in the tumour result in the development of novel epitopes or neoepitopes (Durgeau et al. 2018). Thus, targeting non-mutated neoantigens is a viable and potent method to generating specific responses to tumours with low MHC-I expression and TAP subunit downregulation or deletion. Peptides produced from signal sequences are promising options for therapeutic cancer vaccines against TAP-deficient tumour cells (Ubenik 2003). Indeed, these TAP-independent self-peptides are not presented by normal cells with a normal processing status and appear on the surface of tumour cells because of changes in APM components. This could account for their immunogenicity and ability to elicit potent anti-tumour T-cell responses (Durgeau et al. 2011).

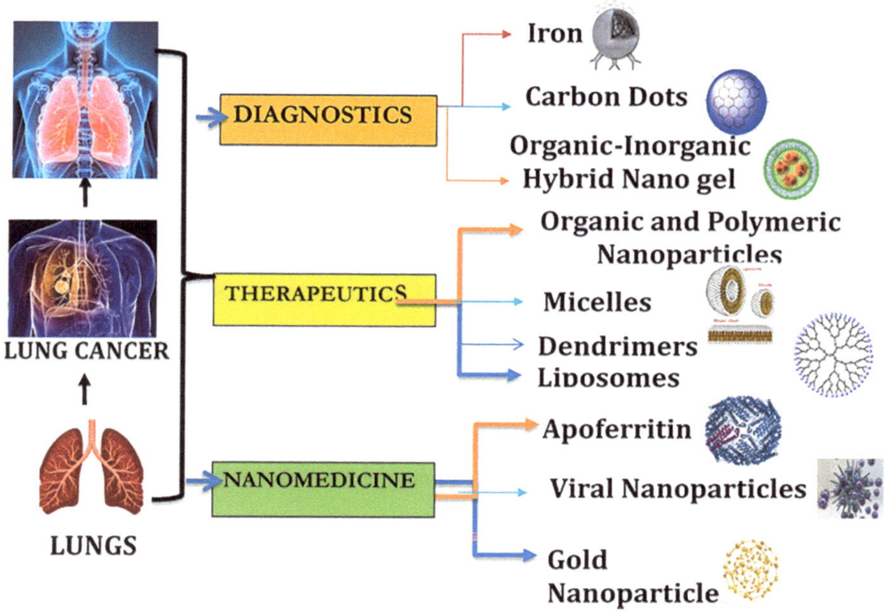

Fig. 4.1 Recent breakthroughs in theranostic in lung cancer

4.8 Revolutionizing Approaches in Lung Cancer Vaccines

The COVID-19 epidemic has prompted the advancement of vaccine technology and refocused public attention on cancer vaccinations. In contrast to antibody-based therapy, cancer vaccines provide a different strategy for fostering anti-tumour immunity. Cancer vaccines function to keep the host immune system and cancer cells interacting at the right level (VanderLaan et al. 2018b). Prophylactic (preventative) and therapeutic (curative) cancer vaccinations are both possible.

However, most tumours that develop in host tissues exhibit "self" antigens, which the immune system has already developed a tolerance for. This makes the production of anti-tumour vaccines problematic. Since these specific to a tissue self-peptide are frequently expressed in many healthy tissues, they are not suitable targets for the development of anti-cancer vaccines (Lindeman et al. 2018).

4.8.1 Prophylactic Vaccines

Human papilloma virus, or HPV, and hepatitis B virus, also known as HBV, prophylactic vaccinations have demonstrated efficacy in reducing the global burden brought on by these two cancer-causing viruses. Vaccines given as a prophylactic are meant to stop cancer before it starts. The US FDA has authorized vaccinations for certain viral infections that are linked to cancer (VanderLaan et al. 2018c).

4.8.2 Therapeutic Vaccines

An immunotherapeutic cancer vaccine falls under several distinct categories. These can take the form of biological (whole tumour/immune cells), viral vectors, or molecular (peptide, DNA, or RNA) components. Numerous innovative immunotherapy approaches have been created because of recent developments in vaccine formulations that successfully boost antigen presentation, stimulate effector T cells, and avoid immunosuppressive pathways brought on by tumours (Baskaran et al. 2018).

Immunological checkpoint inhibitors (ICIs) and cancer vaccines have recently been the subject of several clinical trials to see how well they work together in combating the immunological tolerant milieu present in many solid tumours (Kato et al. 1993). To increase anti-tumour immunity, cancer vaccines present an appealing way to work in conjunction with already existing immunotherapeutic techniques; there are several cytokines, immune checkpoint inhibitors, oncolytic viruses, and other immune modulators. and Patients with advanced lung cancer may benefit from this strategy clinically (Hayata et al. 1982).

4.9 Synergistic Combinations and Innovative Approaches

The clear dynamic of the immune response shows that, as compared to monotherapy, combination therapy may improve cancer patient survival. Chemotherapy, radiation therapy, anti-angiogenic drugs, vaccines, and T-cell modulation are all part of the immunotherapy research. Other hurdles include irAEs, finding adequate biomarkers for immunotherapy response, immunotherapy resistance, and making nonresponders benefit from combo therapy (Hayata et al. 1984). Immunotherapy using anti-angiogenic medicines will improve drug penetration with the tumour while also synergizing with chemotherapy and immunotherapy. Anti-VEGF therapy and bevacizumab-mediated metabolic alterations in the tumour via the LKB1/AMPK pathway will increase survival (Ding et al. 2012).

Durvalumab, Atezolizumab, Pembrolizumab, Ipilimumab, and Nivolumab are the principal immunotherapy medicines used in the chemotherapy of lung cancer in NSCLC and SCLC (Pacilio et al. 2014). In patients with metastatic non-squamous NSCLC, atezolizumab is advised as first-line therapy using the ABCP regimen (atezolizumab + bevacizumab + carboplatin + paclitaxel), Both Nivolumab and Ipilimumab are immune checkpoint inhibitors that work on T cells in complementary ways. Nivolumab inhibits PD-1 receptors, whereas Ipilimumab is an antibody that blocks human CTLA-4. Atezolizumab in combination with etoposide-platinum is recommended as the first-line treatment for patients with Extensive Stage SCLC (Baum et al. 2015). As consolidation immunotherapy, durvalumab has been suggested for patients receiving post-treatment chemoradiation.

Cancer vaccines are an immunotherapy technique that encourages the milieu to boost T-cell or B-cell-mediated anti-tumour responses against tumour-specific entities. There are two types of tumour cell vaccines: autologous (made from the patient's own cancer cells) and allogeneic (made from lines of human tumour cells). These vaccines are categorized into several types according to the target entity, including cell-based (whole tumour vaccines), genetic (DNA vaccines), protein, bacterial, small molecule, and DC-based vaccines (Hollingsworth and Jansen 2019). Either alone or in conjunction with chemotherapy, iCPI anti-angicgenic treatment has synergistic benefits and improves response rates, but some combinations are hazardous. Some targeted medicines, B-RAF and MEK inhibitors, for example, have been associated with immune modulatory activity and might cooperate with iCPIs. BRAF inhibitor Vemurafenib was once combined with an anti-CTLA-4 mAb; however, this pairing produced unfavourable results (Le et al. 2010). In contrast, Vemurafenib was more effective when combined with a PD-L1 inhibitor and kinase/ERK inhibitor. Colony stimulating factor 1, phosphoinositid-3-kinase-g (PI3K-g), and inhibitors of indoleamine (IDO) are other iCPI therapies that, when combined with anti-PD1 therapy, cause cancer to regress (Bezu et al. 2018).

4.9.1 Checkpoint Inhibitor as First-Line Treatment for SCLC

To assess the effectiveness and safety of carboplatin and etoposide combined with atezolizumab as a first-line therapy for extensive-stage small-cell lung cancer (ED-SCLC), a previous research study involved 403 patients from 22 countries. In the IMpower010 trial, 882 patients with stage II-III non-small-cell lung cancer (NSCLC) who had undergone surgery and up to four cycles of adjuvant cisplatin-based chemotherapy were included (Bezu et al. 2018). Among these patients, those randomly assigned to receive 16 cycles of atezolizumab showed improvements in disease-free survival (DFS) compared to those receiving best supportive care. At a median follow-up of 33 months, the median DFS was 42 months in the atezolizumab group versus 35 months in the best supportive care group (HR 0.79, 95%CI, 0.64–0.96). A greater benefit was observed among the 476 patients with PD-L1 expression of ≥1%. The 3-year DFS rates in the overall group were 56% for atezolizumab versus 49% for best supportive care, and among those with PD-L1-positive disease, the rates were 60% versus 48%, respectively. Overall survival (OS) results were not mature, as only approximately 20% of events had been collected at the time of analysis. However, the HR for OS at this early time point among all patients with stage II-III disease was 0.99 (95% CI 0.73–1.33), and 0.77 (95% CI 0.51–1.17) in the subset of patients with PD-L1-positive tumours. Grade 3 or 4 events occurred in 22% of patients receiving atezolizumab and 12% of patients receiving best supportive care (Wu et al. 2019).

Immunomodulatory nanomedicine for the treatment of lung cancer as we have already discussed, immune activation is crucial for the treatment of cancer since it enables the body to identify and get rid of non-self-antigens and create a memory effect for future treatments and represented in (Fig. 4.2). While a variety of immunotherapeutics have achieved remarkable achievements in the treatment of many malignancies, they have also encountered some challenging hurdles, such as low water solubility, poor pharmacokinetic profiles, and ineffectiveness in the treatment

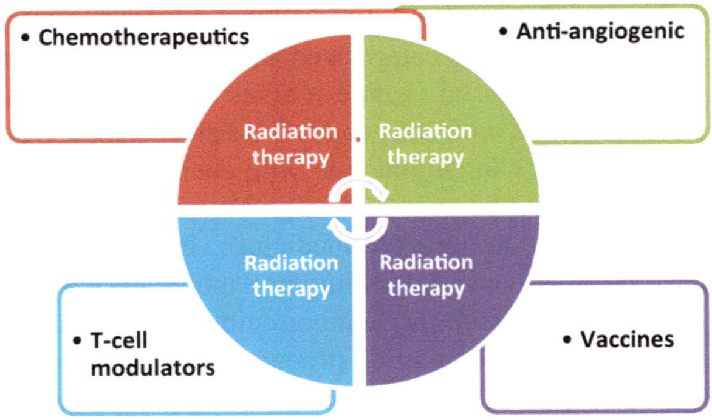

Fig. 4.2 Immune checkpoint inhibitors

of certain tumours Specifically, there is reduced absorption and storage in the tumour site, leading to decreased bioactivity after prolonged circulation and higher immune-mediated off-target damage. To our astonishment, nanotechnology, in all its favourable aspects, is capable of resolving current and emerging problems, achieving the projected degree of achievement in terms of medical benefits (Shi et al. 2019). As we get a better understanding of the tumour microenvironment, smart stimuli-responsive nanocarriers are being developed to take advantage of acidic pH, hypoxia, increased ATP generation, changing redox status of cancer cells, and other characteristics. It turns out that nanoparticles boost the effectiveness of immunotherapy for cancer.

1. delivering antigen and adjuvant protection,
2. concurrent delivery to the APC,
3. TME reprogramming for resumption of immunological surveillance (Mukherjee et al. 2020).

Currently, a plethora of nanomaterials have demonstrated immunomodulatory potential in pre-clinical studies, and a handful of them have advanced through various phases of clinical trials. Oncothyreon Canada Inc. developed a liposomal cancer vaccine (L-BLP25) by incorporating the antigen tecemotide (carcinoma related human MUC-1) and the adjuvant 3-O-Deacyl-4′-monophosphoryl lipid A (MPL) into a lipid bilayer made of 1,2-dipalmitoyl-sn-glycero-3-phosphocholine (DPPC) (Hosomi et al. 2020).

Molecular targeting medicines can trigger immune responses through a variety of ways, including (1) assisting APC in antigen presentation (2) causing ICD in tumour cells, (3) encouraging T cell invasion in TME, (4) activating NK cells, and (5) reducing the number of MDSCs, Tregs, and TAMs in TME. To better molecularly targeted immunomodulation, nanotechnology and nanomaterials were utilized (Travis 2010).

Tumour infiltration of both CD8 + and CD4 + T cells increased, as did NK cell activation, whereas MDSCs and Foxp3 + Treg cells decreased (immune tolerance). A significant amount of research is being undertaken to better understand the role of immunomodulatory nanomedicine in lung cancer immunotherapy, and we believe that their ramifications will expand soon (Paz-Ares et al. 2021). Immunomodulatory nutraceuticals have attracted the interest of researchers worldwide in cancer prevention and supportive treatment, and significant efforts have been made to interpret their therapeutic and immunomodulatory activities (Wang et al. 2023). Because of a paucity of tumour-specific antigens, a hostile TME, and toxicity, cellular therapy is an enticing but unquestionably difficult prospect. Novel therapeutic methods, such as the combination and sequencing of PD-1/PD-L1 inhibitors along with different ICIs and DNA repair targeted medicines, are being tested in clinical trials. Overall, the therapeutic effects of ICIs and ACT have showed promising developments in the therapy of lung cancer (Wang et al. 2023).

Combination drug therapy based on prodrug technology has been employed as a promising treatment strategy to produce synergistic cancer therapy, low medication doses, and fewer side effects. Combination drug therapy based on prodrug technology consists of at least three kinds of systems: two distinct anti-tumour prodrugs, one free anti-cancer drug and another prodrug, and conjugates made up of two different anticancer drugs (D'Andrea 2018). Anti-KIR Natural killer (NK) cells, in addition to improving T-cell-mediated immune responses, are important effectors of the innate immune system and can limit tumour growth. This has been demonstrated in individuals with acute myeloid leukaemia (AML), where number and activity are related to relapse-free survival (RFS). Both stimulatory and inhibitory receptors are found on NK cells. When Ig-like KIRs bind to their ligands, specifically HLA-C molecules, they inhibit NK cell activation (Brandts and Ray 2021).

4.9.2 Other Immunomodulatory and Agonistic Molecules

Immune checkpoints are required for maintaining homeostasis and to avoid incorrect CD8 cytotoxic T cell activation. To avoid detection by the immune system, cancers disrupt immunological checkpoint control. In murine models, retinoid X receptor (RXR) agonists can alter the cancer microenvironment, leading to enhanced anti-cancer and reduced pro-tumour immune populations (American Association for Cancer Research 2021).

The RXR belongs to the nuclear receptor superfamily and functions as a factor that regulates transcription after ligand interaction. RXR interacts with various other members of the nuclear receptor superfamily, including the retinoic acid receptor (RAR), vitamin D receptor (VDR), peroxisome proliferator-activated receptor (PPAR), and liver X receptor (LXR). RXR homodimers or heterodimers regulate monocyte activity, connecting the metabolism of cells and immune function (Sui et al. 2018). RXR agonists can boost the production of cytokines, inhibit viral responses, and stimulate phagocytosis. RXR is a pharmacologically intriguing complement to existing cancer therapies because of its immunomodulatory properties. Bexarotene binds to RAR and has negative consequences on the body (Zhou et al. 2021). Two more RXR agonists, LG100268 and IRX194204, have been created in an effort to enhance pharmacokinetic properties and lessen side effects. In murine models of lung cancer, LG100268 and IRX194204 are active.

4.10 Conclusion

The treatment landscape for lung cancer has undergone a significant transformation with the introduction of immunotherapy. Combining immunotherapy with chemotherapy can enhance the overall response rate (ORR), but it does not necessarily improve long-term survival in patients with high PD-L1 expression. For patients diagnosed with non-small-cell lung cancer (NSCLC) and exhibiting high expression of PD-L1 should receive single-drug immunotherapy. Recently, several immune checkpoint inhibitors (ICIs) have gained approval for the treatment of advanced lung cancer. These inhibitors enhance the body's immune system response against cancer by specifically targeting PD-L1 and PD-1 proteins. Hence, single-drug immunotherapy is recommended for patients with high PD-L1 expression, as these patients have shown long-term survival benefits. While dual immunotherapy combined with chemotherapy is primarily suitable for PD-L1-negative patients, this approach has demonstrated improvements in 5-year survival long-term survival of 18%–20%. In the case of small-cell lung cancer (SCLC), ongoing and upcoming clinical trials are exploring various combinations of immune checkpoint inhibitors (ICIs) with targeted therapies such as PARP inhibitors, AKT1 inhibitors, and ATR inhibitors. Additionally, novel immune-based therapeutic strategies, including CART and BiTES, are being investigated, with the expectation of achieving favourable outcomes.

The combination of these active immune therapies with ICB would promote the expansion of pre-existing antigen-specific T cells and stimulate the development of a broader range of T-cell specificities. This would enhance control over tumour progression, leading to the elimination of most cancer cells, including immune-escaped variants, as well as the eradication of immune deserts or cold tumours that are poorly infiltrated by lymphocytes. Recent research has demonstrated the efficacy of tailored RNA mutanome vaccines and multipeptide neoantigen vaccines as treatments for melanoma patients. In particular, when used alongside an anti-PD-1 monoclonal antibody, active immunotherapies with anticipated tumour neoepitopes showed significantly greater success. However, there have been reports of frequent recurrence of APM faults. In such cases, TEIPP-specific T cells can effectively target immune-edited MHC-I low targets that have developed resistance to immunotherapy. Promising options for therapeutic cancer vaccines that target tumours with downregulated HLA-class I molecules due to TAP expression alterations include peptides derived from signal sequences and their carrier proteins, such as ppCT.

Researchers are currently exploring novel approaches to treating lung cancer that can provide long-term responses to therapy. Immunotherapy represents a promising new treatment modality that can be added to the arsenal of lung cancer treatments, aiming to achieve these goals while minimizing side effects. However, cancer vaccines that rely on non-mutant neoantigens produced by TAP-deficient tumours, which have low levels of MHC-I/peptide complexes and distinct tumour mutanome epitopes, face a significant challenge in treating lung cancer. To overcome this barrier, therapeutic immunization that combines mutant and non-mutant neoepitopes with immune checkpoint blockade (ICB) may prove advantageous for future immunotherapies against cancer.

References

Abele R, Tampe R (2006) Modulation of the antigen transport machinery TAP by friends and enemies. FEBS Lett 580:1156–1163. https://doi.org/10.1016/j.febslet.2005.11.048

American Association for Cancer Research (2021) TROP2 ADC intrigues in NSCLC. Cancer Discov 11(5):OF5. https://doi.org/10.1158/2159-8290.CD-NB2021-0314

Anagnostou V, Cottrell TR, Forde PM, Chaft JE, Smith KN, Hellmann MD et al (2018) Neoadjuvant PD-1 inhibition in lung cancer with curative intent. N Engl J Med 378(21):1976–1986. https://doi.org/10.1056/NEJMoa1716078

Baskaran R, Lee J, Yang SG (2018) Clinical development of photodynamic agents and therapeutic applications. Biomater Res 22:25

Baum RP, Kulkarni HR, Muller D, Satz S, Danthi N, Kim YS, Brechbiel MW (2015) First-in-human study demonstrating tumor-angiogenesis by PET/CT imaging with 68Ga-NODAGA-THERANOST, a high-affinity peptidomimetic for αvβ3 integrin receptor targeting. Cancer Biother Radiopharm 30(4):152–159

Bezu L, Kepp O, Cerrato G, Pol J, Fucikova J, Spisek R, Zitvogel L, Kroemer G, Galluzzi L (2018) Trial watch: peptide-based vaccines in anticancer therapy. Oncoimmunol 7:e1511506. https://doi.org/10.1080/2162402X.2018.1511506

Borghaei H, Gettinger S, Vokes E, Chow LQM, Burgio M, de Castro Carpeno J et al (2021) Results of the randomised, phase III trials CheckMate 017 and 057 comparing docetaxel and nivolumab in previously treated non-small-cell lung cancer at five years. J Clin Oncol 39(7):723–733. https://doi.org/10.1200/JCO.20.016053.2.1

Brandts J, Ray KK (2021) Clinical implications and outcomes of the ORION phase III trials. Futur Cardiol 17(5):769–777. https://doi.org/10.2217/fca-2020-0150

Chen G, Zhou C, Huang Y, Zhou J, Lin L, Feng J (2021) A randomised, open-label, multicenter, phase 3 trial called CameL compared chemotherapy alone to camrelizumab plus carboplatin and pemetrexed in chemotherapy-naive patients with advanced non-squamous non-small-cell lung cancer. Lancet Respir Med 9(3):305–314. https://doi.org/10.1016/S2213-2600(20)30365-9

D'Andrea AD (2018) Mechanisms of PARP inhibitor sensitivity and resistance. DNA Repair 71:172–176. https://doi.org/10.1016/j.dnarep.2018.08.021

Deng L, Liang H, Burnette B et al (2014) Irradiation and anti-PD-L1 treatment synergistically promote antitumor immunity in mice. J Clin Invest 124:687–695. https://doi.org/10.1172/JCI67313

Ding XP, Zhang J, Li BS, Li HS, Wang ZT, Yi Y, Sun HF, Wang DQ (2012) Feasibility of shrinking field radiation therapy through 18F-FDG PET/CT after 40 Gy for stage III non-small cell lung cancers. Asian Pac J Cancer Prev 13:319–323

Domvri K, Petanidis S, Anestakis D, Porpodis K, Bai C, Zarogoulidis P et al (2020) Dual photothermal MDSCs-targeted immunotherapy inhibits lung immunosuppressive metastasis by enhancing T-cell recruitment. Nanoscale 12(13):7051–7062

Durgeau A, El Hage F, Vergnon I, Validire P, de Montpreville V, Besse B et al (2011) Different expression levels of the TAP peptide transporter lead to recognition of different antigenic peptides by tumor-specific CTL. J Immunol 187:5532–5539. https://doi.org/10.4049/jimmunol.1102060

Durgeau A, Virk Y, Gros G, Voilin E, Corgnac S, Djenidi F et al (2018) Human preprocalcitonin self-antigen generates TAP-dependent and -independent epitopes triggering optimised T-cell

responses toward immune-escaped tumours. Nat Commun 9:5097. https://doi.org/10.1038/s41467-018-07603-1
Einstein MH, Leanza S, Chiu LG, Schlecht NF, Goldberg GL, Steinberg BM et al (2009) Genetic variants in TAP are associated with high-grade cervical neoplasia. Clin Cancer Res 15:1019–1023. https://doi.org/10.1158/1078-0432.CCR-08-1207
Felip E, Altorki N, Zhou C, Csszi I, Vynychenko O et al (2021) A randomised, multicenter, open-label, phase 3 trial of adjuvant atezolizumab following adjuvant chemotherapy in resected stage IB-IIIA non-small-cell lung cancer (IMpower010). Lancet 398(10308):1344–1357. https://doi.org/10.1016/S0140-6736(21)02098-5
Garon EB, Ciuleanu TE, Arrieta O, Prabhash K, Syrigos KN, Goksel T et al (2014) Ramucirumab plus docetaxel versus placebo plus docetaxel for second-line treatment of stage IV non-small-cell lung cancer after disease progression on platinum-based therapy (REVEL): a multicentre, double-blind, randomised phase 3 trial. Lancet 384:665–673. https://doi.org/10.1016/S0140-6736(14)60845-X
Hayata Y, Kato H, Konaka C, Ono J, Takizawa N (1982) Hematoporphyrin derivative and laser photoradiation in the treatment of lung cancer. Chest 81:269–277
Hayata Y, Kato H, Konaka C, Amemiya R, Ono J, Ogawa I, Kinoshita K, Sakai H, Takahashi H (1984) Photoradiation therapy with hematoporphyrin derivative in early and stage 1 lung cancer. Chest 86:169–177
Hollingsworth RE, Jansen K (2019) Turning the corner on therapeutic cancer vaccines. NPJ Vaccines 4:7. https://doi.org/10.1038/s41541-019-0103-y
Hosomi Y, Morita S, Sugawara S, Kato T, Fukuhara T, Gemma A et al (2020) Gefitinib alone versus gefitinib plus chemotherapy for non–small-cell lung cancer with mutated epidermal growth factor receptor: NEJ009 study. J Clin Oncol 38(2):115–123
Hottel J, Yin C, Lian Y, Siegel R, Tan X, Fu S (2018) BP1 regulates PI3K/Akt pathway by targeting vascular endothelial growth factor (VEGF) in breast cancer. Oncomedicine 3:67–73
Ilie M, Hofman P (2012) Pitfalls in lung cancer molecular pathology: how to limit them in routine practice? Curr Med Chem 19:2638–2651. https://doi.org/10.2174/092986712800493002
Ishii H, Azuma K, Kawahara A, Yamada K, Imamura Y, Tokito T et al (2015) Significance of programmed cell death-ligand 1 expression and its association with survival in patients with small cell lung cancer. J Thorac Oncol 10(3):426–430
Jett JR, Schild SE, Kesler KA et al (2013) Treatment of small cell lung cancer: diagnosis and management of lung cancer, 3rd ed: American College of Chest Physicians evidence-based clinical practice guidelines. Chest 143:e400S–e419S. https://doi.org/10.1378/chest.12-2363
Kato H, Horai T, Furuse K, Fukuoka M, Suzuki S, Hiki Y, Ito Y, Mimura S, Tenjin Y, Hisazumi H et al (1993) Photodynamic therapy for cancers: a clinical trial of porfimer sodium in Japan. Jpn J Cancer Res 84:1209–1214
Kroemer G, Galluzzi L, Kepp O et al (2013) Immunogenic cell death in cancer therapy. Annu Rev Immunol 31:51–72. https://doi.org/10.1146/annurev-immunol-032712-100008
Le DT, Pardoll DM, Jaffee EM (2010) Cellular vaccine approaches. Cancer J 16:304–310. https://doi.org/10.1097/PPO.0b013e3181eb33d7
Leibowitz MS, Andrade Filho PA, Ferrone S, Ferris RL (2011) Deficiency of activated STAT1 in head and neck cancer cells mediates TAP1-dependent escape from cytotoxic T lymphocytes. Cancer Immunol Immunother 60:525–535. https://doi.org/10.1007/s00262-010-0961-7
Lindeman NI, Cagle PT, Aisner DL et al (2018) Updated molecular testing guideline for the selection of lung cancer patients for treatment with targeted tyrosine kinase inhibitors: guideline from the College of American Pathologists, the International Association for the Study of Lung Cancer, and the Association for Molecular Pathology. J Thorac Oncol 13:323–358. https://doi.org/10.1016/j.jtho.2017.12.001
Marincola FM, Jaffee EM, Hicklin DJ, Ferrone S (2000) Escape of human solid tumors from T-cell recognition: molecular mechanisms and functional significance. Adv Immunol 74:181–273. https://doi.org/10.1016/s0065-2776(08)60911-6
Martoglio B, Dobberstein B (1998) Signal sequences: more than just greasy peptides. Trends Cell Biol 8:410–415. https://doi.org/10.1016/S0962-8924(98)01360-9

Mukherjee S, Madamsetty VS, Bhattacharya D, Roy Chowdhury S, Paul MK, Mukherjee A (2020) Recent advancements of nanomedicine in neurodegenerative disorders theranostics. Adv Funct Mater 30(35):2003054

Naumov GN, Nilsson MB, Cascone T, Briggs A, Straume O, Akslen LA et al (2009) Combined vascular endothelial growth factor receptor and epidermal growth factor receptor (EGFR) blockade inhibits tumor growth in xenograft models of EGFR inhibitor resistance. Clin Cancer Res 15:3484–3494

Ott PA, Hu Z, Keskin DB, Shukla SA, Sun J, Bozym DJ et al (2017) An immunogenic personal neoantigen vaccine for patients with melanoma. Nature 547:217–221. https://doi.org/10.1038/nature22991

Pacilio M, Ventroni G, Basile C, Ialongo P, Becci D, Mango L (2014) Improving the dose-myelotoxicity correlation in radiometabolic therapy of bone metastases with 153Sm-EDTMP. Eur J Nucl Med Mol Imaging 41:238–252

Paz-Ares L, Ciuleanu T-E, Cobo M, Schenker M, Zurawski B, Menezes J et al (2021) First-line nivolumab plus ipilimumab combined with two cycles of chemotherapy in patients with non-small-cell lung cancer (CheckMate 9LA): an international, randomised, open-label, phase 3 trial. Lancet Oncol 22(2):198–211

Reck M, Mok TSK, Nishio M, Jotte RM, Cappuzzo F, Orlandi F et al (2019) Atezolizumab plus bevacizumab and chemotherapy in non-small-cell lung cancer (IMpower150): key subgroup analyses of patients with EGFR mutations or baseline liver metastases in a randomised, open-label phase 3 trial. Lancet Respir Med 7(5):387–401

Reguart N, Remon J (2015) Common EGFR-mutated subgroups (Del19/L858R) in advanced non-small-cell lung cancer: chasing better outcomes with tyrosine kinase inhibitors. Future Oncol 11:1245–1257. https://doi.org/10.2217/fon.15.15

Ren S, Chen J, Xu X, Jiang T, Cheng Y, Chen G et al (2022) Camrelizumab plus carboplatin and paclitaxel as first-line treatment for advanced squamous NSCLC (CameL-Sq): a phase 3 trial. J Thorac Oncol 17(4):544–557. https://doi.org/10.1016/j.jtho.2021.11.018

Rosell R, Dafni U, Felip E, Curioni-Fontecedro A, Gautschi O, Peters S et al (2017) Erlotinib and bevacizumab in patients with advanced non-small-cell lung cancer and activating EGFR mutations (BELIEF): an international, multicentre, single-arm, phase 2 trial. Lancet Respir Med 5:435–444

Rudin CM, Giaccone G, Ismaila N (2016) Treatment of small-cell lung cancer: American Society of Clinical Oncology Endorsement of the American College of Chest Physicians Guideline. J Oncol Pract 12:83–86. https://doi.org/10.1200/JOP.2015.008201

Sahin U, Derhovanessian E, Miller M, Kloke BP, Simon P, Lower M et al (2017) Personalized RNA mutanome vaccines mobilize poly-specific therapeutic immunity against cancer. Nature 547:222–226. https://doi.org/10.1038/nature23003

Saito H, Fukuhara T, Furuya N, Watanabe K, Sugawara S, Iwasawa S et al (2019) Erlotinib plus bevacizumab versus erlotinib alone in patients with EGFR-positive advanced non-squamous non-small-cell lung cancer (NEJ026): interim analysis of an open-label, randomised, multicentre, phase 3 trial. Lancet Oncol 20:625–635

Segovia-Mendoza M, Gonzalez-Gonzalez ME, Barrera D, Diaz L, Garcia-Becerra R (2015) Efficacy and mechanism of action of the tyrosine kinase inhibitors gefitinib, lapatinib and neratinib in the treatment of HER2-positive breast cancer: preclinical and clinical evidence. Am J Cancer Res 5:2531–2561

Setiadi AF, David MD, Seipp RP, Hartikainen JA, Gopaul R, Jefferies WA (2007) Epigenetic control of the immune escape mechanisms in malignant carcinomas. Mol Cell Biol 27:7886–7894. https://doi.org/10.1128/MCB.01547-07

Shi Y-X, Sheng D-Q, Cheng L, Song X-Y (2019) Current landscape of epigenet- ics in lung cancer: focus on the mechanism and application. J Oncol 2019:1–11

Sui H, Ma N, Wang Y, Li H, Liu X, Su Y, Yang J (2018) Anti-PD-1/PD-L1 therapy for non-small-cell lung cancer: toward personalized medicine and combination strategies. J Immunol Res 2018:1

Travis WD (2010) Advances in neuroendocrine lung tumors. Ann Oncol 21(Suppl-7):vii65–vii71

Traxler P (2003) Tyrosine kinases as targets in cancer therapy—successes and failures. Expert Opin Ther Targets 7:215–234. https://doi.org/10.1517/14728222.7.2.215

Ubenik J (2003) Tumour MHC class I downregulation and immunotherapy. Oncol Rep 10:2005–2008. https://doi.org/10.3892/or.10.6.2005

VanderLaan PA, Chen Y, DiStasio M et al (2018a) Molecular testing turnaround time in non-small-cell lung cancer: monitoring a moving target. Clin Lung Cancer 19:e589–e590. https://doi.org/10.1016/j.cllc.2018.04.005

VanderLaan PA, Rangachari D, Costa DB (2018b) Lung cancer with a high tumor mutational burden. N Engl J Med 379:1093. https://doi.org/10.1056/NEJMc1808566

VanderLaan PA, Rangachari D, Majid A et al (2018c) Tumor biomarker testing in non-small-cell lung cancer: a decade of change. Lung Cancer 116:90–95. https://doi.org/10.1016/j.lungcan.2018.01.002

Wang Q, Su C, Zhou C (2023) Recent advances in immunotherapy for lung cancer. Cancer Innov 2:18

Wu J, Wang W, Zhang J, Zhou B, Zhao W, Su Z et al (2019) DeepHLApan: a deep learning approach for neoantigen prediction considering both HLA-peptide binding and immunogenicity. Front Immunol 10:2559

Zhou C, Chen G, Huang Y, Zhou J, Lin L, Feng J et al (2021) Camrelizumab plus carboplatin and pemetrexed versus chemotherapy alone in chemotherapy-naive patients with advanced non-squamous non-small-cell lung cancer (CameL): a randomised, open-label, multicentre, phase 3 trial. Lancet Respir Med 9(3):305–314. https://doi.org/10.1016/S2213-2600(20)30365-9

PD-1/PD-L1 Inhibitors for the Treatment of Lung Cancer

5

Yuvraj Patil, Bariz Dakhni, and Shweta Kolhatkar

5.1 Introduction

Lung cancer is the leading cause of deaths due to cancer across the world, while it ranks third in incidence. As earlier chapters illustrate, multiple factors play a role in the incidence of lung cancer such as behavioral and environmental factors that drive cancer occurrence differentially in diverse geo-cultural regions (Deo et al. 2022; Sung et al. 2021; Ferlay et al. 2020). Lung cancers dominate in males especially in the productive age group, while breast cancer and colorectal cancer precede lung cancer incidence in women. Genetic or metabolic predisposition is not correlated with this observation, supporting the hypothesis of environmental and behavioral factors driving lung cancer in the population. To reconcile the relationship of cancer incidence and mortality in order to put forth a contemporary perspective of the lethality of lung cancer, we present a ratio of deaths due to cancer and the incidence of the disease, described here as a lethality index (Fig. 5.1). The index represents a realistic risk of death due to the cancer type described, based on recently vetted global cancer research data (Sung et al. 2021). As illustrated, lung cancer is the most burdensome neoplastic disease as observed clinically. With this unique perspective of lung cancer, we can appreciate the urgent need for clinical interventions that are superior to current therapy. Chapters in this book detail current clinical interventions for lung cancer. The focus on this chapter is to review the relatively new immunotherapy, which utilizes immune checkpoint inhibition (ICI), specifically inhibition of the PD-1/PD-L1 pathway.

The burden of cancer in lungs is typically classified as small-cell lung cancer (SCLC) and non-small-cell lung cancer (NSCLC). SCLC is considered a more aggressive cancer but accounts for about 15% of total lung cancer cases; NSCLC on

Y. Patil (✉) · B. Dakhni · S. Kolhatkar
School of Health Sciences and Technology, Dr. Vishwanath Karad MIT World Peace University, Pune, Maharashtra, India

S. Bhatt et al. (eds.), *Immunotherapy Against Lung Cancer*,
https://doi.org/10.1007/978-981-99-7141-1_5

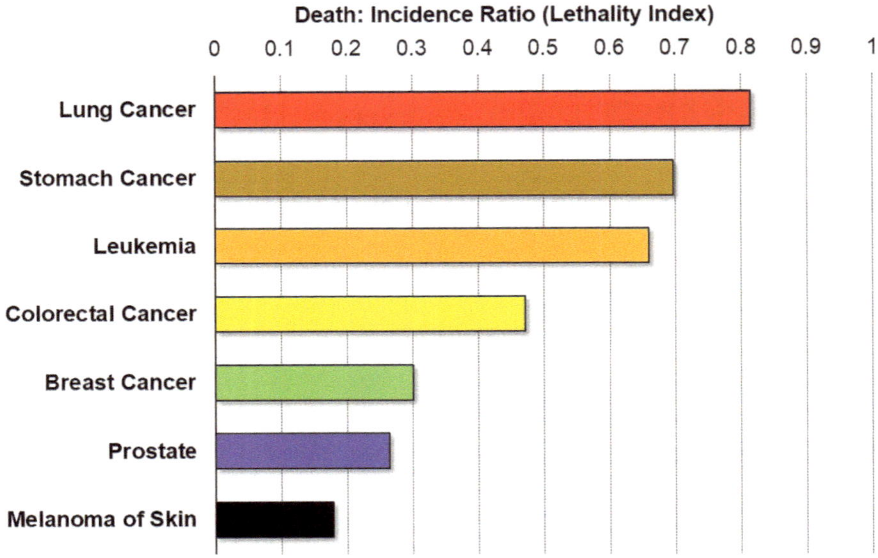

Fig. 5.1 Lethality Index of Selected Cancer Types (2020). The Death: Incidence ratio of cancer reflects the risk of mortality due to the afflicting cancer type (Sung et al. 2021)

the other hand accounts for the remainder and while not regarded as benign, are significantly less aggressive than SCLC. NSCLC bears lung cancer types such as adenocarcinoma, squamous cell carcinoma, and large cell carcinoma (Oser et al. 2015). Due to differences in tumor biology, treatment strategies for SCLC and NSCLC differ in accordance to tumor proliferation; mixed histological results are frequently seen in the two cancer types, for example, 10% large cell carcinomas are noted in SCLC biopsies as well. Treatment strategies are confounded due to the admixture, thus necessitating thorough analysis of subject tumor specimen.

The immunotherapy arsenal in cancer treatment is currently populated with a few potent alternatives. In no particular order of effectiveness, these are (a) chimeric antigen receptor T-cell (CAR-T) therapy, (b) monoclonal antibodies (mABs), (c) immunomodulators and cytokines, (d) oncolytic viruses, (e) cancer vaccines, and (f) immune checkpoint inhibitors (ICIs). While some treatment options are considered mainstream, certain options are still under study for safety and efficacy (Team A 2019).

Early success with immune checkpoint blockade opened the doors for incremental research into the ICI domain, and currently, there are at least nine approved products that act as ICI agents. Besides anti-PD-1 [Pembrolizumab (Keytruda), Nivolumab (Opdivo), Cemiplimab (Libtayo)] and anti-PD-L1 inhibitors [Atezolizumab (Tecentriq), Avelumab (Bavencio), Durvalumab (Imfinzi)], monoclonal antibodies (mABs) for inhibiting CTLA4 [Ipilimumab (Yervoy) and Tremelimumab (Imjuno)] and LAG-3 [Relatlimab] are in continuing clinical trials for over a decade. To the best of our knowledge, there are at least 3777 clinical trials registered involving the use of PD-1/PD-L1 agents, of which at least 798 trials are associated with lung cancer. In total, 195 clinical trials focus on metastatic lung cancer, which implies 3/fourth of all PD-1/PD-L1 trials are carried out in low-mid-grade lung cancer. There are adverse events associated with the administration of ICI, which have resulted in some 3.5% of the studies been withdrawn, suspended or terminated. The chapter will explore the phenomenon behind the poor response to ICI and its implications in immunotherapy for lung cancer.

Furthermore, immune-competency of T cells is influenced by other routes of anticancer therapy. The synergy affecting the gross effectiveness of the combination of therapies is discussed along with the path forward as evidenced by the clinical consensus.

The gender disparity in lung cancer is demonstrated in the 2020 GLOBOCAN cancer report showcasing the disparity in incidence of the disease among men and women (Fig. 5.2).

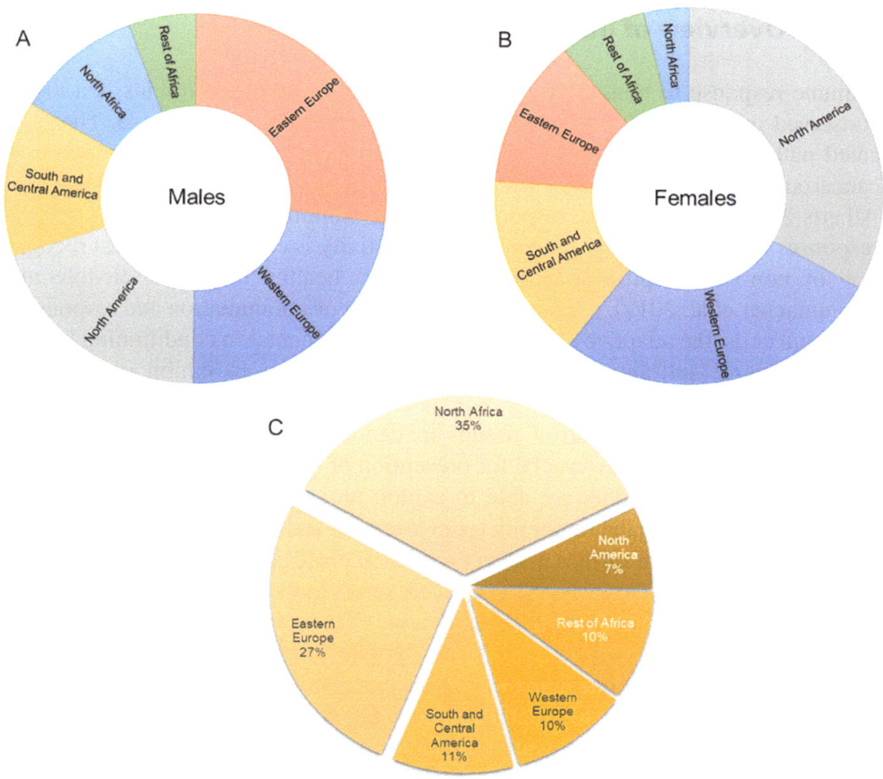

Fig. 5.2 Regiospecific Incidence of Lung Cancer. Age-Normalized Rates by Gender as reported in 2020. Lung Cancer Incidence per 100,000 individuals in (**a**) Males, (**b**) Females, and (**c**) Disparity Index showing greatest rift in incidence rates between men and women

An interesting interpretation of these data are the behavioral traits within a culture that expose females to pro-cancerous stimuli such as smoking and inhaled mutagenic substances. While religious influences in say, North African nations, prevent women from smoking, a more liberated attitude among women from North American nations predisposes them to smoking-related carcinogenic influences (Cornelius et al. 2023). The result is a near-equal distribution of lung cancer distribution between men and women in North America, while on the contrary, the disparity of disease incidence amongst women in northern African nations such as Egypt or Algeria is to the tune of approximately fivefold, compared to men. Observations such as these may well influence the clinical decisions to treat lung cancer in specific populations.

Without over-simplifying the myriad factors that come into account for successful ICI, the present work discusses the origins of immune-blockade, natural responses to T-cell activity, caveats of ICI, its clinical potential and superior patient reception, and a rationale plan for future-wide acceptability of ICI.

5.2 Overview of Immune Checkpoint Signaling

Immune response to non-native epitopes or foreign materials/proteins is a highly conserved mechanism involving innate and adaptive immune response. The dedicated pathway for management of altered cells, as a result of (viral) infection or cancerous changes, is the latter, with a complex regulatory system (Sun et al. 2009; Alberts 2017). Unlike innate response, adaptive immunity is key to highly specific responses to foreign or neo-antigens. This selectivity is crucial for not just recognition of non-native epitopes but also to protect healthy cells via self-tolerance (Schumacher et al. 2019). Specifically, in the event of inflammation and response to abnormal cells, the adaptive immune system is instrumental in conditioning healthy cells to express self-antigens including specific antigens to inhibit potent T-cell response.

The thymus and bone marrow tissues are central to the self-tolerance phenomenon while lymph nodes are crucial for prevention of immune overreaction (Murphy and Weaver 2017). Tumors are able to exploit an aspect of this phenomenon by fundamentally altering the tumor microenvironment and altering the response of the T cells by changing the surface marker expression profiles in the tumor cells (Becker et al. 2013). Central tolerance, as it is termed, refers to the clearance and deletion of clonal populations of auto-reactive lymphocytes before they develop into immune-competent cells and proliferate. This CD4+ lymphocyte-mediated activity typically occurs in the thymus or bone marrow with the end result of fundamentally depressed immune response, leading to T-cell depletion. T-cell clones are systematically programmed for apoptosis, thereby attenuating the anticancer response of the lymphocytes. Binding to appropriate ligands, MHC antigen or self-antigen triggers either survival (stimulatory) signal or apoptosis (inhibitory) event (Morris et al. 2001). Since cancer cells originate from healthy tissue, self-tolerance as an escape mechanism is indeed hijacked by the diseased cells.

Principally, the activated T cell (immuno-competent) is selected by a complex mechanism of co-inhibitory or co-stimulatory signaling systems. Once the naïve T cell is presented with the antigen, it is trained to recognize the presented antigen. Upon perception of foreign antigen, the current understanding portrays a mechanism that upregulates the interaction of a protein termed CD28 (cluster of differentiation 28) with the antigen-presenting cell counterparts of CD80 or CD86 (also known as B7–1 and B7–2, respectively). CD28 is a co-stimulatory protein that codes for T-cell survival and therefore clonal selection. Various pathways triggered by conjugation of CD28 and CD80 or CD86 lead to growth of the T cell and its subsequent proliferation and promotion of immune-competency. The selected T cell clone is thus freely circulated in the system and exacts its T-cell role. As a counteractive pathway, CD 80 or CD86 can also be engaged by an inhibitory protein CTLA4, which is believed to bring down the available content of CD 80/CD 86 leading to depletion of T cells (Lee et al. 1998; Harding et al. 1992; Qureshi et al. 2011). Cytotoxic T-lymphocyte-associated protein 4 or CTLA4 is constitutively expressed in regulatory T cells and activated T cells. The phenomenon also known as T-cell exhaustion leads to a poor immune response and is engaged as a self-tolerance mechanism. This particular mechanism is hijacked by tumors to evade immune-recognition, which relies on upregulation of CTLA4 to negatively influence immune-competency (Krummel and Allison 1995). As the following figure depicts, CD28 and CTLA4 compete to influence outcome for the activated T cell. CD28 is stimulatory in nature and promotes the survival of the T cell, while CTLA4 is responsible for clonal suppression or deletion (Fig. 5.3).

Immune-checkpoint signaling via CTLA4 plays defined roles in the immune response, enumerated in the table below. The particular physiological implications of CTLA4 make it an attractive target for reversing immune-suppression, specifically within a tumor microenvironment.

While CTLA4 undermines the immune poise of the T cells that have been rendered competent, it does not define the nature of cancer cell surface biomarker expression in the tumor microenvironment. As mentioned earlier, while CTLA4 forms one component of the immune-suppressive axis, other proteins have emerged as potent regulators of immune tolerance, such as PD-1 (programmed cell death receptor-1), PD-L1 (programmed cell death receptor ligand-1), TIM-3 (T-cell Immunoglobulin domain and Mucin domain-3), LAG-3 (lymphocyte activation gene-3), and KIR (killer cell immunoglobulin-like receptor). Extensively studied targets for mechanistic understanding and exploration of therapeutic targets for anticancer therapy include PD-1 and its ligand, PD-L1, TIM3, and LAG-3 (Pardoll 2012). Numerous other surface biomarkers have been established with inhibitory and stimulatory roles. While proteins such as TIM3, LAG3, KIR, CTLA4/CD80/86 are predominantly noted in interactions between T cells and APCs, direct interactions with and immune sensing of cancer cells are centered on neo-antigens and PD-1/PD-L1/2 interactions (Fig. 5.4). Neo-antigens are abnormal surface proteins generated by the cancer cell arising from specific mutations or as response to abnormal signaling (Schumacher et al. 2019).

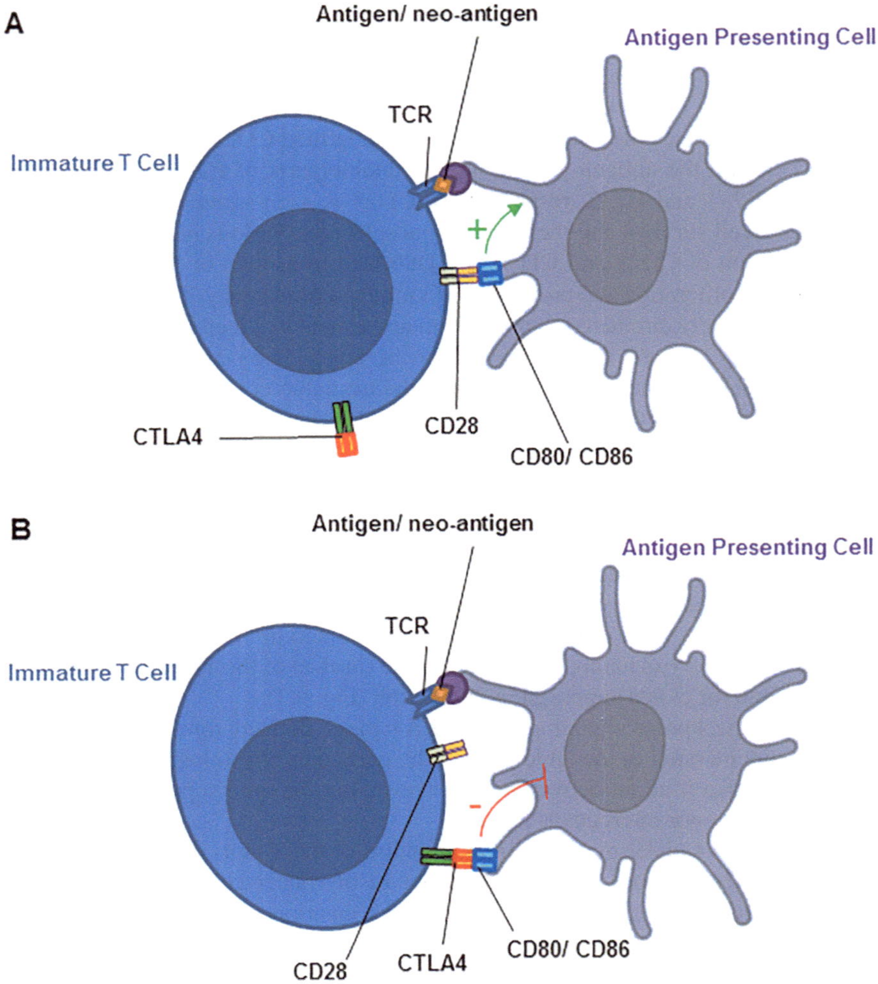

Fig. 5.3 Mechanism of Immune-tolerance Involving Interaction of Antigen-Presenting Cell (APC) with naïve T cell. (**a**) Interaction of CD28 (co-stimulatory) protein with CD80/86 leading to T cell survival, (**b**) Engagement of CD80/86 by CTLA4 resulting in inhibitory signals (T cell apoptosis)

The PD-1/PD-L1 axis of immune response has been studied extensively and has resulted in translational clinical therapeutic advances, which is also the focus of the current chapter. PD-1 or programmed cell death receptor-1 was first noted in the 1990s as a mechanism of programmed cell death (Ishida et al. 1992). Subsequent work has shown evidence of a complex machinery to modulate immune response involving PD-1, which allows for self-tolerance by driving trained T cells to apoptosis and immune-evasion by cancer cells (Becker et al. 2013; Pardoll 2012; Smith et al. 1989; Tumeh et al. 2014). As Fig. 5.4a depicts, PD-1 surface receptor on T

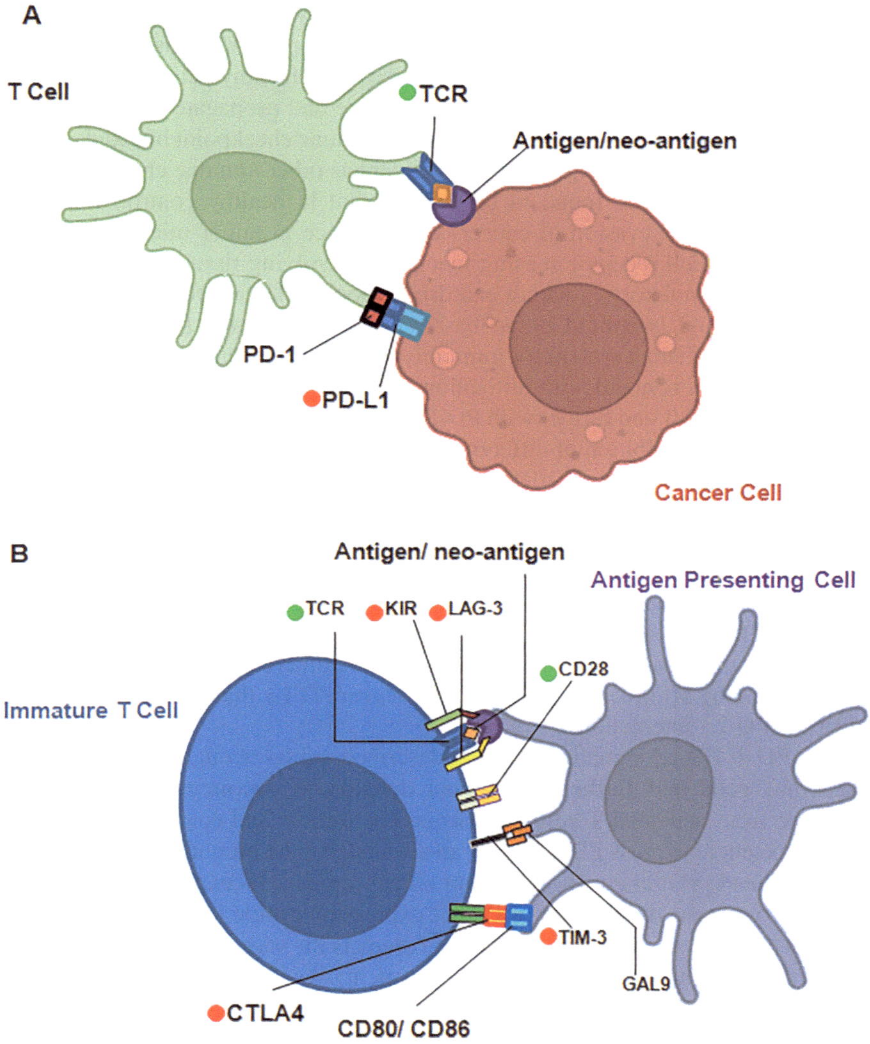

Fig. 5.4 Immune Checkpoint Systems. Regulatory inhibition of T cells in TME (**a**) and in T cell priming tissue systems like the lymph nodes (**b**). Inhibitory signaling molecules (on T cells) are indicated in red circles while stimulatory molecules are identified with green circles

cells is crucial in sensing autologous cells. Diseased cells expressed abnormal cues are tagged for clearance by T cells or NK cells. While toning the immune reaction in order to prevent collateral damage to healthy cells, the body's healthy cells express specific self-recognition antigens such as PD-L1/L2.

The regulatory or activated T cells while recognizing self-antigens within the presented MHC (major histocompatibility complex receptor) are also influenced by the PD-1: PD-L1 interaction between the two cell types. While this evolutionary mechanism developed in mammalian systems to spare widespread damage to healthy cells, cancer cells originating from the same healthy cells are able to take advantage of this escape route to evade clearance and propagate (Schwartz 2012; Chatenoud 2014). The focus of contemporary immune checkpoint blockade therapy rests on this mechanism. Figure 5.4 further depicts other immune checkpoint components that have been found to be instrumental in healthy control of immune response as well as evasion of cancer cell clearance in tumor microenvironment. The primary T-cell receptor sensing machinery involving tissue or cellular MHC molecules is stimulatory in nature and drives clonal selection for the interacting T cell. Thymus and lymphoid tissue–based T-cell proliferation (Table 5.1) further primes the mammalian system for immunity against the specific antigen. The opposite phenomenon is noted with mitigation of the recognition reaction with surface markers like PD-L1 and further with PD-L1/L2 and CTLA4 on APCs. The activated T cell undergoes inhibition of differentiation and proliferation leading ultimately to T-cell depletion (Blank et al. 2019; Zhang et al. 2020b).

Figure 5.5 provides the molecular depictions and interaction of PD-1 and PD-L1. Binding studies show multiple sites on PD-1 that are effective targets for anti-PD-1 antibodies (Lee et al. 2019). Existing antibodies approved by FDA such as nivolumab and pembrolizumab have shown promise in competitive binding to PD-1, thereby inhibiting PD-L1-based T-cell depletion. Similarly, PD-L1 countering FDA-approved antibodies such as atezolizumab, durvalumab, and avelumab also show focused binding affinities for precise locations on PD-L1 that result in interference of PD-1: PD-L1 interactions.

The PD-1: PD-L1 signaling event, as described, brings about immune evasion by cancerous cells and furthermore clonal deletion to downregulate the immune response from activated T cells. Consequently, tumors and cancerous tissues that are competent to express PD-L1 enjoy an advantage to be immunologically selected to survive and proliferate. However, not all cancerous cells express PD-L1 leading to a heterogeneous distribution of PD-L1 expression profile in not only patient tissues but also among individuals. Figure 5.6 depicts the varied distribution of PD-L1 across three human lung cancer (NSCLC) patients. As illustrated, the abundance of PD-L1 changes dramatically from individual to individual over an order of magnitude. The illustration is intended to draw attention to the fact that PD-L1 expression

Table 5.1 Impact of CTLA4 signaling in immune response

Immune Role	Activity	Putative Sites
B cell signaling	–	Bone marrow/thymus
T cell co-stimulation	–	Bone marrow/thymus
T cell co-inhibition	+	Bone marrow/thymus/tumor microenvironment
T_{reg} cell differentiation	–	Thymus
T cell proliferation	–	Lymph nodes/thymus
Immune response	–	Systemic

Activity suppression and enhancement is indicated by "-" and "+" symbols, respectively

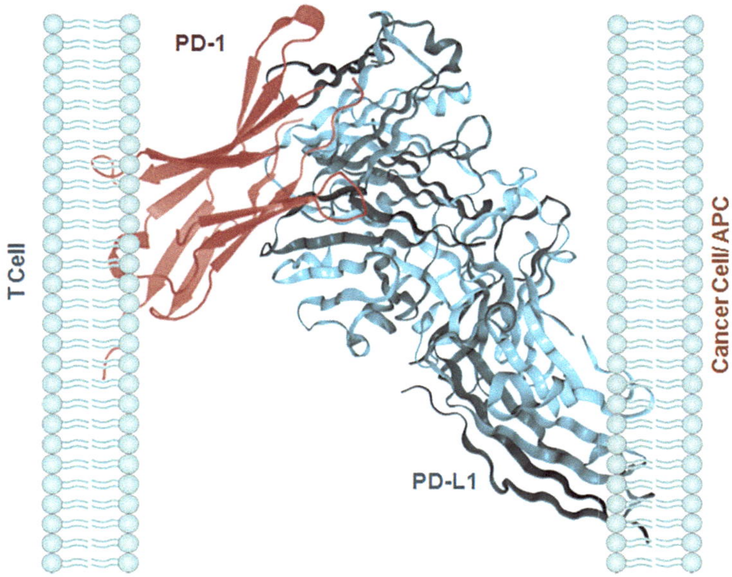

Fig. 5.5 Interaction of PD-1 Receptor and its ligand PD-L1. PD-L1 expressed on cancer cells and borne by antigen-presenting cells is recognized by PD-1 selectively. Protein crystal structures derived and processed from (Berman et al. 2000)

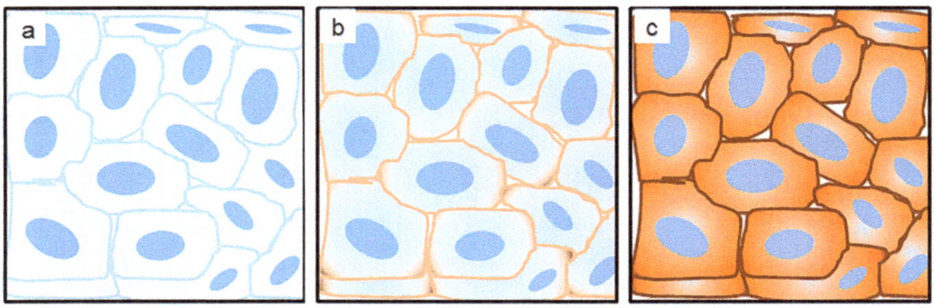

Fig. 5.6 PD-L1 Expression Profile in different clinical subjects with lung cancer (non-small-cell lung cancer, NSCLC). PD-L1 antibody is labeled with (brown) Chromogenic reaction, counterstained with (blue) Hematoxylin. Left to right (**a**–**c**) depicts patients with increasing abundance of PD-L1 in tumor biopsies. (Scheme based on data from (McLaughlin et al. 2016))

is a swing factor for the success of immunotherapy involving PD-L1 therapeutic antibodies. As the subsequent sections elaborate, while anti-PD-L1 antibodies are highly successful in cancer treatment, the low response rate among patients still keeps many cancer clinicians on the fence. The poor response may be explained by the varied PD-L1 expression profiles in the patient population (Liu et al. 2021; Chamoto et al. 2020; Wu et al. 2019; McLaughlin et al. 2016).

Tumor microenvironment (TME) is also noted to demonstrate heterogeneity, which is a major confounding factor for cancer treatment (Fisher et al. 2013; Dagogo-Jack and Shaw 2018; Wu et al. 2022). Mutational changes and DNA repair irregularities as well as microsatellite instabilities create an environment of neo-antigen expression, which promotes lymphocyte infiltration into the TME (Kciuk et al. 2023). Greater expression of PD-L1 by cancerous cells or involved APCs further promotes immune evasion. DNA damage and subsequent neo-antigen presentation drive PD-L1 surface expression (Strickland et al. 2016). As Fig. 5.7 depicts, infiltrating T cells encounter cancerous cells expressing significantly upregulated neo-antigens (A). Activated T cells are primed and trained for recognizing a variety of cancerous biomarkers. Upon presentation to T-cell receptors, positive association (B) leads to clonal selection of activated T cells and further signaling with cytokines such as interferon-γ (IFN-γ). IFN-γ is implicated in defensive roles such as macrophage activation, enhancement of antigen presentation, and activation of immune response (Castro et al. 2018). IFN-γ drives promoters for gene expression in target cells, which include PD-L1 and its L2 variant (Guo et al. 2022; Qian et al. 2018; Abiko et al. 2015; Garcia-Diaz et al. 2017). The resulting gene products are trafficked to the cancer cell surface (C), thereby enabling self-antigen signaling with PD-1 receptors in activated T cells (D). Unlike (B) where a positive recognition between MHC-neo-antigen and T-cell receptor leads to T-cell selection and proliferation, PD-1: PD-L1 interaction inhibits clonal selection and diminishes the T-cell response.

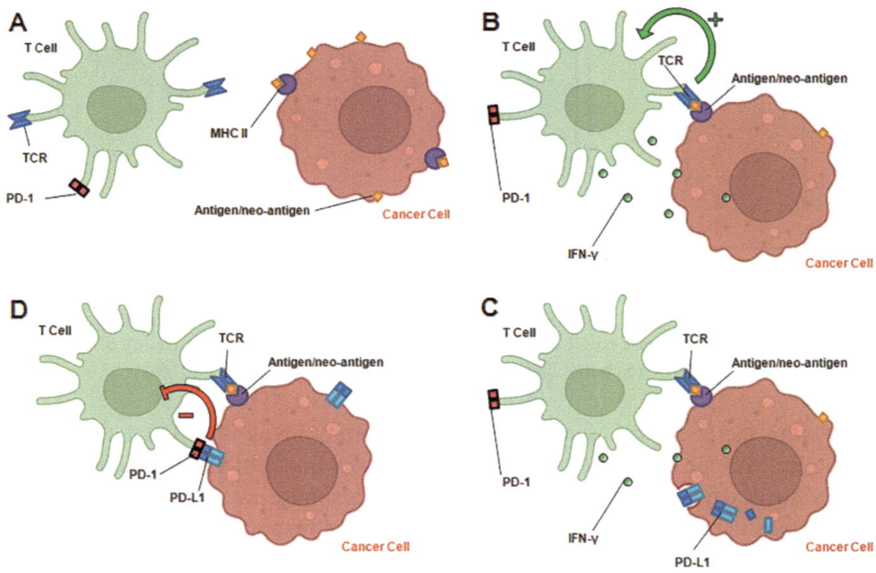

Fig. 5.7 Tumor Microenvironment Adaptation to Activated T cells. IFN-induced PD-L1 expression evades immune response and influences negative T-cell clonal selection

The PD-L1 expression upregulation is primarily driven by the IFN-γ-mediated JAK-STAT-IRS pathway (Garcia-Diaz et al. 2017). PD-L2 expression is alternatively regulated and dually governed by IFN-β and IFN-γ.

The immune checkpoint and cancer cell immune evasion using the checkpoint system make for attractive targets, the therapeutic treatment of which allows proper functioning of the immune system and may provide a better treatment alternative to cytotoxic chemotherapy (Zhao et al. 2020; Zhang et al. 2023).

5.3 First-Generation Immune Checkpoint Blockade (CTLA4 Intervention)

CTLA4 interventions are discussed in detail in a chapter within this volume by Pujari et al. However, the broad understanding of ICI treatment will benefit from a brief review here. CTLA4 as a lymphocyte mediation node involving the immune system alone was considered earlier on, in the mid-1990s as a viable target for anticancer therapy (Kearney et al. 1995; Walunas et al. 1994). Given the infancy of the field, this was a foresighted exploration of immunotherapy. Subsequent to FDA approval of the pioneering anti-CTLA4 antibodies, early breakthrough results promised a paradigm shift in cancer therapy as clinical science knew it at the time (Kearney et al. 1995; Wolchok and Saenger 2008). As depicted in Fig. 5.3, CTLA4 pathway is primarily engaged between cells of the immune system, not involving cancerous cells directly. The targeting of this pathway therefore invites systemic involvement and tuning of the immune response.

The clinically approved antibodies developed against CTLA4, such as ipilimumab and tremelimumab, showed high clinical efficacy, but adverse events emerged soon after, largely centered on self-tolerance. Blockade of CTLA4 with antibodies liberates CD80/86 receptors for signaling with CD28 (Fig. 5.8).

Immune-related toxicity of the skin and gastrointestinal tract appeared as primary reactions to the anti-CTLA4 treatment (Gan et al. 2022; Karimi et al. 2021; Korman et al. 2005). Interestingly, while adverse events are observed in about a fifth of all the treated individuals, only about 11% patients display an objective response in treated patients who do not demonstrate adverse effects. The implied mechanism involves a systematic depletion of Treg cells to have a beneficial anticancer effect (Gan et al. 2022). Not much progress toward development of new antibodies against CTLA4 has been demonstrated in recent years, with the second antibody (tremelimumab) being approved by FDA in 2022 (Keam 2023; Sondak et al. 2011; Abou-Alfa et al. 2022).

A decade of research and clinical interventions with ipilimumab have shown critical improvement as a direct result of the CTLA4 blockade; however, immune-related adverse events are a near-constant accompaniment observed in nearly half of the treated patients. As mentioned earlier, gastrointestinal events are disproportionately high, resulting in the decision to discontinue the therapy. Mortalities from gastrointestinal reactions, triggered auto-immune conditions also abound, despite overall cancer survival noted in patients. Auto-immune reactions are also noted with

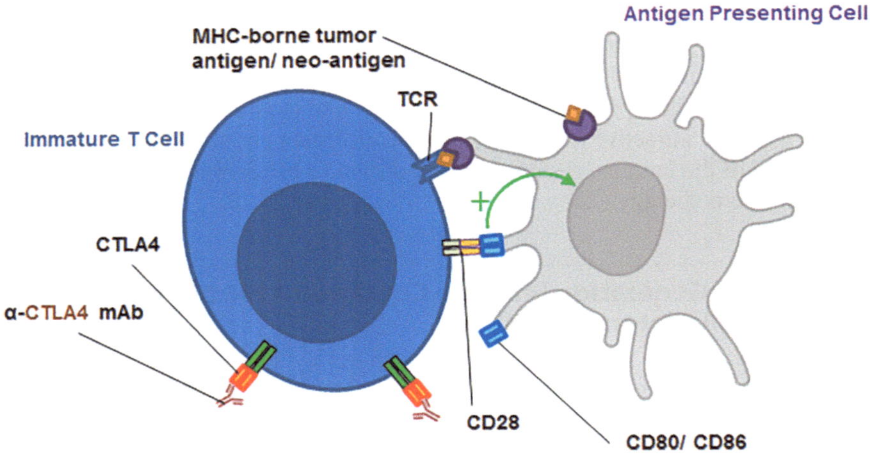

Fig. 5.8 CTLA4 Antibody Interactions with T cells

severe health outcomes. More recently, a gut-immune-cancer axis has been implicated in the persistence of the side effects. The preferential selection of certain microorganisms in the gut, arising due to enhanced clearance of other microorganisms as a result of an activated T–cell-based immune response, has been proposed as a major factor (Guérin et al. 2023; Desilets and Elkrief 2023; Hodi et al. 2010; Graziani et al. 2012).

The approval of tremelimumab in 2022 by FDA in the context of advanced/metastatic cancer regardless of being chemotherapy-naïve is notable in that the drug is recommended as a monotherapy trial. The overall survival and health benefit is considered superior to existing drug treatment, even in metastatic cancer. Furthermore, the binding of tremelimumab is observed to be more robust, compared to ipilimumab, implying more resilient defense of the activated T cells and therefore for a more pronounced anticancer effect (He et al. 2017). Figure 5.9 depicts minor structural changes of the two FDA-approved CTLA4 antibodies; while ipilimumab shows a lateral spread of the light chain, tremelimumab is more constricted. In principle, both antibodies recognize the same epitope (CD80/86 binding domain); however, minor sequence and structure alterations improve the binding capacity of tremelimumab to its target, CTLA4. The decade of work investigating the utility of CTLA4 therapeutic antibodies has revealed mild-to-modest advantage, specifically in overall survival; however, the same is fraught with immune adverse effects, implying the necessity of exploring other avenues of immunotherapy for effective and side-effect-free anticancer therapy. More relevantly, as the next section details, immune blockade therapy may be better served by addressing cancer-specific targets such as the inducible PD-L1 antigen, which appears in certain cancers.

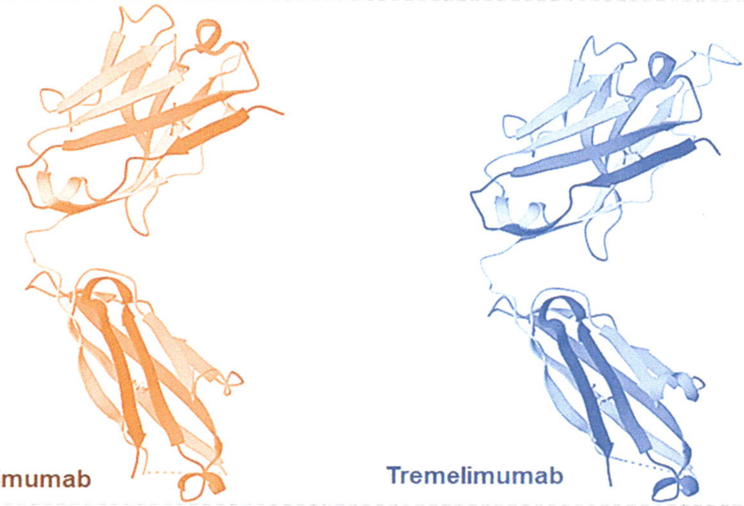

Fig. 5.9 Comparison of Antibody Structures (Fab light chain) for CTLA4. Spatial changes in loop regions on the Fab portion dictate changes in binding affinity and dissociation from CTLA4. Protein crystal structures derived and processed from (Berman et al. 2000)

5.4 PD-1/PD-L1-Driven Immune Checkpoint Inhibition

As described earlier, PD-1: PD-L1/L2 interactions preclude fruitful activation of trained T cells presented with tumor/cancer antigens. It has been shown how PD-1, unlike CTLA4, is directly capable of influencing the immune biology of the tumor microenvironment. For instance, the expression of PD-1 in tumors is inversely correlated with the proportion of infiltrating lymphocytes in a given tumor. Further, reports show PD-1/PD-L1 signaling as crucial for survival of cancer stem cells. PD-L1 expression has been shown to be necessary and sufficient for triggering an EGR-1-mediated tumor angiogenesis and rapid growth of tumors (Yu et al. 2023; Konishi et al. 2004; Akbay et al. 2013; D'Incecco et al. 2015; Xu et al. 2023a). Other growth factors such as EGFR also drive tumors, such as those in lungs, and these are experimentally found to utilize the PD-1 pathway for immune escape. Given PD-1 and its ligand's direct role in tumor sparing and growth, immunotherapy against these two targets appears more viable and direct, compared to CTLA4.

5.4.1 PD-1 Therapeutic Antibodies

Following clinical approvals of the first-generation immune checkpoint blockade antibodies, work carried out on investigation of PD-1 antibodies resulted in dramatic improvement in overall survival of treated patients. Early clinical work was largely focused on melanoma; however, advanced or metastatic lung, colorectal, and breast cancers soon attracted clinical attention for immunotherapy (Table 5.2).

Currently eight monoclonal antibodies directed against PD-1: PD-L1 axis are approved by FDA for treatment in a variety of cancers, usually in advanced or metastatic stages. Pembrolizumab and Nivolumab were the earliest recognized antibodies with a clinical trial record showing significant improvement over standard care in advanced cancer types. While adverse events were noted over 50% of the time in anti-CTLA4 immune checkpoint blockade, with anti-PD-1 blockade, side effects were notably lower (≤30%). The improved patient experience drove anti-PD-1: PD-L1 research resulting in eight marketed drugs not including at least one more anti-PD-1 antibody (Tislelimumab, Novartis) in the clinical trial pipeline, compared to just two marketed CTLA4 antibodies in the past entire decade. While Pembrolizumab, Nivolumab and Cemiplimab have been in the clinical route for a short while, Dostarlimab and Retifanlimab are relatively new. In fact, the newer anti-PD-1 antibodies also lack structural characterization, which impedes their consideration in comparative studies. Figure 5.10 depicts a few protein structures of available PD-1 antibodies in complex with their target, PD-1. The protein epitope (PD-1) is used to align and compare the binding of the various monoclonal antibodies. Figures 5.11 and 5.12 depict the PD-1: PD-L1 interaction, which can be considered for visual reference. PD-1 antibody development has centered largely on the PD-L1/L2 binding domain on PD-1. As seen in Fig. 5.10, all FDA-approved antibodies recognize a specific region on PD-1, while data on Retifanlimab are currently unavailable, ongoing clinical trials with Tislelizumab have yielded new information on potential clinical utility of the new molecule (Xu et al. 2023b).

The crystal structure of PD-1 complexed with Tislelizumab shows a change in target orientation. Figures 5.10 and 5.11 depict a slight shift in axis of antibody binding on PD-1 (Lee et al. 2020). Tislelizumab mimics native PD-1 and PD-L1/L2 binding, implying greater stability of H- and ionic bonds. More importantly, the superior binding may improve the immune checkpoint blockade. The adverse events resulting from unbound antibody in the circulation may be limited by optimizing binding characteristics of antibodies.

FDA has previously approved Nivolumab for a variety of indications such as non-small-cell lung cancer (NSCLC), renal cell carcinoma, bladder cancer (BC),

Table 5.2 List of approved PD-1/PD-L1 antibodies for cancer therapy

IC Target	Name of Antibody	Trade Name	Manufacturer
PD-1	Pembrolizumab	Keytruda	Merck
PD-1	Nivolumab	Opdivo	Bristol Meyer Squibbs
PD-1	Cemiplimab	Libtayo	Regeneron
PD-1	Dostarlimab	Jemperli	GlaxoSmithKline
PD-1	Retifanlimab	Zynyx	Incyte/MacroGenics
PD-L1	Atezolizumab	Tecentriq	Roche
PD-L1	Avelumab	Bavencio	Merck/Pfizer
PD-L1	Durvalumab	Imfinzi	Medimmune/AstraZeneca

IC immune checkpoint (protein)

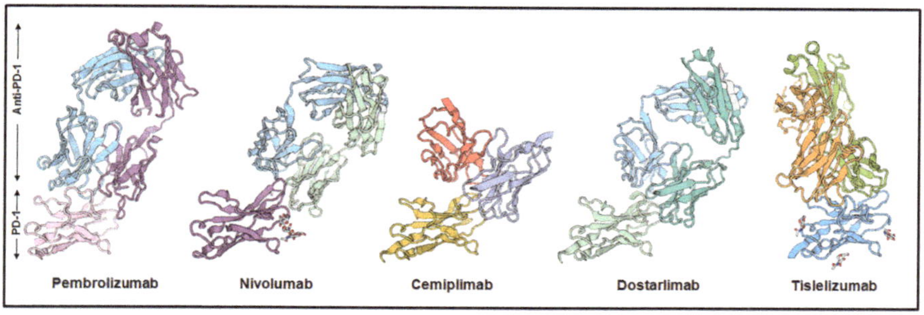

Fig. 5.10 PD-1 Antibodies: Structural Comparison and Epitope Focus. The Protein DataBase images depict Fab/Fv domains of the immunoglobulins, focusing either both on Fab light and heavy chains or light chains alone. All FDA-approved antibodies utilize the same epitope, while Tislelimumab, still in clinical trials, recognizes a slightly offset epitope on the same protein. Unique protein regions or domains are indicated by distinct colors. Protein crystal structures derived and processed from (Berman et al. 2000)

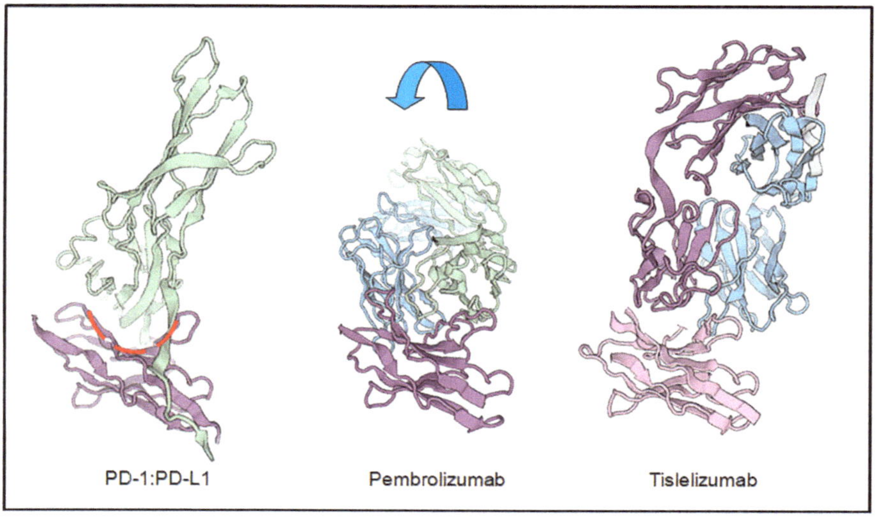

Fig. 5.11 PD-1: Antibody-Binding Dynamics. Binding similarity with native PD-1: PD-L1 is greater with Tislelizumab, implying better binding characteristics. The red labeled pocket is the putative binding site of appropriate ligands for PD-1. Protein crystal structures derived and processed from (Berman et al. 2000)

colon and rectal cancer (CRC) with microsatellite instability (MSI) or mismatch repair (MMR) shortcomings, liver cancer, Hodgkin lymphoma (HL), melanoma, and head and neck squamous cell cancer (HNSCC). Pembrolizumab has been cleared for use in melanoma, HNSCC, cervical cancer, HL, NSCLC, BC, and gastric-esophageal cancers. Additionally, Pembrolizumab is also recommended for use in solid tumors classified as MSI/MMR (Qin et al. 2019).

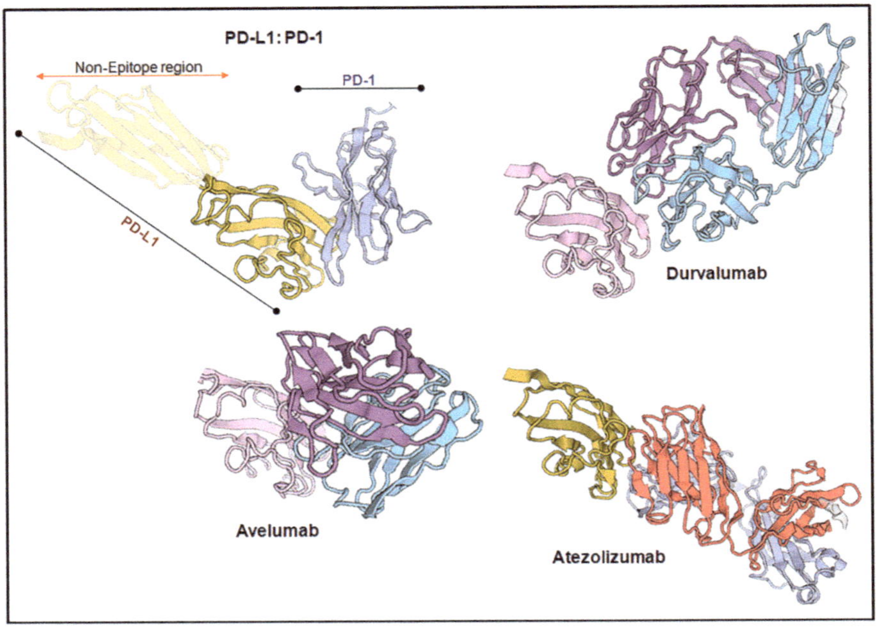

Fig. 5.12 PD-L1 Antibodies: Structural Comparison and Epitope Focus. The Protein DataBase images depict Fab/Fv domains of the immunoglobulins, focusing either both on Fab light and heavy chains or light chains alone. Unique protein regions or domains are indicated by distinct colors. Protein crystal structures derived and processed from (Berman et al. 2000)

Cemiplimab is a recently approved antibody, indicated by FDA in adults for advanced NSCLC with no concomitant EGF, lymphoma kinase, and ROS-1 abnormalities (Akinboro et al. 2022). Dostarlimab was cleared by the FDA in 2021 to treat MMR and advanced endometrial cancer in adults (Markham 2021; Shuvo et al. 2022).

5.4.2 PD-L1 Antibodies

Interestingly, PD-L1 targeting antibodies are significantly more effective at blocking the PD-1/PD-L1 signaling axis that PD-1 antibodies (De Sousa et al. 2019). While PD-1 is expressed mostly on T cells, PD-L1/L2 is expressed by cancer cells and infrequently by APCs (Sun et al. 2009; Becker et al. 2013; Morris et al. 2001; Tumeh et al. 2014; Schwartz 2012; Zhang et al. 2020b). Influencing the signaling by blocking PD-1 will subject the T cells to regulation, but not necessarily inhibit the cancer cells from interacting with and downregulating additional T cells (see Fig. 5.4). Furthermore, studies have shown the nature of PD-1: PD-L1 axis to be reminiscent of antibody–receptor interactions with beta-sheet and loop architecture of both PD-1 and PD-L1 conducive toward highly specific interactions (De Sousa et al. 2019; Lin et al. 2008; Zak et al. 2017). Consequently, a focus diversion toward PD-L1 as a target has resulted in at least three FDA-approved therapeutic antibodies. Currently, FDA has approved Atezolizumab and Durvalumab for the treatment of NSCLC. Avelumab has been recently cleared by the FDA for urothelial cancer and renal cell cancer; however, it is being used in a variety of cancer types including NSCLC, HNSCC, solid tumors, etc. An additional advantage of PD-L1 antibodies is the observed antibody-dependent cell-mediated cytotoxicity (ADCC). The value-added feature of such therapeutic options is the potential to reduce tumor growth, on top of immune-modulation in the treatment of cancer.

An interesting feature of the approved PD-L1 antibodies is their spatial orientation on the precise epitope, as depicted in Fig. 5.12. The epitope domain is schematically demonstrated as a constant motif, while the antibody-complex formation, based on crystal structures of individual antibodies, is displayed relative to the epitope.

While the loop interactions are highly specific, the diverse spatial placements of the Fab domains of antibodies show flexibility of the epitope. Given the more robust binding of PD-L1 epitope to its antibodies, compared to antibodies for PD-1, it may be hypothesized that the PD-L1 blockade could be non-competitive in nature (Lee et al. 2017). Monotherapy using immune checkpoint blockade is efficacious in individuals with a PD-L1 expressing tumor poise; however, as described earlier, due to the tumor and patient PD-L1 expression heterogeneity, monotherapy is effective in a relative small proportion of treated individuals. To overcome this phenomenon, combination of ICI can be recommended and is under active clinical investigation (Zhao et al. 2020; Abou-Alfa et al. 2022; Guérin et al. 2023; Zhang et al. 2020a). Interestingly, while combinations of CTLA4 and PD-1 or PD-L1 antibodies are being utilized in cancer therapy, combinations of PD-1 and PD-L1 antibodies have not been noted in clinical studies. Dual biomarker knockdown of PD-1 and PD-L1 could conceivably abolish the PD-1: PD-L1 axis; since the putative roles of these proteins are broadly distributed affecting physiological functions in the mammalian body (see Table 5.1).

Adverse events, although significantly less severe than conventional anticancer therapy, are altogether frequent in immune checkpoint blockade. As described for CTLA4 blockade, anti-PD-1/PD-L1 blockade raises adverse reactions including but not limited to gastrointestinal issues, auto-immune events, inflammatory issues in the skin and other tissues, as well as rare fatalities arising from complications. ICI therapy has been observed to affect multiple tissue/organ systems in the context of anticancer therapy (Johnson et al. 2022; Tuerxun et al. 2023). While clinical trials reveal lesser collateral damage due to ICI therapy in mono or combination therapies, the effects are nonetheless widespread and potentially long-lasting (Zhang et al. 2023). Multiple reports cite damage to the reproductive system by ICI (Tuerxun et al. 2023; Cosci et al. 2023). ICI is rapidly getting integrated into conventional anticancer therapy and thereby pervading across socioeconomic and age-gradient groups. As a growing number of individuals sexually mature, having being treated for cancer in their adolescence, it is observed that sexual health is compromised in the said individuals. Effects of ICI on the hypothalamus and direct effects on the reproductive organs have been implicated and are a current area of investigation. Similarly, endocrine consequences have been observed as a direct result of ICI (Cosci et al. 2023; Liao et al. 2023; Dudzińska et al. 2020). ICI has been blamed for induction of diabetes mellitus, which is a serious consequence, given the underlying pathology of cancer. A major factor in such immune-related adverse events (irAEs) is the re-enabling or even enhancement of antigen recognition, which leads to sensitizing of the immune cells. Urinary system organs have also been reported to have ICI-related toxicity; bladder cancer and cancers of diverse etiologies treated with ICI have shown emergence of kidney-associated irAEs (Lumlertgul et al. 2023; Davaro et al. 2023). More recently, gastrointestinal injuries arising from ICI therapy have been document (Mitchell and Karamchandani 2023).

5.5 ICI Combination Therapy

The poor response rate (~20%) of patients to immune checkpoint blockade with anti-PD-1 or anti-PD-L1 antibodies is largely attributed to diversity and heterogeneity of PD-L1 expression in patients or even tumors. As PD-1/PD-L1-based antibodies are primarily indicated in advanced or metastatic cancers, it is interesting to note that at such a late development stage, the clinical benefit may not emerge after all. A study in lung cancer patients involving survival in KRAS mutated context clinically staged at IV showed that ICI therapy may not bring relief to the patient in terms of overall survival. The present case had a baseline brain metastasis as a complication of Stage IV lung cancer (Swart et al. 2023). Furthermore, the positive impact of ICI therapy, especially monotherapy, diminishes with age (Nie et al. 2021; Suazo-Zepeda et al. 2023).

An interesting take on tumor physiology is the concept of a (PD-L1) cold tumor versus a "hot" tumor that leads to a better response for immunotherapy. These are also better infiltrated with macrophages and T cells, less prone to clonal deletion (T cell exhaustion) (Makuku et al. 2021; Zheng et al. 2022). A variety of existing anticancer treatments have a diverse bouquet of physiological responses, which may well enhance the productivity of ICI treatment. Cytotoxic chemotherapy with anthracyclines, platinums, alkylating agents, or anti-metabolites have profound effects on the immune system including expanding T-cell population, suppression of tumor-associated macrophages, etc. (Galluzzi et al. 2015; Vincent et al. 2010; Obeid et al. 2007). As clinical trials demonstrated, these are directly complementary to the activity of ICI agents. Tumors are also widely treated with radiation for better control in combination or continuation with chemotherapy. ICI therapy has been shown to be synergistic with radiotherapy as a result of selective T-cell population promotion and overall benefit in tumor size reduction (Crittenden et al. 2018). Radiation has also been well tolerated in combination with PD-1/PD-L1 ICI (Hu et al. 2017). Androgen blockade in combination with ICI therapy is being actively explored with benefits in overall survival and reduction in tumor size noted as well (Graff et al. 2016). Similar strategies have evolved using other anticancer agents with an active role in immune cell modulation (Page et al. 2019). Taken together, a large body of work to date shows a benefit that is statistically superior when combination of anticancer therapies is used including ICI administration, compared to ICI monotherapy or conventional anticancer treatments (Zhang et al. 2020a, 2023; Xu et al. 2023b; Nie et al. 2021; Zheng et al. 2022; Page et al. 2019; Yi et al. 2022; Robert 2020).

5.6 Current Perspective and Path Forward

Clinical networks are increasingly relying on ICI therapy, and there are increasingly more products in the clinical trial pipeline for use in immune checkpoint blockade. ICI therapy with PD-1/PD-L1 antibodies, while appearing potent and efficacious in selective cancer patients, does not work as a generalized strategy for anticancer treatment. The primary physiological factor behind this selectivity is the capability of tumors in expression of PD-L1. As clinical indications are now refined for drugs such as Pembrolizumab, Durvalumab, and Atezolizumab, clinical verification of PD-L1 expression of 1–49% tumor mass has now become a parametric requirement for anti-PD-1/PD-L1 therapy, regardless of combination used. Personalized medication approach is key in enabling ICI therapy for maximum effect, as potential adverse reactions also need to be balanced. A few studies have also shown benefit from non-steroidal anti-inflammatory drugs (NSAIDs) in curbing immune reactions arising from PD-1/PD-L1 treatment.

Interestingly, the growing consensus in the medical and biological research community regarding synergy of conventional chemo/radiotherapy and ICI therapy may lead the trend in future clinical trials and effective treatment regimen. In terms of therapeutic antibody development, the emerging market is establishing the role of PD-1/PD-L1 antibodies. The recent FDA approvals of ICIs are bringing these drugs into the mainstream of clinical options for cancer treatment. Given lung cancer's colossal footprint, having a growing arsenal or new agents is a welcome development. A majority of clinical studies involving PD-1/PD-L1 have centered on NSCLC. A greater focus on addressing multiple lung cancer types is currently required to observe the efficacy of PD-related ICI treatments, as well as safety and incidence of irAEs. While personalized cancer therapy is already in practice with single-cell genomics and CTC analysis, etc., PD-L1 prevalence can be viewed as a worthy addition to the panel for clinical decision. The effectiveness of ICI in reduction of tumor size and overall survival benefit is a clinical edge, which is currently superior to conventional chemotherapy, especially considering the relative burden of specific adverse events. With the growing prevalence of lung cancers, which is mostly environmentally driven, ICIs may well provide the golden mean to balance clinical outcome with impact on quality of life for the patient.

References

Abiko K, Matsumura N, Hamanishi J, Horikawa N, Murakami R et al (2015) Br J Cancer 112:1501–1509

Abou-Alfa GK, Lau G, Kudo M, Chan SL, Kelley RK et al (2022) NEJM Evidence 1:EVIDoa2100070

Akbay EA, Koyama S, Carretero J, Altabef A, Tchaicha JH et al (2013) Cancer Discov 3:1355–1363

Akinboro O, Larkins E, Pai-Scherf LH, Mathieu LN, Ren Y et al (2022) Clin Cancer Res 28:2221–2228

Alberts B (2017) Molecular biology of the cell. In: Norton WW (ed) Garland science, p 1464

Becker JC, Andersen MH, Schrama D, thor Straten P. (2013) Cancer Immunol Immunother 62:1137–1148

Berman HM, Westbrook J, Feng Z, Gilliland G, Bhat TN et al (2000) Nucleic Acids Res 28:235–242

Blank CU, Haining WN, Held W, Hogan PG, Kallies A et al (2019) Nat Rev Immunol 19:665–674

Castro F, Cardoso AP, Gonçalves RM, Serre K, Oliveira MJ (2018) Front Immunol 9:9

Chamoto K, Hatae R, Honjo T (2020) Int J Clin Oncol 25:790–800

Chatenoud L (2014) Science 344:1343–1344

Monica Cornelius, Caitlin Loretan, Ahmed Jamal, Brittny Davis Lynn, Margaret Mayer, et al. (2023) Tobacco product use among adults–United States, centers for disease control and prevention, United States

Cosci I, Grande G, Di Nisio A, Rocca MS, Del Fiore P et al (2023) Int J Mol Sci 24:599

Crittenden MR, Zebertavage L, Kramer G, Bambina S, Friedman D et al (2018) Sci Rep 8:7012

Dagogo-Jack I, Shaw AT (2018) Nat Rev Clin Oncol 15:81–94

Davaro F, Jain R, Li R (2023) Eur Urol Focus 9:579–581

De Sousa LA, Battin C, Jutz S, Leitner J, Hafner C et al (2019) Sci Rep 9:11472

Deo SVS, Sharma J, Kumar S (2022) Ann Surg Oncol 29:6497–6500

Desilets A, Elkrief A (2023) Curr Opin Oncol 35:35

D'Incecco A, Andreozzi M, Ludovini V, Rossi E, Capodanno A et al (2015) Br J Cancer 112:95–102

Dudzińska M, Szczyrek M, Wojas-Krawczyk K, Świrska J, Chmielewska I, Zwolak A (2020) Cancers 12:2314

Ferlay J, Ervik M, Lam F, Colombet M, Mery L et al (2020) Global cancer observatory: cancer today. WHO, International Agency for Research on Cancer, Lyon

Fisher R, Pusztai L, Swanton C (2013) Br J Cancer 108:479–485

Galluzzi L, Buqué A, Kepp O, Zitvogel L, Kroemer G (2015) Cancer Cell 28:690–714

Gan X, Shan Q, Li H, Janssens R, Shen Y et al (2022) Proc Natl Acad Sci 119:e2200879119

Garcia-Diaz A, Shin DS, Moreno BH, Saco J, Escuin-Ordinas H et al (2017) Cell Rep 19:1189–1201

Graff JN, Alumkal JJ, Drake CG, Thomas GV, Redmond WL et al (2016) Oncotarget 7:7

Graziani G, Tentori L, Navarra P (2012) Pharmacol Res 65:9–22

Guérin C, Laramas M, Bettega F, Bocquet A, Berton E et al (2023) Bull Cancer 110:825–835

Guo L, Tang X, Wong SW, Guo A, Lin Y, Kwok HF (2022) Front Pharmacol 13:13

Harding FA, McArthur JG, Gross JA, Raulet DH, Allison JP (1992) Nature 356:607–609

He M, Chai Y, Qi J, Zhang CWH, Tong Z et al (2017) Oncotarget 8:8

Hodi FS, O'Day SJ, McDermott DF, Weber RW, Sosman JA et al (2010) N Engl J Med 363:711–723

Hu ZI, McArthur HL, Ho AY (2017) Curr Breast Cancer Rep 9:45–51

Ishida Y, Agata Y, Shibahara K, Honjo T (1992) EMBO J 11:3887–3895

Johnson DB, Nebhan CA, Moslehi JJ, Balko JM (2022) Nat Rev Clin Oncol 19:254–267

Karimi A, Alilou S, Mirzaei HR (2021) Front Oncol 11:11

Kciuk M, Kołat D, Kałuzińska-Kołat Ż, Gawrysiak M, Drozda R et al (2023) Cell 12:530

Keam SJ (2023) Drugs 83:93–102

Kearney ER, Walunas TL, Karr RW, Morton PA, Loh DY et al (1995) J Immunol 155:1032–1036

Konishi J, Yamazaki K, Azuma M, Kinoshita I, Dosaka-Akita H, Nishimura M (2004) Clin Cancer Res 10:5094–5100

Korman A, Yellin M, Keler T (2005) Curr Opin Investig Drugs 6:582–591
Krummel MF, Allison JP (1995) J Exp Med 182:459–465
Lee K-M, Chuang E, Griffin M, Khattri R, Hong DK et al (1998) Science 282:2263–2266
Lee HT, Lee JY, Lim H, Lee SH, Moon YJ et al (2017) Sci Rep 7:5532
Lee HT, Lee SH, Heo Y-S (2019) Molecules 24:1190
Lee SH, Lee HT, Lim H, Kim Y, Park UB, Heo Y-S (2020) Biochem Biophys Res Commun 527:226–231
Liao D, Liu C, Chen S, Liu F, Li W et al (2023) Int Immunopharmacol 122:110414
Lin DY-W, Tanaka Y, Iwasaki M, Gittis AG, Su H-P et al (2008) Proc Natl Acad Sci USA 105:3011–3016
Liu J, Chen Z, Li Y, Zhao W, Wu J, Zhang Z (2021) Front Pharmacol 12:12
Lumlertgul N, Vassallo P, Tydeman F, Lewis N, Hobill A et al (2023) Eur J Cancer 191:112967
Makuku R, Khalili N, Razi S, Keshavarz-Fathi M, Rezaei N (2021) J Immunol Res 2021:6661406
Markham A (2021) Drugs 81:1213–1219
McLaughlin J, Han G, Schalper KA, Carvajal-Hausdorf D, Pelekanou V et al (2016) JAMA Oncol 2:46–54
Mitchell JM, Karamchandani DM (2023) Surg Pathol Clin 16:703
Morris PJ, Wood KJ, Sprent J, Kishimoto H (2001) Philos Trans R Soc Lond B Biol Sci 356:609–616
Murphy KM, Weaver C (2017) Janeway's Immunobiology. Garland Science/Taylor & Francis Group, LLC
Nie R-C, Chen G-M, Wang Y, Zhou J, Duan J-L et al (2021) Front Oncol 11:11
Obeid M, Tesniere A, Ghiringhelli F, Fimia GM, Apetoh L et al (2007) Nat Med 13:54–61
Oser MG, Niederst MJ, Sequist LV, Engelman JA (2015) Lancet Oncol 16:e165–e72
Page DB, Bear H, Prabhakaran S, Gatti-Mays ME, Thomas A et al (2019) Npj Breast Cancer 5:34
Pardoll DM (2012) Nat Rev Cancer 12:252–264
Qian J, Wang C, Wang B, Yang J, Wang Y et al (2018) J Neuroinflammation 15:290
Qin W, Hu L, Zhang X, Jiang S, Li J et al (2019) Front Immunol 10:10
Qureshi OS, Zheng Y, Nakamura K, Attridge K, Manzotti C et al (2011) Science 332:600–603
Robert C (2020) Nat Commun 11:3801
Schumacher TN, Scheper W, Kvistborg P (2019) Annu Rev Immunol 37:173–200
Schwartz RH (2012) Cold Spring Harb Perspect Biol 4:a006908
Shuvo PA, Tahsin A, Rahman MM, Emran TB (2022) Ann Med Surg 81:81
Smith CA, Williams GT, Kingston R, Jenkinson EJ, Owen JJT (1989) Nature 337:181–184
Sondak VK, Smalley KSM, Kudchadkar R, Grippon S, Kirkpatrick P (2011) Nat Rev Drug Discov 10:411–412
Strickland KC, Howitt BE, Shukla SA, Rodig S, Ritterhouse LL et al (2016) Oncotarget 7:13587
Suazo-Zepeda E, Vinke PC, Heuvelmans MA, Sidorenkov G, Hiltermann TJN, de Bock GH (2023) Lung Cancer 176:89–97
Sun JC, Beilke JN, Lanier LL (2009) Nature 457:557–561
Sung H, Ferlay J, Siegel RL, Laversanne M, Soerjomataram I et al (2021) CA Cancer J Clin 71:209–249
Swart EM, Noordhof AL, Damhuis RAM, Kunst PWA, De Ruysscher DKM et al (2023) Lung Cancer 182:107290
Team A (2019) How immunotherapy is used to treat cancer. ed. TAC Society. Atlanta, GA: The American Cancer Society
Tuerxun H, Zhao Y, Li Y, Liu X, Wen S et al (2023) Crit Rev Oncol Hematol 188:104064
Tumeh PC, Harview CL, Yearley JH, Shintaku IP, Taylor EJM et al (2014) Nature 515:568–571
Vincent J, Mignot G, Chalmin F, Ladoire S, Bruchard M et al (2010) Cancer Res 70:3052–3061
Walunas TL, Lenschow DJ, Bakker CY, Linsley PS, Freeman GJ et al (1994) Immunity 1:405–413
Wolchok JD, Saenger Y (2008) Oncologist 13:2–9
Wu Y, Chen W, Xu ZP, Gu W (2019) Front Immunol 10:10
Wu H-J, Temko D, Maliga Z, Moreira AL, Sei E et al (2022) Cell Genom 2:100165
Xu X, Zhang W, Xuan L, Yu Y, Zheng W et al (2023a) Nat Cell Biol 25:170–182

Xu J, Kato K, Raymond E, Hubner RA, Shu Y et al (2023b) Lancet Oncol 24:483–495
Yi M, Zheng X, Niu M, Zhu S, Ge H, Wu K (2022) Mol Cancer 21:28
Yu J, Zhuang A, Gu X, Hua Y, Yang L et al (2023) Cell Discov 9:33
Zak KM, Grudnik P, Magiera K, Dömling A, Dubin G, Holak TA (2017) Structure 25:1163–1174
Zhang J-y, Yan Y-y, Li J-j, Adhikari R, Fu L-w (2020a) Front Pharmacol 11:11
Zhang Z, Liu S, Zhang B, Qiao L, Zhang Y (2020b) Front Cell Develop Biol 8:17
Zhang Y, Yao Q, Pan Y, Fang X, Xu H et al (2023) Cancers 15:682
Zhao B, Zhao H, Zhao J (2020) Ther Adv Med Oncol 12:1758835920937612
Zheng J, Shao M, Yang W, Ren J, Chen X, Yang H (2022) Int Immunopharmacol 112:109244

CTLA-4 Inhibitors for the Treatment of Lung Cancer

6

Shvetank Bhatt, Shreya Sharma, Shubham Patil, and Rohini Pujari

6.1 Introduction

With an estimated two million new cases and 176 million deaths each year, lung cancer is one of the most frequently diagnosed malignancies and the main cause of cancer-related deaths globally (Sung et al. 2021). In the last 20 years, there has been a great advancement in disease biology knowledge, the use of predictive biomarkers, and changes in therapy that have changed outcomes for many patients (Carbone et al. 2015).

Only a small portion of NSCLC patients in clinical practice receive an early diagnosis, and the majority already have locally advanced or metastatic disease at the time of diagnosis, which contributes to the disease's poor 5-year survival rate of 4–17% (Carbone et al. 2015; Hirsch et al. 2017). For individuals with early-stage NSCLC, surgical resection continues to be the therapy of choice (Postmus et al. 2017; Osmani et al. 2018). However, following surgery, 58–73% of patients with stage I illness and roughly 40% of those with stage II disease relapse, which lowers their chances of surviving for 5 years (Liang and Wakelee 2013; Gao et al. 2020). In contrast, NSCLC patients are receiving a variety of treatments depending on their general health and the size of their tumours. Although platinum-based chemotherapy and radiation therapy are the traditional treatments for such tumours, the last decade has seen the emergence of molecular targeted therapies, such as tyrosine kinase inhibitors (TKIs) targeting the epidermal growth factor receptor (EGFR) and immune checkpoint inhibitors (ICIs), which have helped improve the outcome of patients with NSCLC (Hanna et al. 2017; Tabchi et al. 2017).

S. Bhatt · S. Sharma · S. Patil · R. Pujari (✉)
School of Health Sciences and Technology, Dr. Vishwanath Karad MIT World Peace University, Pune, Maharashtra, India

S. Bhatt et al. (eds.), *Immunotherapy Against Lung Cancer*,
https://doi.org/10.1007/978-981-99-7141-1_6

When the immune system is weak, cancer, especially lung cancer, is more likely to occur. Cancer cells have the potential to become immune system–resistant, which opens the door to unchecked growth (Swann and Smyth 2007). This phenomenon can be explained in terms of the cancer immunoediting theory, which holds that transformed cells may evade immune surveillance in the third and final phase of a three-phase control process: elimination, equilibrium, and escape. In the first stage, tumours are found and removed by suppressor mechanisms before they manifest clinically. The following stage is equilibrium, which is a stage of tumour quiescence during which the immune system and the tumour are brought into a dynamic balance that controls the progression of the malignancy. Last but not least, the point of escape is where cancer cells first appear. These cells either exhibit decreased immunogenicity or set off a variety of potential immunosuppressive processes that compromise the anti-tumour immune response, resulting in the creation of gradually larger tumours (Yu et al. 2019).

Immune checkpoints, often referred to as inhibitory receptors, can function during both immune activation and continuing immunological responses. PD-1, CTLA-4, T-cell immunoglobulin and mucin-domain containing-3 (TIM-3), lymphocyte-activation gene 3 (LAG-3), and T-cell immunoreceptor with Ig and ITIM domains (TIGIT) are just a few examples of non-redundant inhibitory receptors that T cells are known to upregulate during chronic inflammation in particular and that reduce their effectiveness. Therefore, exhaustion serves as both a physiological check on immunopathology during prolonged infection and a significant impediment to anti-tumour immune responses (Khoja et al. 2017; Singh et al. 2020).

A member of the B7/CD28 family, CTLA-4 (CD152), blocks T-cell activity. The production of CTLA-4 and other inhibitory receptors is another feature of exhausted T cells. By subtly reducing signalling through the co-stimulatory receptor CD28, CTLA-4 promotes immunosuppression. Although both receptors have the ability to bind CD80 and CD86, CTLA-4 does so with a far greater affinity than CD28 (Leung et al. 1995).

Patients with lung cancer, particularly those who have lung cancer, benefit greatly from immunotherapy. Immunotherapy, more especially immune checkpoint inhibitors, has changed the standard of care for treating a number of tumour types in recent years, including non-small-cell lung cancer (NSCLC), and it is currently being aggressively tested in patients with small-cell lung cancer (SCLC) (Beatty and Gladney 2015).

A new form of immunotherapy for the treatment of cancer, immune checkpoint inhibitors (ICIs), including CTLA-4 inhibitors, has made significant strides by improving the prognosis for patients with neoplasms like small-cell lung cancer (SCLC) and non-small-cell lung cancer (NSCLC). Awareness of the toxicities and their treatment is essential while administering this medication to patients as these drugs have specific adverse events (AEs) (Chen and Mellman 2013).

6.2 Association Between Lung Cancer and the Immune System

Lung cancer cells, like other cancers, are genetically unstable, which contributes to their unchecked growth and the development of immune system–recognisable antigens. These antigens comprise both new proteins produced by mutation and gene rearrangement and regular proteins that cancer cells overexpress. Immune cells known as cytotoxic CD8+ T cells are particularly good in mediating anti-tumour immune responses (Chen and Mellman 2017). These cells could develop the ability to identify the tumour-specific antigens displayed on MHC class I molecules and destroy specific tumour cells as a result. After being appropriately stimulated by antigen-presenting cells that have gathered antigens at the tumour site, CD8+ T cells develop into licenced effector cells (Blank et al. 2016). For efficient T-cell activation, antigen-presenting cells must also provide co-stimulatory signals via surface receptors such as CD28 and cytokines such as interleukin (IL)-12 in addition to the antigen peptides anchored on the MHC molecules (McGranahan et al. 2016).

Different strategies are used by tumour cells to evade immune detection and immunological-mediated death. Immunoediting, a method of selecting clones that can avoid the immune system, is frequently assumed to be the source of established tumours (Kawakami 2016). By downregulating characteristics that render them susceptible, such as tumour antigens or MHC class I, tumour cells may directly elude immune identification. Alternately, tumours could elude immune responses by utilising the negative feedback systems that the body has developed to stop immunopathology (Wei et al. 2019). These include metabolic regulators like indoleamine 2,3-dioxygenase (IDO), inhibitory receptors like PD-1 and CTLA-4, inhibitory cytokines like IL-10 and tumour growth factor (TGF)-, and inhibitory cell types like regulatory T cells (Tregs), regulatory B cells (Bregs), and myeloid-derived suppressor cells (MDSCs) (Singh et al. 2020).

6.3 Immune Checkpoints in Lung Cancer

Immune checkpoints, or inhibitory receptors, are present on a variety of cell types, including those of the lungs. They are crucial for both central and peripheral tolerance because they block co-stimulatory molecules' simultaneous activation signalling. Both immune activation and continuing immunological responses may trigger the action of inhibitory receptors. T cells are known to become worn out and to upregulate a variety of non-redundant inhibitory receptors or immunological checkpoints that restrict their function, especially during chronic inflammation (Carbone et al. 2015).

Research efforts are currently concentrated on immune checkpoints, including cytotoxic T lymphocyte-associated protein 4 (CTLA4), programmed cell death protein 1 (PD1), programmed death ligand 1 (PDL1), T-cell immunoglobulin and mucin domain containing protein 3 (TIM3), lymphocyte activation gene 3 (LAG3), and T-cell immunoreceptor with Ig and ITIM domains (TIGIT) (Singh et al. 2020).

CTLA 4: The human chromosome 2q33 contains the gene for CTLA4, a member of the immunoglobulin superfamily. Similar in structure to CD28, CTLA4 has two ligands in common with CD28: CD80 and CD86. Through a number of mechanisms, including the inhibition of T-cell differentiation, proliferation, and cell cycle progression, CTLA4 also modifies T-cell activation. As a result, CTLA4 is crucial to immunotherapy and has demonstrated promising therapeutic advantages (Vinay et al. 2015).

PD1/PD L1: PD1 belongs to the CD28 superfamily and is connected to programmed cell death. Although dendritic cells, natural killer (NK) cells, and monocytes are also known to contain it, T and B cells are known to express it preferentially. PDL1 is the primary ligand for PD1, which forms conjugates with PDL1 and PDL2, both proteins belonging to the B7 protein family. To reduce T-cell activation and improve immunological escape, PD1 interacts with PDL1 (Zaretsky et al. 2016).

LAG3: Ig-like domains 14 are present in LAG3, also known as CD223. The 'extra loop', a 30 amino acid region, is part of domain 1. Although it is also found on plasmacytoid dendritic cells, regulatory T cells (Tregs), activated B cells, and NK T cells, LAG3 is primarily expressed on CD4+ and CD8+ T cells (Anderson et al. 2016).

TIM 3: TIM3 belongs to the TIM family of immunoregulatory proteins. T cells, B cells, NK cells, dendritic cells (DCs), and monocytes all include the type I transmembrane protein known as TIM3 (Anderson et al. 2016).

TIGIT: TIGIT is a key player in limiting immunological activity and is a member of a rapidly expanding family of poliovirus receptor-like proteins (Anderson et al. 2016; Chen and Mellman 2017).

6.4 CTLA-4 and Their Ligands in Cancer

Both cancer cells themselves and infiltrating Tregs or worn-out conventional T cells may express CTLA-4 in tumour lesions. Despite CTLA-4's immunosuppressive function, it is unclear if it affects disease prognosis; nevertheless, it should be emphasised that only a small number of research studies have examined the prognostic significance of CTLA-4 levels in the cancer site. As of now, nasopharyngeal carcinoma and non-small-cell lung cancer have both shown enhanced survival when CTLA-4 is expressed on tumours (Salvi et al. 2012; Huang et al. 2016).

6.5 Mechanism and Functions of CTLA 4 Pathway in Cancer

CTLA-4 is an immunological checkpoint mechanism that regulates the activity of T lymphocytes, a subgroup of immune cells crucial for locating and eliminating cancer cells. The CTLA-4 receptor and its ligands, CD80 and CD86, are found on antigen-presenting cells (APCs) and certain cancer cells, and together they form the pathway (Huang et al. 2016).

Lung cancer is a complicated illness with several subtypes, and CTLA-4 may have a different effect in each subtype. The CTLA-4 pathway lowers T-cell activation and proliferation in normal physiology, which lowers the likelihood of autoimmune diseases (Salvi et al. 2012). When T cells come into touch with antigen-presenting APCs, such as cancer cells, they become activated and grow, which triggers an immune response against the antigen. Although CTLA-4's interaction with CD80 and CD86 on APCs inhibits T-cell activation and proliferation, this avoids an excessive or unnecessary immune response (Qureshi et al. 2011). The most common form of lung cancer, non-small-cell lung cancer (NSCLC), has been shown to have elevated CTLA-4 expression in tumour-infiltrating T cells, suggesting that the CTLA-4 pathway may be implicated in immune suppression and tumour progression (Vétizou et al. 2015).

Malignant tumour cells can exploit the CTLA-4 pathway to evade immune surveillance and prevent eradication. The capacity of cancer cells to express CD80 and CD86 can impair the immune system's ability to combat the tumour by binding to CTLA-4 on T cells and reducing T-cell activation and proliferation. This stops cancer cells from being attacked by the immune system, allowing them to grow and spread. The CTLA-4 pathway has been investigated as a possible lung cancer immunotherapy target. Uncertainty exists over CTLA-4's role in small-cell lung cancer (SCLC), a more aggressive subtype of lung cancer with a poor prognosis. Some studies suggest that CTLA-4 may not be as important in SCLC as it is in NSCLC (Salvi et al. 2012; Huang et al. 2016).

6.6 Anti-CTLA-4 Agents in Anticancer Therapy

In order to counteract this immune suppression, immunotherapy drugs that block the CTLA-4 pathway allow T cells to activate and attack cancer cells. Anti-CTLA-4 therapeutic experience has made it clear from the start that patients need to get interdisciplinary medical care. The first ICI tested in oncological patients that showed potential efficacy was anti-CTLA-4. Because it has been shown that CTLA-4 inhibitors like ipilimumab improve patient survival, the FDA has authorised its use in the treatment of lung cancer. More research is being done to see whether combining CTLA-4 inhibitors with other immunotherapies, such as PD-1/PD-L1 inhibitors, might improve cancer outcomes (Robert et al. 2011) (Fig. 6.1).

6.7 Ipilimumab

One such drug is ipilimumab, a monoclonal antibody that binds to CTLA-4 and prevents it from interacting with CD80 and CD86. By blocking CTLA-4, ipilimumab enhances T-cell activation and proliferation, enhancing the immune system's capacity to combat malignancies. In actuality, ipilimumab was the first antibody to receive FDA approval and be used on a regular basis in clinical settings with cancer patients (Qureshi et al. 2011).

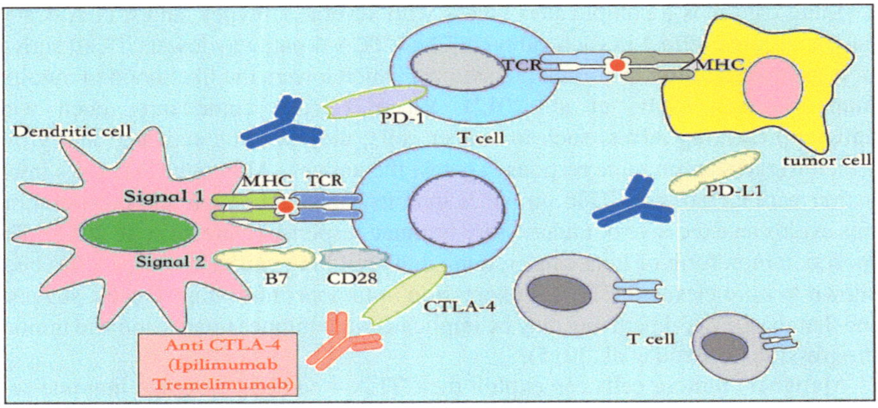

Fig. 6.1 Mechanism of action of CTLA-4 inhibitors

Preclinical research has shown that blocking CTLA-4 with ipilimumab can increase survival and the anti-tumour immune response in mouse models of NSCLC.

In studies involving SCLC, ipilimumab and chemotherapy were used. Patients with end-stage SCLC who had not previously received treatment were randomised to receive doublet chemotherapy (carboplatin/paclitaxel) alone or in conjunction with ipilimumab. The immune-related PFS was 5.7 against 6.4 versus 5.3 months (HR 0.64; $p = 0.03$) for the phased combination when compared with the control, providing a little indication of enhanced effectiveness with the regimen (Reck et al. 2013). The median OS was 11 versus 10.9 months (HR 0.94; 95% CI, 0.81–1.09), indicating that the phased combination of ipilimumab, platinum/etoposide, and maintenance ipilimumab did not prolong survival compared to chemotherapy alone (Reck et al. 2016). Additionally, median PFS did not significantly increase (4.6 vs. 4.4 months; HR 0.85; 95% CI, 0.75–0.97), and ORR remained unchanged at 62% in each arm. Treatment discontinuation rates (18% vs. 2%) and mortality (5% vs. 2%) were greater in patients who had immune-related toxicity, which included diarrhoea, dermatitis, and colitis. There is currently no place for the use of ipilimumab combined chemotherapy in the treatment of patients with SCLC due to the disappointing results of this confirmatory phase III (Reck et al. 2013; Reck et al. 2016).

In clinical research, ipilimumab in conjunction with chemotherapy has been explored for people with advanced NSCLC. In a phase II study, it was shown that ipilimumab with chemotherapy improved progression-free survival in patients with advanced NSCLC compared to chemotherapy alone. Despite this improvement, there was no discernible rise in overall survival. In a phase III study for individuals with extensive-stage cancer, the addition of ipilimumab to chemotherapy did not significantly increase patient survival (Antonia et al. 2016).

In general, the CTLA-4 pathway has shown promise as a target for lung cancer immunotherapy, particularly for NSCLC. The optimum way to use CTLA-4 inhibitors in the treatment of lung cancer is still being discovered, and continuing research is looking into the idea of combining CTLA-4 inhibitors with other immunotherapies, notably PD-1/PD-L1 inhibitors, to improve results (Hellmann et al. 2018).

Prior to this, consideration was also given to the large increase in overall survival, despite the relatively low rate of objective responses to therapy (about 10% of patients) and the modest number of patients (20–25%) who saw long-term improvements. Additionally, the peculiar profile of side effects associated with ipilimumab therapy such as primarily skin and gastrointestinal reactions was reported (Vétizou et al. 2015).

6.8 Tremelimumab

Tremelimumab research has not yet yielded encouraging findings, in contrast to ipilimumab, which would discourage its broad usage in monotherapy (Ribas et al. 2013). Response rates of 15% and 30%, respectively, were observed in trials that used tremelimumab and nivolumab to treat HCC patients. The use of tremelimumab and durvalumab in combination therapy is still being studied, though (Rizvi et al. 2020).

6.9 Efficacy and Mode of Action of CTLA-4 Inhibitors

When compared to standard chemotherapies, CTLA-4 inhibitors have improved patient survival in several trials, including those on melanoma, renal cell carcinoma, squamous cell carcinoma, and non-small-cell lung cancer (Snyder et al. 2014).

The independent inhibition of CD3/CD28-dependent signalling by CTLA-4 raises the possibility that underlying immunological responses are necessary for checkpoint inhibitor therapy to be effective. When T cells are infiltrating a tumour, or it has a high mutation rate, it is more immunogenic and consequently more responsive to CTLA-4 blockades. Most studies on the direct immunological effects of anti-CTLA-4 therapy have focused on T cells (Curran et al. 2010). When CTLA-4-expressing Tregs remove CD80/CD86 from the surface of antigen-presenting cells, decreasing their capacity to effectively excite tumour-specific T cells, the stage of T-cell activation in the draining lymph nodes is hypothesised to be affected by the inhibition of CTLA-4 (24). As worn-out CTLA-4-expressing T cells and Tregs might aggregate inside the cancer microenvironment, CTLA-4 inhibition may also have an impact at the tumour site (Salvi et al. 2012).

Effective anti-tumour immune responses depend on type I immune responses, which also include IFN- production and cytotoxic T-cell activities. Type I immune responses are also linked to greater responses to anti-CTLA-4 therapies (Huang et al. 2016).

Given that effector memory T cells readily produce cytotoxic molecules like perforin and granzyme B, it may be tempting to hypothesise that immune checkpoint inhibitors selectively enhance the activity of these cells. The co-stimulatory receptor CD28, via which CTLA-4 inhibits T-cell activity, is absent from these cells (Qureshi et al. 2011).

The effectiveness of anti-CTLA-4 therapy may also be influenced by the features of a tumour itself. Tumour cells' mutational load may make them more immunogenic while simultaneously improving their capacity to thwart immunological reactions brought on by therapy (Vétizou et al. 2015).

Commensal bacteria could potentially have an impact on how well immune checkpoint drugs work. Anti-CTLA-4 therapy was shown to have no impact on mice raised in sterile environments, but it did cause a change in the intestinal flora of conventionally raised mice. Additional research revealed that the presence of certain bacterial strains, specifically Bacteroides fragilis, boosted Th1 polarisation in the animals and was linked to an enhanced anti-tumour immune response (Vétizou et al. 2015).

6.10 Biomarkers of CTLA-4 Inhibitor Treatment Efficacy

To prevent unnecessary medication exposure, biomarkers are required both before and during therapy to determine whether individuals are most or least likely to react to CTLA-4 inhibitor therapies. A reduction in tumour size during therapy is referred to as a therapeutic response. Immune checkpoint inhibitor response rates are correlated with a variety of variables related to illness prognoses in untreated individuals (Sharma et al. 2017).

Neo-antigens on altered cancer cells increase anti-tumour immunogenicity, which promotes therapeutic efficiency. Therefore, a high genetic difference between host cells and cancer cells is a sign of a successful checkpoint inhibitor therapy. This was especially observed in melanoma patients receiving anti-CTLA-4 therapy when their tumours showed neo-antigens (Snyder et al. 2014).

High levels of CD8+ T cells infiltrating the tumour or present at the tumour margin, high eosinophil and lymphocyte blood counts, and elevated serum TGF levels in melanoma patients receiving anti-PD-1 therapy are additional pre-treatment immunological factors linked to better treatment responses. In responder patients with various solid tumours who were treated with anti-PD-L1, it was also shown that increased Th1 and CTLA-4 gene expression levels, but not FoxP3 levels, were present (Herbst et al. 2016).

Improved immune checkpoint inhibitor responses have also been linked to a variety of post-treatment immunological findings. For instance, patients with higher numbers of ICOS-expressing T cells and lower neutrophil-to-lymphocyte ratios were more likely to react to anti-CTLA-4 therapy. Treatment response was also correlated with an increase in Th9 cell frequency in the blood of the patient and an increase in CD8+ T-cell proliferation inside the tumour lesion.

Together, these trials show that individuals who already have anti-tumour immune responses before treatment are more likely to benefit from CTLA-4 inhibitors (Im et al. 2016). In spite of opposing biomarker-based predictions, patients may still react to treatment since not all biomarkers are necessarily equally effective.

Additionally, many patients may have trouble obtaining tumour tissue, especially after therapy, thus less invasive blood-based 'liquid biopsies' could be more appropriate. Importantly, it has been demonstrated that combining the investigation of many biomarkers might enhance therapeutic foresight. A particularly intriguing possibility for a biomarker appears to be the recently found ctDNA (Calapre et al. 2017).

6.11 Adverse Events Associated with CTLA-4 Therapy

In order to effectively administer this medication to patients, it is essential to be aware of the specific adverse events (AEs) that CTLA-4 might cause as well as how to manage them. These adverse events (AEs) are brought on by organ-specific immune-mediated tissue destruction. In many cases, T cells are involved in this tissue damage, although other cytokines and humoral immune activation may also cause toxicities. There is hypothesis that host variables like genetic variability may control the occurrence of these toxicities as they only affect a small fraction of individuals (Larkin et al. 2015). There was, however, no correlation between the risk of AEs and genetic markers, at least according to one study. To determine variables that may forecast for AEs, more research is required. It's possible that various toxicities are influenced by different circumstances. More frequent side effects of anti-CTLA-4 medications include colitis and hypophysitis (Robert et al. 2011).

Under physiological circumstances, CTLA-4 inhibits autoimmunity and restricts immune activation to prevent bystander injury. Therefore, therapeutic antibody inhibition of these receptors for the treatment of cancer is linked to a variety of adverse events that mimic autoimmune responses. Studies and treatments had very different rates of serious side effects. Clinical trials that directly contrasted various immune checkpoint inhibitors and their combinations found that anti-CTLA-4 treatment resulted in a higher rate of adverse events (27.3%). When both were used in the treatment process, even more patients (55%) were impacted (Chae et al. 2017).

Immune checkpoint inhibitors, such as anti-CTLA-4, almost often cause moderate adverse effects in patients, such as diarrhoea, tiredness, pruritus, rash, nausea, and reduced appetite. Colitis, severe diarrhoea, elevated alanine aminotransferase levels, inflammatory pneumonitis, and interstitial nephritis are examples of severe adverse responses. There have also been cases of people getting type 1 diabetes or seeing their pre-existing autoimmune disorders like psoriasis go worse (Mullangi et al. 2021). Patients who experience particularly severe adverse effects may need to stop receiving medication, but they may recover later. It is interesting to note that several treatment-related auto-immune reactions, such rash and vitiligo, have been demonstrated to correlate with a better prognosis for the illness, indicating a possible overlap between auto-immune and anti-tumour immune responses (Freeman-Keller et al. 2016).

6.12 Limitations of CTLA-4 Inhibitors

Although the use of CTLA-4 inhibitors may be initially beneficial, many patients may eventually experience recurrence and tumour development. Therefore, several research studies have tried to figure out how anti-CTLA-4 therapies lose their effectiveness (Gao et al. 2017).

Other inhibitory receptors may also be upregulated by anti-CTLA-4 therapy. Even patients who initially react well to CTLA-4 blocking drugs sometimes relapse, demonstrating the need for more effective or different therapy (Koyama et al. 2016).

Anti-CTLA-4 combinations with other immune checkpoint inhibitors are also being investigated. In comparison to individual administration, the combination of anti-CTLA-4 and anti-PD-1 therapies demonstrated higher effectiveness, but it was also linked to an increase in adverse effects. As a result, several intriguing novel directions are now being investigated, albeit ongoing and upcoming clinical trials are still needed to prove their clinical effectiveness (Arlauckas et al. 2017).

6.13 Conclusion

CTLA-4-targeted medicines have increased the average life expectancy of cancer patients, especially those with lung cancer. Advanced-stage patients continue to have a high death rate, underscoring the need for more advancements in the area. Anti-CTLA-4 medicines tend to be more successful in individuals who already have anti-tumour immunity, indicating that these medications cannot generate anti-tumour immune responses from scratch in patients who lack such immunity. However, as our knowledge of the mechanisms underlying these medications expands, opportunities are opening up to better utilise them by not only focusing on patients who are most likely to respond through appropriate biomarker screening techniques, but also by combining currently prescribed immune checkpoint inhibitors with other complementary medications to help patients who are not responding to the regimens as prescribed.

References

Anderson AC, Joller N, Kuchroo VK (2016) Lag-3, Tim-3, and TIGIT: co-inhibitory receptors with specialized functions in immune regulation. Immunity 44(5):989–1004

Antonia SJ, López-Martin JA, Bendell J, Ott PA, Taylor M, Eder JP, Jäger D, Pietanza MC, Le DT, de Braud F, Morse MA, Ascierto PA, Horn L, Amin A, Pillai RN, Evans J, Chau I, Bono P, Atmaca A, Sharma P, Harbison CT, Lin CS, Christensen O, Calvo E (2016) Nivolumab alone and nivolumab plus ipilimumab in recurrent small-cell lung cancer (CheckMate 032): a multicentre, open-label, phase 1/2 trial. Lancet Oncol 17(7):883–895

Arlauckas SP, Garris CS, Kohler RH, Kitaoka M, Cuccarese MF, Yang KS, Miller MA, Carlson JC, Freeman GJ, Anthony RM, Weissleder R, Pittet MJ (2017) In vivo imaging reveals a tumor-associated macrophage-mediated resistance pathway in anti-PD-1 therapy. Sci Transl Med 9(389):eaal3604

Beatty GL, Gladney WL (2015) Immune escape mechanisms as a guide for cancer immunotherapy. Clin Cancer Res 21(4):687–692

Blank CU, Haanen JB, Ribas A, Schumacher TN (2016) Cancer immunology. The "cancer immunogram". Science 352(6286):658–660

Calapre L, Warburton L, Milward M, Ziman M, Gray E (2017) Circulating tumour DNA (ctDNA) as a liquid biopsy for melanoma. Cancer Lett 404:62

Carbone DP, Gandara DR, Antonia SJ, Zielinski C, Paz-Ares L (2015) Non-small-cell lung cancer: role of the immune system and potential for immunotherapy. J Thorac Oncol 10(7):974–984

Chae YK, Chiec L, Mohindra N, Gentzler R, Patel J, Giles F (2017) A case of pembrolizumab-induced type-1 diabetes mellitus and discussion of immune checkpoint inhibitor-induced type 1 diabetes. Cancer Immunol Immunother 66(1):25–32

Chen DS, Mellman I (2013) Oncology meets immunology: the cancer-immunity cycle. Immunity 39(1):1–10

Chen DS, Mellman I (2017) Elements of cancer immunity and the cancer-immune set point. Nature 541(7637):321–330

Curran MA, Montalvo W, Yagita H, Allison JP (2010) PD-1 and CTLA-4 combination blockade expands infiltrating T cells and reduces regulatory T and myeloid cells within B16 melanoma tumors. Proc Natl Acad Sci U S A 107(9):4275–4280

Freeman-Keller M, Kim Y, Cronin H, Richards A, Gibney G, Weber JS (2016) Nivolumab in resected and Unresectable metastatic melanoma: characteristics of immune-related adverse events and association with outcomes. Clin Cancer Res 22(4):886–894

Gao S, Li N, Gao S, Xue Q, Ying J, Wang S, Tao X, Zhao J, Mao Y, Wang B, Shao K, Lei W, Wang D, Lv F, Zhao L, Zhang F, Zhao Z, Su K, Tan F, Gao Y, Sun N, Wu D, Yu Y, Ling Y, Wang Z, Duan C, Tang W, Zhang L, He S, Wu N, Wang J, He J (2020) Neoadjuvant PD-1 inhibitor (Sintilimab) in NSCLC. J Thorac Oncol 15(5):816–826

Gao J, Ward JF, Pettaway CA, Shi LZ, Subudhi SK, Vence LM, Zhao H, Chen J, Chen H, Efstathiou E, Troncoso P, Allison JP, Logothetis CJ, Wistuba MA II, Sepulveda J, Sun J, Wargo JB, Sharma P (2017) VISTA is an inhibitory immune checkpoint that is increased after ipilimumab therapy in patients with prostate cancer. Nat Med 23(5):551–555

Hanna N, Johnson D, Temin S, Baker S Jr, Brahmer J, Ellis PM, Giaccone G, Hesketh PJ, Jaiyesimi I, Leighl NB, Riely GJ, Schiller JH, Schneider BJ, Smith TJ, Tashbar J, Biermann WA, Masters G (2017) Systemic therapy for stage IV non-small-cell lung cancer: American Society of Clinical Oncology clinical practice guideline update. J Clin Oncol 35(30):3484–3515

Hellmann MD, Ciuleanu TE, Pluzanski A, Lee JS, Otterson GA, Audigier-Valette C, Minenza E, Linardou H, Burgers S, Salman P, Borghaei H, Ramalingam SS, Brahmer J, Reck M, O'Byrne KJ, Geese WJ, Green G, Chang H, Szustakowski J, Bhagavatheeswaran P, Healey D, Fu Y, Nathan F, Paz-Ares L (2018) Nivolumab plus Ipilimumab in lung cancer with a high tumor mutational burden. N Engl J Med 378(22):2093–2104

Herbst RS, Baas P, Kim DW, Felip E, Pérez-Gracia JL, Han JY, Molina J, Kim JH, Arvis CD, Ahn MJ, Majem M, Fidler MJ, de Castro G Jr, Garrido M, Lubiniecki GM, Shentu Y, Im E, Dolled-Filhart M, Garon EB (2016) Pembrolizumab versus docetaxel for previously treated, PD-L1-positive, advanced non-small-cell lung cancer (KEYNOTE-010): a randomised controlled trial. Lancet 387(10027):1540–1550

Hirsch FR, Scagliotti GV, Mulshine JL, Kwon R, Curran WJ Jr, Wu YL, Paz-Ares L (2017) Lung cancer: current therapies and new targeted treatments. Lancet 389(10066):299–311

Huang PY, Guo SS, Zhang Y, Lu JB, Chen QY, Tang LQ, Zhang L, Liu LT, Zhang L, Mai HQ (2016) Tumor CTLA-4 overexpression predicts poor survival in patients with nasopharyngeal carcinoma. Oncotarget 7(11):13060–13068

Im SJ, Hashimoto M, Gerner MY, Lee J, Kissick HT, Burger MC, Shan Q, Hale JS, Lee J, Nasti TH, Sharpe AH, Freeman GJ, Germain RN, Nakaya HI, Xue HH, Ahmed R (2016) Defining CD8+ T cells that provide the proliferative burst after PD-1 therapy. Nature 537(7620):417–421

Kawakami Y (2016) Introduction: cancer immunology special issue-immunotherapy. Int Immunol 28(7):317

Khoja L, Day D, Wei-Wu Chen T, Siu LL, Hansen AR (2017) Tumour- and class-specific patterns of immune-related adverse events of immune checkpoint inhibitors: a systematic review. Ann Oncol 28(10):2377–2385

Koyama S, Akbay EA, Li YY, Herter-Sprie GS, Buczkowski KA, Richards WG, Gandhi L, Redig AJ, Rodig SJ, Asahina H, Jones RE, Kulkarni MM, Kuraguchi M, Palakurthi S, Fecci PE, Johnson BE, Janne PA, Engelman JA, Gangadharan SP, Costa DB, Freeman GJ, Bueno R, Hodi FS, Dranoff G, Wong KK, Hammerman PS (2016) Adaptive resistance to therapeutic PD-1 blockade is associated with upregulation of alternative immune checkpoints. Nat Commun 7:10501

Larkin J, Chiarion-Sileni V, Gonzalez R, Grob JJ, Cowey CL, Lao CD, Schadendorf D, Dummer R, Smylie M, Rutkowski P, Ferrucci PF, Hill A, Wagstaff J, Carlino MS, Haanen JB, Maio M, Marquez-Rodas I, McArthur GA, Ascierto PA, Long GV, Callahan MK, Postow MA, Grossmann K, Sznol M, Dreno B, Bastholt L, Yang A, Rollin LM, Horak C, Hodi FS, Wolchok JD (2015) Combined Nivolumab and Ipilimumab or monotherapy in untreated melanoma. N Engl J Med 373(1):23–34

Leung HT, Bradshaw J, Cleaveland JS, Linsley PS (1995) Cytotoxic T lymphocyte-associated molecule-4, a high-avidity receptor for CD80 and CD86, contains an intracellular localization motif in its cytoplasmic tail. J Biol Chem 270(42):25107–25114

Liang Y, Wakelee HA (2013) Adjuvant chemotherapy of completely resected early stage non-small cell lung cancer (NSCLC). Transl Lung Cancer Res 2(5):403–410

McGranahan N, Furness AJ, Rosenthal R, Ramskov S, Lyngaa R, Saini SK, Jamal-Hanjani M, Wilson GA, Birkbak NJ, Hiley CT, Watkins TB, Shafi S, Murugaesu N, Mitter R, Akarca AU, Linares J, Marafioti T, Henry JY, Van Allen EM, Miao D, Schilling B, Schadendorf D, Garraway LA, Makarov V, Rizvi NA, Snyder A, Hellmann MD, Merghoub T, Wolchok JD, Shukla SA, Wu CJ, Peggs KS, Chan TA, Hadrup SR, Quezada SA, Swanton C (2016) Clonal neoantigens elicit T cell immunoreactivity and sensitivity to immune checkpoint blockade. Science 351(6280):1463–1469

Mullangi S, Ponnam S, Lekkala MR, Koya S (2021) A case of De novo psoriasis secondary to Nivolumab in a patient with metastatic renal cell carcinoma. Cureus 13(6):e15703

Osmani L, Askin F, Gabrielson E, Li QK (2018) Current WHO guidelines and the critical role of immunohistochemical markers in the subclassification of non-small cell lung carcinoma (NSCLC): moving from targeted therapy to immunotherapy. Semin Cancer Biol 52(Pt 1):103–109

Postmus PE, Kerr KM, Oudkerk M, Senan S, Waller DA, Vansteenkiste J, Escriu C, Peters S (2017) Early and locally advanced non-small-cell lung cancer (NSCLC): ESMO clinical practice guidelines for diagnosis, treatment and follow-up. Ann Oncol 28(suppl_4):iv1–iv21

Qureshi OS, Zheng Y, Nakamura K, Attridge K, Manzotti C, Schmidt EM, Baker J, Jeffery LE, Kaur S, Briggs Z, Hou TZ, Futter CE, Anderson G, Walker LS, Sansom DM (2011) Trans-endocytosis of CD80 and CD86: a molecular basis for the cell-extrinsic function of CTLA-4. Science 332(6029):600–603

Reck M, Bondarenko I, Luft A, Serwatowski P, Barlesi F, Chacko R, Sebastian M, Lu H, Cuillerot JM, Lynch TJ (2013) Ipilimumab in combination with paclitaxel and carboplatin as first-line therapy in extensive-disease-small-cell lung cancer: results from a randomized, double-blind, multicenter phase 2 trial. Ann Oncol 24(1):75–83

Reck M, Luft A, Szczesna A, Havel L, Kim SW, Akerley W, Pietanza MC, Wu YL, Zielinski C, Thomas M, Felip E, Gold K, Horn L, Aerts J, Nakagawa K, Lorigan P, Pieters A, Kong Sanchez T, Fairchild J, Spigel D (2016) Phase III randomized trial of Ipilimumab plus etoposide and platinum versus placebo plus etoposide and platinum in extensive-stage small-cell lung cancer. J Clin Oncol 34(31):3740–3748

Ribas A, Kefford R, Marshall MA, Punt CJ, Haanen JB, Marmol M, Garbe C, Gogas H, Schachter J, Linette G, Lorigan P, Kendra KL, Maio M, Trefzer U, Smylie M, McArthur GA, Dreno B, Nathan PD, Mackiewicz J, Kirkwood JM, Gomez-Navarro J, Huang B, Pavlov D, Hauschild A (2013) Phase III randomized clinical trial comparing tremelimumab with standard-of-care chemotherapy in patients with advanced melanoma. J Clin Oncol 31(5):616–622

Rizvi NA, Cho BC, Reinmuth N, Lee KH, Luft A, Ahn MJ, van den Heuvel MM, Cobo M, Vicente D, Smolin A, Moiseyenko V, Antonia SJ, Le Moulec S, Robinet G, Natale R, Schneider J, Shepherd FA, Geater SL, Garon EB, Kim ES, Goldberg SB, Nakagawa K, Raja R, Higgs BW, Boothman AM, Zhao L, Scheuring U, Stockman PK, Chand VK, Peters S (2020) Durvalumab with or without Tremelimumab vs standard chemotherapy in first-line treatment of metastatic non-small cell lung cancer: the MYSTIC phase 3 randomized clinical trial. JAMA Oncol 6(5):661–674

Robert C, Thomas L, Bondarenko I, O'Day S, Weber J, Garbe C, Lebbe C, Baurain JF, Testori A, Grob JJ, Davidson N, Richards J, Maio M, Hauschild A, Miller WH Jr, Gascon P, Lotem M, Harmankaya K, Ibrahim R, Francis S, Chen TT, Humphrey R, Hoos A, Wolchok JD (2011) Ipilimumab plus dacarbazine for previously untreated metastatic melanoma. N Engl J Med 364(26):2517–2526

Salvi S, Fontana V, Boccardo S, Merlo DF, Margallo E, Laurent S, Morabito A, Rijavec E, Dal Bello MG, Mora M, Ratto GB, Grossi F, Truini M, Pistillo MP (2012) Evaluation of CTLA-4 expression and relevance as a novel prognostic factor in patients with non-small cell lung cancer. Cancer Immunol Immunother 61(9):1463–1472

Sharma P, Hu-Lieskovan S, Wargo JA, Ribas A (2017) Primary, adaptive, and acquired resistance to cancer immunotherapy. Cell 168(4):707–723

Singh S, Hassan D, Aldawsari HM, Molugulu N, Shukla R, Kesharwani P (2020) Immune checkpoint inhibitors: a promising anticancer therapy. Drug Discov Today 25(1):223–229

Snyder A, Makarov V, Merghoub T, Yuan J, Zaretsky JM, Desrichard A, Walsh LA, Postow MA, Wong P, Ho TS, Hollmann TJ, Bruggeman C, Kannan K, Li Y, Elipenahli C, Liu C, Harbison CT, Wang L, Ribas A, Wolchok JD, Chan TA (2014) Genetic basis for clinical response to CTLA-4 blockade in melanoma. N Engl J Med 371(23):2189–2199

Sung H, Ferlay J, Siegel RL, Laversanne M, Soerjomataram I, Jemal A, Bray F (2021) Global cancer statistics 2020: GLOBOCAN estimates of incidence and mortality worldwide for 36 cancers in 185 countries. CA Cancer J Clin 71(3):209–249

Swann JB, Smyth MJ (2007) Immune surveillance of tumors. J Clin Invest 117(5):1137–1146

Tabchi S, Kassouf E, Rassy EE, Kourie HR, Martin J, Campeau MP, Tehfe M, Blais N (2017) Management of stage III non-small cell lung cancer. Semin Oncol 44(3):163–177

Vétizou M, Pitt JM, Daillère R, Lepage P, Waldschmitt N, Flament C, Rusakiewicz S, Routy B, Roberti MP, Duong CP, Poirier-Colame V, Roux A, Becharef S, Formenti S, Golden E, Cording S, Eberl G, Schlitzer A, Ginhoux F, Mani S, Yamazaki T, Jacquelot N, Enot DP, Bérard M, Nigou J, Opolon P, Eggermont A, Woerther PL, Chachaty E, Chaput N, Robert C, Mateus C, Kroemer G, Raoult D, Boneca IG, Carbonnel F, Chamaillard M, Zitvogel L (2015) Anticancer immunotherapy by CTLA-4 blockade relies on the gut microbiota. Science 350(6264):1079–1084

Vinay DS, Ryan EP, Pawelec G, Talib WH, Stagg J, Elkord E, Lichtor T, Decker WK, Whelan RL, Kumara H, Signori E, Honoki K, Georgakilas AG, Amin A, Helferich WG, Boosani CS, Guha G, Ciriolo MR, Chen S, Mohammed SI, Azmi AS, Keith WN, Bilsland A, Bhakta D, Halicka D, Fujii H, Aquilano K, Ashraf SS, Nowsheen S, Yang X, Choi BK, Kwon BS (2015) Immune evasion in cancer: mechanistic basis and therapeutic strategies. Semin Cancer Biol 35(Suppl):S185–s198

Wei Z, Zhou C, Zhang Z, Guan M, Zhang C, Liu Z, Liu Q (2019) The landscape of tumor fusion neoantigens: a pan-cancer analysis. iScience 21:249–260

Yu JX, Hubbard-Lucey VM, Tang J (2019) Immuno-oncology drug development goes global. Nat Rev Drug Discov 18(12):899–900

Zaretsky JM, Garcia-Diaz A, Shin DS, Escuin-Ordinas H, Hugo W, Hu-Lieskovan S, Torrejon DY, Abril-Rodriguez G, Sandoval S, Barthly L, Saco J, Homet Moreno B, Mezzadra R, Chmielowski B, Ruchalski K, Shintaku IP, Sanchez PJ, Puig-Saus C, Cherry G, Seja E, Kong X, Pang J, Berent-Maoz B, Comin-Anduix B, Graeber TG, Tumeh PC, Schumacher TN, Lo RS, Ribas A (2016) Mutations associated with acquired resistance to PD-1 blockade in melanoma. N Engl J Med 375(9):819–829

Adoptive T-Cell Therapy for the Treatment of Lung Cancer

7

Jayaraman Rajangam, Vasanth Raj Palanimuthu, Dinesh Kumar Upadhyay, Lucy Mohapatra, Navanita Sivaramakumar, Narahari N. Palei, and Priyal Soni

Abbreviations

ACT	Adoptive cellular immune treatment
CAR	Chimeric antigen receptor
CAR-T	Chimeric Antigen Receptor T
CD	Cluster of differentiation
CEA	Carcinoembryonic antigen
CRC	Colorectal cancer
DC	Dendritic cells
DLL3	Delta-like ligand 3
EGFR	Epidermal growth factor receptor
GD2	Disialoganglioside
GPC3	Glypican-3
HER2	Human epidermal growth factor receptor 2
HEV	High endothelial venules
IL-2	Interleukin-2
LC	Lung cancer
LC	Lung cancer
mDC	Mature Dendritic cells

J. Rajangam (✉)
Shri Venkateshwara College of Pharmacy, Ariyur, Puducherry, India

V. R. Palanimuthu · N. Sivaramakumar
JSS College of Pharmacy, JSS Academy of Higher Education & Research, Ooty, Tamil Nadu, India

D. K. Upadhyay
School of Pharmaceutical Sciences, Jaipur National University, Jaipur, India

L. Mohapatra · N. N. Palei · P. Soni
AMITY Institute of Pharmacy, AMITY University, Lucknow, Uttar Pradesh, India

S. Bhatt et al. (eds.), *Immunotherapy Against Lung Cancer*,
https://doi.org/10.1007/978-981-99-7141-1_7

MSLN	Mesothelin (MSLN)
MUC1	Mucin 1
NK cell	Natural Killer cell
NSCLC	Non-small cell lung cancer
ROR1	Receptor tyrosine kinase-like orphan receptor 1 (ROR1)
ScFv	Single-chain variable fragments
SD	Stable disease
T cell	T Lymphocyte cell
TAA	Target tumor-associated antigens
TCR	T cell receptor
Tem	Effect memory T cell
TIL	Tumor-Infiltrating Lymphocyte
TLS	Tertiary lymphoid structures

7.1 Introduction

Lung cancer is the most prevalent cause of death around the globe, and it develops when lung cells start mutating or proliferate. In most cases, this is due to inhalation or exposure to harmful substances. In many cases, lung cancer can develop in individuals without exposure to harmful chemicals. Cancer cells multiply uncontrollably, forming malignant tumors and destroying the normal healthy tissues of the lung. Clinical manifestations usually start during metastasis to other organs and interfere with their function. But smoking causes 80% of lung cancer fatalities and is the primary risk factor for illness, whereas persons who have never smoked account for 20% of lung cancer fatalities. Exposure to radon gas, family history and genetic factors, intake of arsenic-containing drinking water, and processed meat may have a role in the development of LC (Centers For Disease Control And Prevention and National Center For Health Statistics 2017). Small-cell LC (SCLC) and non-small-cell LC (NSCLC) are the two primary histological types of lung cancer, with the latter subclassified into a large number of diverse subgroups (Inamura 2017; The Cancer Genome Atlas Research Network 2014). Smoking-related lung cancers (SCLCs) are aggressive tumors that make up 15–25% of all primary lung cancers (Peifer et al. 2012). SCLC is characterized by paraneoplastic illnesses and MYC gene amplifications (Darnell 1996). Lung adenocarcinoma (LUAD), lung squamous cell carcinoma (LUSC), big cell carcinoma, and bronchial carcinoid tumor are the four subtypes of NSCLC.

LUAD is the most common primary lung tumor, particularly prevalent among female nonsmokers. It exhibits glandular histology and is characterized by activating mutations in driver genes like KRAS, EGFR, and BRAF. The development of tumors, both at their primary location and in metastatic sites, is heavily influenced by the surrounding environment known as the tumor microenvironment. This environment comprises various stromal cells, including T cells, B cells, natural killer (NK) cells, fibroblasts, adipocytes, vascular endothelial cells, and pericytes, which envelop the growing tumor (Fig. 7.1). These cells release signaling molecules that play crucial roles in tumor survival, growth, invasion, migration, and the alteration of cancer cell behavior, a phenomenon referred to as onco-modulation (Anderson and Simon 2020). Some of the important signaling molecules involved include TNF-α (tumor necrosis factor-alpha), mTOR (mammalian target of rapamycin), FASL (Fas ligand), PDL1/L2 (programmed cell death protein ligand 1/ligand2), TGF-β (transforming growth factor beta), STAT (signal transducer and activator of transcription), IL-1β (interleukin-1beta), EGF (epidermal growth factor), IL-6 (interleukin-6), sRAGE (soluble receptor for the advanced glycation end product), IFN-γ (Interferon-gamma), HIF1A1 (hypoxia-inducible factor 1A1alpha), IGF2 (insulin-like growth factor-2), MMP14 (matrix metalloproteinase 14), VEGF (vascular endothelial growth factor), CXCL1 (C-X-C motif chemokine ligand (1), HMMR (hyaluronan mediated motility receptor), CXCR2 (C-X-C motif chemokine

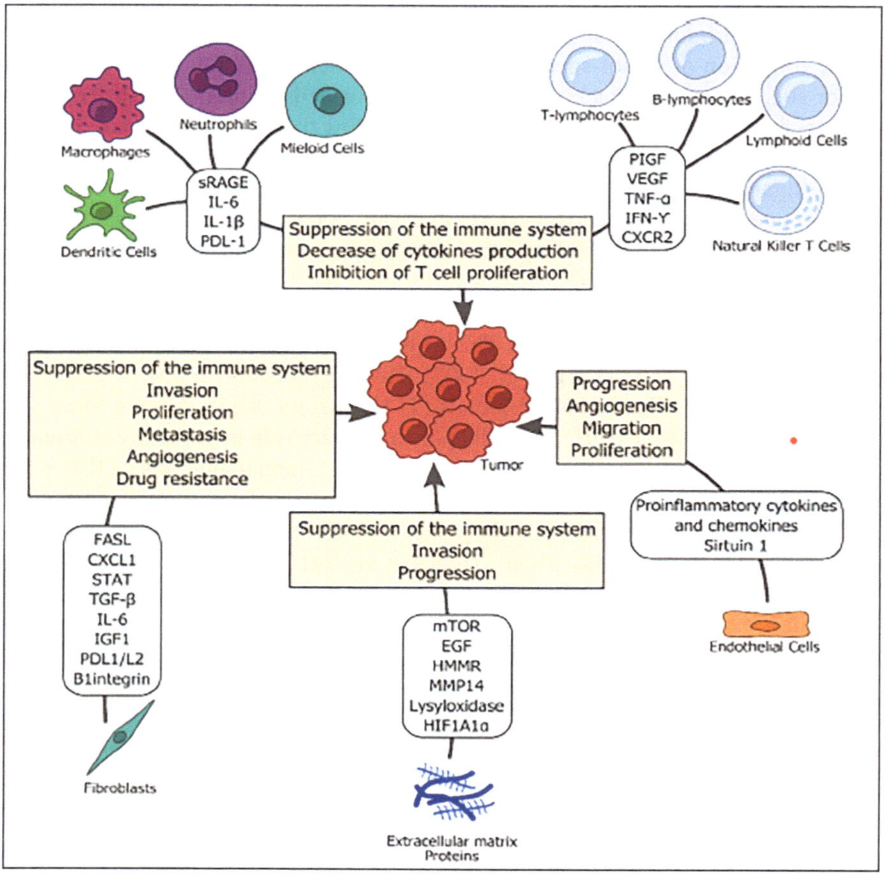

Fig. 7.1 The tumor microenvironment in lung cancer

receptor (2), and PIGF (placental growth factor) (Budisan et al. 2021; Cheng and Hao 2017) (Fig. 7.1).

7.2 Cancer Immunology

CD8+ cytotoxic lymphocytes (CTLs) are regarded as the cornerstone of the immunological protective reactions against tumors (Zitvogel et al. 2008; Liu and Zeng 2012). Numerous findings indicated that within human solid tumors, there are abundant CTLs found, which are mono-nuclear cells originating from the chronic-inflammatory infiltration. The identification of specific tumor antigens by T lymphocytes is essential for generating an effective anticancer immune response (Clark Jr et al. 1989; Gao et al. 2007; Gonzalez-Rodriguez et al. 2010). Tumor antigen presentation can occur in two ways: directly through tumor cells in lymph nodes draining the tumor or through cross-presentation by specialized antigen-presenting cells known as pAPC (Van Mierlo et al. 2004).

The cross-priming of naive CD8+ T cells by pAPC initiates a process that results in the formation of tumor-specific CTLs, which then proliferate and travel to the tumor site, eventually attacking and killing tumor cells (Kurts et al. 2010). CTLs used several ways to eradicate cancer cells, including the use of granzymes, perforin (Shresta et al. 1998; Cullen and Martin 2008; Cullen et al. 2010), and TNF superfamily ligands (Nagata and Golstein 1995). Additionally, activated CD8+ T cells secrete interferon-gamma (IFN-γ) (Qin et al. 2003) and TNF-alpha (TNF-α) (Stoelcker et al. 2000), both of which contribute to an anti-tumor effect. The role of CD4+ T cells in the anti-tumor immune response has become more understood in recent years. When naive CD4+ T cells become activated, they differentiate into various subsets, including Th1, Th2 (Mosmann and Coffman 1989), Tregs (Sakaguchi 2005), Th17 (Korn et al. 2007), Th9 (Végran et al. 2015), Th22 (Trifari et al. 2009), and follicular helper T cells (TFH) (Crotty 2011). Among these sub-populations of CD4+ T cells, Th1 cells play a primary role in anticancer immunity by promoting the proliferation and production of substantial amounts of IFN-γ and chemokines (Bos and Sherman 2010). Significantly, the IFN-γ produced by Th1 cells exerts anti-proliferative, pro-apoptotic, and anti-angiogenic effects on tumor cells independently of CD8+ T cells (Ikeda et al. 2002). Th1 cells also attract and activate inflammatory cells within the tumor microenvironment (Galaine et al. 2015; Haabeth et al. 2014).

In recent times, NK cells found to be effective in cancer immunotherapy. They directly eliminate tumor cells through various mechanisms, including:

- Releasing cytoplasmic granules containing perforin and granzymes (Trapani et al. 2000),
- Triggering apoptosis via death receptor-mediated pathways (Cretney et al. 2002; Sutlu and Alici 2009), or.
- NK cells destroy tumor cells by using antibody-dependent cellular cytotoxicity through the expression of CD16 and the secretion of TNF (Smyth et al. 2002).

Additionally, NK cells exert an indirect anticancer effect by generating cytokines, chemokines, and growth factors. IFN-γ produced by NK cells plays a crucial role in initiating the differentiation of CD8+ T cells into CTLs and directing CD4+ T cells toward a Th1 response (Martin-Fontecha et al. 2004). NK cells also initiate inflammatory responses, influence the proliferation and differentiation of monocytes, dendritic cells (DCs), and granulocytes, and boost future adaptive immune responses by releasing cytokines (Wu and Lanier 2003; Prehn 1970; Wortzel and Philipps 1983).

7.3 Epidemiological Incidences of Lung cancer

As per recent reports, the number of fatalities globally attributable to lung cancer alone was 1,761,000 globally (Fig. 7.2). High rates of LC are observed in countries where smoking habits are more irrespective of gender differences but caused mortality of men alone in 93 different countries. In contrast, female lung cancer fatalities have been documented in 28 different countries. In the United States, a projected 238,340 LC individuals in 2023 with every 16 males and one in every 17 females ratio. Furthermore, according to statistics, over 127,070 Americans die each year (International Agency for Research on Cancer 2020; American Cancer Society 2023).

The greatest risk factor for lung cancer is air pollution, which is caused by carcinogens produced during the combustion of fossil fuels. According to studies, lung

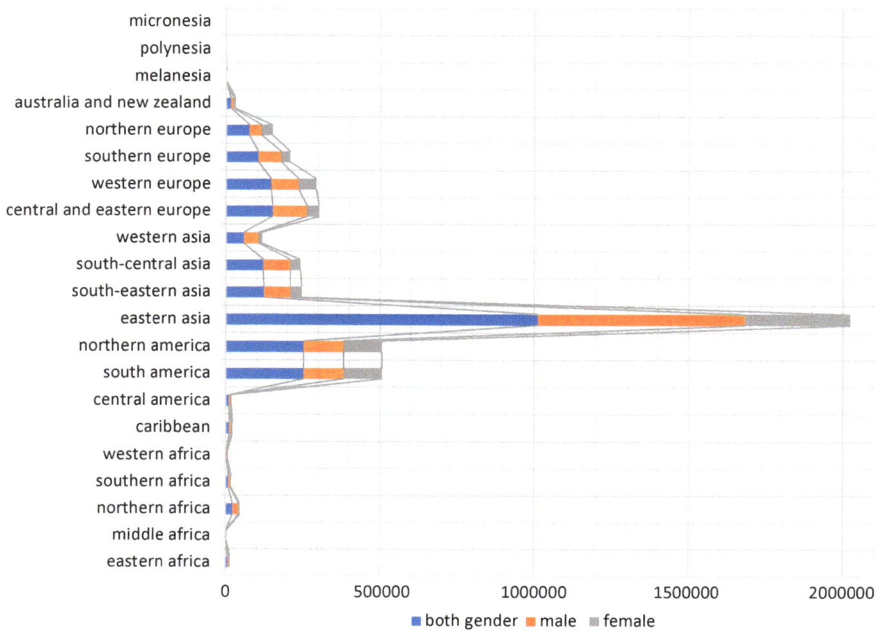

Fig. 7.2 Incidence of lung cancer worldwide among individuals

cancer cases have increased since the pandemic COVID-19. In the year 2020, more than 2.2 million fresh cases of lung cancer were diagnosed (Fig. 7.3). Survival rates improved in nations with better access to diagnostic and treatment options. Lung cancer is diagnosed at an average age of 70 years old in both genders in the United States; 53% of cases occurred between the ages of 55 and 74, with 37% occurring in those over the age of 75. The advanced carcinomas were seen in young female patients aged 20–46 years (Thandra et al. 2021; WCRF International 2022).

As depicted in Fig. 7.4, there are two types of LC, namely small-cell lung cancer (SCLC) and non-small-cell lung cancer (NSCLC). NSCLC affects 80–85% of people, SCLC affects 10–15% (Torre et al. 2016). The percentage of male and female mortality in the USA in 2022 was 68,820 and 61,360, respectively (Zhou et al. 2022). In 2018, lung cancer was responsible for 18.4% of all deaths worldwide (Jenkins et al. 2023). The incidence rate of lung cancer based on the types and global incidences was as follows (Cancerresearchuk.org 2023; Deshpand et al. 2022; The Global Cancer Observatory WHO 2020).

7.4 Signaling Molecules of Lung Cancer

The complex disease of LC is influenced by a number of genomic and environmental variables. The deregulation of signaling molecules is one of the main elements involved in the initiation and spread of lung cancer. Signaling molecules are molecules that are produced by cells and act as messengers to communicate with other

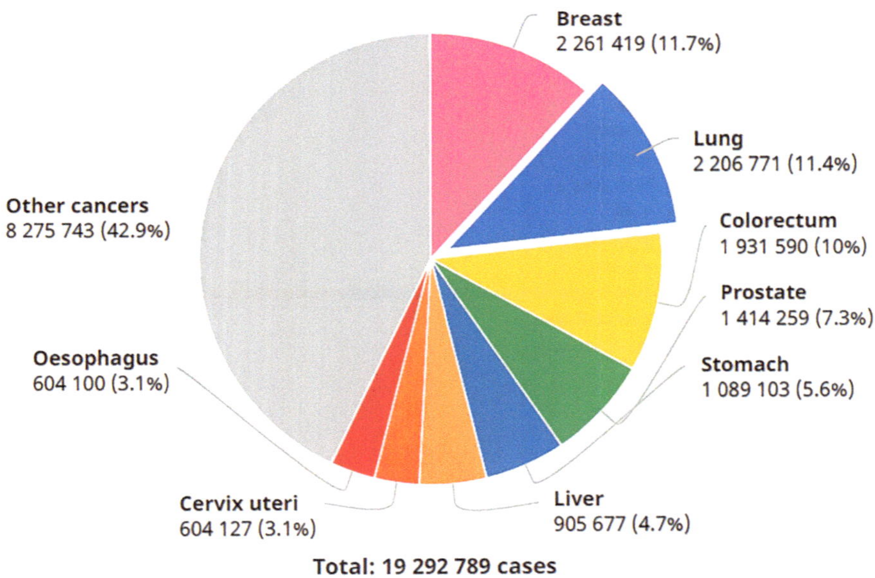

Fig. 7.3 No. of new cases in 2020, Both Sexes—all ages (Source: Globacan –2020)

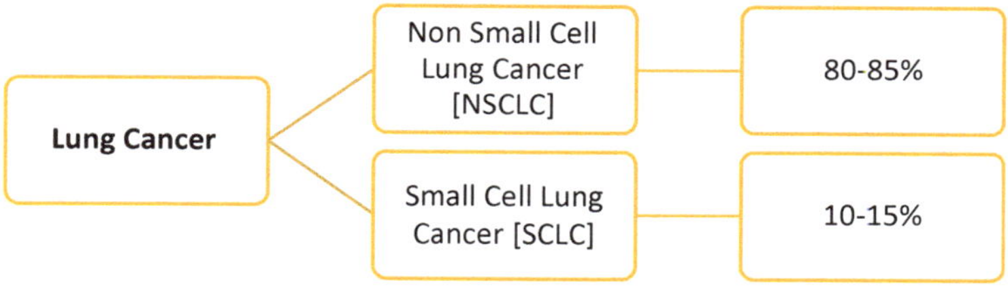

Fig. 7.4 Incidence rate of LC

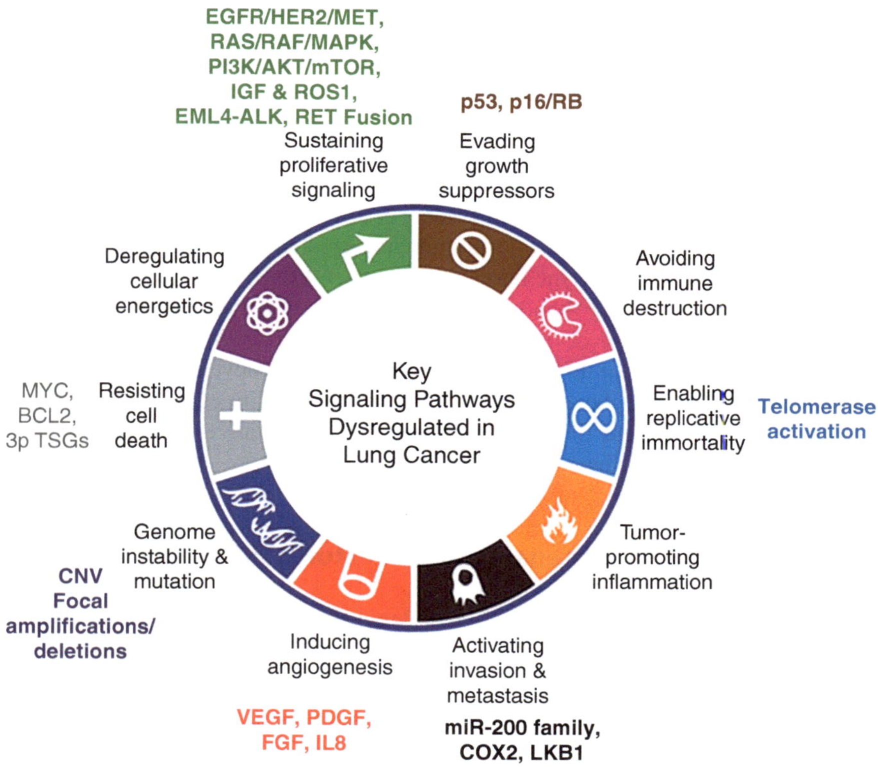

Fig. 7.5 Signaling pathways for lung cancer

cells, tissues, and organs in the body. In lung cancer, these signaling molecules can promote the growth of cancer cells (Fig. 7.5).

EGFR and VEGF are two crucial signaling molecules in LC that can promote cancer cell growth, survival, migration, angiogenesis, and metastasis (Hanahan and Weinberg 2011). EGFR is overexpressed in NSCLC, and mutations in its gene lead to constitutive activation of the receptor, which is associated with chemotherapy and targeted therapy resistance, and VEGF is involved in angiogenesis and its inhibition.

MKP-1 expression is found in NSCLC and is related to increased survival; yet, it suppresses cisplatin-induced apoptosis in NSCLC cells.

7.5 Epidermal Growth Factor Receptor (EGFR)

EGFR is found to be overexpressed in many types of lung cancer. Mutations cause resistance to chemotherapies (Gschwind et al. 2004). EGFR plays a critical role in lung carcinogenesis, as it is overexpressed in approximately 45% of NSCLC cases due to mutations (Da Cunha et al. 2011). However, such mutations are limited to a subset of NSCLC cases (Lynch et al. 2004; Paez et al. 2004), including those in nonsmokers (Pao et al. 2004). Additionally, EGFR tyrosine kinase domain mutations are nearly always present in lung cancer (Yatabe and Mitsudomi 2007). Gefitinib and erlotinib are examples of tyrosine kinase inhibitors that directly inhibit intracellular kinase activity; alternatively, anti-EGFR antibodies that target the extracellular domain of the receptor can indirectly inhibit EGFR ligand binding (Ray et al. 2009; Gridelli et al. 2009; Fischel et al. 2005). However, acquired resistance to EGFR inhibitors poses a significant challenge to effective treatment (Wheeler et al. 2010). Given the interaction between EGFR and Src family kinases (SFKs), targeting both EGFR and SFKs with combination therapy may offer a viable open for patients who develop resistance to cetuximab (Wheeler et al. 2009). Furthermore, PTEN instability has been implicated in the development of acquired cetuximab resistance in the HCC827 NSCLC cell line (Kim et al. 2010), whereas IGFRs with gefitinib and ERRs have shown anti-proliferative effects (Kim et al. 2010; Choi et al. 2010; Shen et al. 2010; Yang et al. 2010).

7.6 Vascular Endothelial Growth Factor (VEGF)

VEGF is a kind of cytokine and essential molecule in lung cancer involved in angiogenesis, which is required for tumor development and spread. In lung cancer, targeting VEGF and its receptors has been demonstrated to be a successful treatment technique. Vascular endothelial growth factors (VEGFs) are crucial regulators of angiogenesis, creating new blood vessels (Shibuya and Claesson-Welsh 2006; Gotink and Verheul 2010). The VEGF-VEGFR system is a promising target for anticancer treatment (Kim et al. 1993; Sandler et al. 2006; Gandhi et al. 2009). This category of drugs, like bevacizumab, have shown to decrease tumor development in NSCL (De Braganca et al. 2010). However, drug resistance remains a significant barrier to employing these anti-angiogenic medicines against NSCLC (Bergers and Hanahan 2010). Combinatorial treatment with EGFR and VEGFR inhibitors may overcome EGFR inhibitor resistance (Naumov et al. 2009).

7.7 Mitogen-Activated Protein Kinase Phosphatase 1 (MKP-1)

MKP-1 expression is observed to be substantially greater in NSCLC than in SCLC. According to the findings of Vicent et al. (Vicent et al. 2004), increased MKP-1 levels are often related with enhanced lung cancer patient survival. MKP-1, however, shields NSCLC cells against cisplatin-induced apoptosis. Cisplatin is a platinum-based chemotherapeutic agent that induces cellular death and apoptosis in various malignancies, but it can also modify this pathway leading to apoptosis. Additionally, to sensitize NSCLC to chemotherapy using NF-kB and PI(3)K inhibitors, MKP-1 inhibition is indispensable (Oliver et al. 2010; Cortes-Sempere et al. 2009).

7.8 Peroxisome Proliferator-Activated Receptor

A class of transcription factors called PPARs is a subfamily of nuclear hormone receptors. As a potential biomarker, increased PPAR-g expression has been connected to lung cancer. Elevated levels of PPAR-g expression in lung adenocarcinoma seem to correlate with the stage of maturation, differentiated phenotype, tumor histological type, and grade (Keshamouni et al. 2004; Theocharis et al. 2002). Other signaling molecules that have been connected to lung cancer include TGF, IGF, and FGF. These chemicals can enhance cell proliferation, migration, and invasion while also regulating the tumor microenvironment.

7.9 Treatment Strategies

For many years, conventional lung cancer treatment methods included surgery, chemotherapy, radiation therapy, and targeted therapy (Kobayashi et al. 2005). However, recent attention in lung cancer therapy has been directed toward tumor immunotherapy, which seeks to enhance the body's inherent anticancer defenses. This approach encompasses passive and active immune-therapies. Passive immunotherapy involves the administration of drugs that directly target tumors, such as monoclonal type antibodies or ACTs (Morgan et al. 2006; Schuster et al. 2006). Conversely, active immunotherapy strives to activate the body's immune system to combat cancer by utilizing approaches such as tumor antigen vaccination, nonspecific immune-modulation using bacterial substances, or addressing inhibitory receptors that dampen the immune response against tumors (Gabrilovich and Nagaraj 2009). In the end, successful tumor immunotherapy should trigger a strong antitumor immune response while mitigating the inhibitory impact of tumor-induced immune-suppression (Inamura 2017).

7.10 Lung Cancer Vaccines

In the last 15 years, vaccines with specific tumor-associated antigens have led to various endeavors in anti-tumor responses. Even though many trials have not met their primary objectives, subgroup analyses suggested that such vaccinations could be a viable treatment option for various malignancies, including lung cancer. Still, research has shown that combining therapeutic vaccinations with immune checkpoint inhibitors may be beneficial in lung cancer treatment. Crucially, a significant aspect of immunotherapy involves creating vaccines for strong immune and therapeutic responses. Therapeutic vaccinations for lung cancer are being tested in clinical studies, including MAGE-A3 (Vansteenkiste et al. 2013), BLP25 (Butts et al. 2005, 2007, 2014), Belagenpumatucel-L (Giaccone et al. 2015), CIMAvax EGF (NeningerVinageras et al. 2008), and TG4010 (Quoix et al. 2011).

7.11 Tumor-Infiltrating Lymphocyte [TIL] Therapy

TIL treatment is a kind of autologous cell therapy that employs the patient's personalized immune system to combat carcinomas. During TIL therapy, a significant amount of TIL is activated and grown as in-vitro using one of interleukin-2 (IL-2) and is subsequently reintroduced into the patient's body as depicted in Fig. 7.6. TIL is isolated from the site of the tumor using surgery or resection. The pre-rapid expansion phase, in which TIL breaks down or otherwise emigrates from tumor fragments and experiences early amplifying, is when the process of producing TIL usually commences (Rosenberg et al. 1988). After that, TIL proceeds to expand in a period called the rapid expansion phase in reaction to stimuli like IL-2 and/or feeder cells. TIL formation commonly involves 6–8 weeks and is investigated for specific

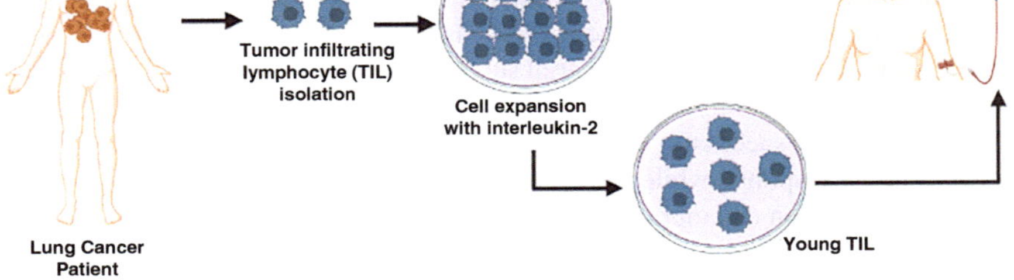

Fig. 7.6 An illustration of the TIL therapy production technique

tumor identification (Huang et al. 2005; Powell Jr et al. 2005). T cells, macrophages, and mast cells constitute most of the immune cells in lung cancer microenvironments, whereas plasma cells, NK cells, and suppressor cells derived from myeloid cells are somewhat rare (Kataki et al. 2002; Salgaller 2002). More recently, the influence of T cells on the clinical results of a diversity of solid cancers as well as a strong infiltration of TILs proved to be connected with a beneficial clinical trials conclusion in several malignancies including LC. More specifically, T cells, particularly cytotoxic T cells, memory T cells, and T helper cells, were shown to have the most constant favorable prognostic effects (Dudley et al. 2005). There has been discussion over the root cause of the positive correlation between TILs and the outcome of LC patients (Gajewska et al. 2001; Moyron-Quiroz et al. 2004; Tesar et al. 2004), even though immune cells usually spread randomly within malignancies. The formation of tertiary lymphoid structures (TLSs), also known as ectopic lymph nodes, in NSCLC tumors (Dieu-Nosjean et al. 2008; Remark et al. 2015). Antigen presentation occurs in these, which appear and behave like secondary lymphoid (Neyt et al. 2012; Martinet et al. 2012). High endothelial venules (HEVs), an unusual kind of blood vessel that is in contact with cells and a germinal center, surround TLSs, which have dendritic cells (DCs), T- and B-cell zones, and additional characteristics that are indicative of working immunological sites. Clusters of T cells and mature DCs (mDCs) make up the T-cell region (Radvanyi et al. 2012). The efficacy of TIL therapy is largely dependent on T cells' capacity to identify and eliminate tumor cells (Andersen et al. 2016; Schumacher and Schreiber 2015).

In TIL, a single-cell solution after surgical removal and IL-2 is then used to develop it in-vitro. The "selected TIL" technique selects enlarged cells based on their capacity to recognize autologous cancer cells, while the "young TIL" strategy skips this selection phase. The TIL colony is subsequently raised to an amount that is beneficial for therapy and returned to the patient. Accordingly, in solid tumors with high mutation loading, such melanoma, TIL has so demonstrated greater clinical effectiveness to CAR-T (Titov et al. 2021; Bedognetti et al. 2013). Second, effect memory T (Tem) cells with the chemokine receptors CCR5 and CXCR3 expressed on their surface appear to make up the majority of TIL after being triggered by tumor proteins in-vivo (Mikucki et al. 2015). The development of a next-generation TIL product is currently underway to lessen the adverse effects brought on by high doses of IL-2 as well as enhance the in vivo durability and function of the current TIL treatment. Next-generation TIL is modified genetically TIL that either employs transmission of viruses to excessively express a gene of interest or uses CRISPR or TALEN to entirely eradicate the target gene (Forget et al. 2017).

Due to the high mutational complexity during LC, TIL treatment may be a suitable therapeutic strategy. It has especially produced positive results for NSCLC that is resistant to immune inhibitors of checkpoints. TILs must be given and developed ex vivo under a particular scenario, which restricts their application (Nowroozi et al. 2022).

7.12 Chimeric Antigen Receptor T-Cell [CAR-T] Therapy in Lung Cancer

With almost two million new diagnoses and more than one million deaths from the disease worldwide in 2020 (Morgan et al. 2023), LC is one of the most common diseases. Recent studies focused on CAR-T-cell therapy as a potential innovative anticancer treatment, particularly for hematologic malignancies such as LC. The goal of the CAR-T strategy is to purify T cells from the peripheral blood of patients or other volunteers and genetically alter them with a CAR structure that enables them to recognize antigens on the surface of cancer cells. These enhanced T cells recognize and destroy cancer cells that produce target antigens after being injected back into patients as shown in Fig. 7.1. An external hinge, a domain of the transmembrane membrane, an antigen-binding site, and an intracellular domain constitute the four primary components of the molecular framework of CARs (Hirsch et al. 2017). The antigen-binding sites of CARs usually target tumor-associated antigens (TAAs) employing single-chain variable fragments (scFv) that enable MHC-independent stimulating immune cells (T cells) (Singh and McGuirk 2020). Adoptive T-cell immunotherapy, which includes CAR-T cell therapy, is currently an area of study as it has proved successful in managing cancer. To produce CAR on the patient's autologous T cells, CAR-T cell immunotherapy mainly makes use of technology for gene editing. Cytotoxic T cells subsequently facilitate the immediate eradication of cancer cells by this CAR-expressing T-cell pool. The efficacy of CAR-T cell therapy in treating a range of solid tumors and blood-related conditions has been demonstrated in previous studies (Koneru et al. 2015; Song et al. 2011). CAR-T cells are currently being used successfully to treat blood cancer (Zetterberg and Öfverholm 1999; Park et al. 2016) and are anticipated in the attempts of humans to eradicate cancerous tumors (Kunert et al. 2017; Hay and Turtle 2017). CAR-T cells (Fig. 7.7) are made through gene transfer and can identify and eradicate tumor cells with specificity (Morgan et al. 2010). The University of Pennsylvania–developed CTL019 CD19-CAR-T cell treatment got the FDA's novel classification in the United States on July 1, 2014 (Gill and June 2015; Ruella and Kenderian 2017).

Initially, the autologous lymphocytes from the lung cancer patient is collected. Then, the T cells are isolated and activated in order to engineer and attach T cells with CAR gene. The elements like spacer, transmembrane domain and CD28 domain are targeted to get the desired effect. The expansion of CAR-T cell takes place, and afterward, the manufactured CAR-T cells are infused back into the lung cancer patient and activity takes place (Neelapu et al. 2017b). The lung TAAs examined in current clinical trials are mainly CEA, HER2, EGFR, MSLN, GD2, ROR1, MUC1, GPC3, and DLL3. The use of CAR-T cell therapy is now being investigated in human studies to treat lung cancer (Hammarström 1999). But Phase II (NCT02674568) and Phase III (NCT03061812, NCT03033511) research investigations produced negative findings, with an elevated rate of complications and minimal benefits for survival (Morgensztern et al. 2019). To treat patients with EGFR-positive (>50% overexpression) relapsed/refractory NSCLC, a Phase I clinical study of EGFR-targeting CAR-T cell therapy has seen promptly outcomes.

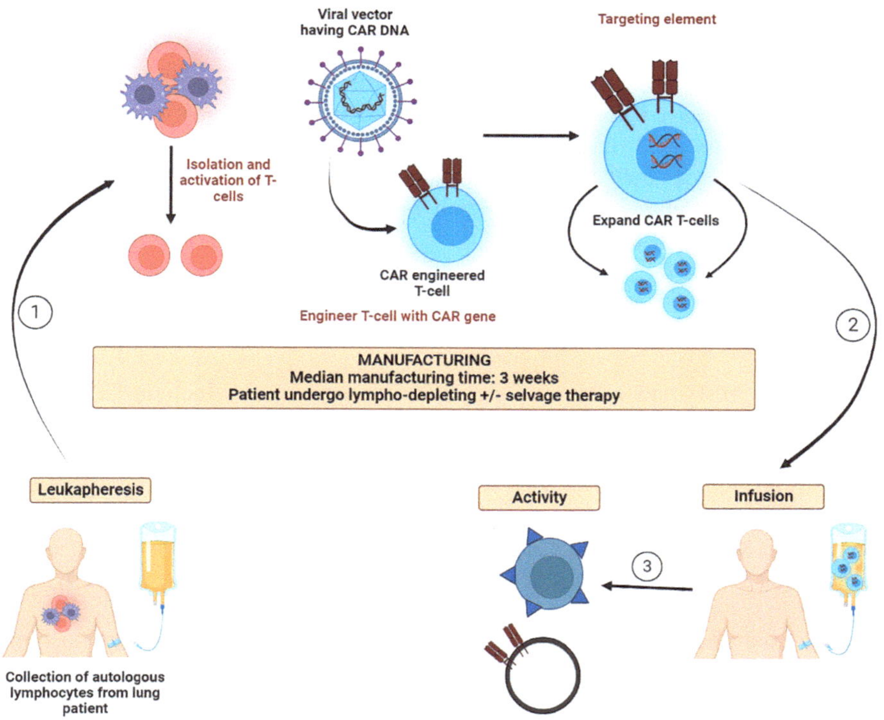

Fig. 7.7 Procedure for the production of CAR-T cell

(NCT01869166). After receiving dose-escalating CAR-T cell treatments, some patients encountered minor skin toxicity and discomfort with some patients experiencing a shrinkage of EGFR-positive tumors. Statistically, among 11 voluntary patients, two displayed a partial reaction, and continued to have SD (Feng et al. 2016; Yan et al. 2019; Wei et al. 2017). Using second-generation CAR-T cell, a CT (NCT02349724) targeting CEA in LC and other solid tumors has produced promising findings in patients with CEA-positive metastasized CRC (Zhang et al. 2017b). An independent prognostic indicator for overall mortality, the receptor tyrosine kinase ROR1 is an oncofetal antigen that has been elevated in lung ADC (Zheng et al. 2016). Although therapy will be carried at accredited treatment centers in the USA with staff who are properly trained on a thorough risk mitigation tactics, the advances in cell production and manufacturing, and the facilities for clinical execution of CAR-T cell therapy are currently well established. The field of CAR-T cell therapy is expanding rapidly, and we expect that improvements in CAR-T cell therapy and their effective use in various kinds of tumors will result from the advancements in biotechnology and immunology for cancer (Sheridan 2017).

7.13 Tackling of T-Cell Therapy–Related Consequences

Therapeutic vaccination and passive immunization are two fundamentally dissimilar methods that have been studied in people over the last 50 years to promote anti-tumor immunity. ACT is a recently developed medical procedure that entails extracting cancerous cells from a person's body, reconfiguring them to fight a specific target, multiplying them, and then reinfusing them back into the patient (Fig. 7.8) (Baxter 2014).

7.14 Tackling the Challenges in ACT

Some of the ACTs now being considered for cancer treatment include TIL therapy, CAR-T or T-cell receptors (TCRs), cytotoxic indigenous lymphocytes, etc. Despite groundbreaking achievements in identifying cancerous cells to attack, ACT's therapeutic efficacy in treating cancer is limited by difficulties in gathering enough tumor-reactive T (TRT) cells as well as the immunosuppressive tumor microenvironment (TME) (Patel et al. 2019; Mills et al. 2021; Ngo Trong et al. 2020). Advantages and disadvantages of various adoptive T-cell-based therapies are given in Table 7.1.

The labor-intensive and costly procedures required for ACT, the lack of high-level data to indicate effectiveness, and the treatment's toxicities in the absence of reliable indicators of response are its main barriers to wider use. Although innovative systemic drugs used in immunotherapy are more expensive and labor-intensive than ACT, various collaborative initiatives between academic institutions and

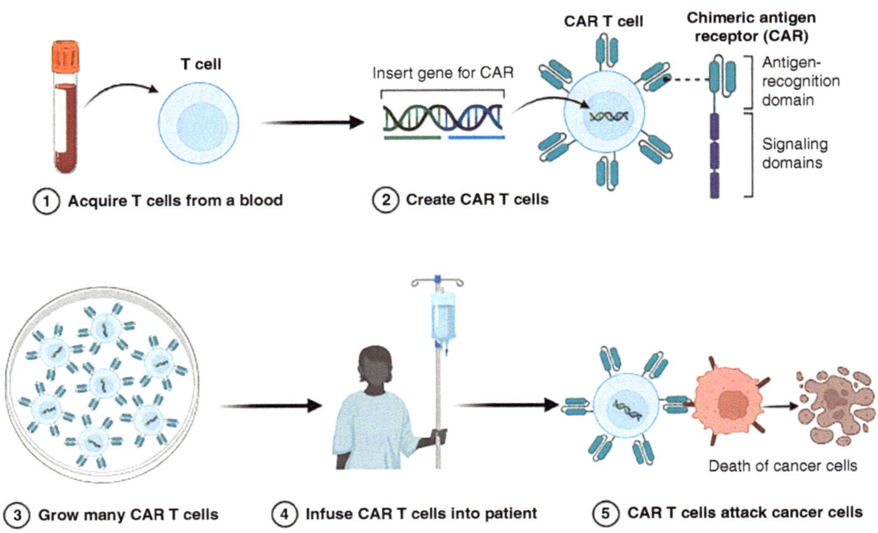

Fig. 7.8 An overview of CAR-T cell therapy, a type of ACT

Table 7.1 Different types of adoptive T-cell therapies

Adoptive cell therapy	Advantages	Disadvantages
CAR-modified T cells	• Does not depend on MHC; • Counteract the suppression of the tumor MHC molecule • Powerful in identifying any peptide, carbohydrate, or glycolipid cytoplasmic membrane antigen • Suited to a wide variety of individuals and T cell types. • Large-scale tumor-specific cell generation in a reasonably short time	• Limited to only cellular surface antigens • Reports of lethal toxicity brought on by a cytokine storm
T cell receptor (TCR) transduced T cells	• Selecting the customized population (effector stage, kind, and differentiation); • Gene insertion enhancing effectiveness, usefulness, and polarization	• Monoclonal specificity predominates • Incapable of preventing tumor escape variations • Surprising toxicity brought on by the mismatch between endogenous and transfected α and β TCR chains
Tumor infiltrating lymphocytes (TILs)	• Strictly aimed towards tumor-specific antigens • Effective use in individuals with melanoma	• Inactive in the face of immunoediting-induced tumor alterations • Difficulty in quantifying tumor isolation • Extended ex vivo expansion leading to therapeutic latency • Surrounded by an immunosuppressive TME

business have lately been established in an effort to commercialize these technologies and so widen access to them (Fig. 7.9).

The toxicity of CAR-T cells in clinical settings is still an issue, despite the fact that they provide a potential method for addressing NSCLC. Since so many TAAs lack specificity, on-target/off-tumor toxicities are brought on when CAR-T cells connect to a specific antigen on a healthy (off-tumor) tissue. Different individuals and antigens have varying degrees of the on-target/off-tumor impact, which may lead to disease affecting different major organs. Combinatorial antigen detecting techniques assigned to provide detection of onco-tissue to tumor-targeted T lymphocytes that have been programmed with a TCR or a CAR in order to avoid such on-target toxicities. Several of these techniques are covered by Geldres et al., regarding the application of iCAR (CAR designed to send an inhibitory signal) and AND-gate CAR T cells (T cells co-transduced using two independent CARs: one that delivers subpar activation and the other identifying an unique antigen, which produces a costimulatory signal) (Geldres et al. 2016). Ideally, a safer approach would be to target antigens that are more specifically produced by tumors. Debets et al. explore the qualities of an ideal target antigen and balance the advantages and

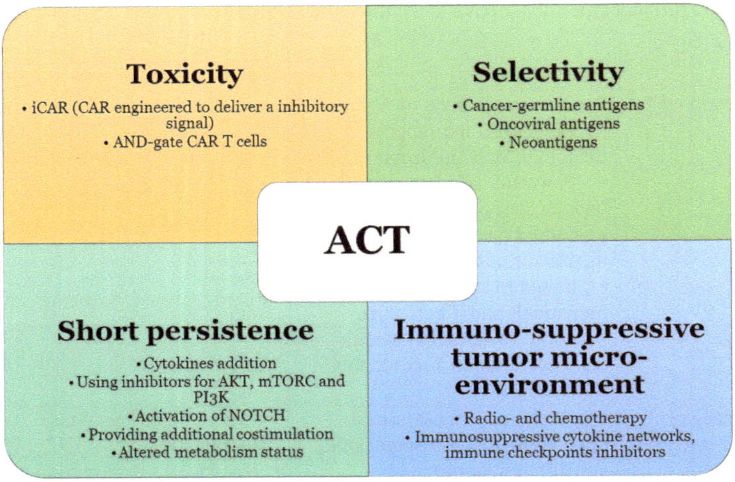

Fig. 7.9 Approaches to tackle challenges associated with ACT therapy. *iCAR* inhibitory chimeric antigen receptor, *mTORC* mammalian target of rapamycin complex, *P13K* phosphoinositide 3-kinases

disadvantages of targeting every one of these kinds of antigens. The studies emphasized that important factors in choosing an antigen should include its immunogenicity, tumor specificity of expression, and maybe even its participation in oncogenic pathways. The ability to proactively detect tumor neoantigens by TILs had previously been regarded to be an uphill task, but breakthroughs in bioinformatic analysis and the next-generation sequencing revolution have made this potential a reality (Debets et al. 2016).

Debets et al. outline the many approaches that may be used to improve the expression and functioning of the TCR. When utilizing TCRs with supra-physiological affinities, the researchers issue an advisory regarding the counterintuitive functional deterioration that may be seen. By blocking crucial stages in the catecholamine production pathway using metyrosine, the toxicity of CRS in mice was successfully minimized (Staedtke et al. 2018). Clinical studies have mostly used TRT cells produced from entire mononuclear cells from peripheral blood, despite an abundance of evidence supporting the use of these less-differentiated, stem memory T cells (Tscm). Pre-selection of immature or Tscm is used as productive method for producing T cells that are stronger and more effective. When employing TILs that are frequently discovered in a state of aging and functional fatigue, it is difficult to isolate less-differentiated T-cell subsets, even though it may be a useful technique for producing improved TCR or CAR-engineered T cells from patients' blood. Karagiannis et al. highlight the potential for repopulating TILs cell populations using induced pluripotent stem cell (iPSC) technology (Karagiannis et al. 2016). Ji et al. show how particular miRNA might be used to fine-tune TCR signaling, improve T cell fitness, and increase T-cell effector capabilities. They also provide an overview of our present knowledge of miRNA biology in T cells (Ji et al.

2016). Long-term efficiency of cytotoxic T lymphocytes (CTLs) is varied because of the complicated immunosuppressive TME. Nevertheless, CTLs are successful for suppressing tumors in the short term. High-affinity T-cell engraftment is believed to be related to the effectiveness of early tumor suppression by ACT; however, if long-term anti-tumor T-cell persistence is needed, this association may not hold true. Activating NOTCH, weak TCR signaling upon activation, altering metabolic status, inhibiting AKT, mTORC, and PI3K pathways, and adding of cytokines are current methods to produce Tscm-like ACT to manage the malignancy and recurrence (Kondo et al. 2017; Presotto et al. 2017; Sukumar et al. 2016; van der Waart et al. 2014; Abdelsamed et al. 2017). The various methods that may be used to alter the TME in order to improve T-cell-based immunotherapies have been described (Arina et al. 2016; Beavis et al. 2016). These approaches vary from imprecise molecular manipulations to targeting immunosuppressive cytokine circuits, inhibition of immunological checkpoints, and metabolic enzymes with regulatory functions to poorly specified procedures like radiotherapy and chemotherapy to enhance tumor cell recognition and decrease immunosuppressive types. According to accumulated data from clinical studies, the tumor mutation burden (TMB) is an indicator that predicts how well ACT and immune checkpoint inhibitor (ICI) therapy will work as a treatment (Sadelain et al. 2017; Steuer and Ramalingam 2018). The so-called "first generation" of CAR attached the scFv tumor antigen-recognition motif to either the CD3ζ or FcγR signaling domain. While these cells were capable of inducing anti-tumor immune responses, their effectiveness was quite constrained due to the absence of costimulatory signaling pathway. As a result, second-generation CARs were engineered to integrate the CD28 or 4-1BB signaling domains (Carpenito et al. 2009; Zhong et al. 2010).

7.15 Trends, Challenges, and Future Directions of T-Cell Therapy

Cell therapy, notably CAR-T cell therapy, has transformed cancer treatment by employing immune cells to specifically target cancer cells. While early successes have been remarkable and challenging. Moreover, as the field evolves, new trends and considerations are emerging, including the use of allogeneic T cells, CAR-T cell therapies, and the exploration of combination therapies. With continued attempts to broaden the use of these treatments to other diseases, and create novel strategies to combat resistance, the future of T-CT is still bright despite these trends and obstacles (Maude et al. 2018; Schuster et al. 2017; Bonifant et al. 2016; Adusumilli et al. 2020; Dotti et al. 2014).

7.16 Trends in T-Cell Therapy

7.16.1 CAR-T Cell Therapy

CAR-T cell treatment is a type of immunotherapy that entails genetically modifying a patient's own T cells to produce CARs, which can recognize and bind to particular cancer cells. These CARs are programmed to identify specific antigen such as CD19, CD20, or HER2 and may detect and eliminate cancer cells with extraordinary efficacy in treating carcinomas including blood carcinomas (Maude et al. 2018; Neelapu et al. 2017a).

7.16.2 Personalized T-Cell Therapy

With personalized T-CT, a patient's T cells are modified to specifically target their own cancer cells. This approach could potentially improve the effectiveness of T-CT and reduce side effects. One strategy for personalized T-CT involves using neoantigens, which are antigens that are specific to a patient's tumor cells and are not present on normal cells. Researchers can identify these neoantigens by sequencing the patient's tumor DNA and then design T cells to target these antigens. Another strategy involves using T cells that are engineered to recognize the patient's own cancer-specific proteins (Schumacher and Schreiber 2015; Kalaitsidou et al. 2018).

7.16.3 Combination Therapies

T-CT is combined with other medications, such as checkpoint inhibitors (CPIs), as combination therapy to boost the anticancer immune response. To prevent detection, CPI drugs block the inhibitory signals. The effectiveness and longevity of T-cell treatment may be increased by combining it with checkpoint inhibitors (Ribas and Wolchok 2018; June et al. 2017).

7.16.4 Solid Tumors

Solid tumors are a difficult type of cancer to treat with T-CT, as the tumor can evade the immune system. However, efforts have been made to overcome this challenge by developing new techniques and strategies to target solid tumors. One strategy involves using T cells, which are modified to recognize tumor-specific mutations. Another strategy involves using combination therapies to overcome the immunosuppressive environment of solid tumors (Ribas et al. 2016; Brown and Mackall 2019).

7.16.5 Off-the-Shelf T-Cell Therapy

Off-the-shelf T-CT is a new approach being developed to provide readily available T-cell therapies for multiple patients. T-CT now necessitates the extraction of a patient's own T cells, which are subsequently manipulated and reintroduced into the patient. However, off-the-shelf T-cell therapies could make T-cell therapy more accessible and cost-effective. One strategy for off-the-shelf T-CT involves using T cells from healthy donors that are engineered to recognize and attack cancer cells. Another strategy involves using iPSCs to generate T cells that can be used for multiple patients (Shah and Fry 2019; Kebriaei et al. 2016).

7.17 Challenges

7.17.1 CAR-T Cell Therapy

Regardless of its success in treating certain blood malignancies, this therapy confronts certain demerits. One challenge is the potential for toxicity and side effects, which can include cytokine release syndrome (CRS), neurotoxicity, and infections. Another challenge is the development of antigen-negative relapses, where cancer cells lose the antigen targeted by the CAR-T cells and are no longer recognized by the therapy (Neelapu et al. 2018).

7.17.2 Personalized T-Cell Therapy

Personalized T-CT faces many challenges related to the logistics of manufacturing and delivering the therapy. Because each patient's T cells are unique, the manufacturing process can be time-consuming and expensive. In addition, the therapy must be delivered to the patient within a short timeframe, which can be challenging for patients who live far from the manufacturing facility (Wang and Rivière 2016).

7.17.3 Combination Therapies

Combination therapies face several challenges related to the immune system reactions followed by toxicity. Because the immune system is highly regulated, combining different therapies can result in unpredictable and potentially harmful interactions. In addition, some combination therapies can cause severe toxicity, such as severe immune-related adverse events.

7.17.4 Solid Tumors

T-CT faces several challenges in treating solid tumors, which have a more complex and immunosuppressive microenvironment compared to blood cancers. One challenge is non-availability of tumor-specific antigens targeting T cells. Another challenge is the presence of inhibitory signals that can suppress the immune response and prevent T cells from infiltrating the tumor. Furthermore, solid tumors can have heterogeneous antigen expression, making it challenging to create T cells capable of recognizing all cancer cells (Hegde et al. 2016).

7.17.5 Off-the-Shelf T-Cell Therapy

Off-the-shelf T-CT faces several challenges related to the production and quality (QC) of the therapy. Because these cells are derived from normal healthy volunteers, there is a risk of immune rejection and transmission of infections. In addition, the manufacturing process must ensure the safety and efficacy of T cells in multiple patients, which can be challenging due to the heterogeneity of T cells and their potential to cause adverse reactions (Zhang et al. 2017a).

7.18 Future Directions

7.18.1 CAR-T Cell Therapy

The future of this therapy involves improving the safety and efficacy in diverse set of patients. One direction is to develop next-generation CAR-T cells that can recognize multiple antigens or bypass antigen-negative relapses. Another direction is to develop less toxic and have a lower risk of side effects. Researchers are also exploring ways to improve the potency, such as using gene editing to modify the T cells or combined immunotherapies (Heczey et al. 2015).

7.18.2 Personalized T-Cell Therapy

Success of personalized T-CT involves improving the manufacturing and delivery of the therapy. One direction is to develop faster and more cost-effective methods for manufacturing patient-specific T cells. Another direction is to develop methods for delivering the therapy to patients who live far from the manufacturing facility. Researchers are also exploring ways to improve the specificity, potency of personalized T cells using editing of genes to accelerate the T cells or for targeting neoantigens.

7.18.3 Combination Therapies

The future of combination therapies involves optimizing the combination of different immunotherapies to improve the response rate and durability of the therapy. One approach would be to create predictive biomarkers that might identify right target beneficiary people from combo medication. Another approach is to devise algorithms for determining the best mix of medicines for each patient. Researchers are also exploring ways to minimize toxicity and adverse events associated with combination therapy.

7.18.4 Solid Tumors

The future of T-CT for solid tumors involves developing new strategies to overcome the immunosuppressive microenvironment of solid tumors. One direction is to develop T cells that are engineered to recognize multiple tumor-specific antigens or that can overcome inhibitory signals in the tumor microenvironment. Another direction is to combine T-CT with other immunotherapies or targeted therapies to enhance the anticancer immune response. Researchers are also exploring new ways such as using nanoparticles or other targeted delivery methods.

7.18.5 Off-the-Shelf T-Cell Therapy

The future of off-the-shelf T-cell therapy involves improving the therapeutic safety and treatment efficacy. One direction is to establish multiple methods for generating T cells from induced pluripotent stem cells (iPSCs) that can be used for multiple patients. Another direction is to develop methods for selecting the optimal T cells for each patient, such as using biomarkers or gene editing to modify the T cells. Researchers are also exploring ways to minimize host rejection response and transmission of infections related with off-the-shelf T-CT.

7.19 Conclusion

The most typical form of LC, NSCL, accounts for the majority of cancer-related fatalities worldwide. In addition to known signaling molecules, a growing body of evidence suggests that non-coding riboneuleic acids play important roles in the development and progression of lung cancer. Signaling molecule dysregulation is a common hallmark of lung cancer, and understanding their involvement in tumor growth and progression is crucial for creating effective therapeutics for this lethal illness. Tumor immunotherapy is getting increased attention as a viable treatment strategy despite standard treatment approaches.

To battle cancer, both passive and active immunotherapies aim to either directly target tumors or activate the immune system. CTLs are regarded to constitute the foundation of the immune response to tumors, and innate immunity and adaptive immunity both play important roles in the antitumor immune response. By encouraging the growth, activation, and infiltration of CD8+ T cells into the tumor site and by producing substantial quantities of IFN, Th1 cells coordinate cell-mediated immunity responses against cancer cells. An effective tumor immunotherapy method demonstrates a strong anti-tumor immune response as well as the reversal of tumor immune-suppression.

To realize the full promise of ACT-based immunotherapies, a more progressive approach that treats a smaller sample of patients with T cells engineered to specifically target tumor antigens may be required. Although ACT's capacity to target both internal and membrane antigens broadens its potential applications, its efficacy may limit its safe administration to tumor-specific or highly tissue-restricted antigens. Because it is a promising strategy, the application of ACT as a cancer therapy is becoming increasingly evident to us. However, various hurdles must be overcome in order to overcome therapeutic and economic constraints. In conclusion, T-cell therapy has emerged as a feasible technique for treating cancer and other illnesses by utilizing the capabilities of the immune system. CAR-T cell therapy has shown outstanding efficacy in treating several blood cancers, while personalized T-cell therapy and combination therapies are being researched for a number of diseases and illnesses. T-cell therapy, on the other hand, has a variety of challenges, including toxicity and side effects, manufacturing and delivery logistics, immunosuppressive tumor microenvironments, and T-cell heterogeneity. T-cell therapy's future includes the development of next-generation CAR-T cells, faster and more cost-effective manufacturing procedures, predictive biomarkers, and methods for overcoming immunosuppressive tumor microenvironments. Overall, T-cell therapy has significant potential for cancer treatment and tailored medicine in the future.

References

Abdelsamed HA, Moustaki A, Fan Y, Dogra P, Ghoneim HE, Zebley CC, Triplett BM, Sekaly RP, Youngblood B (2017) Human memory CD8 T cell effector potential is epigenetically preserved during in vivo homeostasis. J Exp Med 214(6):1593–1606

Adusumilli PS, Zauderer MG, Rusch VW, O'Cearbhaill D, Zhu A, Ngai DA (2020) Regional delivery of mesothelin-targeted CAR T cell therapy generates potent and long-lasting CD4-dependent tumor immunity. Sci Transl Med 12(532):eaaz1736. https://doi.org/10.1126/scitranslmed.aaz1736

American Cancer Society (2023) Cancer facts and figures 2023. American Cancer Society, Atlanta

Andersen R, Donia M, Ellebaek E, Borch TH, Kongsted P, Iversen TZ, Hölmich LR, Hendel HW, Met Ö, Andersen MH, thorStraten P. (2016) Long-lasting complete responses in patients with metastatic melanoma after adoptive cell therapy with tumor-infiltrating lymphocytes and an attenuated IL2 regimen. Clin Cancer Res 22(15):3734–3745

Anderson NM, Simon MC (2020) The tumor microenvironment. Curr Biol 30(16):R921–R925. https://doi.org/10.1016/j.cub.2020.06.081. PMID: 32810447; PMCID: PMC8194051

Arina A, Corrales L, Bronte V (2016) Enhancing T cell therapy by overcoming the immunosuppressive tumor microenvironment. In: Seminars in immunology, vol 28. Academic, Cambridge, MA, pp 54–63

Baxter D (2014) Active and passive immunization for cancer. Hum Vaccin Immunother 10(7):2123–2129. https://doi.org/10.4161/hv.29604. PMID: 25424829; PMCID: PMC4370360
Beavis PA, Slaney CY, Kershaw MH, Gyorki D, Neeson PJ, Darcy PK (2016) Reprogramming the tumor microenvironment to enhance adoptive cellular therapy. In: Seminars in immunology, vol 28. Academic, Cambridge, MA, pp 64–72
Bedognetti D, Spivey TL, Zhao Y, Uccellini L, Tomei S, Dudley ME, Ascierto ML, De Giorgi V, Liu Q, Delogu LG, Sommariva M (2013) CXCR3/CCR5 pathways in metastatic melanoma patients treated with adoptive therapy and interleukin-2. Br J Cancer 109(9):2412–2423
Bergers G, Hanahan D (2010) Modes of resistance to antiangiogenic therapy. Nat Rev Cancer 8:592–601
Bonifant CL, Jackson HJ, Brentjens RJ, Curran KJ (2016) Toxicity and management in CAR T-cell therapy. Mol Ther Oncolytics 3:16011. https://doi.org/10.1038/mto.2016.11
Bos R, Sherman LA (2010) CD4+ T-cell help in the tumor milieu is required for recruitment and cytolytic function of CD8+ T lymphocytes. Cancer Res 70(21):8368–8377
Brown CE, Mackall CL (2019) CAR T cell therapy: inroads to response and resistance. Nat Rev Immunol 19(2):73–74. https://doi.org/10.1038/s41577-018-0108-z
Budisan L, Zanoaga O, Braicu C, Pirlog R, Covaliu B, Esanu V, Korban SS, Berindan-Neagoe I (2021) Links between infections, lung cancer, and the immune system. Int J Mol Sci 22(17):9394. https://doi.org/10.3390/ijms22179394
Butts C, Maksymiuk A, Goss G, Soulieres D, Marshall E, Cormier Y et al (2007) A multicentre phase IIB randomized controlled study of BLP25 liposome vaccine (LBLP25 or Stimuvax) for active specific immunotherapy of non-small cell lung cancer (NSCLC): updated survival analysis. Thorac Oncol 2(8):s332–s333
Butts C, Murray N, Maksymiuk A, Goss G, Marshall E, Soulières D et al (2005) Randomized phase IIB trial of BLP25 liposome vaccine in stage IIIB and IV non–small-cell lung cancer. Clin Oncol 23(27):6674–6681
Butts C, Socinski MA, Mitchell PL, Thatcher N, Havel L, Krzakowski M et al (2014) Tecemotide (L-BLP25) versus placebo after chemoradiotherapy for stage III non-small-cell lung cancer (START): a randomised, double-blind, phase 3 trial. Lancet Oncol 15(1):59–68
Cancerresearchuk.org (2023) Types of lung cancer [Internet]. [cited 2023 Apr 5]. https://www.cancerresearchuk.org/about-cancer/lung-cancer/stages-types-grades/types
Carpenito C, Milone MC, Hassan R, Simonet JC, Lakhal M, Suhoski MM, Varela-Rohena A, Haines KM, Heitjan DF, Albelda SM, Carroll RG (2009) Control of large, established tumor xenografts with genetically retargeted human T cells containing CD28 and CD137 domains. Proc Natl Acad Sci 106(9):3360–3365
Centers For Disease Control And Prevention. National Center For Health Statistics (2017) CDC WONDER On-Line Database, Compiled from Compressed Mortality File 1999–2016 Series 20 No. 2V
Cheng KY, Hao M (2017) Mammalian target of rapamycin (mTOR) regulates transforming growth factor-β1 (TGF-β1)-induced epithelial-mesenchymal transition via decreased pyruvate kinase M2 (PKM2) expression in cervical cancer cells. Med Sci Monit 23:2017–2028. https://doi.org/10.12659/msm.901542. PMID: 28446743; PMCID: PMC5417590
Choi YJ, Rho JK, Jeon BS et al (2010) Combined inhibition of IGFR enhances the effects of gefitinib in H1650: a lung cancer cell line with EGFR mutation and primary resistance to EGFR-TK inhibitors. Cancer Chemother Pharmacol 66:381–388
Clark WH Jr, Elder DE, Guerry D, Braitman LE, Trock BJ, Schultz D et al (1989) Model predicting survival in stage I melanoma based on tumor progression. Natl Cancer Inst 81(24):1893–1904
Cortes-Sempere M, Chattapadhyay S, Rovira A et al (2009) MKP1 repression is required for the chemosensitizing effects of NF-kappaB and PI(3)K inhibitors to cisplatin in nonsmall cell lung cancer. Cancer Lett 286:206–216
Cretney E, Takeda K, Yagita H, Glaccum M, Peschon JJ, Smyth MJ (2002) Increased susceptibility to tumor initiation and metastasis in TNF related apoptosis inducing ligand-deficient mice. Immunology 168(3):1356–1361
Crotty S (2011) Follicular helper CD4 T cells (TFH). Annu Rev Immunol 29:621–663

Cullen SP, Brunet M, Martin SJ (2010) Granzymes in cancer and immunity. Cell Death Differ 17(4):616–623
Cullen SP, Martin SJ (2008) Mechanisms of granule-dependent killing. Cell Death Differ 15(2):251–262
Da Cunha SG, Shepherd FA, Tsao MS (2011) EGFR mutations and lung cancer. Annu Rev Pathol 6:49–69
Darnell RB (1996) Onconeural antigens and the paraneoplastic neurologic disorders: at the intersection of cancer, immunity, and the brain. Proc Natl Acad Sci U S A 93:4529–4536. https://doi.org/10.1073/pnas.93.10.4529
De Braganca KC, Janjigian YY, Azzoli CG et al (2010) Efficacy and safety of bevacizumab in active brain metastasis from nonsmall cell lung cancer. J Neuro Oncol 100:443–447
Debets, R., Donnadieu, E., Chouaib, S. and Coukos, G., 2016, TCR-engineered T cells to treat tumors: seeing but not touching?. In Seminars in immunology 28, 1, pp. 10–21. Academic, Cambridge, MA
Deshpand R, Chandra M, Rauthan A (2022) Evolving trends in lung cancer: epidemiology, diagnosis, and management. Indian J Cancer 59(Suppl 1):S90
Dieu-Nosjean MC, Antoine M, Danel C, Heudes D, Wislez M, Poulot V, Rabbe N, Laurans L, Tartour E, de Chaisemartin L, Lebecque S (2008) Long-term survival for patients with non–small-cell lung cancer with intratumoral lymphoid structures. J Clin Oncol 26(27):4410–4417
Dotti G, Gottschalk S, Savoldo B, Brenner MK (2014) Design and development of therapies using chimeric antigen receptor-expressing T cells. Immunol Rev 257(1):107–126. https://doi.org/10.1111/imr.12131
Dudley ME, Wunderlich JR, Yang JC, Sherry RM, Topalian SL, Restifo NP, Royal RE, Kammula U, White DE, Mavroukakis SA, Rogers LJ (2005) Adoptive cell transfer therapy following non-myeloablative but lymphodepleting chemotherapy for the treatment of patients with refractory metastatic melanoma. J Clin Oncol 23(10):2346
Feng K, Guo Y, Dai H, Wang Y, Li X, Jia H, Han W (2016) Chimeric antigen receptor-modified T cells for the immunotherapy of patients with EGFR-expressing advanced relapsed/refractory non-small cell lung cancer. Sci China Life Sci 59:468–479
Fischel JL, Formento P, Milano G (2005) Epidermal growth factor receptor double targeting by a tyrosine kinase inhibitor (Iressa) and a monoclonal antibody (cetuximab). Impact on cell growth and molecular factors. Br J Cancer 92:1063–1068
Forget MA, Tavera RJ, Haymaker C, Ramachandran R, Malu S, Zhang M, Wardell S, Fulbright OJ, Toth CL, Gonzalez AM, Thorsen ST (2017) A novel method to generate and expand clinical-grade, genetically modified, tumor-infiltrating lymphocytes. Front Immunol 8:908
Gabrilovich DI, Nagaraj S (2009) Myeloid-derived suppressor cells as regulators of the immune system. Nat Rev Immunol 9(3):162–174
Gajewska BU, Alvarez D, Vidric M, Goncharova S, Stämpfli MR, Coyle AJ, Gutierrez-Ramos JC, Jordana M (2001) Generation of experimental allergic airways inflammation in the absence of draining lymph nodes. J Clin Invest 108(4):577–583
Galaine J, Borg C, Godet Y, Adotévi O (2015) Interest of tumor-specific CD4 T helper 1 cells for therapeutic anticancer vaccine. Vaccines 3(3):490–502. Disis ML (Nora), ed
Gandhi L, McNamara KL, Li D et al (2009) Sunitinib prolongs survival in genetically engineered mouse models of lung cancinogenesis. Cancer Prev Res (Phila) 2:330–337
Gao Q, Qiu SJ, Fan J, Zhou J, Wang XY, Xiao YS et al (2007) Intratumoral balance of regulatory and cytotoxic T cells is associated with prognosis of hepatocellular carcinoma after resection. Clin Oncol 25(18):2586–2593
Geldres C, Savoldo B, Dotti G (2016) Chimeric antigen receptor-redirected T cells return to the bench. In: Seminars in immunology, vol 28. Academic, Cambridge, MA, pp 3–9
Giaccone G, Bazhenova LA, Nemunaitis J, Tan ME, Ramlau JR, Heuvel MM et al (2015) A phase III study of belagenpumatucel-L, an allogeneic tumour cell vaccine, as maintenance therapy for non-small cell lung cancer. Eur J Cancer 51(16):2321–2329
Gill S, June CH (2015) Going viral: chimeric antigen receptor T-cell therapy for hematological malignancies. Immunol Rev 263(1):68–89

Gonzalez-Rodriguez AP, Contesti J, Huergo-Zapico L, Lopez-Soto A, Fernandez-Guizan A, Acebes-Huerta A et al (2010) Prognostic significance of CD8 and CD4 T cells in chronic lymphocytic leukemia. Leuk Lymphoma 51(10):1829–1836

Gotink KJ, Verheul HMW (2010) Antiangiogenic tyrosine kinase inhibitors: what is their mechanism of action? Angiogenesis 13:1–14

Gridelli C, Maione P, Ferrara ML et al (2009) Cetuximab and other antiepidermal growth factor receptor monoclonal antibodies in the treatment of nonsmall cell lung cancer. Oncologist 14:601–611

Gschwind A, Fischer OM, Ullrich A (2004) The discovery of receptor tyrosine kinases: targets for cancer therapy. Nat Rev Cancer 4:361–370

Haabeth OW, Tveita AA, Fauskanger M, Schjesvold F, Lorvik KB, Hofgaard PO et al (2014) How do CD4+ T cells detect and eliminate tumor cells that either lack or express MHC class II molecules? Front Immunol 5:174

Hammarström S (1999) The carcinoembryonic antigen (CEA) family: structures, suggested functions and expression in normal and malignant tissues. In: Seminars in cancer biology, vol 9. Academic, Cambridge, MA, p 67

Hanahan D, Weinberg RA (2011) Hallmarks of cancer: the next generation. Cell 144:646–674

Hay KA, Turtle CJ (2017) Chimeric antigen receptor (CAR) T cells: lessons learned from targeting of CD19 in B-cell malignancies. Drugs 77:237–245

Heczey A, Louis CU, Savoldo B, Dotti G (2015) Harnessing the potential of CAR-T cell therapy for high-risk childhood cancers. Pediatr Clin N Am 62(5):1091–1104. https://doi.org/10.1016/j.pcl.2015.05.014

Hegde PS, Karanikas V, Evers S (2016) The where, the when, and the how of immune monitoring for cancer immunotherapies in the era of checkpoint inhibition. Clin Cancer Res 22(8):1865–1874. https://doi.org/10.1158/1078-0432.CCR-15-1507

Hirsch FR, Scagliotti GV, Mulshine JL, Kwon R, Curran WJ, Wu YL, Paz-Ares L (2017) Lung cancer: current therapies and new targeted treatments. Lancet 389(10066):299–311

Huang J, Khong HT, Dudley ME, El-Gamil M, Li YF, Rosenberg SA, Robbins PF (2005) Survival, persistence, and progressive differentiation of adoptively transferred tumor-reactive T cells associated with tumor regression. J Immunother 28(3):258. (Hagerstown, Md.: 1997)

Ikeda H, Old LJ, Schreiber RD (2002) The roles of IFN in protection against tumor development and cancer immunoediting. Cytokine Growth Factor Rev 13(2):95–109

Inamura K (2017) Lung cancer: understanding its molecular pathology and the 2015 WHO classification. Front Oncol 7:193. https://doi.org/10.3389/fonc.2017.00193

International Agency for Research on Cancer (2020) GLOBOCAN lung cancer facts sheet

Jenkins R, Walker J, Roy UB (2023) 2022 cancer statistics: focus on lung cancer. Future Oncol

Ji Y, Hocker JD, Gattinoni L (2016) Enhancing adoptive T cell immunotherapy with microRNA therapeutics. In: Seminars in immunology, vol 28. Academic, Cambridge, MA, pp 45–53

June CH, Warshauer JT, Bluestone JA (2017) Is autoimmunity the Achilles' heel of cancer immunotherapy? Nat Med 23(5):540–547. https://doi.org/10.1038/nm.4331

Kalaitsidou M, Kueberuwa G, Schanz A et al (2018) T cell-mediated immunotherapy for cancer: harnessing the power of trained immunity. Front Immunol 9:2931. https://doi.org/10.3389/fimmu.2018.02931

Karagiannis P, Iriguchi S, Kaneko S (2016) Reprogramming away from the exhausted T cell state. In: Seminars in immunology, vol 28. Academic, Cambridge, MA, pp 35–44

Kataki A, Scheid P, Piet M, Marie B, Martinet N, Martinet Y, Vignaud JM (2002) Tumor infiltrating lymphocytes and macrophages have a potential dual role in lung cancer by supporting both host-defense and tumor progression. J Lab Clin Med 140(5):320–328

Kebriaei P, Singh H, Huls MH et al (2016) Phase I trials using sleeping beauty to generate CD19-specific CAR T cells. J Clin Invest 126(9):3363–3376. https://doi.org/10.1172/JCI86721

Keshamouni VG, Reddy RC, Arenberg DA et al (2004) Peroxisome proliferatoractivated receptor-gamma activation inhibits tumor progression in nonsmall cell lung cancer. Oncogene 23:100–108

Kim SM, Kim JS, Kim JH et al (2010) Acquired resistance to cetuximab is mediated by increased PTEN instability and leads cross-resistance to gefitinib in HCC827 NSCLC. Cancer Lett 296:150–159

Kim KJ, Li B, Winer J et al (1993) Inhibition of vascular endothelial growth factor induced angiogenesis suppresses tumor growth in vivo. Nature 362:841–844

Kobayashi S, Boggon TJ, Dayaram T, Janne PA, Kocher O, Meyerson M et al (2005) EGFR mutation and resistance of non-small-cell lung cancer to gefitinib. N Engl J Med 352:786–792

Kondo T, Morita R, Okuzono Y, Nakatsukasa H, Sekiya T, Chikuma S, Shichita T, Kanamori M, Kubo M, Koga K, Miyazaki T (2017) Notch-mediated conversion of activated T cells into stem cell memory-like T cells for adoptive immunotherapy. Nat Commun 8(1):15338

Koneru M, O'Cearbhaill R, Pendharkar S, Spriggs DR, Brentjens RJ (2015) A phase I clinical trial of adoptive T cell therapy using IL-12 secreting MUC-16 ecto directed chimeric antigen receptors for recurrent ovarian cancer. J Transl Med 13:1–1

Korn T, Oukka M, Kuchroo V, Bettelli E (2007) Th17 cells: effector T cells with inflammatory properties. Semin Immunol 19(6):362–371

Kunert A, Obenaus M, Lamers CH, Blankenstein T, Debets R (2017) T-cell receptors for clinical therapy: in vitro assessment of toxicity risk in vitro selection of safe T-cell receptors. Clin Cancer Res 23(20):6012–6020

Kurts C, Robinson BW, Knolle PA (2010) Cross-priming in health and disease. Nat Rev Immunol 10(6):403–414

Liu Y, Zeng G (2012) Cancer and innate immune system interactions: translational potentials for cancer immunotherapy. Immunotherapy 35(4):299–308

Lynch TJ, Bell DW, Sordella R et al (2004) Activating mutations in the epidermal growth factor receptor underlying responsiveness of non small cell lung cancer to gefitinib. N Engl J Med 350:2129–2139

Martinet L, Le Guellec S, Filleron T, Lamant L, Meyer N, Rochaix P, Garrido I, Girard JP (2012) High endothelial venules (HEVs) in human melanoma lesions: major gateways for tumor-infiltrating lymphocytes. Onco Targets Ther 1(6):829–839

Martin-Fontecha A, Thomsen LL, Brett S, Gerard C, Lipp M, Lanzavecchia SF (2004) Induced recruitment of NK cells to lymph nodes provides IFNgamma for T(H)1 priming. Nat Immunol 5(12):1260–1265

Maude SL, Laetsch TW, Buechner J et al (2018) Tisagenlecleucel in children and young adults with B-cell lymphoblastic leukemia. N Engl J Med 378(5):439–448. https://doi.org/10.1056/NEJMoa1709866

Mikucki ME, Fisher DT, Matsuzaki J, Skitzki JJ, Gaulin NB, Muhitch JB, Ku AW, Frelinger JG, Odunsi K, Gajewski TF, Luster AD (2015) Non-redundant requirement for CXCR3 signalling during tumoricidal T-cell trafficking across tumour vascular checkpoints. Nat Commun 6(1):7458

Mills JK, Henderson MA, Giuffrida L, Petrone P, Westwood JA, Darcy PK, Neeson PJ, Kershaw MH, Gyorki DE (2021) Generating CAR T cells from tumor-infiltrating lymphocytes. Ther Adv Vaccines Immunother 9:25151355211017119. https://doi.org/10.1177/25151355211017119. PMID: 34159293; PMCID: PMC8186112

Morgan E, Arnold M, Gini A, Lorenzoni V, Cabasag CJ, Laversanne M, Vignat J, Ferlay J, Murphy N, Bray F (2023) Global burden of colorectal cancer in 2020 and 2040: incidence and mortality estimates from GLOBOCAN. Gut 72(2):338–344

Morgan RA, Dudley ME, Wunderlich JR, Hughes MS, Yang JC, Sherry RM et al (2006) Cancer regression in patients after transfer of genetically engineered lymphocytes. Science 314:126–129

Morgan RA, Yang JC, Kitano M, Dudley ME, Laurencot CM, Rosenberg SA (2010) Case report of a serious adverse event following the administration of T cells transduced with a chimeric antigen receptor recognizing ERBB2. Mol Ther 18(4):843–851

Morgensztern D, Besse B, Greillier L, Santana-Davila R, Ready N, Hann CL, Glisson BS, Farago AF, Dowlati A, Rudin CM, Le Moulec S (2019) Efficacy and safety of Rovalpituzumab Tesirine in third-line and beyond patients with DLL3-expressing, relapsed/refractory small-cell lung cancer: results from the phase II TRINITY StudyPhase II study results of Rova-T in DLL3-expressing SCLC. Clin Cancer Res 25(23):6958–6966

Mosmann TR, Coffman RL (1989) TH1 and TH2 cells: different patterns of lymphokine secretion lead to different functional properties. Annu Rev Immunol 7:145–173

Moyron-Quiroz JE, Rangel-Moreno J, Kusser K, Hartson L, Sprague F, Goodrich S, Woodland DL, Lund FE, Randall TD (2004) Role of inducible bronchus associated lymphoid tissue (iBALT) in respiratory immunity. Nat Med 10(9):927–934

Nagata S, Golstein P (1995) The Fas death factor. Science 267(5203):1449–1456

Naumov GN, Nilsson MB, Cascone T et al (2009) Combined vascular endothelial growth factor receptor and epidermal growth factor receptor (EGFR) blockade inhibits tumor growth in xenograft models of EGFR inhibitor resistance. Clin Cancer Res 15:3484–3494

Neelapu SS, Locke FL, Bartlett NL, Lekakis LJ, Miklos DB, Jacobson CA, Braunschweig I, Oluwole OO, Siddiqi T, Lin Y, Timmerman JM (2017b) Axicabtagene ciloleucel CAR T-cell therapy in refractory large B-cell lymphoma. N Engl J Med 377(26):2531–2544

Neelapu SS, Locke FL, Bartlett NL et al (2017a) AxicabtageneCiloleucel CAR T-cell therapy in refractory large B-cell lymphoma. N Engl J Med 377(26):2531–2544. https://doi.org/10.1056/NEJMoa1707447

Neelapu SS, Tummala S, Kebriaei P et al (2018) Chimeric antigen receptor T-cell therapy - assessment and management of toxicities. Nat Rev Clin Oncol 15(1):47–62. https://doi.org/10.1038/nrclinonc.2017.148

NeningerVinageras E, de la Torre A, Osorio Rodriguez M, Catalá Ferrer M, Bravo I, Mendoza del Pino M et al (2008) Phase II randomized controlled trial of an epidermal growth factor vaccine in advanced non-small-cell lung cancer. Clin Oncol 26:1452–1458

Neyt K, Perros F, GeurtsvanKessel CH, Hammad H, Lambrecht BN (2012) Tertiary lymphoid organs in infection and autoimmunity. Trends Immunol 33(6):297–305

Ngo Trong H, Le Van Manh H, Thanh Dang V, Ho-Thao Nguyen N, Vu Thanh B, Pham P (2020) Current strategies for adoptive immunotherapy for cancer: Off-the-shelfâ immune cells. Biomed Res Ther 7(12):4170–4189. https://doi.org/10.15419/bmrat.v7i12.655

Nowroozi A, Khalili N, Razi S, Keshavarz-Fathi M, Rezaei N (2022) Tumor-infiltrating lymphocyte therapy for lung cancer and its future paradigms. Expert Opin Biol Ther 22(6):735–745

Oliver TG, Mercer KL, Sayles LC et al (2010) Chronic cisplatin treatment promotes enhanced damage repair and tumor progression in mouse model of lung cancer. Genes Dev 24:837–852

Paez JG, Janne PA, Lee JC et al (2004) EGFR mutation in lung cancer: correlation with clinical response to gefitinib therapy. Science 304:1497–1500

Pao W, Miller V, Zakowski M et al (2004) EGF receptor gene mutations are common in lung cancer from ‘never smokers’ and are associated with sensitivity of tumours to gefitinib and erlotinib. Proc Natl Acad Sci U S A 101:13306–13311

Park JH, Geyer MB, Brentjens RJ (2016) CD19-targeted CAR T-cell therapeutics for hematologic malignancies: interpreting clinical outcomes to date. Blood 127(26):3312–3320

Patel S, Burga RA, Powell AB, Chorvinsky EA, Hoq N, McCormack SE, Van Pelt SN, Hanley PJ, Cruz CRY (2019) Beyond CAR T cells: other cell-based immunotherapeutic strategies against cancer. Front Oncol 9:196. https://doi.org/10.3389/fonc.2019.00196. PMID: 31024832; PMCID: PMC6467966

Peifer M, Fernandez-Cuesta L, Sos ML, George J, Seidel D, Kasper LH et al (2012) Integrative genome analyses identify key somatic driver mutations of small-cell lung cancer. Nat Genet 44:1104–1110. https://doi.org/10.1038/ng.2396

Powell DJ Jr, Dudley ME, Robbins PF, Rosenberg SA (2005) Transition of late-stage effector T cells to CD27+ CD28+ tumor-reactive effector memory T cells in humans after adoptive cell transfer therapy. Blood 105(1):241–250

Prehn RT (1970) Analysis of antigenic heterogeneity within individual 3- methylcholanthrene-induced mouse sarcomas. Natl Cancer Inst. 45(5):1039–1045

Presotto D, Erdes E, Duong MN, Allard M, Regamey PO, Quadroni M, Doucey MA, Rufer N, Hebeisen M (2017) Fine-tuning of optimal TCR signaling in tumor-redirected CD8 T cells by distinct TCR affinity-mediated mechanisms. Front Immunol 8:1564

Qin Z, Schwartzkopff J, Pradera F, Kammertoens T, Seliger B, Pircher H, Blankenstein T (2003) A critical requirement of interferon gamma-mediated angiostasis for tumor rejection by CD8+ T cells. Cancer Res 63(14):4095–4100
Quoix E, Ramlau R, Westeel V, Papai Z, Madroszyk A, Riviere A et al (2011) Therapeutic vaccination with TG4010 and first-line chemotherapy in advanced non-small-cell lung cancer: a controlled phase 2B trial. Lancet Oncol 12:1125–1133
Radvanyi LG, Bernatchez C, Zhang M, Fox PS, Miller P, Chacon J, Wu R, Lizee G, Mahoney S, Alvarado G, Glass M (2012) Specific lymphocyte subsets predict response to adoptive cell therapy using expanded autologous tumor-infiltrating lymphocytes in metastatic melanoma patients tumor-infiltrating lymphocyte therapy for melanoma. Clin Cancer Res 18(24):6758–6770
Ray M, Salgia R, Vokes EE (2009) The role of EGFR inhibition in the treatment of nonsmall cell lung cancer. Oncologist 14:1116–1130
Remark R, Becker C, Gomez JE, Damotte D, Dieu-Nosjean MC, Sautes-Fridman C, Fridman WH, Powell CA, Altorki NK, Merad M, Gnjatic S (2015) The non–small cell lung cancer immune contexture. A major determinant of tumor characteristics and patient outcome. Am J Respir Crit Care Med 191(4):377–390
Ribas A, Shin DS, Zaretsky J et al (2016) PD-1 blockade expands Intratumoral memory T cells. Cancer Immunol Res 4(3):194–203. https://doi.org/10.1158/2326-6066.CIR-15-0210
Ribas A, Wolchok JD (2018) Cancer immunotherapy using checkpoint blockade. Science 359(6382):1350–1355. https://doi.org/10.1126/science.aar4060
Rosenberg SA, Packard BS, Aebersold PM, Solomon D, Topalian SL, Toy ST, Simon P, Lotze MT, Yang JC, Seipp CA, Simpson C (1988) Use of tumor-infiltrating lymphocytes and interleukin-2 in the immunotherapy of patients with metastatic melanoma. N Engl J Med 319(25):1676–1680
Ruella M, Kenderian SS (2017) Next-generation chimeric antigen receptor T-cell therapy: going off the shelf. BioDrugs 31(6):473–481
Sadelain M, Rivière I, Riddell S (2017) Therapeutic T cell engineering. Nature 545(7655):423–431
Sakaguchi S (2005) Naturally arising Foxp3-expressing CD25 + CD4+ regulatory T cells in immunological tolerance to self and non-self. Nat Immunol 6(4):345–352
Salgaller ML (2002) The development of immunotherapies for non-small cell lung cancer. Expert Opin Biol Ther 2(3):265–278
Sandler A, Gray R, Perry MC et al (2006) Palcitaxel–carboplatin alone or with bevacizumab for nonsmall cell lung cancer. N Engl J Med 355:2542–2550
Schumacher TN, Schreiber RD (2015) Neoantigens in cancer immunotherapy. Science 348(6230):69–74
Schuster M, Nechansky A, Kircheis R (2006) Cancer immunotherapy. Biogeosciences 1(2):138–147
Schuster SJ, Svoboda J, Chong EA et al (2017) Chimeric antigen receptor T cells in refractory B-cell lymphomas. N Engl J Med 377(26):2545–2554. https://doi.org/10.1056/NEJMoa1708566
Shah NN, Fry TJ (2019) Mechanisms of resistance to CAR T cell therapy. Nat Rev Clin Oncol 16(6):372–385. https://doi.org/10.1038/s41571-019-0184-6
Shen H, Yuan Y, Sun J et al (2010) Combined tamoxifen and gefinitib in small cell lung cancer shows antiproliferative effects. Biochem Pharmacother 64:88–92
Sheridan C (2017) First approval in sight for Novartis' CAR-T therapy after panel vote. Nat Biotechnol 35(8):691
Shibuya M, Claesson-Welsh L (2006) Signal transduction by VEGF receptors in regulation of angiogenesis and lymphangiogenesis. Exp Cell Res 312:549–560
Shresta S, Pham CT, Thomas DA, Graubert TA, Ley TJ (1998) How do cytotoxic lymphocytes kill their targets? Curr Opin Immunol 10(5):581–587
Singh AK, McGuirk JP (2020) CAR T cells: continuation in a revolution of immunotherapy. Lancet Oncol 21(3):e168–e178
Smyth MJ, Hayakawa Y, Takeda K, Yagita H (2002) New aspects of natural killer-cell surveillance and therapy of cancer. Nat Rev Cancer 2(11):850–861

Song DG, Ye Q, Carpenito C, Poussin M, Wang LP, Ji C, Figini M, June CH, Coukos G, Powell DJ Jr (2011) In vivo persistence, tumor localization, and antitumor activity of CAR-engineered T cells is enhanced by costimulatory signaling through CD137 (4-1BB). Cancer Res 71(13):4617–4627
Staedtke V, Bai RY, Kim K, Darvas M, Davila ML, Riggins GJ, Rothman PB, Papadopoulos N, Kinzler KW, Vogelstein B, Zhou S (2018) Disruption of a self-amplifying catecholamine loop reduces cytokine release syndrome. Nature 564(7735):273–277
Steuer CE, Ramalingam SS (2018) Tumor mutation burden: leading immunotherapy to the era of precision medicine? J Clin Oncol Off J Am Soc Clin Oncol 36(7):631–632
Stoelcker B, Ruhland B, Hehlgans T, Bluethmann H, Luther T, Mannel DN (2000) Tumor necrosis factor induces tumor necrosis via tumor necrosis factor receptor type 1-expressing endothelial cells of the tumor vasculature. Am J Pathol 156(4):1171–1176
Sukumar M, Liu J, Mehta GU, Patel SJ, Roychoudhuri R, Crompton JG, Klebanoff CA, Ji Y, Li P, Yu Z, Whitehill GD (2016) Mitochondrial membrane potential identifies cells with enhanced stemness for cellular therapy. Cell Metab 23(1):63–76
Sutlu T, Alici E (2009) Natural killer cell-based immunotherapy in cancer: current insights and future prospects. Intern Med 266(2):154–181
Tesar BM, Chalasani G, Smith-Diggs L, Baddoura FK, Lakkis FG, Goldstein DR (2004) Direct antigen presentation by a xenograft induces immunity independently of secondary lymphoid organs. J Immunol 173(7):4377–4386
Thandra KC, Barsouk A, Saginala K, Aluru JS, Barsouk A (2021) Epidemiology of lung cancer. Contemp Oncol (Pozn) 25(1):45–52. https://doi.org/10.5114/wo.2021.103829. Epub 2021 Feb 23. PMID: 33911981; PMCID: PMC8063897
The Cancer Genome Atlas Research Network (2014) Comprehensive molecular profiling of lung adenocarcinoma. Nature 511:543–550. https://doi.org/10.1038/nature13385
The Global Cancer Observatory WHO (2020) International agency for research on cancer
Theocharis S, Kanelli H, Politi E et al (2002) Expression of peroxisome proliferator activated receptor-gamma in non small cell lung carcinoma: correlation with histological type and grade. Lung Cancer 36:249–255
Titov A, Zmievskaya E, Ganeeva I, Valiullina A, Petukhov A, Rakhmatullina A, Miftakhova R, Fainshtein M, Rizvanov A, Bulatov E (2021) Adoptive immunotherapy beyond CAR T-cells. Cancers 13:743
Torre LA, Siegel RL, Jemal A (2016) Lung cancer statistics. Adv Exp Med Biol 893:1–19. https://www.cancer.org/cancer/lung-cancer/about/key-statistics.html
Trapani JA, Davis J, Sutton VR, Smyth MJ (2000) Proapoptotic functions of cytotoxic lymphocyte granule constituents in vitro and in vivo. Curr Opin Immunol. 12(3):323–329
Trifari S, Kaplan CD, Tran EH, Crellin NK, Spits H (2009) Identification of a human helper T cell population that has abundant production of interleukin 22 and is distinct from TH-17, TH1 and TH2 cells. Nat Immunol 10(8):864–871
van der Waart AB, van de Weem NM, Maas F, Kramer CS, Kester MG, Falkenburg JF, Schaap N, Jansen JH, van der Voort R, Gattinoni L, Hobo W (2014) Inhibition of Akt signaling promotes the generation of superior tumor-reactive T cells for adoptive immunotherapy. Blood 124(23):3490–3500
Van Mierlo GJ, Boonman ZF, Dumortier HM, den Boer AT, Fransen MF, Nouta J et al (2004) Activation of dendritic cells that cross-present tumor-derived antigen licenses CD8+ CTL to cause tumor eradication. Immunology 173(11):6753–6759
Vansteenkiste J, Zielinski M, Linder A, Dahabreh J, Gonzalez EE, Malinowski W et al (2013) Adjuvant MAGE-A3 immunotherapy in resected non-small-cell lung cancer: phase II randomized study results. Clin Oncol 31(19):2396–2403
Végran F, Apetoh L, Ghiringhelli F (2015) Th9 cells: a novel CD4 T-cell subset in the immune war against cancer. Cancer Res 75(3):475–479
Vicent S, Garayoa M, Lopez-Picazo JM et al (2004) Mitogen activated protein kinase phosphatase-1 is overexpressed in nonsmall cell lung cancer and is an independent predictor of outcome in patients. Clin Cancer Res 10:3639–3649

Wang X, Rivière I (2016) Clinical manufacturing of CAR T cells: foundation of a promising therapy. Mol Ther Oncolytics 3:16015. https://doi.org/10.1038/mto.2016.15
WCRF International (2022) Lung cancer statistics [internet] [cited 2023 Apr 4]. https://www.wcrf.org/cancer-trends/lung-cancer-statistics/
Wei X, Lai Y, Li J, Qin L, Xu Y, Zhao R, Li B, Lin S, Wang S, Wu Q, Liang Q (2017) PSCA and MUC1 in non-small-cell lung cancer as targets of chimeric antigen receptor T cells. Onco Targets Ther 6(3):e1284722
Wheeler DL, Dunn EF, Harari PM (2010) Understanding resistance to EGFR inhibitors: impact on future treatment strategies. Nat Rev Clin Oncol 7:493–507. Understanding EGFR mutation and drug resistance is important for future chemotherapy
Wheeler DL, Lida M, Kruser TJ et al (2009) Epidermal growth factor receptor cooperates with Src family kinases in acquired resistance to cetuximab. Cancer Biol Ther 8:696–703
Wortzel RDC, Philipps HS (1983) Multiple tumor-specific antigens expressed on a single tumour cell. Nature 304:165–167
Wu J, Lanier LL (2003) Natural killer cells and cancer. Adv Cancer Res 90:127–156
Yan W, Hu H, Tang B (2019) Advances of chimeric antigen receptor T cell therapy in ovarian cancer. Onco Targets Ther 12:8015
Yang J, Wang Y, Wong C (2010) Estrogen related receptor alpha inverse agonist XCT-790 arrests A549 lung cancer cell population growth by inducing mitochondrial reactive oxygen species production. Cell Prolif 43:103–113
Yatabe Y, Mitsudomi T (2007) Mutation of the epidermal growth factor receptor gene and related genes as determinant of growth factor receptor tyrosine kinase inhibitors sensitivity in lung cancer. Cancer Sci 98:1817–1824
Zetterberg C, Öfverholm T (1999) Carpal tunnel syndrome and other wrist/hand symptoms and signs in male and female car assembly workers. Int J Ind Ergon 23(3):193–204
Zhang C, Liu J, Zhong JF, Zhang X (2017a) Engineering CAR-T cells. Biomark Res 5:22. https://doi.org/10.1186/s40364-017-0102-y
Zhang C, Wang Z, Yang Z, Wang M, Li S, Li Y, Zhang R, Xiong Z, Wei Z, Shen J, Luo Y (2017b) Phase I escalating-dose trial of CAR-T therapy targeting CEA+ metastatic colorectal cancers. Mol Ther 25(5):1248–1258
Zheng YZ, Ma R, Zhou JK, Guo CL, Wang YS, Li ZG, Liu LX, Peng Y (2016) ROR1 is a novel prognostic biomarker in patients with lung adenocarcinoma. Sci Rep 6(1):36447
Zhong XS, Matsushita M, Plotkin J, Riviere I, Sadelain M (2010) Chimeric antigen receptors combining 4-1BB and CD28 signaling domains augment PI3kinase/AKT/Bcl-XL activation and CD8+ T cell–mediated tumor eradication. Mol Ther 18(2):413–420
Zhou B, Zang R, Zhang M, Song P, Liu L, Bie F, Peng Y, Bai G, Gao S (2022) Worldwide burden and epidemiological trends of tracheal, bronchus, and lung cancer: a population-based study. EBioMedicine 78:103951
Zitvogel L, Apetoh L, Ghiringhelli F, André F, Tesniere A, Kroemer G (2008) The anticancer immune response: indispensable for therapeutic success? Clin Invest 118(6):1991–2001

LAG-3 Inhibitors for the Treatment of Lung Cancer

8

Kaustubhi Sankpal, Saurabh Morparia, Vasanti Suvarna, and Manikanta Murahari

8.1 Introduction

Lung cancer is largely renowned as the leading cancer death contributor in the globe (Bray et al. 2018). Both small-cell lung cancer (SCLC) and non-small-cell lung cancer (NSCLC) are included in lung cancers. These are mainly over 85% cases of NSCLC. Despite there being certain improvements, however, statistics indicate that not greater than two in every ten cases of children with NSCLS live for up to 5 years after being diagnosed—implying a remarkably high rate of deaths, which are associated with this cancer disease (Li et al. 2019). With the help of modern techniques such as next-generation sequencing, mouse models of lung cancer, and human tumor databases, our understanding of the nature of the disease becomes more accurate. These methods ensure easier understanding since they are more advanced than what would be required to examine tissue specimen using a microscope (Li et al. 2019). There are several treatment options that can be applied in NSCLC including radiation therapy, chemotherapy, surgery, and targeted therapies. Yet, its effects on patient results have been limited. The term "immunotherapy" was used in a new approach that aimed at increasing our understanding of tumor immunology (Bray et al. 2018; Li et al. 2019).

The recent breakthroughs in immunotherapy focus on hitting specifically defined immune checkpoints, which are key determinants for whether any foreign body will be accepted or not by the immune system of a person (Li et al.

K. Sankpal · S. Morparia · V. Suvarna
Department of Pharmaceutical Analysis, Dr. Bhanuben Nanavati College of Pharmacy, Mumbai, Maharashtra, India

M. Murahari (✉)
Department of Pharmacy, Koneru Lakshmaiah Education Foundation, Vaddeswaram, Andhra Pradesh, India

S. Bhatt et al. (eds.), *Immunotherapy Against Lung Cancer*,
https://doi.org/10.1007/978-981-99-7141-1_8

2019). Intervention effectivity has been demonstrated in reducing immunosuppression and enhancing tumor killing capacity of T lymphocytes among lung cancer victim population. Suppression of suppressor receptors like CTLA-4 and PD-1 are immune checkpoint molecules that produce immune response against neoplasma/cancer cells (Bray et al. 2018). Recently, lymphocyte activation gene-3 (LAG −3) or CD223/FDC protein was discovered to be an immune checkpoint receptor. The initial findings were discovered by prominent French immunologist, Frederic Triebel, and his research party in 1990 (Triebel et al. 1990). This type I integral membrane protein plays a vital role within the IgSF family found on chromosome 12. It has various compartments including membrane, extracellular, and cytosol domains (Triebel 2003). Several human tumor types exhibited a correlation between the expression of LAG −3 and prognosis. Increased expression of LAG-3 was detected in clear cell leukemia, NSCLC, primary neuroendocrine lymphoma (PCNSL), hepatocellular carcinoma (HCC), and tumors to the nervous system. There is evidence that it may indicate emotions (Darvin et al. 2018).

Both effector and regulatory T cells show LAG-3 on their surface. It is known that such cell types play great role in the regulation of signaling pathways between T lymphocytes and APCs involved into adaptation immune response working (Maruhashi et al. 2020). LAG-3 along with CTLA-4 and PD-1/PD-L1 was found expressed in CD8 and CD4 T cells when subjected to long-term antigenic stimulation; however, naive T cells did not show such induction (Qin et al. 2019).

Since LAG-3 acts as an inhibitor within immune cells, it necessitates the use of antibody medications or small chemical inhibitors. However, prolonged infection may lead to chronic exposure to antigen resulting in elevated expression of LAG-3 and some other inhibitory core receptors on both CD8 and CD4 T cells (Anderson et al. 2016).

When T cells are exhausted, they show significant reduction in their powerful effector function, which, as a consequence, results in lowering tumor-associated mortality rate and response, as well as increase in immunosuppressive activity of regulatory T cells (Tregs) (Anderson et al. 2016). Study demonstrated that preventing the expression of LAG −3 resulted into normalcy of T-cell cytotoxicity and decreased immunosuppression by regulatory T cells, which consequently increased effectiveness during the fight against cancer. An additive inhibitory effect results when LAG-3 blockade is administered simultaneously with anti-PD-1/PD-L1 in cancer cells. It is such an impact that includes suppression of Treg functioning, enhancement of dendritic cell mature stage, and normalization of CD4+ or CD8+ T cells. LAG-3 is known as a prognostic tumor marker that is already undergoing clinical trials in association with other well-established targets such as PD-1/PD-L1, and CTLA-4 making it applicable for other than established targets (Ruffo et al. 2019; Puhr and Ilhan-Mutlu 2019).

8.2 Structure and Functions of LAG-3

LAG3 proteins are in lipid rafts, which are unique intracellular microdomains, containing multiple factors such as CD4, CD8, and CD3. LAG-3 molecule consists of three distinct domains, namely the transmembrane, extracellular region, and cytoplasmic regions. LAG-3, a protein found in the cytoplasm, is secreted from the cell by the enzymatic activity of the metalloproteinase ADAM10/17 in its transmembrane domain. LAG-3 extracellular domain is involved in the interaction with ligands and causes the formation of four immunoglobulin superfamily (IgSF) domains, namely D1, D2, D3, and D4. Particularly, D1 belonging to the V immunoglobulin superfamily is distinguished by a proline-rich loop domain and a disulfide link in the chain. This region exhibits specific characteristics. D2, D3, and D4 are members of the C2 family. The cytoplasmic domain of LAG-3 contains three essential elements: the serine phosphorylation site S454, a conserved motif called "KIEELE," and the EP sequence, which serves as a target for protein kinase C (Huard et al. 1997; Wang et al. 2001).

The KIEELE motif plays a key role in the operation of LAG-3; nevertheless, any mutation occurring in the gene results in a full obstruction of its activity. The LAG-3 protein is found on the external membrane of T cells, NK cells, B cells, and DCs, and it exerts a negative regulatory influence on T-cell function under physiological circumstances (Workman et al. 2002). Research has indicated that there is a restricted number of lymphocytes expressing LAG-3 (lymphocyte-activation gene 3) in inflamed lymphoid organs, such as tonsils or lymph nodes (Huard et al. 1994). The presence of LAG-3 on lymphocytes that have infiltrated tumors, a pathological state, has been observed to have a clear correlation with the development and advancement of human tumors such as NSCLC and HCC (McLane et al. 2019; Ma et al. 2017; Hald et al. 2018). LAG-3 protein plays a significant role in the regulation of T-cell function, thus contributing to immune homeostasis and facilitating autoimmune evasion of tumor cells in the diseases. Consequently, it has important potential as a useful alternative for the treatment of resistant tumors (Fig. 8.1, Table 8.1).

There are four major LAG ligands in the tumor microenvironment, namely galectin-3, MHC II, FGL1, and LSECtin (Huard et al. 1997). Major histocompatibility complex II abbreviated as MHC II is an important ligand with higher affinity for LAG-3 binding than CD4. This observation suggests that competitive binding occurs between CD4 and LAG −3 molecules. In accordance with previous studies, the intracellular domain of LAG −3 was shown to function to suppress signal transduction. It does this by transmission of inhibitory signals to the cytoplasmic domain and not by disrupting the association between MHC II and CD4 (Huard et al. 1995; Weber and Karjalainen 1993). Galectin-3, a soluble lectin, has a molecular weight of 31 kilodaltons (kDa) and acts as a ligand for LAG −3. This particular lectin has the ability to interact with LAG −3 to regulate T-cell responses. The results of

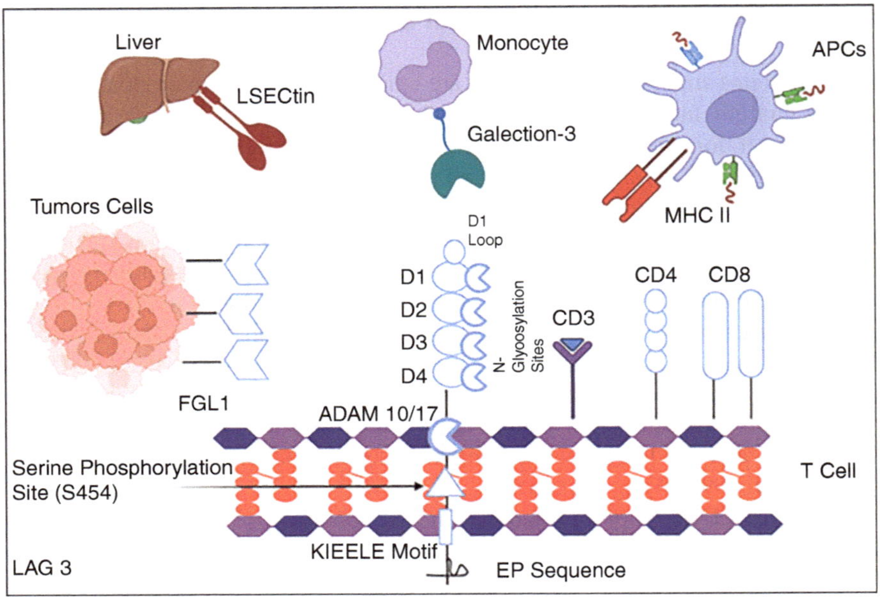

Fig. 8.1 LAG-3 Structure and Ligands

Table 8.1 Analysis of the emergence of immunological checkpoint molecules and their corresponding ligands

Proteins	Location of the gene (human)	Cell Expression	Ligand	Presenting cell	Effect on immune system
LAG-3	Chromosome 12p13.32 is a crucial chromosome in the human genome	T cells NK B-cells DCs	MHC II Galactine-3 LSECtin FGL-1	APC Soluble Tumor cells Soluble	Decreased Th1 cell activation, proliferation, and cytokine secretion

in vitro experiments show a significant impact of LAG −3 on the suppression of IFN-g production by CD8+ T lymphocytes through the involvement of galectin-3 (Liu et al. 2004; Dumic et al. 2006). LSECtin, a putative ligand for LAG −3, shows predominant expression in hepatic organs and malignant melanoma cells (Liu et al. 2004). The contact of LSECtin and LAG-3 initiates tumor development by attenuating the immunological response of anti-tumor T lymphocytes in melanoma-type cells (Xu et al. 2014). FGL1, a ligand for LAG-3, shows efficacy in inhibiting immune responses without interference by muscle homologous complex II (MHC II), and this inhibition is achieved through specific interactions between FGL1 and D1 and D2 domains of LAG-3 (Wang et al. 2019). A new study provided evidence that the association between LAG-3 and MHC II inhibits T-cell function, thereby activating tumor body immunity. Ligands not yet identified for LAG-3 may be involved in this interaction (Maruhashi et al. 2020).

8.2.1 Expression of LAG-3

The LAG3 protein is present on activated T and NK-type cells in humans (Triebel et al. 1990). The marker induces activation of CD4 and CD8 T cells, which become detectable within 24 h following stimulation. The levels of activated T cells reach their highest point at 48 h and subsequently decline by the eighth day in mice (Workman et al. 2002). Chronic inflammatory situations, such as tumors or viral infections, have the capacity to elicit T-cell malfunction through the activation of LAG3 and other immunological checkpoint receptors (Zarour 2016). In the quiescent state, regulatory T cells (Tregs) originating from the thymus exhibit minimal expression of LAG3, which subsequently rises upon their activation. According to one study, transfer of HA TCR transgenic CD4-specific T cells into C3-HA mice resulted in the generation of HA-CD4 T-cell tolerance, which exhibited properties of induced regulatory T cells (Tregs). These Tregs showed high expression of LAG3 and proved to be strong regulatory (Huang et al. 2004). The expression of LAG3 has been seen to be more pronounced in tumors among individuals diagnosed with human cancer, hence aiding in the selective elimination of regulatory T cells (Tregs) in various subtypes of tumors. The disputed nature of the role played by LAG3 and other immunological checkpoint receptors on regulatory T cells (Tregs) in relation to fatigue and functionality has prompted extensive research aimed at figuring out its translational significance. The proposed definition of a subpopulation of IL10 CD4 type-1 T regulatory cells involves the utilization of LAG3 and CD49b markers (Gagliani et al. 2013). Cells can produce interleukin-10 (IL-10), a cytokine that shows a key function in the immune system. LAG3/CD49b, a specific marker used to identify and study these cells, is commonly used to detect IL-10 secretion. Recent research has revealed that there is a dynamic expression of LAG3 and other immune checkpoint receptors. The role of LAG3 in Tr1 function is to negate its suppressive effect upon inhibition (Gagliani et al. 2013; White and Wraith 2016). A significant proportion (18%) of γδ T cells exhibit the expression of LAG3, while TCRγδ intraepithelial lymphocytes (IEL) contain considerable levels of LAG3 mRNA (Workman et al. 2002; Fahrer et al. 2001). The expression of LAG3 in TCRαβCD8αα intraepithelial lymphocytes (IEL) remains undetermined; however, it is observed to be higher compared to TCRαβCD8αβ IEL or spleen. The expression of LAG3 is contingent upon T-cell activation by B cells (Kisielow et al. 2005).

LAG3 is a protein found on various hematopoietic type cells, containing plasmacytoid dendritic cells (pDCs), which express it at higher levels than other subset (Workman et al. 2009). Resting pDCs show a 70-fold growth in Lag3 mRNA related to T cells, but CpG activation does not increase Lag3 mRNA expression in pDCs (Workman et al. 2002; Fahrer et al. 2001). LAG3 mRNA was found in the red pulp of the spleen, expressed on NK type cells and invariant NKT cells, even though its implication remains unclear (Workman et al. 2002).

Lag3 mRNA is present in the thymic medulla and cerebellum, where it shows binding affinity toward α-synuclein fibrils, thereby starting endocytosis within neurons (Mao et al. 2016). The pathogenesis of Parkinson's disease may be due to propagation of misfolded α-synuclein fibers between neighboring cells. Inhibition of LAG3 is currently under investigation as a potential treatment for Parkinson's disease.

8.2.2 The LAG3 Signaling

Unlike other IRs, LAG3 possesses a cytoplasmic domain with a pattern of glutamic acid and proline dipeptide repeats; this may be important in its signal transduction process (Mastrangeli et al. 1996). Researchers have found evidence that LAG3-associated protein (LAP) binds to LAG3 and facilitates its co-localization along with CD3, CD4, and/or CD8 inside lipid rafts (Iouzalen et al. 2001; Macon-Lemaitre and Triebel 2005). Lipid rafts partition co-stimulatory molecules to enhance TCR signaling, potentially preventing excessive activation. Categorization with IRs, counting LAG3, may avoid activation, but EP motif-less LAG3 mutants keep activity (Workman et al. 2002).

The KIEELE motif, a conserved lysine residue in primates, mice, and rats, is crucial for LAG3 activity (Workman et al. 2002). The unique motif in LAG3 could potentially activate an unknown signaling molecule or mechanism, prompting a top priority to understand the potential intracellular binding associates, and signaling mechanism.

LAG3 mediates bidirectional signaling to interacting APCs, and binding of MHC class-II to LAG3-expressing Tregs inhibits DC activation and suppresses their maturation (Liang et al. 2008). The ITAM inhibitory pathway, concerning FcγRγ and ERK, inhibits CD86 upregulation and IL-12 secretion. A LAG3 mutant suppresses DC function, allowing Tregs to enforce tolerance. This reverse signaling mechanism is clear in the interaction among DC and melanoma-type cells, where MHC class-II expressing melanoma-type cells are anti to Fas-mediated apoptosis through MAPK/ERK and PI3K/Akt survival pathways when unprotected to LAG3-transfected type cells (Hemon et al. 2011).

8.2.3 Immunological Functions of LAG 3

LAG-3 is a cytokine molecule that controls T-cell function by binding to MHC II, thereby reducing cytokine secretion and CD4 T-cell proliferation. Antibodies against LAG-3 can reactivate these cells, but the exact mechanism is unknown (Liu et al. 2004; Zhang et al. 2019). LAG-3 selectively binds pMHC II and inhibits CD4 T-cell reactivity to pMHC II (Maruhashi et al. 2018; Hoffmann and Slansky 2020). LAG-3 negatively affects mitochondrial function in naive CD4 T cells, important to T-cell enervation and antitumor effect (Previte et al. 2019). Fig. 8.2 shows that LAG-3 is upregulated in CD8 T cells enhanced by tumor antigens (Ascione et al. 2019). A protein called LAG-3 suppresses CD8 T cells in mice, making them more active than normal mice. This inhibition is independent of MHC II and CD4 T-type cells. Also, LAG-3 can increase activity of Treg cells and decrease the activity of T cells. It can activate Treg cells and accelerate their immune function. LAG-3 can interact with additional suppressor molecules to increase suppressive Treg cells, resulting in immune tolerance. DCs also play a vital role in tumor immune escape by promoting cell growth and activation. It can also activate NK cells (Huang et al. 2004; Okamura et al. 2018; Camisaschi et al. 2010).

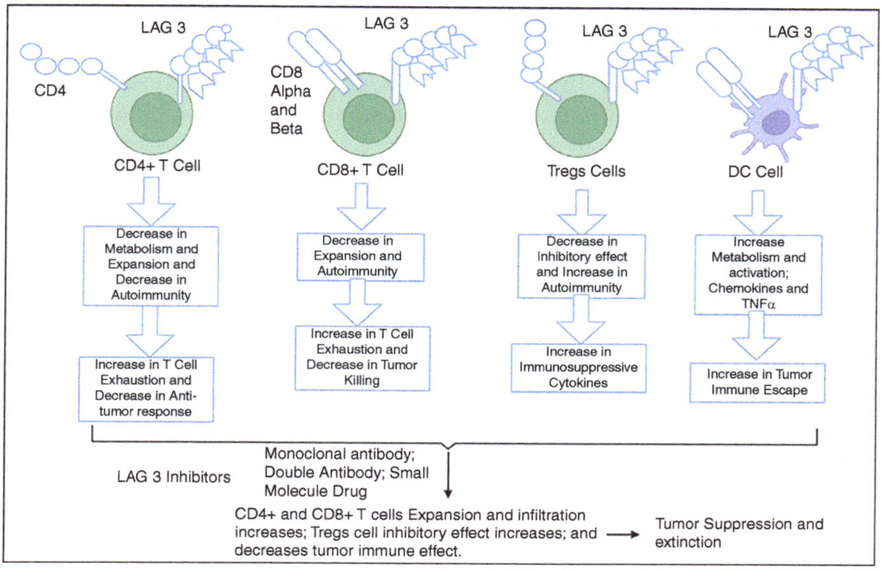

Fig. 8.2 The present research explores the functional contributions of LAG-3 in diverse cellular populations, encompassing CD4+, CD8+, Treg cells, and DC cells, within the context of tumor microenvironments

8.2.4 Roles of LAG-3 Inhibitors in Tumors

LAG-3 is a protein found on tumor-infiltrating lymphocytes (TILs) and regulates activation of T-cell, proliferation, and homeostasis. It is co-expressed along with PD-1 in the microenvironment of tumor cells, thereby suppressing T-cell function through various mechanisms. Inhibition of PD1 along with LAG3 on CD8 and CD4 TILs enhances anticancer activity in various mouse models. LAG3 brings the generation of TGF-b1 and IL-10, which contribute to tumor immune discharge (Workman and Vignali 2003). Studies have shown that inhibition of LAG-3 can reestablish T-cell activation, reactivates the immune system, reduces the immune function of Treg cells, and enhances tumor apoptosis (Melaiu et al. 2022).

Hindering LAG-3 activity and anti-PD-1 or PD-L1 on cancer cells has double inhibitory properties, i.e., slowing Treg function, inducing DC maturation, and releasing dysfunctional CD4/CD8 T cells (Jiang et al. 2021). LAG-3 is identified as a promising target for the therapy of autoimmune tumors and has proceeded to more than 80 clinical trials. LAG-3 inhibitors, including monoclonal antibodies and small molecules, target LAG-3 molecules, restore T-cell activation, and inhibit Treg cell function (Wang et al. 2019; Jiang et al. 2021; Bagchi et al. 2021).

8.3 Anti-LAG-3 Antibody-Based Therapies

Therapies targeting LAG-3 include anti-LAG-3 monoclonal antibodies, bispecific LAG-3, and Ig (Ig) immunoglobulin fusion proteins, which inhibit IL-12 and IFN generation in T-cell co-cultures (Avice et al. 1999). A monoclonal antibody against LAG −3 blocks the contact between monocytes and MHC class II, suppressing the positive signal and inhibiting the T-cell impact to IL-12. Blocking LAG-3 only cannot be the most effective treatment approach as cancer cells might evade antitumor immune responses through various molecules (Chocarro et al. 2022). Bispecific antibodies (BsAbs) are a promising area of research and medical advancement due to their flexible pathways. These antibodies direct two uncommon antigens or epitopes of the similar antigen, and full-length BsAbs with Fc-mediated immune activity demonstrate higher potential for antitumor therapy (Gandhi et al. 2006).

Clinical trials show that combining anti-LAG-3 and anti-PD-1 therapies can significantly improve antitumor effects, as LAG-3 is co-expressed along with PD-1 on CD8+ T cells, and antibody co-blockade increases cell proliferation and cytokine production (Chen and Chen 2014). A mouse study established that twin blockade of LAG −3 and PD-1 in vivo led to a substantial increase in antigen-specific CD8 T-cell numbers and purpose and a significant reduction in viral titer (Nurgalieva et al. 2021). Combining treatment with both anti-PD-1 and anti-LAG3 monoclonal antibodies showed potent antitumor activity in MHC-II expressing tumors. LAG-3 suppresses the antineoplastic effect by inhibition of CD4 T-cell effect. Treatment with ABVD has slight therapeutic benefit with increased penetration of LAG-3TILs. Clinical studies indicate that IMP321 is the simply soluble LAG-3 recombinant (Maruhashi et al. 2020; Dirix and Triebel 2019).

IMP321 is a fusion protein that joins the extracellular domain of LAG-3 to human Fc domain of immunoglobulin, interacts with MHC-II, and triggers antigen-presenting cells (APCs). This interaction induces upregulation of CD80/CD86, IL-12, TNF, and dendritic projections, unlike antagonistic LAG-3 antibodies that block this interaction. Monotherapy IMP321 with limited therapeutic benefit showed promising results when combined with cytotoxic chemotherapy and vaccination strategy. The study investigated the potential for adoptive T-cell transfer and immune modulation, with expression of TB hallmarks decreased in patients treated with IMP321. IMP321 immunization enhanced antigen-specific T lymphocyte responses and function, while selectively inhibiting Treg expansion, suggesting that an improved CD8-to-Treg effector ratio might describe positive immune effetcs (Poorebrahim et al. 2021; Sordo-Bahamonde et al. 2021) (Fig. 8.3).

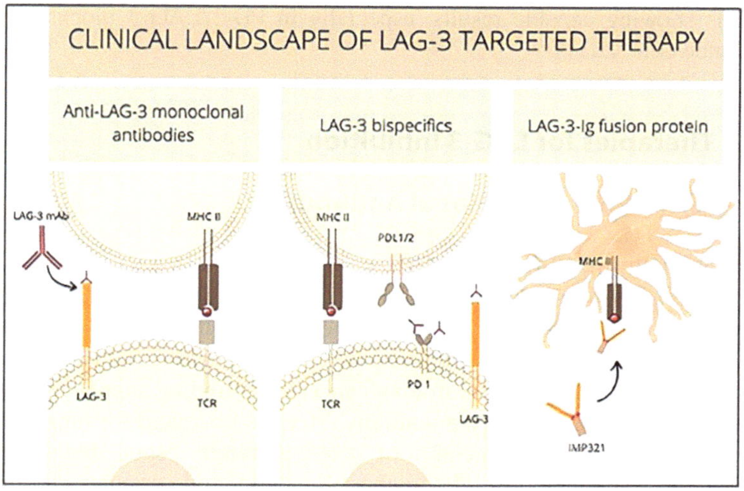

Fig. 8.3 LAG-3-targeted therapies

8.4 Anti-LAG-3 Cell-Based Therapies

The medical research community is gaining excitement about the potential of genetically engineered immune cells, specifically CAR-T cells, as a new cancer treatment method.

Researchers successfully generated LAG-3 knockout T and CAR-T cells without compromising viability and immunophenotype using the CRISPR-Cas9 system, introduced through electroporation. LAG-3 was effectively removed from both T and CAR-T cells that are strong in the essential region. The LAG-3 knockout CAR-T cells proved antigen-specific cytokine issue and antitumor strength in vitro and in vivo (Zhang et al. 2019). Blocking PD-1 and LAG-3, along with other immune checkpoint receptors, enhances CAR-T cell effector functions, suggesting that LAG-3 signaling pathways suppress antitumor effects in dysfunctional CAR-T cells (Poorebrahim et al. 2021).

Genetic modification of LAG-3 does not affect CD8 T-cell functionality, but removing expression leads to sustained antitumor activity, reduced tumor growth, and increased survival. MGD013 enhances T-cell responses beyond benchmark antibodies (Wang et al. 2019).

8.5 LAG-3 Clinical Trials with Experimental Medicine

Clinical research has shown that CD15 is expressed in various pathological conditions, including monoclonal antibodies, LAG-3-Ig fusion proteins, and specific anti-LAG-3 antibodies. Clinical Trials lists 115 trials worldwide investigating LAG-3 safety and efficacy, with IMP321 being the simply soluble recombinant LAG-3 on which trials are being conducted. Research on bispecific drugs targeting

LAG-3 is showing capable results, especially in PD-1/LAG-3 blockade (Sordo-Bahamonde et al. 2021).

8.6 Therapies for LAG-3 Inhibition

8.6.1 Anti-LAG-3 Monoclonal Antibodies

8.6.1.1 Relatlimab (BMS-986016)

Relatlimab is a new antibody that has the potential to restore T and NK cell responses in lung cancer patients by promoting cytokine production (Sordo-Bahamonde et al. 2021). The enhanced antitumor response of LAG-3 inhibitory signaling disruption has been seen in NK and T cells in lung cancer. This finding supports monoclonal antibodies targeting LAG-3 as a potentially effective treatment for lung cancer. By effectively decreasing the expression of Bcl-2, a protein responsible for stopping apoptosis, the combination of relatlimab with lenalidomide dramatically improves leukemic cells removal. Despite not directly affecting the cytotoxicity of these cells, the research shows that co-administering LAG-3 inhibitors with lenalidomide boosts the way natural killer (NK) cells derived from cancer individuals use their antibody-dependent cellular cytotoxicity (ADCC) function. This added boost comes with no surprise to researchers, as combining lenalidomide and interleukin-2 (IL-2) has already been shown to make T cells generate more IL-2 and ease ADCC. To patients with metastatic tumors who did not have any other treatments, the combination of relatlimab and nivolumab showed great results. When it came to progression-free survival, it showed better efficacy than monotherapy, which only targeted PD-1. Trials are currently underway for people with stomach or gastroesophageal junction cancer in relation to this medication mix (Brignone et al. 2009).

8.6.1.2 Nivolumab

Nivolumab is a human IgG4 antibody that specifically targets the programmed death-1 (PD-1) receptor found on T cells. By doing this, it stops the negative signaling pathways that allow PD-1 to interact with its inhibitors, PD-L1 and PD-L2. Consequently, restoration of T-cell effector function by the antibody is weak. Nivolumab has demonstrated efficacy in cancer prevention, and the breadth of evidence exceeds expectations. Patients who relapsed or demonstrated resistance to PD-1 therapy showed evidence of sustained objective response. Although it was used for treatment in patients suffering through advanced lung cancer (NSCLC), it showed a good response and was safe. Even better, they stayed longer than those on docetaxel. The main reason for this was the rapid response and tolerability of nivolumab. It is authorized for the therapy of patients suffering from metastatic NSCLC. However, there is still a need for those seeking nivolumab as a treatment. Disease progression is indeed shown following platinum-based chemotherapy and targeted therapy with tyrosine kinase inhibitors (TKIs). In addition, their genomic tumor abnormality must involve EGFR or ALK genes. Nivolumab, a therapeutic agent sanctioned by the European Union for the treatment of advanced or metastatic Non-Small Cell Lung Cancer (NSCLC), has been rigorously evaluated for its safety and efficacy. The potential benefits of Nivolumab, either as a standalone treatment or as a combination of existing standard therapies, have been assessed in the context of initial-line treatment for advanced NSCLC. This underscores its potential role in enhancing therapeutic outcomes in this patient population (Dirix and Triebel 2019; Anagnostou and Brahmer 2015).

8.6.1.3 Ipilimumab

The drug ipilimumab, which is a human immunoglobulin G and anti-CTLA-4 monoclonal antibody, was thought to increase vaccine-specific T-cell effects blocking CTLA-4 on CD8 T cells. However, no rise in the number of CD3 or CD8 T-type cells or vaccine-specific CD8 T-type cells was found in the peripheral blood. This study suggests that the enhanced CD8 T-cell effect resulting from CTLA-4 signaling blockade does not seem to be the main reason for tumor regression. Due to its unique mechanism of action and potential efficacy in NSCLC, ipilimumab may be investigated for adjuvant or neoadjuvant treatment option in early stages of the disease. It could also be considered for maintenance therapy after induction chemotherapy or for unresectable stage III disease. Future research should explore ipilimumab in early or later stage of advanced lung cancer, alongside other immunotherapies targeting LAG-3 and consider biomarker research for personalized and optimized use in NSCLC (Anagnostou and Brahmer 2015).

8.6.1.4 Pembrolizumab (MK-3475)

Pembrolizumab is a type of medication known to be selective, humanized IgG4 kappa isotype monoclonal antibody. It targets PD-1, a protein found on certain cells in immune system. By blocking PD-1, pembrolizumab helps to activate the body's immune response with tumor cells. It is commonly used as a first choice of treatment for non-squamous cancer that has metastasized and does not have specific gene mutations. Additionally, pembrolizumab can be combined with other drugs such as carboplatin and paclitaxel or an albumin-stabilized nanoparticle formulation for the treatment of squamous cell cancer or used alone for cancers expressing the PD-L1 protein. It may also be prescribed for patients with stage III cancer who are unable to undergo surgery, chemotherapy, or radiation therapy, as well as those whose cancer has spread to other parts of the body (Anagnostou and Brahmer 2015).

8.6.2 Anti-LAG-3 Bispecific

8.6.2.1 Tebotelimab (Formerly MGD013)

Tebotelimab (MGD013) is a bispecific antibody, which specifically targets the PD-1 and LAG-3 genes on chronically activated T type cells (Wang et al. 2020; Wang-Gillam et al. 2013). Tebotelimab treatment significantly boosts serum IFN levels, resulting in increased circulating CD3CD8 and CD3CD4-CD8 T-cell subpopulations and cytolytic markers like perforin and granzyme B (Jenkins et al. 2021). Tebotelimab is an experimental DART molecule that blocks LAG −3 and PD-1 checkpoint molecules to restore T-cell function in lung cancer treatment. Combination with monoclonal antibodies targeting these immune checkpoints may enhance clinical activity. Tebotelimab is a drug that targets LAG −3 and PD-1 to disrupt non-redundant inhibitory pathways, restoring function to depleted T cells (Wang et al. 2020; Wang-Gillam et al. 2013).

8.6.2.2 RO7247669

RO7247669 is a novel PD1-LAG3 bispecific antibody that offers dual checkpoint block through great affinity for monovalent binding to both PD-1 and LAG-3, enhancing avidity-mediated selectivity improvement (Brignone et al. 2010). This IgG1 bispecific antibody, with a silent Fc region, blocks the communication of PD-1 with PD-L1, PD-L2 and LAG-3 with MHCII, reviving damaged T cells and overcoming LAG3-assisted resistance to checkpoint blockers, resulting in a cytotoxic T lymphocyte–persuaded immune response alongside tumor cells (Jiang et al. 2021).

8.6.3 Soluble LAG-3–Ig Fusion Proteins: Eftilagimod Alpha

Eftilagimod alpha, a solvable form of LAG-3, is an unfamiliar immune checkpoint blocker that directs APCs, induces an MHC-II-facilitated feedback signal. IMP321 boosts T-cell proliferation, and induces a fully Tc1-activated phenotype, resulting in the generation of various cytokines (Brignone et al. 2009; Brignone et al. 2010). It enhances the production of CCL4 and TNF- by myeloid cells, as well as IFN- and TNF- by CD8 and NK cells. Efti binds to MHC class molecules II in lipid rafts of plasma membrane on immature human dendritic cells, causing rapid morphological changes, dendritic projection formation, and upregulating costimulatory molecules expression and IL-12 and TNF- production. Efti has been found to keep the formation and expansion of tumor antigen-specific CD8 T lymphocytes in lung cancer patients, thereby enhancing their ex vivo CD8 T-cell memory response. Pembrolizumab, an immune checkpoint inhibitor, aims to enhance activity by combining efti's activating effect on immune cells with its inhibitory effects by disrupting the PD-1/PD-L1 axis (Brignone et al. 2010).

8.7 LAG3 Inhibition and Evaluation of Targeting Agents in Lung Cancer Trials

Figure 8.4 verifies that LAG3 regulates T-cell proliferation, cytokine assembly, and cytolytic activity through its cytoplasmic domain. Despite its complexity, its function is known to depend on the recognition of complex complexes of peptide-MHC-II (Maruhashi et al. 2018). LAG3 expression indicates an active immune response in inflammatory environments such as the tumor microenvironment. Targeting LAG3 is important because of preexisting immune responses. \Peptide-MHC-II complexes form after IFN release activation, and LAG3 expression depends on activation, forming the basis for clinical targeting (Lui & Davis. 2018). Combining LAG3 with anti-PD-1 or anti-PD-L1 agents in cancer subjects has been shown to inhibit Treg activities, promote DC maturation, and rescue dysfunctional CD4 Th TIL and CD8 CTL TIL, as shown in Fig. 8.5.

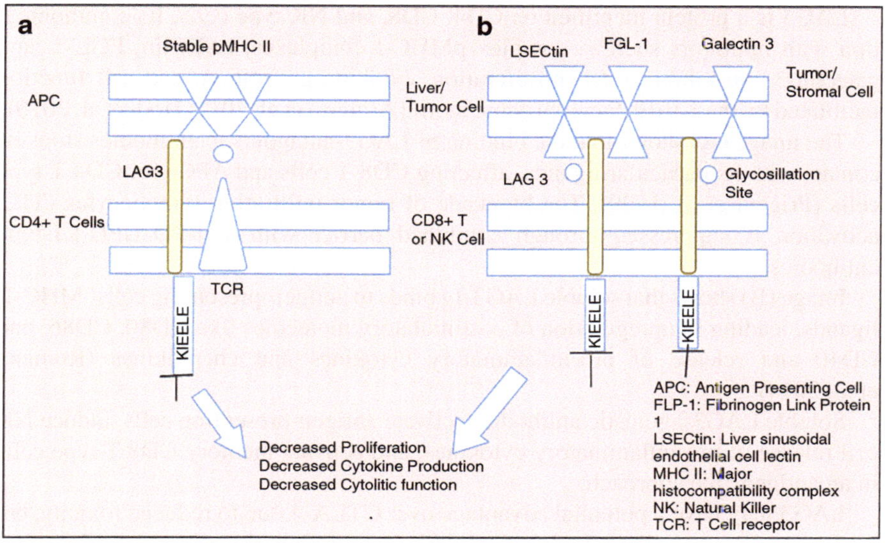

Fig. 8.4 The study delves into the molecular mechanisms of the function of LAG3

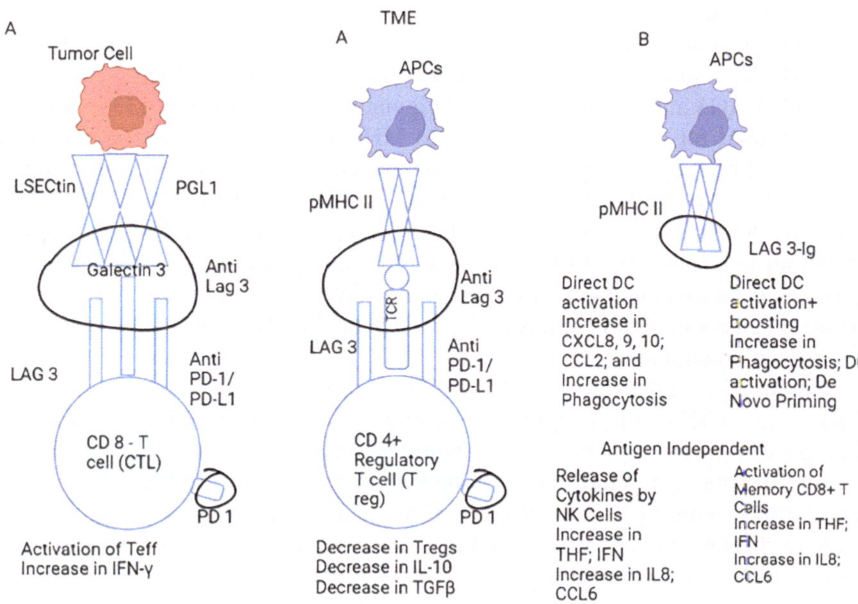

Fig. 8.5 The figure shows the activation of antigen-presenting cells by LAG3 antagonistic antibodies and soluble LAG3 immunoglobulin (Ig) targeting effector-regulatory T cells

LAG3 is a protein identified on CD4, CD8, and NK type cells. Its communication with inhibitors such as complex pMHC-I complexes, LSECtin, FGL-1, and galectin-3 can inhibit T-cell proliferation, cytokine generation, and cell function facilitated by the KIEELE cytoplasmic motif (Ascierto et al. 2017; Hodi et al. 2010).

The image (A) shows that the binding of LAG3-antagonistic antibodies stops its contact with its particular ligands, affecting CD8 T cells and APCs for CD4 T type cells (Prigent et al. 1999). The blockade of tumor-infiltrating lymphocytes (TIL) activation is suppressed through combined barrier with anti-PD-1/PD-L1-type antibodies.

Image (B) shows that soluble LAG3-Ig binds to antigen-presenting cells' MHC-II ligands, leading to upregulation of costimulatory molecules like CD80, CD86, and CD40 and release of pro-inflammatory cytokines and chemokines (Romano et al. 2014).

Soluble LAG3-agonistic antibodies activate antigen-presenting cells, induce NK cell release of pro-inflammatory cytokines, and activate memory CD8 T-type cells in an antigen-free approach.

LAG3 may have a potential advantage over CTLA-4 due to reduced toxicity, but further studies and clinical trials are needed to confirm this. Currently, LAG3 is under clinical investigation in patients cured with PD-1/PD-L1 antagonists, and pilot data in cancer affected patients have demonstrated the efficacy of these two agents. Further research and clinical trials are needed to compare these targets. The combination of CTLA-4 and nivolumab, an anti-PD-1 agent, shows greater activity and efficacy in immunocompromised patients, but also increases the incidence of immune-related adverse events.

Table 8.2 shows several clinical trials of agents targeting LAG −3, including the first IMP321, a soluble recombinant dimer protein with four extracellular domains in soluble LAG3 immunoglobulin (Ig). Originally developed as a LAG3 antagonist, it is now used for high-affinity binding to MHC-II of antigen-presenting cells. It serves as an immunoadjuvant for activation, which is expressed in mature dendritic cells. Preliminary studies indicate that LAG3-Ig, which interacts with MHC-II in immature dendritic cells, upregulates CD80/86, produces IL2 and TNF, and induces deviations in metabolism IMP321, a receptor for antigens cross-demonstration to T cells was enhanced and CD8 Ma T-cell activation retorts were evaluated as monotherapy or in combination with pembrolizumab or chemotherapy, and showed little activity with monotherapy.

Immunoassay targets such as PD-1, PD-L1, CTLA-4, and LAG-3 can be used alone or in combination with a LAG-3 inhibitor, where their inhibitory molecules are blocked immune response LAG-3 inhibitors orally, in which both LAG-3 and its ligand block the interaction, they can replace the purpose of depleted T-type cells and restore immunity to cancer cells. Combination therapies targeting multiple immune checkpoints, like LAG-3 and PD-1, may have higher clinical activity compared to targeting a single checkpoint (Wang-Gillam et al. 2013).

EMB-02 is a Phase I/II clinical trial measuring the safety and tolerability of a bispecific monoclonal antibody targeting PD -1/LAG −3 for metastatic colorectal cancer patients. This study has been initiated aiming at determining MTD and

Table 8.2 Presents a clinical trial involving LAG-3 inhibitors for treating lung cancer

Agents	Phase	Tumor type	Primary end point
Combination of IMP321 and pembrolizumab (anti-PD-1)	II	Untreated, unresectable, or metastatic NSCLC is a serious health issue that requires immediate attention and treatment	Objective response rate
EMB-02 is a bispecific mAb that specifically targets PD-1/LAG-3	I/II	Advanced solid tumors are a growing concern in the medical field	Adverse effects, objective response rate
Combination of Relatlimab (anti-LAG-3 mAb), Nivolumab, and BMS-986205 (IDO1 inhibitor) or Ipilimumab	I/II	Advanced malignant tumors are a growing concern in the medical field	The study examines the impact of adverse effects, the objective response rate, and the median duration of response
RO7247669 is a bispecific antibody that specifically targets PD-1/LAG3	I	Advanced and/or metastatic NSCLC	The objective response rate, duration of response, and progression-free survival are crucial factors to consider
SRF388 is an anti-IL-27 mAb	I/Ib	Advanced NSCLC is a type of cancer treatment that involves the use of advanced technology to treat several types of cancer	The objective response rate is a crucial factor to consider when evaluating the potential negative effects of a particular action.
Combination of Eftilagimod alpha and Pembrolizumab	II	Untreated, unresectable, or metastatic NSCLC is a type of cancer that cannot be treated or resectable	Objective response rate
The antibody TSR-033 is a combination of anti-LAG-3 and anti-PD-1	I	Advanced NSCLC is a type of cancer treatment that involves the use of advanced technology to treat several types of cancer	Safety, objective response rate, dose-limiting toxicities

RP2D for these advanced tumor patients. The study will also assess the immunogenicity and antitumor activity of the antibody.

Early exploratory data on the combination of LAG3 and PD –1 showed 11% response rate among those with metastatic cancer who were unsuccessful at PD-1/PD-L1 treatment. The data indicate that LAG3 may be an effective biomarker for selecting patients for treatment. Relatlimab, an investigating drug, has been showing great improvement in progression-free survival (PFS) when used alongside nivolumab for treating NSCLC. At present, therefore, this drug is under investigation for its use as the first treatment option in advanced cases of NSCLC (Sordo-Bahamonde et al. 2021).

Results from a large-scale clinical trial have shown promising efficacy of combination therapy for lung cancer. The study evaluated four different treatment options: nivolumab, ipilimumab, nivolumab monotherapy, and chemotherapy. Patients who received any of these treatments had a median overall survival (OS) of 17.1 months for PD-L1 positive NSCLC. It is worth noting that the combination therapy was approved by the FDA, indicating its superiority over chemotherapy alone. The trial also included patients with NSCLC who had not received prior therapy, regardless of their PD-L1 expression or tumor histology. This comprehensive approach involved dual checkpoint blockade alongside chemotherapy to maximize effectiveness. The trial group achieved a median overall survival (OS) of 15.6 months, prolonged progression-free survival (PFS), and improved response rate (RR). Furthermore, in 2020, the Food and Drug Administration approved this treatment but is not used in patients.

This study was designed to measure the efficacy, safety, and pharmacokinetics of RO7247669 in grouping with pembrolizumab in patients with untreated, locally advanced, non-small-cell lung cancer.

The study is a phase 1/1b clinical trial, which is an open-label study. The study was conducted to evaluate the safety and efficacy of SRF388, a monoclonal antibody specifically targeting IL-27. This is the first human study to include a subsequent dosing and expansion phase. The study was conducted in three phases, focusing on the efficacy of monotherapy and in grouping for subjects with solid tumors. The study was conducted to assess the safety, tolerability, drug delivery bioactivity (PK), pharmacokinetics, and efficacy of SRF388 as monotherapy in patients with advanced lung cancer.

The objective of the phase B observation was to evaluate protection, efficacy, tolerability, and pharmacokinetics as monotherapy in subjects with clean mobile renal cell carcinoma (ccRCC), hepatocellular carcinoma (HCC), and NSCLC in specific subgroup.

Phase C was steered to evaluate the safety, efficacy, tolerability, and pharmacokinetics (PK) of SRF388 in combination with pembrolizumab on patients with advanced lung cancer (NSCLC).

The safety and efficacy of soluble fusion protein LAG −3 eftilagimod alpha were assessed in combination with pembrolizumab in the therapy of patients with NSCLC which showed a remarkable response, suggesting a potentially compelling treatment combination. The first phase of the study, Phase 1, gradually ramps up the dose to determine the optimal dose of TSR-033 in Phase 2, as stand-alone therapy and in combination with dostarlimab.

The objective of phase 2A is to investigate the antitumor efficacy of the combination of TSR-033 and dostarlimab in subjects with advanced cancer. Phase 2B was conducted to measure the safety and efficacy for combination of TSR-033-dostarlimab and bevacizumab in humans with advanced or metastatic lung cancer.

The potential of LAG3 antagonists as drug conjugates in immunotherapy trials aimed at blocking the PD-1/PD-L1 molecular pathway is currently being explored by proof-of-concept pretreatment showing synergy with PD -1 inhibitors supporting this approach. A number of Fc domain–containing antibodies can specifically bind LAG3 in humans and mice. This binding ability allows for effective inhibition of the interface involving LAG3 and MHC-II molecules. In addition, these antibodies have demonstrated to stimulate IL-2 making upon activation of T cells.

8.8 Conclusion

The potential of LAG3 inhibitors as effective targets for cancer immunity is noteworthy because of their ability to increase tumor-infiltrating lymphocytes (TILs) proliferation and cytokine secretion. This enhances the immune response against tumors against lung cancer. An important role is highlighted. Several LAG3 inhibitors are currently being developed and are being investigated in clinical trials. However, our understanding of the functional properties of LAG-3 is incomplete and requires further exploration in cancer immunotherapy. The limited benefit of monotherapy with anti-LAG3 therapy has been demonstrated, thus demonstrating the potential for synergistic approaches involving the addition of inhibitors, which is good. The use of LAG-3 inhibitors has been extensively studied in lung cancer clinical trials, typically in combination with CTLA-4 or PD-1/PD-L1 antagonists. Based on clinical data, initial treatment responses to the monoclonal antibody LAG-3 have been found to be poor.

Clinical data from phase I trials of the LAG-3 monoclonal antibody reveal a relatively low objective response rate of 6% in patients with solid tumors who experienced treatment failure with therapies and have been previously internalized in addition to a 17% diagnosis rate. The principal objective of this study was to measure the efficacy of combination strategies involving LAG-3 and PD-1 in combination with a bifunctional monoclonal antibody. This study is particularly important due to short-term reports for combination therapies specifically targeting these proteins.

Concomitant use of anti-LAG3 antibodies with PD-1 and LAG3 has been shown to increase tolerance, increase objective response rate (ORR), extend progression-free survival, and reduce the risk of death. However, further investigation is essential to comprehend the precise efficacy related to this treatment.

The comprehension of the functional characteristics of LAG-3 holds the potential to ease the advancement of innovative therapeutic approaches for lung cancer. More investigation is crucial to gain a comprehensive interpretation of the biology and functionality of LAG-3. This entails further exploration into its existence, the specific signaling pathways it engages in, as well as the underlying mechanisms that contribute to the constructive collaboration between LAG-3 and PD-1. The long-term implementation of a personalized therapeutic approach for lung cancer patients could be eased by the identification of certain combination immunotherapy treatments that are most effective based on the microenvironment or antigens associated with different forms of lung cancer.

References

Anagnostou VK, Brahmer JR (2015) Cancer Immunotherapy: a future paradigm shift in the treatment of non–small cell lung cancer. Clin Cancer Res 21(5):976–984. https://doi.org/10.1158/1078-0432.CCR-14-1187

Anderson AC, Joller N, Kuchroo VK (2016) Lag-3, Tim-3, and TIGIT: co-inhibitory receptors with specialized functions in immune regulation. Immunity 44(5):989–1004. https://doi.org/10.1016/j.immuni.2016.05.001

Ascierto PA, Bono P, Bhatia S, Melero I, Nyakas MS, Svane I-M, Larkin J, Gomez-Roca C, Schadendorf D, Dummer R, Marabelle A, Hoeller C, Maurer M, Harbison CT, Mitra P, Suryawanshi S, Thudium K, Muñoz Couselo E (2017) Efficacy of BMS-986016, a monoclonal antibody that targets lymphocyte activation gene-3 (LAG-3), in combination with nivolumab in Pts with melanoma who progressed during prior anti–PD-1/PD-L1 therapy (Mel Prior IO) in all-comer and biomarker-enriched populations. Ann Oncol 28:v611–v612. https://doi.org/10.1093/annonc/mdx440.011

Ascione A, Arenaccio C, Mallano A, Flego M, Gellini M, Andreotti M, Fenwick C, Pantaleo G, Vella S, Federico M (2019) Development of a novel human phage display-derived anti-LAG3 ScFv antibody targeting CD8+ T lymphocyte exhaustion. BMC Biotechnol 19(1):67. https://doi.org/10.1186/s12896-019-0559-x

Avice M-N, Sarfati M, Triebel F, Delespesse G, Demeure CE (1999) Lymphocyte activation Gene-3, a MHC class II ligand expressed on activated T cells, stimulates TNF-α and IL-12 production by monocytes and dendritic cells. J Immunol 162(5):2748–2753. https://doi.org/10.4049/jimmunol.162.5.2748

Bagchi S, Yuan R, Engleman EG (2021) Immune checkpoint inhibitors for the treatment of cancer: clinical impact and mechanisms of response and resistance. Annu Rev Pathol Mech Dis 16(1):223–249. https://doi.org/10.1146/annurev-pathol-042020-042741

Bray F, Ferlay J, Soerjomataram I, Siegel RL, Torre LA, Jemal A (2018) Global cancer statistics 2018: GLOBOCAN estimates of incidence and mortality worldwide for 36 cancers in 185 countries. CA Cancer J Clin 68(6):394–424. https://doi.org/10.3322/caac.21492

Brignone C, Escudier B, Grygar C, Marcu M, Triebel F (2009) A phase I pharmacokinetic and biological correlative study of IMP321, a novel MHC class II agonist, in patients with advanced renal cell carcinoma. Clin Cancer Res 15(19):6225–6231. https://doi.org/10.1158/1078-0432.CCR-09-0068

Brignone C, Gutierrez M, Mefti F, Brain E, Jarcau R, Cvitkovic F, Bousetta N, Medioni J, Gligorov J, Grygar C, Marcu M, Triebel F (2010) First-line Chemoimmunotherapy in metastatic breast carcinoma: combination of paclitaxel and IMP321 (LAG-3Ig) enhances immune responses and antitumor activity. J Transl Med 8(1):71. https://doi.org/10.1186/1479-5876-8-71

Camisaschi C, Casati C, Rini F, Perego M, De Filippo A, Triebel F, Parmiani G, Belli F, Rivoltini L, Castelli C (2010) LAG-3 expression defines a subset of CD4+CD25highFoxp3+ regulatory T cells that are expanded at tumor sites. J Immunol 184(11):6545–6551. https://doi.org/10.4049/jimmunol.0903879

Chen J, Chen Z (2014) The effect of immune microenvironment on the progression and prognosis of colorectal cancer. Med Oncol 31(8):82. https://doi.org/10.1007/s12032-014-0082-9

Chocarro L, Blanco E, Arasanz H, Fernández-Rubio L, Bocanegra A, Echaide M, Garnica M, Ramos P, Fernández-Hinojal G, Vera R, Kochan G, Escors D (2022) Clinical landscape of LAG-3-targeted therapy. Immuno Oncol Technol 14:100079. https://doi.org/10.1016/j.iotech.2022.100079

Darvin P, Toor SM, Sasidharan Nair V, Elkord E (2018) Immune checkpoint inhibitors: recent Progress and potential biomarkers. Exp Mol Med 50(12):1–11. https://doi.org/10.1038/s12276-018-0191-1

Dirix L, Triebel F (2019) AIPAC: a phase IIb study of Eftilagimod alpha (IMP321 or LAG-3Ig) added to weekly paclitaxel in patients with metastatic breast cancer. Future Oncol 15(17):1963–1973. https://doi.org/10.2217/fon-2018-0807

Dumic J, Dabelic S, Flögel M (2006) Galectin-3: an open-ended story. Biochim Biophys Acta BBA-Gen Subj 1760(4):616–635. https://doi.org/10.1016/j.bbagen.2005.12.020

Fahrer AM, Konigshofer Y, Kerr EM, Ghandour G, Mack DH, Davis MM, Chien Y (2001) Attributes of γδ intraepithelial lymphocytes as suggested by their transcriptional profile. Proc Natl Acad Sci U S A 98(18):10261

Gagliani N, Magnani CF, Huber S, Gianolini ME, Pala M, Licona-Limon P, Guo B, Herbert DR, Bulfone A, Trentini F, Di Serio C, Bacchetta R, Andreani M, Brockmann L, Gregori S, Flavell RA, Roncarolo M-G (2013) Coexpression of CD49b and LAG-3 identifies human and mouse T regulatory type 1 cells. Nat Med 19(6):739–746. https://doi.org/10.1038/nm.3179

Gandhi MK, Lambley E, Duraiswamy J, Dua U, Smith C, Elliott S, Gill D, Marlton P, Seymour J, Khanna R (2006) Expression of LAG-3 by tumor-infiltrating lymphocytes is coincident with the suppression of latent membrane antigen–specific CD8+ T-cell function in Hodgkin lymphoma patients. Blood 108(7):2280–2289. https://doi.org/10.1182/blood-2006-04-015164

Hald SM, Rakaee M, Martinez I, Richardsen E, Al-Saad S, Paulsen E-E, Blix ES, Kilvaer T, Andersen S, Busund L-T, Bremnes RM, Donnem T (2018) LAG-3 in non–small-cell lung cancer: expression in primary tumors and metastatic lymph nodes is associated with improved Survival. Clin Lung Cancer 19(3):249–259.e2. https://doi.org/10.1016/j.cllc.2017.12.001

Hemon P, Jean-Louis F, Ramgolam K, Brignone C, Viguier M, Bachelez H, Triebel F, Charron D, Aoudjit F, Al-Daccak R, Michel L (2011) MHC class II engagement by its ligand LAG-3 (CD223) contributes to melanoma resistance to apoptosis. J Immunol 186(9):5173–5183. https://doi.org/10.4049/jimmunol.1002050

Hodi FS, O'Day SJ, McDermott DF, Weber RW, Sosman JA, Haanen JB, Gonzalez R, Robert C, Schadendorf D, Hassel JC, Akerley W, van den Eertwegh AJM, Lutzky J, Lorigan P, Vaubel JM, Linette GP, Hogg D, Ottensmeier CH, Lebbé C, Peschel C, Quirt I, Clark JI, Wolchok JD, Weber JS, Tian J, Yellin MJ, Nichol GM, Hoos A, Urba WJ (2010) Improved survival with ipilimumab in patients with metastatic melanoma. N Engl J Med 363(8):711–723. https://doi.org/10.1056/NEJMoa1003466

Hoffmann MM, Slansky JE (2020) T-cell receptor affinity in the age of cancer immunotherapy. Mol Carcinog 59(7):862–870. https://doi.org/10.1002/mc.23212

Huang C-T, Workman CJ, Flies D, Pan X, Marson AL, Zhou G, Hipkiss EL, Ravi S, Kowalski J, Levitsky HI, Powell JD, Pardoll DM, Drake CG, Vignali DAA (2004) Role of LAG-3 in regulatory T cells. Immunity 21(4):503–513. https://doi.org/10.1016/j.immuni.2004.08.010

Huard B, Mastrangeli R, Prigent P, Bruniquel D, Donini S, El-Tayar N, Maigret B, Dréano M, Triebel F (1997) Characterization of the major histocompatibility complex class II binding site on LAG-3 protein. Proc Natl Acad Sci 94(11):5744–5749. https://doi.org/10.1073/pnas.94.11.5744

Huard B, Prigent P, Tournier M, Bruniquel D, Triebel F (1995) CD4/major histocompatibility complex class II interaction analyzed with CD4- and lymphocyte activation Gene-3 (LAG-3)-Ig fusion proteins. Eur J Immunol 25(9):2718–2721. https://doi.org/10.1002/eji.1830250949

Huard B, Tournier M, Hercend T, Triebel F, Faure F (1994) Lymphocyte-activation gene 3/major histocompatibility complex class II interaction modulates the antigenic response of CD4+ T lymphocytes. Eur J Immunol 24(12):3216–3221. https://doi.org/10.1002/eji.1830241246

Iouzalen N, Andreae S, Hannier S, Triebel F (2001) LAP, a lymphocyte activation gene-3 (LAG-3)-associated protein that binds to a repeated EP motif in the intracellular region of LAG-3, may participate in the downregulation of the CD3/TCR activation pathway. Eur J Immunol 31(10):2885–2891. https://doi.org/10.1002/1521-4141(2001010)31:10<2885::aid-immu2885>3.0.co;2-2

Jenkins S, Wesolowski R, Gatti-Mays ME (2021) Improving breast cancer responses to immunotherapy—a search for the Achilles heel of the tumor microenvironment. Curr Oncol Rep 23(5):55. https://doi.org/10.1007/s11912-021-01040-y

Jiang H, Ni H, Zhang P, Guo X, Wu M, Shen H, Wang J, Wu W, Wu Z, Ding J, Tang R, Zhou S, Chen B, Yu M, Jing H, Liu J (2021) PD-L1/LAG-3 bispecific antibody enhances tumor-specific immunity. Onco Targets Ther 10(1):1943180. https://doi.org/10.1080/2162402X.2021.1943180

Kisielow M, Kisielow J, Capoferri-Sollami G, Karjalainen K (2005) Expression of lymphocyte activation gene 3 (LAG-3) on B cells is induced by T cells. Eur J Immunol 35(7):2081–2088. https://doi.org/10.1002/eji.200526090

Li Q, Huang Q, Cheng S, Wu S, Sang H, Hou J (2019) Circ_ZNF124 promotes non-small cell lung cancer progression by abolishing MiR-337-3p mediated downregulation of JAK2/STAT3 signaling pathway. Cancer Cell Int 19(1):291. https://doi.org/10.1186/s12935-019-1011-y

Liang B, Workman C, Lee J, Chew C, Dale BM, Colonna L, Flores M, Li N, Schweighoffer E, Greenberg S, Tybulewicz V, Vignali D, Clynes R (2008) Regulatory T cells inhibit dendritic cells by lymphocyte activation Gene-3 engagement of MHC class II. J Immunol 180(9):5916–5926. https://doi.org/10.4049/jimmunol.180.9.5916

Liu W, Tang L, Zhang G, Wei H, Cui Y, Guo L, Gou Z, Chen X, Jiang D, Zhu Y, Kang G, He F (2004) Characterization of a novel C-type lectin-like gene, LSECtin. J Biol Chem 279(18):18748–18758. https://doi.org/10.1074/jbc.M311227200

Lui Y, Davis SJ (2018) LAG-3: a very singular immune checkpoint. Nat Immunol 19(12):1278–1279. https://doi.org/10.1038/s41590-018-0257-1

Ma Q-Y, Huang D-Y, Zhang H-J, Wang S, Chen X-F (2017) Function and regulation of LAG3 on CD4+CD25- T cells in non-small cell lung cancer. Exp Cell Res 360(2):358–364. https://doi.org/10.1016/j.yexcr.2017.09.026

Macon-Lemaitre L, Triebel F (2005) The negative regulatory function of the lymphocyte-activation Gene-3 co-receptor (CD223) on human T cells. Immunology 115(2):170–178. https://doi.org/10.1111/j.1365-2567.2005.02145.x

Mao X, Ou MT, Karuppagounder SS, Kam T-I, Yin X, Xiong Y, Ge P, Umanah GE, Brahmachari S, Shin J-H, Kang HC, Zhang J, Xu J, Chen R, Park H, Andrabi SA, Kang SU, Gonçalves RA, Liang Y, Zhang S, Qi C, Lam S, Keiler JA, Tyson J, Kim D, Panicker N, Yun SP, Workman CJ, Vignali DAA, Dawson VL, Ko HS, Dawson TM (2016) Pathological α-Synuclein transmission initiated by binding lymphocyte-activation gene 3. Science 353(6307):aah3374. https://doi.org/10.1126/science.aah3374

Maruhashi T, Okazaki I, Sugiura D, Takahashi S, Maeda TK, Shimizu K, Okazaki T (2018) LAG-3 inhibits the activation of CD4+ T cells that recognize stable PMHCII through its conformation-dependent recognition of PMHCII. Nat Immunol 19(12):1415–1426. https://doi.org/10.1038/s41590-018-0217-9

Maruhashi T, Sugiura D, Okazaki I, Okazaki T (2020) LAG-3: from molecular functions to clinical applications. J Immunother Cancer 8(2):e001014. https://doi.org/10.1136/jitc-2020-001014

Mastrangeli R, Micangeli E, Donini S (1996) Cloning of murine LAG-3 by magnetic bead bound homologous probes and PCR (GENE-CAPTURE PCR). Anal Biochem 241(1):93–102. https://doi.org/10.1006/abio.1996.0382

McLane LM, Abdel-Hakeem MS, Wherry EJ (2019) CD8 T cell exhaustion during chronic viral infection and cancer. Annu Rev Immunol 37(1):457–495. https://doi.org/10.1146/annurev-immunol-041015-055318

Melaiu O, Lucarini V, Giovannoni R, Fruci D, Gemignani F (2022) News on immune checkpoint inhibitors as immunotherapy strategies in adult and pediatric solid tumors. Semin Cancer Biol 79:18–43. https://doi.org/10.1016/j.semcancer.2020.07.001

Nurgalieva AK, Safina S, Shakirova E, Filonenko V, Skripova V, Bulatova L, Savenkova D, Bogdanov M, Kiyamova R (2021) 53P expression of sodium-dependent phosphate transporter NaPi2b is downregulated in malignant ovarian tumors after neoadjuvant chemotherapy. Ann Oncol 32:S1361–S1362. https://doi.org/10.1016/j.annonc.2021.08.2049

Okamura T, Yamamoto K, Fujio K (2018) Early growth response gene 2-expressing CD4+LAG3+ regulatory T cells: the therapeutic potential for treating autoimmune diseases. ("early growth response gene 2-expressing CD4 - Frontiers"). Front Immunol 9:340. https://doi.org/10.3389/fimmu.2018.00340

Poorebrahim M, Melief J, Pico de Coaña Y, Wickström LS, Cid-Arregui A, Kiessling R (2021) Counteracting CAR T Cell Dysfunction. ("TCR-like CARs and TCR-CARs targeting neo-epitopes: an emerging ...—nature"). Oncogene 40(2):421–435. https://doi.org/10.1038/s41388-020-01501-x

Previte DM, Martins CP, O'Connor EC, Marre ML, Coudriet GM, Beck NW, Menk AV, Wright RH, Tse HM, Delgoffe GM, Piganelli JD (2019) Lymphocyte activation Gene-3 maintains mitochondrial and metabolic quiescence in naive CD4+ T cells. Cell Rep 27(1):129–141.e4. https://doi.org/10.1016/j.celrep.2019.03.004

Prigent P, El Mir S, Dréano M, Triebel F (1999) Lymphocyte activation Gene-3 induces tumor regression and antitumor immune responses. Eur J Immunol 29(12):3867–3876. https://doi.org/10.1002/(SICI)1521-4141(199912)29:12<3867::AID-IMMU3867>3.0.CO;2-E

Puhr HC, Ilhan-Mutlu A (2019) New emerging targets in cancer immunotherapy: the role of LAG3. ESMO Open 4(2):e000482. https://doi.org/10.1136/esmoopen-2018-000482

Qin S, Xu L, Yi M, Yu S, Wu K, Luo S (2019) Novel immune checkpoint targets: moving beyond PD-1 and CTLA-4. Mol Cancer 18(1):155. https://doi.org/10.1186/s12943-019-1091-2

Romano E, Michielin O, Voelter V, Laurent J, Bichat H, Stravodimou A, Romero P, Speiser DE, Triebel F, Leyvraz S, Harari A (2014) MART-1 peptide vaccination plus IMP321 (LAG-3Ig fusion protein) in patients receiving autologous PBMCs after Lymphodepletion: results of a phase I trial. J Transl Med 12(1):97. https://doi.org/10.1186/1479-5876-12-97

Ruffo E, Wu RC, Bruno TC, Workman CJ, Vignali DAA (2019) Lymphocyte-activation gene 3 (LAG3): the next immune checkpoint receptor. Semin Immunol 42:101305. https://doi.org/10.1016/j.smim.2019.101305

Sordo-Bahamonde C, Lorenzo-Herrero S, González-Rodríguez AP, Payer ÁR, González-García E, López-Soto A, Gonzalez S (2021) LAG-3 blockade with Relatlimab (BMS-986016) restores anti-leukemic responses in chronic lymphocytic leukemia. Cancers 13(9):2112. https://doi.org/10.3390/cancers13092112

Triebel F (2003) LAG-3: a regulator of T-cell and DC responses and its use in therapeutic vaccination. Trends Immunol 24(12):619–622. https://doi.org/10.1016/j.it.2003.10.001

Triebel F, Jitsukawa S, Baixeras E, Roman-Roman S, Genevee C, Viegas-Pequignot E, Hercend T (1990) LAG-3, a novel lymphocyte activation gene closely related to CD4. J Exp Med 171(5):1393–1405. https://doi.org/10.1084/jem.171.5.1393

Wang J, Asch AS, Hamad N, Weickhardt A, Tomaszewska-Kiecana M, Dlugosz-Danecka M, Pylypenko H, Bahadur S, Ulahannan S, Koucheki J, Sun J, Li H, Chen F, Zhang X, Muth J, Kaminker P, Moore P, Sumrow BJ (2020) A phase 1, open-label study of MGD013, a bispecific DART® molecule binding PD-1 and LAG-3 in patients with relapsed or refractory diffuse large B-cell lymphoma. Blood 136(Supplement 1):21–22. https://doi.org/10.1182/blood-2020-139868

Wang J, Meijers R, Xiong Y, Liu J, Sakihama T, Zhang R, Joachimiak A, Reinherz EL (2001) Crystal structure of the human CD4 N-terminal two-domain fragment complexed to a class II MHC molecule. Proc Natl Acad Sci U S A 98:10799

Wang J, Sanmamed MF, Datar I, Su TT, Ji L, Sun J, Chen L, Chen Y, Zhu G, Yin W, Zheng L, Zhou T, Badri T, Yao S, Zhu S, Boto A, Sznol M, Melero I, Vignali DAA, Schalper K, Chen L (2019) Fibrinogen-like protein 1 is a major immune inhibitory ligand of LAG-3. Cell 176(1–2):334–347.e12. https://doi.org/10.1016/j.cell.2018.11.010

Wang-Gillam A, Plambeck-Suess S, Goedegebuure P, Simon PO, Mitchem JB, Hornick JR, Sorscher S, Picus J, Suresh R, Lockhart AC, Tan B, Hawkins WG (2013) A phase I study of IMP321 and gemcitabine as the front-line therapy in patients with advanced pancreatic adenocarcinoma. Investig New Drugs 31(3):707–713. https://doi.org/10.1007/s10637-012-9866-y

Weber S, Karjalainen K (1993) Mouse CD4 binds MHC class II with extremely low affinity. ("the structural basis of CD4 — MHC class II interactions …—springer"). Int Immunol 5(6):695–698. https://doi.org/10.1093/intimm/5.6.695

White AM, Wraith DC (2016) Tr1-like T cells–an enigmatic regulatory T cell lineage. Front Immunol 7:7. https://doi.org/10.3389/fimmu.2016.00355

Workman CJ, Dugger KJ, Vignali DAA (2002) Cutting edge: molecular analysis of the negative regulatory function of lymphocyte activation Gene-3. J Immunol 169(10):5392–5395. https://doi.org/10.4049/jimmunol.169.10.5392

Workman CJ, Rice DS, Dugger KJ, Kurschner C, Vignali DAA (2002) Phenotypic analysis of the murine CD4-related glycoprotein, CD223 (LAG-3). Eur J Immunol 32(8):2255. https://doi.org/10.1002/1521-4141(200208)32:8<2255::AID-IMMU2255>3.0.CO;2-A

Workman CJ, Vignali DAA (2003) The CD4-related molecule, LAG-3 (CD223), regulates the expansion of activated T cells. Eur J Immunol 33(4):970–979. https://doi.org/10.1002/eji.200323382

Workman CJ, Wang Y, El Kasmi KC, Pardoll DM, Murray PJ, Drake CG, Vignali DAA (2009) LAG-3 regulates Plasmacytoid dendritic cell homeostasis. J Immunol 182(4):1885–1891. https://doi.org/10.4049/jimmunol.0800185

Xu F, Liu J, Liu D, Liu B, Wang M, Hu Z, Du X, Tang L, He F (2014) LSECtin expressed on melanoma cells promotes tumor progression by inhibiting antitumor T-cell responses. Cancer Res 74(13):3418–3428. https://doi.org/10.1158/0008-5472.CAN-13-2690

Zarour HM (2016) Reversing T-cell dysfunction and exhaustion in cancer. Clin Cancer Res 22(8):1856–1864. https://doi.org/10.1158/1078-0432.CCR-15-1849

Zhang J, Liu W, Xie T, Huang L, Hu Y, Wen B, Tang P, Guo F, Jin K, Zhang P, Niu L, Liu Z, Qu X (2019) Elevated LAG-3 on CD4+ T cells negatively correlates with neutralizing antibody response during HCV infection. Immunol Lett 212:46–52. https://doi.org/10.1016/j.imlet.2019.06.003

IDO and TGF-β Inhibitors for the Treatment of Lung Cancer

9

Thangaraj Devadoss, Yeole Kalpesh Rajendra, Ranmale Bhavesh Rajesh, and Borse Chetan Sambhaji

This chapter comprises two major sections: Sect. 9.1. discusses about the IDO inhibitors, and Sect. 9.2. describes about TGF-β inhibitors.

9.1 IDO Inhibitors

9.1.1 Introduction

Indoleamine-2,3-dioxygenase (IDO) is a metalloenzyme that falls under the category of oxygenase enzyme. The metal part of the indoleamine-2,3-dioxygenase enzyme is heme. This enzyme exists in two forms: IDO1 and IDO2. The IDO catalyzes the conversion of tryptophan to *N*-formylkynurenine, and it is the rate-limiting step in the kynurenine pathway (Fang et al. 2018). Like IDO, TDO (tryptophan-2,3-dioxygenase) helps in the formation of *N*-formylkynurenine from tryptophan. TDO is stereospecific, and it acts only on L-tryptophan. On the other hand, IDO acts on both L and D forms of tryptophan (Knox and Mehler 1950). It also catalyzed the degradation of indole derivatives like serotonin and tryptamine (Shimizu et al. 1978). In the rate-limiting step, IDO introduces two oxygen atoms across the double bond located at the second and third position of tryptophan, which results in the breaking of the indole nucleus and affords *N*-formylkynurenine (an anthranilic acid derivative). Figure 9.1 represents the metabolic pathway of tryptophan.

IDO1 is a cytosolic enzyme located in the lung, spleen, liver, kidney, and brain (Capece et al. 2020). It is a monomeric enzyme activated by the ferrous form of the metal. Further, the enzyme activity is controlled by

T. Devadoss (✉) · Y. K. Rajendra · R. B. Rajesh · B. C. Sambhaji
Department of Pharmaceutical Chemistry, Shri Vile Parle Kelavani Mandal's Institute of Pharmacy, Behind Gurudwara, Mumbai Agra National Highway, Dhule, Maharashtra, India

S. Bhatt et al. (eds.), *Immunotherapy Against Lung Cancer*,
https://doi.org/10.1007/978-981-99-7141-1_9

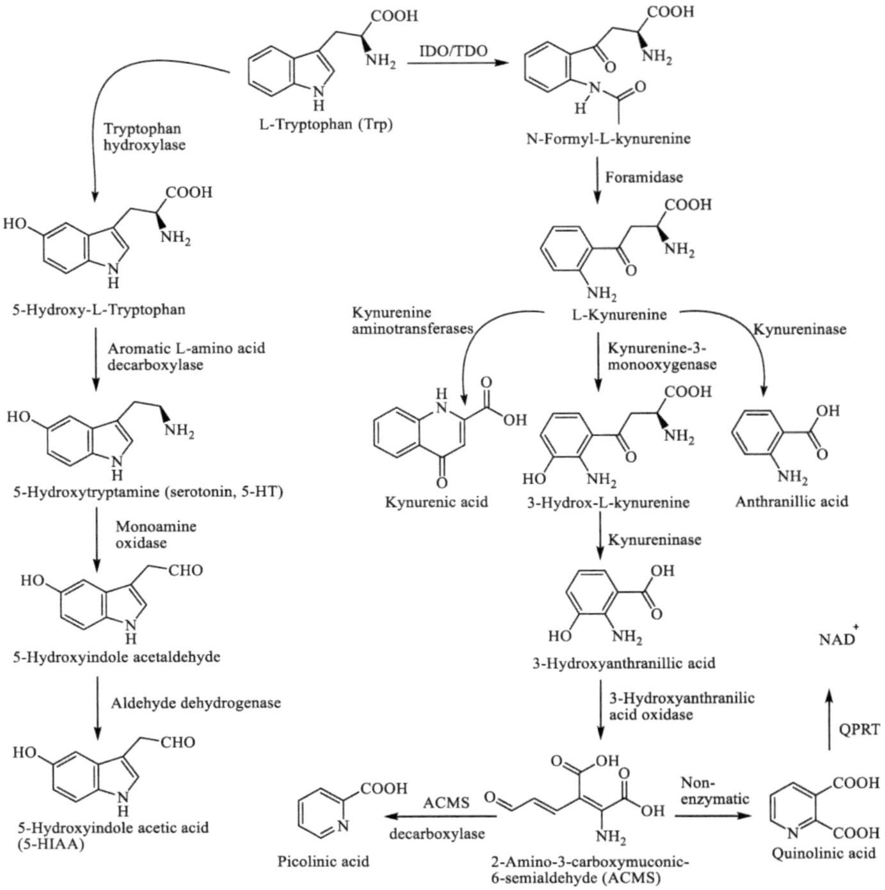

Fig. 9.1 Metabolic pathway of tryptophan

phosphorylatable tyrosine residues Tyr115 and Tyr253 (Hornyák et al. 2018). Change in the conformation of IDO1 occurs when any one of these amino acid residues is phosphorylated, which results in blockage of the catalytic activity of the IDO1 enzyme. Hence, targeting these sites may prolong or reduce the half-life of the IDO1 enzyme (Pallotta et al. 2014).

The enzyme IDO1 is expressed in various cells including astrocytes, macrophages, dendritic cells, and tumor cells. The enzyme IDO1 is induced by a wide range of substances, and it includes transforming growth factor-β, tumor necrosis factor-α, interferon-gamma, prostaglandin E2, etc. (Muller et al. 2008; Li et al. 2016; Smith et al. 2012; Liu et al. 2018). The increased IDO activity is well correlated with many diseases and disorders. The condition includes inflammation, liver disease, diabetes, cancer, depression, HIV, and rejection of organ transplantation (Moon et al. 2015).

The IDO acted like an immune suppressive agent by promoting the tolerogenicity of antigen-presenting cells (APCs) and the death of immune cells. One of the possible factors implicated in this phenomenon is the kynurenine pathway.

9.1.2 IDO and Proliferation of Cancer Cells

Depletion of tryptophan and formation of kynurenine by IDO significantly inhibit T-cell differentiation and proliferation and activate the proliferation of T-regulatory cells (Ye et al. 2019). All these processes inhibit the antitumor immune responses (Ye et al. 2019).

The depletion of tryptophan leads to the accumulation of uncharged tryptophan-transfer RNA. It activates the general control non-derepressible 2 (GCN2) by binding at the allosteric site, which leads to phosphorylation of eIF-2. The phosphorylated eIF-2 limits protein translation, which leads to the suppression of T-cell proliferation (Munn et al. 2005).

The activated form of mTORC1 inhibits the autophagy process. The diminished level of tryptophan suppresses the mTORC1 via the blockade of amino acid sensing kinase glucokinase1 (GLK1). This leads to autophagy and increased T-effector cell apoptosis (Ye et al. 2019).

The metabolite kynurenine formed from tryptophan is an endogenous substrate of the aryl hydrocarbon receptor (AhR). The binding of kynurenine with AhR favors the T-regulatory cells' (Tregs) differentiation, thus inhibiting the antitumor immune responses (Ye et al. 2019).

9.1.3 Structure of Active Site of IDO Enzyme

The human IDO enzyme comprises a large *C*-terminal domain and a small *N*-terminal domain. The cofactor heme is present in the C-terminal region and is responsible for the catalytic activity of the enzyme. The *N*-terminal domain contains two small domains involved in signaling functions and is defined as an immunoreceptor tyrosine-based inhibiting motif (Feng et al. 2020).

The active site of the region consists of three pockets: Pocket A, Pocket B, and Pocket C. At the entrance of the active site pocket B is located, while pocket A is located in the deeper hydrophobic region, and pocket C is located at the distal region. The interaction between the ligands and pocket A and/or pocket B is well explored.

9.1.4 Pharmacophore of IDO Inhibitors

Through docking studies/fragment-based approaches, pharmacophore elements of IDO inhibitors are identified. As a molecule to display better IDO inhibitor activity, it should possess the following features, an aromatic ring (in a bicyclic system), an atom with lone pair of electrons (nitrogen, sulfur, and oxygen), a large alkyl group, and a group able to form hydrogen bonding (Röhrig et al. 2010).

The aryl system interacts with the hydrophobic region of pocket A, the lone pair electrons of the electronegative atoms (nitrogen, sulfur, and oxygen) bind with the cofactor of the enzyme (pocket A region), the large alkyl portion of the inhibitor binds with pocket B of the enzyme through van der Waals interaction (Röhrig et al. 2010). In a study, Smith and co-researchers indicated that compounds with ester imidamide linkage between two aryl systems displayed potent IDO inhibitor activity (Smith et al. 2012).

9.1.5 Classification of IDO Inhibitors

Based on the difference in binding modes, the IDO inhibitors are classified into four types (Röhrig et al. 2019). The type I category compounds bind with oxygen-bound ferrous holoIDO1, while in the type II category, compounds bind to free ferrous holoIDO1. The type III and IV category compounds bind to free ferric holoIDO1 (type III) and apoIDO1, respectively.

9.1.6 Well-Known IDO Inhibitors

In the past two decades, a wide range of chemical classes of molecules are synthesized and studied for their IDO inhibitor properties by academic or industrial scientists. The chemical classes of the molecule include indole, quinoline, oxadiazole, imidazoisoindole, imidazole, tetrazole, and triazole with quinone or hydroxylamine derivatives. In this section, the most studied IDO inhibitors are discussed, and chemical structures are presented in Fig. 9.2.

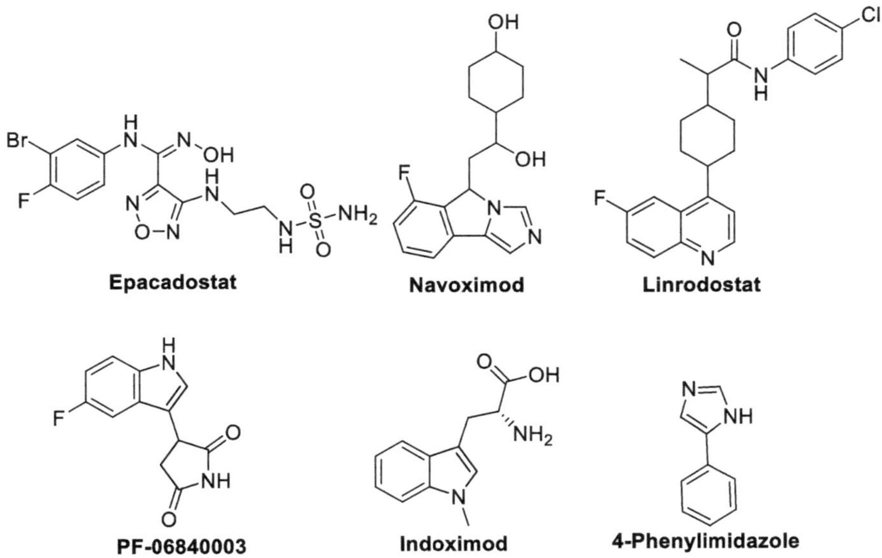

Fig. 9.2 Chemical structures of most widely studied IDO inhibitors

9.1.6.1 Epacadostat

Epacadostat (INCB024360) is developed by Incyte Corporation. It is a derivative of hydroxylamidine and an orally active IDO inhibitor. In cell-based assays, epacadostat selectively inhibits the IDO1 with the IC_{50} value of 10 nM and has little affinity toward IDO2 and TDO1 (Prendergast et al. 2018). In in vitro studies, it promoted T cell and NK cell proliferation, increased number of CD86 high DCs, and reduced the Treg cells. In the tumor cells, kynurenine levels are reduced by 90%. Epacadostat has 1000 times more selectivity toward IDO1 over IDO2 and TDO. Many preclinical and clinical studies displayed antitumor activity. The half-life of epacadostat is 2.4–3.9 h.

In the clinical studies, three principal metabolites are identified for the epacadostat (Boer et al. 2016). The metabolite **M9** (INCB-056867) is formed as a result of conjugation with glucuronic acid, an amidine metabolite **M11** (INCB056868) is formed due to the action of gut microbiota, and the metabolite **M12** is the secondary metabolite of amidine metabolite (*N*-alkylated derivative, INCB052101). The proposed metabolic pathway of epacadostat is presented in Fig. 9.3 (Boer et al. 2016).

In the clinical studies, epacadostat displayed synergistic effects when administered along with immune checkpoint blockades (pembrolizumab, ipilimumab, nivolumab) (Liu et al. 2018). In some clinical trials, negative results are observed, which led to the withdrawal/termination of several phase III clinical trials. In monotherapy clinical studies, it showed fatigue, nausea, loss of appetite, vomiting, and constipation (Beatty et al. 2017).

9.1.6.2 Navoximod (NLG919, GDC-0919)

The part of the navoximod possesses structural similarity with 4-phenylimidazole. The kynurenine levels are reduced to 50% in mice treated with navoximod (Tang et al. 2021). It is also one of the orally effective IDO inhibitors. Navoximod and indoximod are considered IDO modulators rather than IDO inhibitors, because it exerts the actions by mimicking the tryptophan. In clinical studies, it is given along with atezolizumab, a checkpoint inhibitor targeting PD-L1.

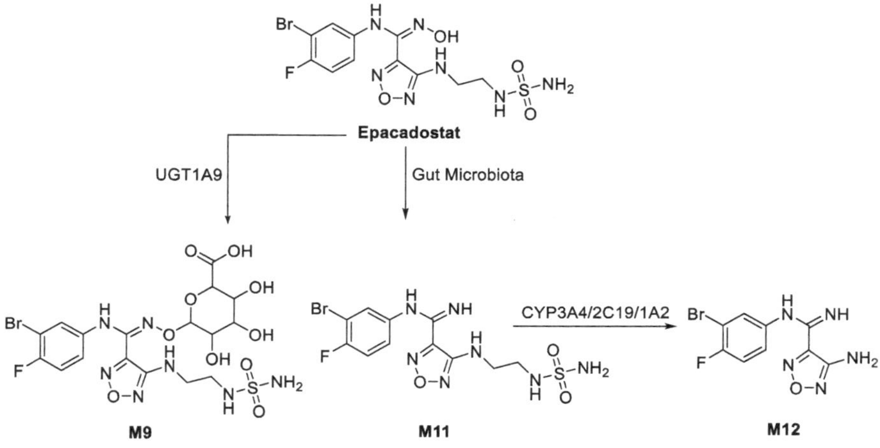

Fig. 9.3 Proposed metabolic pathway of epacadostat (Boer et al. 2016)

Navoximod is safe, rapidly absorbed, and well tolerated up to 800 mg twice daily, and only around 6% of the administrated molecule is not metabolized (Jung et al. 2019). Glucuronidation is the principal metabolic pathway of navoximod (Ma et al. 2019). Fatigue, pruritus, and nausea are the common adverse effects associated with the navoximod treatment (Nayak-Kapoor et al. 2018).

9.1.6.3 Linrodostat (BMS-986205)

Linrodostat is an irreversible IDO inhibitor with an IC_{50} value of 1.7 nM (Prendergast et al. 2018). It is also an orally effective IDO inhibitor, available mesylate salt. Linrodostat selectively inhibits the IDO1 over IDO2 or TDO. It reduces the kynurenine levels in tumor cells (Davar and Bahary 2018). The efficacy and pharmacokinetic property of the lindrostat are better than those of Epacadostat (Prendergast et al. 2018). In the clinical studies, it co-administered with nivolumab, ipilimumab, or relatlimab. It reversed immunosuppression in cancer patients. The maximum tolerable and recommended doses are 200 mg and 100 mg, respectively (Liu et al. 2018).

9.1.6.4 PF-06840003 (Synonyms EOS200271)

It is an orally active and selective IDO1 inhibitor. It reduces the kynurenine level by more than 80% in the mice model (Gomes et al. 2018). As it crosses the blood–brain barrier, it is used for treating brain metastases. A single dose is sufficient because of the long half-life. It is a non-heme-binding IDO1 inhibitor. It can be combined with PD-1 OR PDL1 inhibitors to get a synergistic effect on the treatment of cancer. The IC_{50} value of PF-06840003 is 0.4 μM for the hIDO1. It is well tolerated up to 500 mg twice daily (Reardon et al. 2020).

9.1.6.5 Indoximod (1-Methyl-D-Tryptophan, 1-MT, NLG-8189)

It is a derivative of tryptophan amino acid having an additional methyl group at first position of the indole nucleus. It is also called *N*-methyltryptophan, and it is a non-proteinogenic amino acid. The DL form of 1-methyltryptophan is found in *Aspergillus fumigatus*. The IDO inhibitor of the 1-methyltryptophan is studied for all three stereoisomers (1-methyl-D-tryptophan, 1-methyl-L-tryptophan, and 1-methyl-DL-tryptophan). In many preclinical studies, D-stereoisomer displayed better IDO inhibitor properties compared to other stereoisomers. It is also an orally effective IDO inhibitor. Monotherapy of indoximod exhibits little antitumor activity. On the other hand, in combination with a vaccine or immune checkpoint inhibitor (pembrolizumab/ nivolumab/ ipilimumab), it showed a synergistic anticancer effect (Tang et al. 2021; Liu et al. 2018).

Indoximod did not alter the ratio of kynurenine to tryptophan level at any dose (Soliman et al. 2016). Indoximod is well tolerated at the maximum dose of 0.2 g twice daily (Brochez et al. 2017). The half-life of indoximod is 10.5 h, and 20% of the molecule is renally excreted (Soliman et al. 2016). The most common adverse events associated with indoximod treatment were fatigue, anemia, anorexia, dyspnea, cough, and nausea (Soliman et al. 2016).

9.1.6.6 4-Phenylimidazole (4-PI, PIM, 4PI)

It is a non-competitive inhibitor of the IDO enzyme; it binds to the IDO enzyme at an inactive ferric state (Röhrig et al. 2019). The X-ray structure of IDO-bound PIM gave clarity for understanding the intermolecular force of attraction between the enzyme and PIM (Sugimoto et al. 2006). The phenyl ring of the molecule interacts with the pocket-A, and the nitrogen atom of the imidazole has coordination with heme.

9.1.7 Natural IDO Inhibitors

Very recently, Tan and co-researchers (Tan et al. 2022) reviewed IDO inhibitors of natural products. Based on chemical class, they categorized the natural IDO inhibitors into four types: quinones, alkaloids, polyphenols, and others. Table 9.1 represents chemical classes of IDO inhibitors from natural products. The chemical structures of selected natural products with IDO inhibitor properties are depicted in Fig. 9.4.

Table 9.1 Natural products with IDO inhibitor properties (Tan et al. 2022)

Chemical class	Name/code of the molecule	IDO inhibition in IC_{50} or Ki value
Quinones	Coenzyme Q	$IC_{50} = 1.30\ \mu M$
	Vitamin K3	$IC_{50} = 1.00\ \mu M$
	Shikonin	$IC_{50} = 0.98\ \mu M$
	Nanaomycin	Ki = 950 nM
	Mitomycin C	Ki = 24.6 μM
	Annulin B	Ki = 0.12 μM
	Exiguamine	Ki = 40.0 nM
	NSC255109	Ki = 24.6 μM
	β-Lapachone	$IC_{50} = 97.0\ nM$
	Saprorthoquinone	$IC_{50} = 1.76\ \mu M$
	Dihydrotanshinone	$IC_{50} = 2.80\ \mu M$
Alkaloids	Tryptanthrin	Ki = 4.81 μM
	NSC111041	Ki = 4.30 μM
	Brassinin	Ki = 27.9 μM
	3-Deazaguanine	Ki = 21.4 μM
	PQA26	$IC_{50} = 32.0\ \mu M$
	Berberine	$IC_{50} = 9.30\ \mu M$
	Lysicamine	$IC_{50} = 6.22\ \mu M$
	Albogrisin D	$IC_{50} = 12.2\ \mu M$
	Cinnabarinic acid	$IC_{50} = 0.46\ \mu M$
	Plectosphaeroic acid A	$IC_{50} = 2.00\ \mu M$
Polyphenols	Kushenol F	$IC_{50} = 28.3\ \mu M$
	Kushenol E	$IC_{50} = 4.40\ \mu M$
	Herqueinone	$IC_{50} = 19.1\ \mu M$
	(2S)-2′-Methoxykurarinone	$IC_{50} = 23.8\ \mu M$
	Ent-12-Methoxyisoherqueinone	$IC_{50} = 32.6\ \mu M$
	Ent-Peniciherquinone	$IC_{50} = 24.2\ \mu M$
Others	NSC401366	Ki = 1.50 μM
	Benzomalvin E	$IC_{50} = 21.4\ \mu M$
	Thielavin Q	$IC_{50} = 26.5\ \mu M$
	Halicloic acid A	$IC_{50} = 11.0\ \mu M$

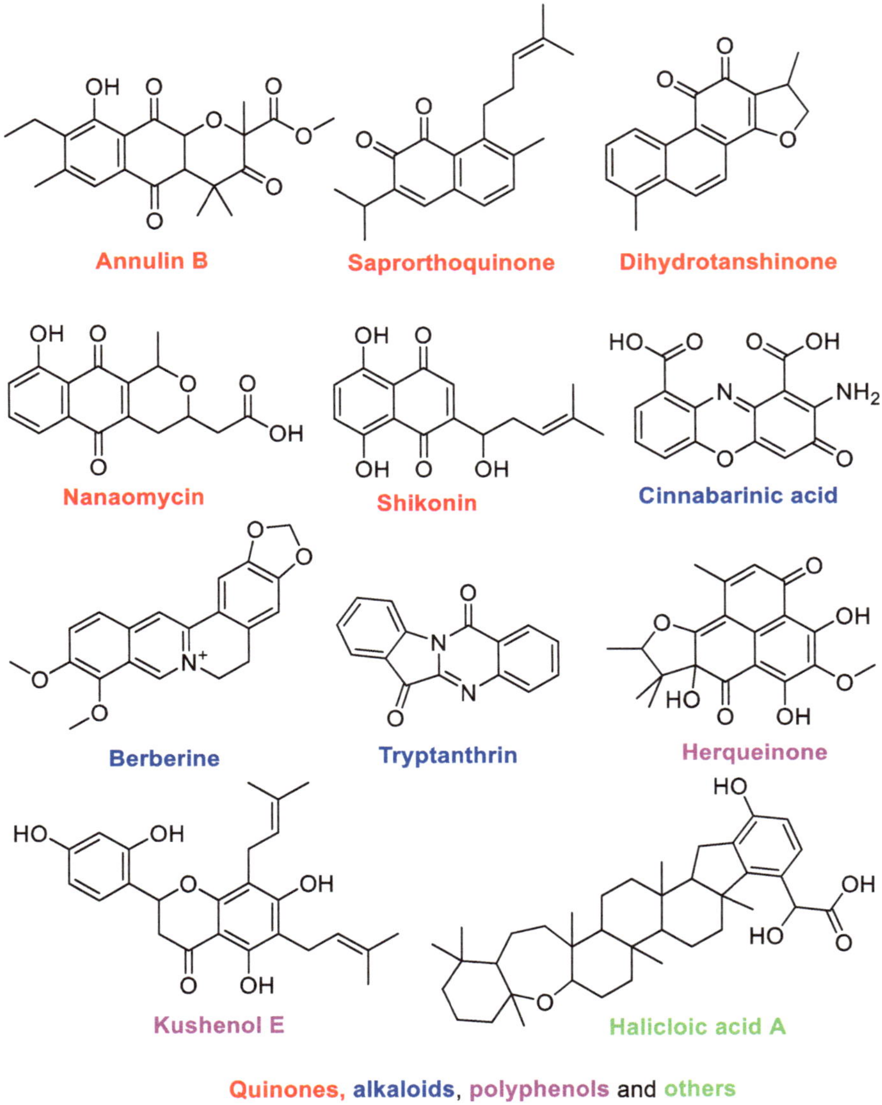

Fig. 9.4 Chemical structures of selected natural products with IDO inhibitor properties

9.1.8 IDO Inhibitors for Lung Cancer

The enzyme IDO is one of the targets for treating various diseases and disorders. In the last few decades, research teams are extensively working to discover the new IDO inhibitors for one or more pathological conditions. This section aimed to overview the discovery and development of new IDO inhibitors to treat lung cancer.

Huang and their team members (Huang et al. 2011) studied IDO inhibitor activity for a series of triazole derivatives. Among the synthesized compounds, compounds **1, 2,** and **3** displayed good IDO inhibitor activity compared to 1-methyltryptophan. The Ki values of **1, 2, 3,** and 1-MT (a standard IDO inhibitor) were 22.5 μM, 18 μM, 14.5 μM, and 34 μM, respectively. In the T-cell proliferation assay, compounds **1, 2,** and **3** increased the T-cell proliferation in the presence of Lewis Lung Cancer (LLC) cells. Compared to 1-methyltryptophan, compound **3** displayed two- to threefold increased T-cell proliferation. The structure–activity relationship indicates that the compound bearing the electron-withdrawing substituents with low steric hindrance (chlorine) in the vicinity of NH of triazoles favors better IDO inhibition.

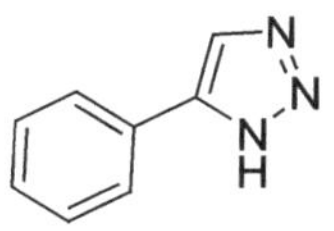

1

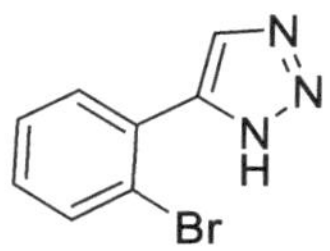

2

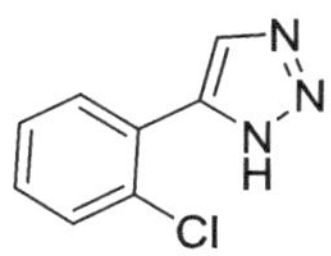

3

Two years later, Yang and co-researchers (Yang et al. 2013) reported IDO inhibitor properties of tryptanthrin-based derivatives. Structure–activity relationship analysis helps to identify the potent IDO inhibitor (**4**), which displayed IDO inhibitory activity at nanomolar concentration. Compound **4** significantly increased the proliferation of T cells in vitro study. Similarly, it suppresses the growth of the Lewis lung cancer cells in mice by inhibiting the IDO-1 activity.

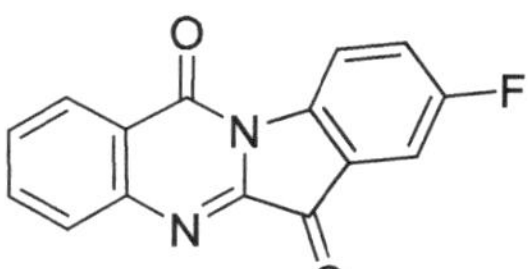

4

In 2018, Luo and co-researchers (Luo et al. 2018) investigated the mechanism of action for the beneficial effects of Feiji Recipe (Compound Chinese herbal medicine) in lung cancer. In cancer patients, this herbal medicine stabilizes the lesions and prolongs their survival. The Feiji Recipe significantly reduced the formation of kynurenine from tryptophan and suppressed the apoptosis of T cells. This result indicates that the anticancer effect of Feiji Recipe may be due to the inhibition of the IDO enzyme.

In the same year, Chauhan and coworkers (Chauhan et al. 2018) demonstrated the design, synthesis, and anticancer activity of aroyl/aryliminotryptamine derivatives as IDO inhibitors. The synthesized molecules are screened on four cancer cell lines, human non-small-cell lung adenocarcinoma (A549), cervical cancer (HeLa), breast cancer (MCF7), and liver cancer (HePG2) cells. The compounds **5** and **6** displayed potent (IC_{50} of 6 μM) antiproliferative effect against human non-small-cell lung adenocarcinoma cells. These compounds (**5** and **6**) displayed IDO inhibition (IC_{50}) at 2.01 and 0.74 μM, respectively. The aroyl-substituted tryptamines displayed better activity than aryliminotryptamines.

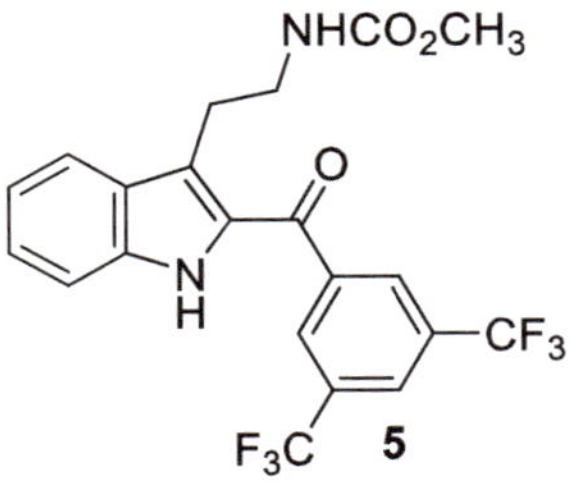

5

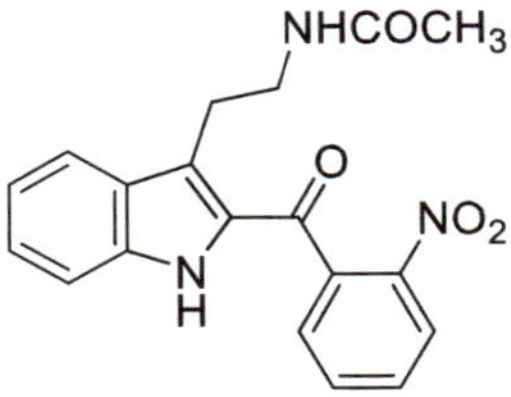

6

Fang and co-researchers designed dual inhibitors by hybridizing pharmacophoric elements of IDO inhibitor (epacadostat) and histone decatylase (HDAC) inhibitor (mocetinostat) (Fang et al. 2018), Fig. 9.5. All the designed compounds displayed inhibitory activity on both inhibitors. Among the designed molecule, one compound (compound **7**) displayed equal inhibitory activity on IDO (IC_{50} = 69.0 nM) and HDAC (IC_{50} = 66.5 nM).

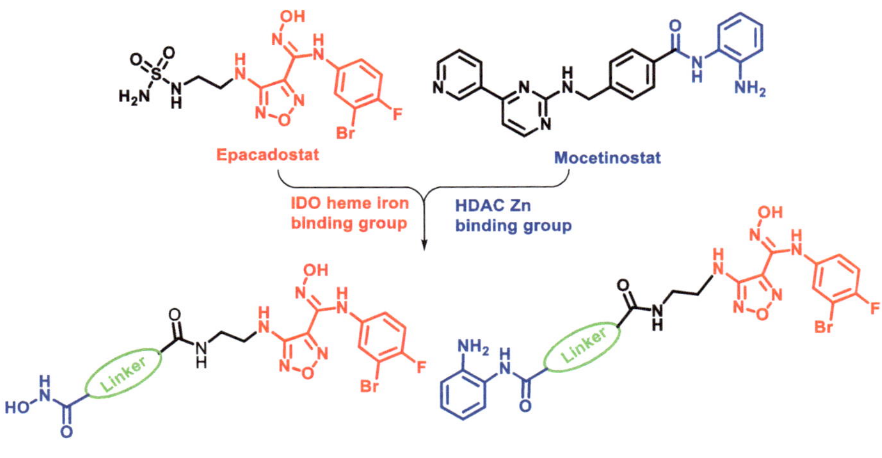

Fig. 9.5 Design of dual IDO1 and HDAC inhibitors (Fang et al. 2018)

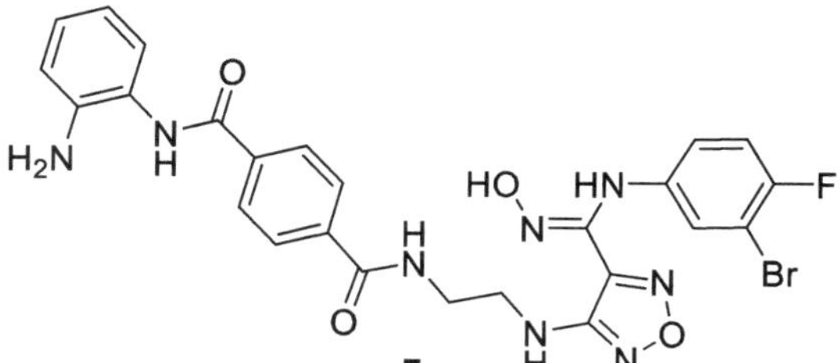

7

The designed molecules are screened for their antiproliferative activities against LLC (Lewis lung cancer), CT-26 (mouse colon cancer), A549 (human lung cancer), HCT-116 (human colon cancer), and HT-29 (human colon cancer) cell lines by the CCK8 (Cell Counting Kit-8) assay. Compound **7** displayed IC_{50} values of 15.13 ± 1.85 μM and 20.65 ± 5.66 μM against LLC and A549, respectively (Fang et al. 2018).

In 2019, Du and their co-researcher (Du et al. 2019) demonstrated the design, synthesis, and biological activities of a series of phosphonamidate esters. Among the synthesized compounds, three compounds (**8, 9,** and **10**) showed good inhibitory activity against IDO1 (hIDO1 IC_{50} = 78–121 nM). Compound **8** displayed a better antiproliferation effect on Lewis Lung cells in vivo.

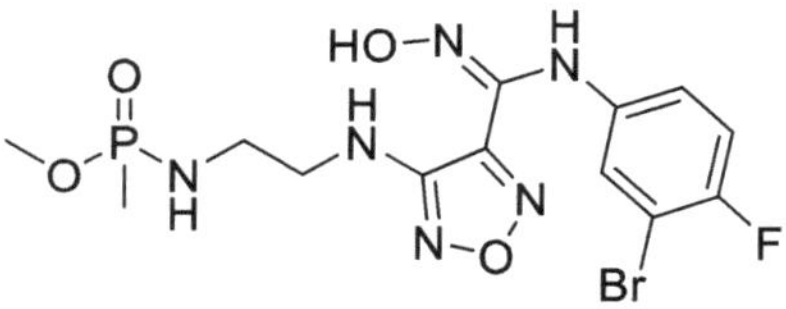

8

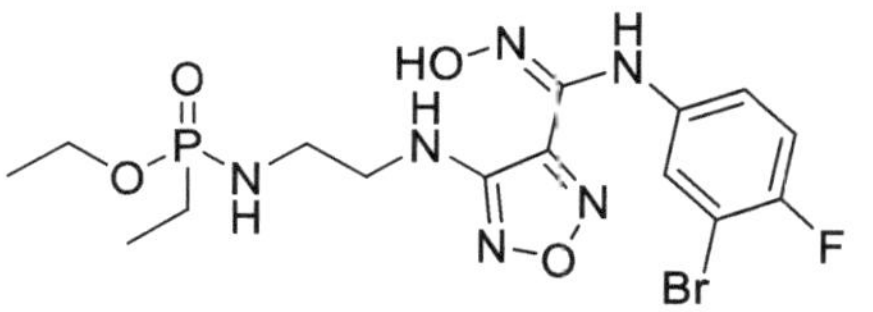

9

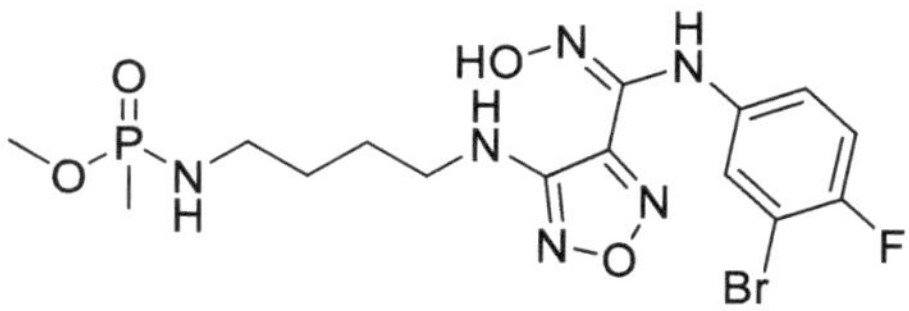

10

Recently, Wang and co-researchers (Wang et al. 2023) reported the discovery of dual inhibitors to target Nicotinamide Phosphoribosyltransferase (NAMPT) and IDO1 enzymes for the treatment of drug-resistant non-small-cell lung cancer (Wang et al. 2023). The dual inhibitors consist of an imidazopyridine ring connected to the oxadiazole-bearing oxime group via a linker.

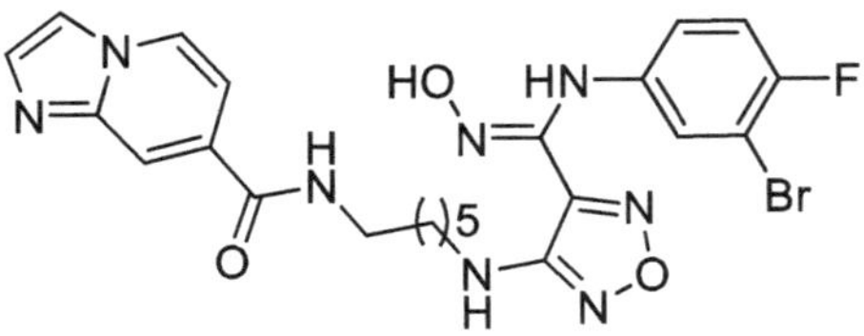

11

Among the synthesized compounds, compound **11** showed good inhibitor activities against both the targets IC_{50} values of 57.7 ± 2.8 nM and 233 ± 45.5 nM for NAMPT and IDO1, respectively. The compounds with alkyl chain as linker afforded inhibitory activity than respective aryl linker. The compound **11** showed more robust antiproliferative activity (IC_{50} = 5.35 μM) against A549/R cells relative to FK866 and epacadostat. The antiproliferative effect of **11** is due to NAD^+ reduction and reactive oxygen species (ROS) accumulation.

9.2 Transforming Growth Factor-β Inhibitors

9.2.1 Introduction

Transforming growth factor-β (TGF-β) is a group of polypeptide molecules acting like hormones or like local mediators (Massaous and Hata 1997). They are present in both vertebrates and invertebrates. This superfamily includes prototype TGF-βs, bone morphogenetic proteins (BMPs), the activins, and growth and differentiation factors (GDFs). TGF-β exists in five isoforms, namely TGF-β1-TGF-β5. In the mammalian, the first three isoforms (TGF-β1, TGF-β2, and TGF-β3) are identified (Wang et al. 2020).

A variety of cells secrete the TGF-β. In humans, platelets contribute a major role. TGF-β is secreted as an inactive form (homodimeric polypeptide bounded with extracellular proteins) from the cells. The proteolytic cleavage affords the active form of TGF-β (Katz et al. 2013). This active form of the ligand binds with the receptor complex (heteromeric complex of type II, and type I receptors). The TGF-β receptor II phosphorylates and activates the TGF-β receptor I. The phosphorylated type I receptor transfers the phosphate group to SMAD2/SMAD3 and activates them. The activated SMADs detached from the type I receptors and formed a new complex with SMAD4. The formed trimeric complex migrated to the nucleus, where it interacts with DNA-binding transcription factors and produces biological effects (Katz et al. 2013).

The transforming growth factor-β (TGF-β) is involved in a variety of biological processes like cell growth, cell proliferation, cell differentiation, autophagy, apoptosis, epithelial–mesenchymal transition (EMT), immune responses, angiogenesis, inflammation, and maintenance of adult tissue homeostasis (Liu et al. 2021; Yang et al. 2021).

Dysregulation of the TGF-β pathway leads to the development of several diseases and disorders. It includes immune dysfunction, fibrosis, cerebrovascular diseases, and cancer (Liu et al. 2021). In cancer, TGF-β plays two different roles; it inhibits the cancer cell growth in the early stages of cancer. On the other hand, in the advanced stages of cancer, it promotes the proliferation of cancer cells (van den Bulk et al. 2021). In the disease and disorder conditions, inhibiting the TGF-β signaling pathway affords beneficial effects.

9.2.2 Different Targets of TGF-β Signaling Pathway

The signaling pathway can be targeted by any one of the following strategies.

9.2.2.1 In the Ligand Level

The antisense oligonucleotides promote degradation of TGF-β mRNA, which leads to decreased biosynthesis of the ligand (TGF-β) (Fan et al. 2019). Examples of this category include Trabedersen (AP12009), ISTH0036, and AP1104/AP15012 (Haque and Morris 2017).

9.2.2.2 Ligand Traps and Neutralizing Antibodies

Soluble receptors TβRII and TβRIII (βglycan) serve as TGF-β ligand traps. This trapping process prevents the interaction between the receptors and ligands (Haque and Morris 2017).

The monoclonal antibodies are used to neutralize the ligands (TGF-β1, TGF-β2, and TGF-β1) thereby interfering with the signaling pathway. The following monoclonal antibodies extensively studied for this purpose are fresolimumab (GC1008), 2G7, 1D11, metelimumab, and lerdelimumab. These antibodies are also known as anti-TGF-β antibodies (Arteaga et al. 1993) and TGF-β–neutralizing antibodies (Tabe et al. 2013).

9.2.2.3 Combined Vaccine/Antisense

Belagenpneumatucel–L (Lucanix) is a combination of anticancer vaccine and antisense oligonucleotides prepared from non-small-cell lung cancer lines (Haque and Morris 2017).

9.2.2.4 Peptide Aptamers

Signaling molecules (SMADs) are targeted to inhibit the TGF-β signaling pathway. Small peptide molecules are employed to inhibit the TGF-β signaling pathway. The peptide molecules behave like antibodies and specifically interact with epitopes of SMADs (SMAD2/SMAD3). This protein (aptamer)–protein (SMADs) interaction prevents the heterotrimeric complex (SMAD 2/3-SMAD 4) formation with SMAD 4, leading to a defective TGF-β signaling pathway (Huang et al. 2021).

9.2.2.5 TGF-β Receptor Kinase Inhibitors

Small molecules are designed to inhibit the kinase activity and thereby block the TGF-β signaling pathway. Most of the small molecules developed for this purpose are inhibiting the type 1 receptors of TGF-β. Alternatively, this receptor is named activin receptor-like kinase-5, ALK5 (Jeon and Jen 2010).

9.2.3 Most Widely Studied TGF-β Receptor Kinase Inhibitors

In this section, we will see elaborately about small-molecule inhibitors, which target the type I receptors of transforming growth factor-β.

Based on the core chemical moiety, the most widely studied small-molecule inhibitors can be classified into three types. The imidazole-based molecules, pyrazole, and pteridine-based molecules. Regardless of the category, a minimum of two cyclic moieties are attached to the core chemical moiety. Most of these molecule targets the TGF-β type I receptor at ATP (adenosine-5-triphosphate) binding site. This binding process inhibits the phosphorylation of SMADs (SMAD2/SMAD3), which leads to the inhibition of the TGF-β signaling pathway. The chemical structures of imiadazole and pyrazole/pteridine-based TGF-β type I receptor inhibitors are depicted in Figs. 9.6 and 9.7.

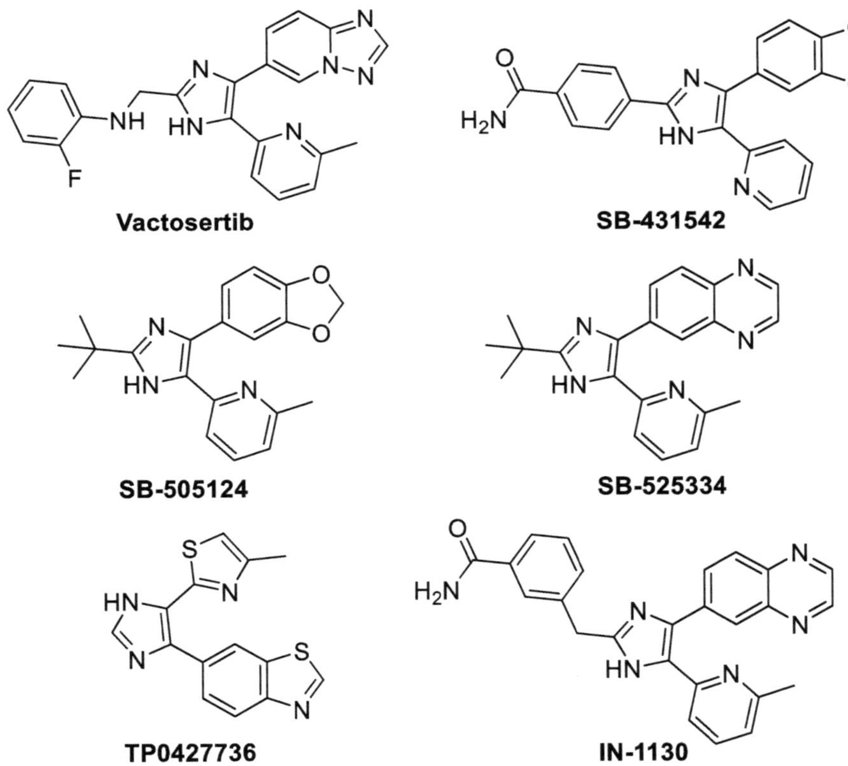

Fig. 9.6 Chemical Structures of Imidazole-based TGF-β Receptor I inhibitors

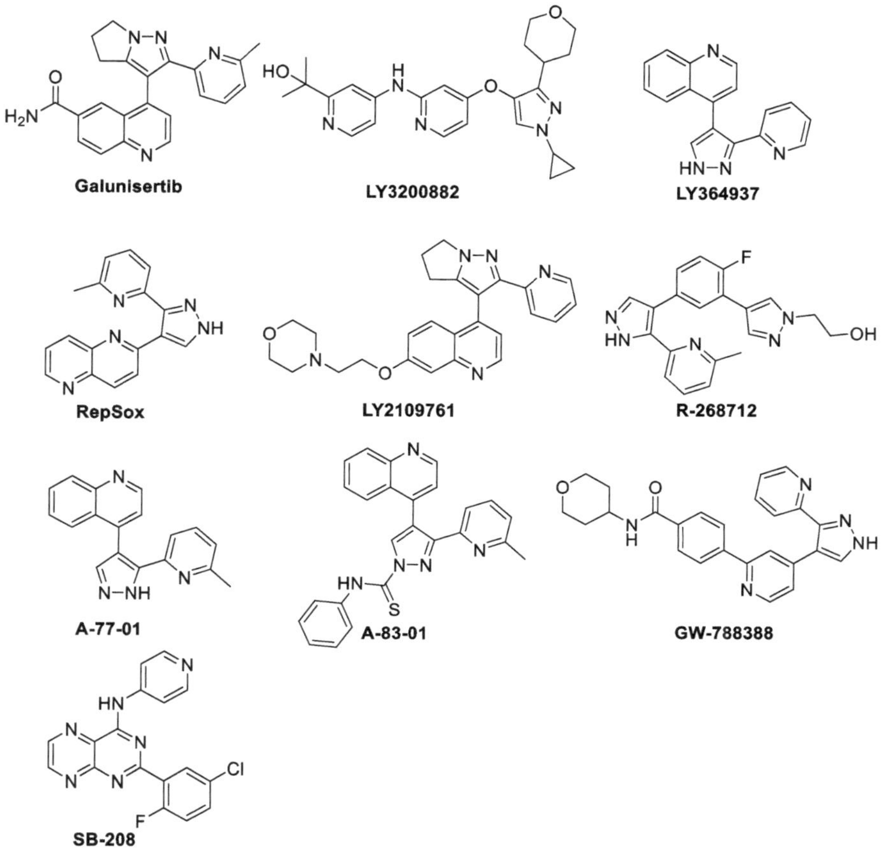

Fig. 9.7 Chemical Structures of Pyrazole/Pteridine-based TGF-β Receptor I inhibitors

9.2.3.1 Vactosertib

Vactosertib was discovered by MedPacto, Seoul, South Korea. It is previously identified with the code TEW-7197 and EW-7197. It inhibits the transforming growth factor-β type I receptor with an IC_{50} value of 12.9 nM (Jung et al. 2020). It also inhibits ALK2 and ALK-4. The median terminal half-life of vactosertib is 3.2 h (Jung et al. 2020), and it is more effective than galunisertib against melanoma. Co-administration of vactosertib with immune checkpoint inhibitors is one of the best strategies to treat cancer (Kim et al. 2021). The most common adverse effects of vactosertib are anemia, loss of appetite, fatigue, and urticaria.

9.2.3.2 Sb-431542

SB-431542 was discovered by GlaxoSmithKline. SB-431542 inhibits the kinase activity of transforming growth factor-β receptor type I with the IC_{50} value of 94 nM. It did not show any effects on other signaling pathways like ERK, JNK, and p38 MAPK (Wang et al. 2020).

9.2.3.3 Sb-505124

In the in vitro study, SB-505124 did not show any toxicity to renal epithelial A498 cells for up to 3 days at a concentration of 100 μM. It is a less potent inhibitor of ALK4 with an IC_{50} value of 129 nM compared to ALK5. This molecule did not show any inhibition for ALK2 at concentrations up to 10 μM (DaCosta et al. 2004).

9.2.3.4 Sb-525334

SB-525334 was discovered by GlaxoSmithKline. It is a potent and selective inhibitor of transforming growth factor-beta type I receptor. SB-525334 is a more selective inhibitor toward ALK5 kinase (IC_{50} = 14.3 nM) than ALK4 kinase (IC_{50} = 58.5 nM), and it is inactive toward ALK2, ALK3, and ALK6 (Grygielko et al. 2005).

9.2.3.5 TP0427736

TP0427736 was discovered by Taisho Pharmaceutical. TP0427736 inhibits TGF-β receptor-I with an IC_{50} value of 2.72 nM (Naruse et al. 2017).

9.2.3.6 IN-1130 (In2Gen)

The pharmacokinetic study showed that IN-1130 gave the oxidized metabolite as a major metabolite (Kim et al. 2008). This molecule is relatively nontoxic and more potent than SB-431542 or SB-505124 (Kim et al. 2008). IN-1130 is metabolized by multiple enzymes (human CYP2C8, CYP3A4, CYP2C19, and CYP2D6*1); hence, drug–drug interaction would be low (Kim et al. 2008).

9.2.3.7 Galunisertib

Galunisertib was discovered by Eli Lilly & Co. It is formerly identified with code number LY21557299. The plasma half-life of galunisertib is 8.6 h, and in the form of 14C, its half-life is 10 h. In the systemic circulation, seven metabolites are detected. Among the metabolites, the oxidized form (LSN3199597) and glucuronide conjugated metabolite (LSN3199607) are the major metabolites of galunisertib. The major metabolite (LSN3199597) displayed less potency compared to the parent molecule in the pharmacological studies (Cassidy et al. 2018).

Galunisertib displayed antiproliferative activity in three in vivo non-small-cell lung cancer models and two breast cancer models (Wick et al. 2020). In the clinical studies, galunisertib exhibited anticancer activity by reducing the growth of lung and breast cancer cells (Kim et al. 2021). However, in one of Phase II clinical studies, the combination of galunisertib with lomustine failed to improve the overall survival compared to lomustine with a placebo (Brandes et al. 2016).

9.2.3.8 LY3200882

LY3200882 was discovered by Eli Lilly. It is a potent, safe, and highly selective ATP competitive inhibitor of the TGF-βRI. Monotherapy or combination therapy LY3200882 showed anticancer activity (Yap et al. 2021). The most common adverse effects associated with the LY3200882 are fatigue, headache, and increased level of alanine aminotransferase (Yap et al. 2021). LY3200882 is absorbed within 2.16 h and has a half-life of 7.44 h, and the molecule is completely eliminated in 48 h.

9.2.3.9 LY364937

LY364937 is a potent and selective competitive inhibitor of TGFβR-I, discovered by Eli Lilly. It displays TGFβR-I inhibitory property with an IC50 value of 59 nM. It exhibits seven times high selectivity toward TGFβR-I over TGFβR-II (Kim et al. 2021).

9.2.3.10 RepSox

RepSox is a selective inhibitory property toward the TGF-β type I receptor (Gellibert et al. 2004). Chemically it is known as 2-(3-(6-methylpyridin-2-yl)-1H-pyrazol-4-yl)-1,5-naphthyridine.

9.2.3.11 LY2109761

LY2109761 was discovered by Eli Lilly Pharmaceuticals. It is a dual inhibitor and it inhibits both TβRI and TβRII with the *K*i value of 38 nmol/L and 300 nmol/L in vitro kinase assay, respectively (Melisi et al. 2008). In the in vivo study, the combination of LY2109761 and gemcitabine (a nucleoside metabolic inhibitor) reduced the tumor burden significantly and prolonged the survival (Melisi et al. 2008).

9.2.3.12 R-268712

R-268712 was discovered by Daiichi Sankyo. R-268712 is a potent inhibitor of transforming growth factor-β receptor I with an IC_{50} of 2.5 nM (Terashima et al. 2014).

9.2.3.13 A-77-01

This molecule was discovered by the Japanese Foundation for Cancer Research. It is also one of the potent inhibitors of TGF-β receptor type-I with an IC_{50} value of 25 nM.

9.2.3.14 A-83-01

A-83-01 was discovered by the Japanese Foundation for Cancer Research. The chemical structure of the A-83-01 is shown in Fig. 9.7 (Tojo et al. 2005).

9.2.3.15 GW 788388

GW 788388 was discovered by GlaxoSmithKline. GW 788388 is a selective inhibitor of transforming growth factor-β (TGF-β) type 1 receptor (IC_{50} = 18 nM) (Bhide et al. 2006).

9.2.3.16 Sb-208

SB-208 was discovered by Scios (Johnson & Johnson). It is a derivative of pteridine. It displayed transforming growth factor-β receptor I inhibition with an IC_{50} value of 48 nM.

9.2.4 Natural Products with TGF-β Receptor I Antagonistic/Inhibitor Properties

The natural products that displayed TGF-β receptor I inhibition are presented in Table 9.2, and their chemical structures are presented in Figs. 9.8 and 9.9.

Table 9.2 Natural Products with TGF-β receptor I inhibitor properties

S. No.	Natural product	Chemical class/biological source	References
1	Betanin	Betacyanin, present in fruits of *Opuntia elatior mill*	Esatbeyoglu et al. (2015), Avila-Carrasco et al. (2019)
2	Codonolactone	Sesquiterpene lactone, found in rhizomes of *Atractylodes lancea*	Fu et al. (2016)
3	Cryptotanshinone	Diterpenoid, present in dry root and rhizome of *salvia miltiorrhiza*	Kim et al. (2014), Li et al. (2015)
4	Curcumin	Polyphenol, found in the rhizomes of *Curcuma longa*	Hewlings and Kalman (2017), Avila-Carrasco et al. (2019)
5	Gambogic acid	Xanthonoid, resin obtained from *Garcinia hanburyi* tree	Hatami et al. (2020), Avila-Carrasco et al. (2019)
6	Genistein	Isoflavone, found in the seeds of Glycine max	Bagchi et al. (2011), Avila-Carrasco et al. (2019)
7	Gentiopicroside	Secoiridoid glycoside, present in the root of *Gentiana lutea*	Tchimene et al. (2013), Avila-Carrasco et al. (2019)
8	Hesperetin	Flavanone, present in citrus fruits like lemon, limes, oranges, tangerines and also found in grapes	Choi et al. (2020)
9	Ligustrazine	Pyrazine nucleus-based alkaloid, found in the root of *Ligusticum chuanxiong* Hort	Ma et al. (2022), Avila-Carrasco et al. (2019)
10	Osthole	Coumarin derivative, obtained from fruits of *Cnidium monnieri*	Yang et al. (2022), Avila-Carrasco et al. (2019)
11	Oxymatrine	Alkaloid, present in the roots of Sophora flavescens	Wei et al. (2014), Avila-Carrasco et al. (2019)
12	Paeoniflorin	Monoterpene glycoside, found in roots of *Paeonia lactiflora*	Zhang et al. (2022), Avila-Carrasco et al. (2019)
13	Resveratrol	Polyphenol derivative of stilbene, present in the fruits of grapes, blueberries, raspberries, etc.	Adedokun et al. (2023), Avila-Carrasco et al. (2019)
14	Tannic acid	Polyphenol, found in gall nuts and leaves of *Caesalpinia spinosa*, *Rhus semialata*, etc.	Cabezas et al. (2015), Avila-Carrasco et al. (2019)

9.2.5 Structure of TβRI and Pharmacophoric Elements of TGF-β1 Receptor Inhibitors

Ogunjimi et al. (2012) reported the interaction between the SB-431542 and transforming growth factor-β receptor I. The co-crystal of SB-431542 and TβR-I reveals the composition of the TβR-I: it consists of a small N-terminal lobe and a large

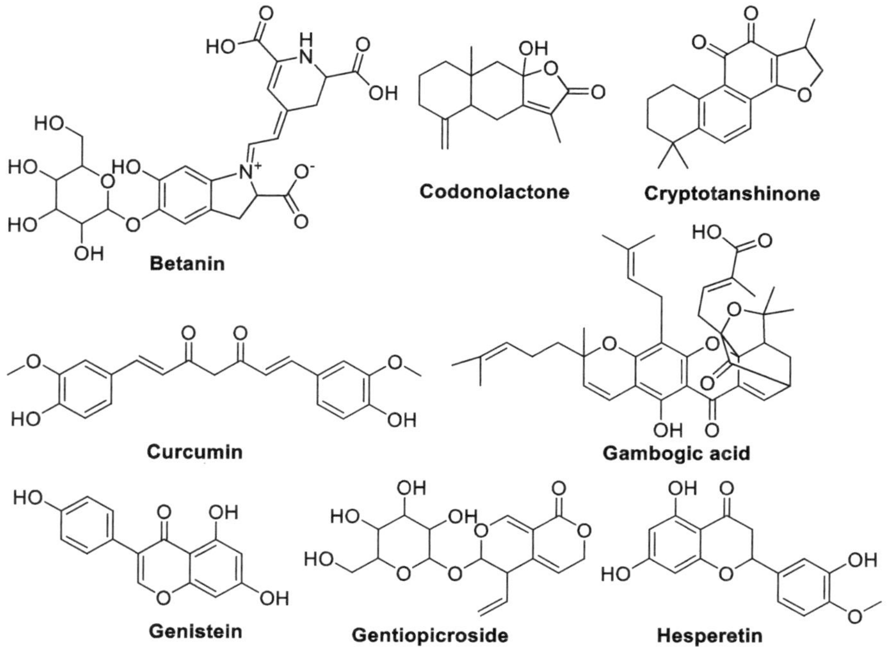

Fig. 9.8 Chemical structures of natural products with TGF-β Receptor I Inhibitors

C-terminal lobe, and these regions are connected through a linker also known as a hinge region. The N-terminal lobe is mainly composed of β-sheets, while the C-terminal is composed of α-helices (Ogunjimi et al. 2012).

Similarly, solving the co-structure of SB-431542 and TβR-I discloses the types of intermolecular interaction between the small molecule and the macromolecule. Like other kinase inhibitors, this molecule occupies the ATP binding site, which is close to the site of the linker (hinge region). The pyridinyl and benzodioxol rings are having hydrophobic interactions with TβR-I. The oxygen atom of the benzodioxol system involves in hydrogen bond interaction with amide nitrogen of H283 from the hinge region of the TβRI (Ogunjimi et al. 2012).

The imidazole ring of SB-431542 has direct hydrogen bond interaction with K232 of TβRI and indirect hydrogen bond interaction with TβRI through a water molecule. Another hydrogen bond interaction was also observed between SB-431542 and TβRI, an amide portion of SB-431542 with D351 residue of TβRI. Except for the benzamide ring, all other ring systems of SB-431542 strongly interacted with the TβRI (Ogunjimi et al. 2012).

The analysis of co-crystal structure of another imidazole-based TβRI inhibitor (IN-1130) indicates that binding modes of IN-1130 with TβRI are like SB-431542. However, compound IN-1130 has an additional hydrogen bond interaction with the D351 residue of TβRI (Wang et al. 2020).

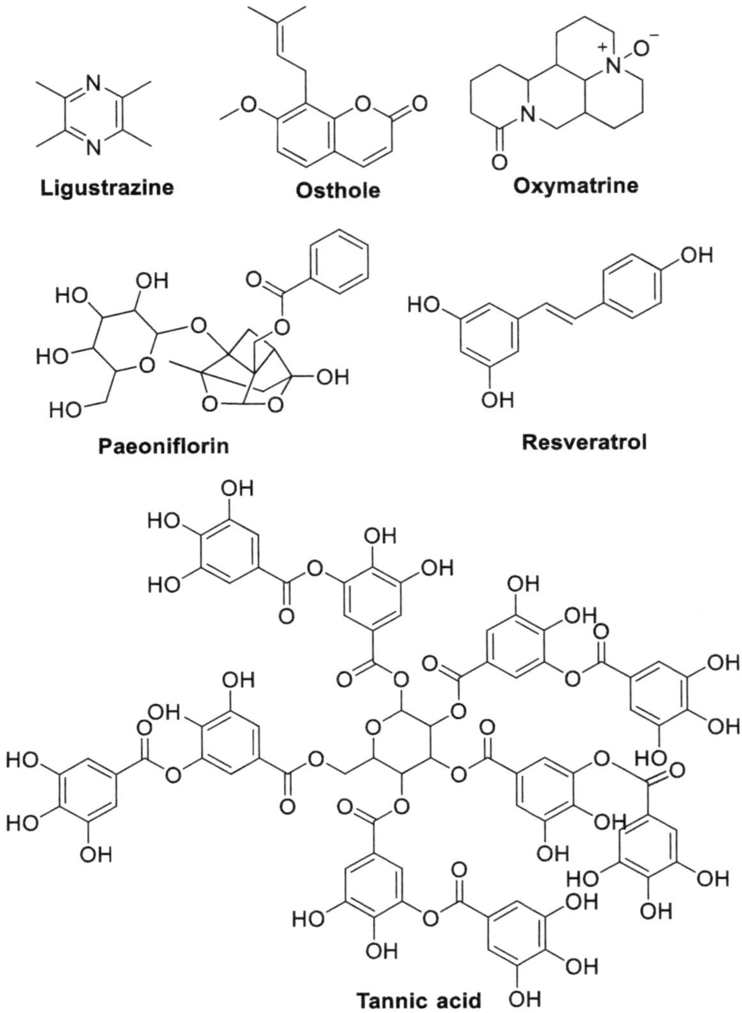

Fig. 9.9 Chemical structures of natural products with TGF-β Receptor I Inhibitors

9.2.6 New TGF-β Receptor I Inhibitors for Treating Lung Cancer

The currently available kinase inhibitors often lack specificity (Wu et al. 2020). Therefore, discovering new molecules with high selectivity/specificity will afford safer anticancer agents. This section overviews the discovery of TGF-β receptor I inhibitors for treatment of lung cancer.

Geraniin is a natural product obtained from *Phyllanthus amarus* and falls under the chemical class of polyphenols. It possesses a wide range of pharmacological properties including antitumor activity. To identify the role of geraniin, Ko (2015) investigated the effect of geraniin on EMT (epithelial–mesenchymal transition). This study revealed that geraniin suppressed the EMT by inhibiting the transforming growth factor-β receptor I in A549 lung cancer cells (Wu et al. 2020).

Dioscin is another natural product that belongs to the category of the same polyphenols obtained from *Phyllanthus amarus* and displayed the antitumor property by inhibiting the transforming growth factor-β receptor I in A549 lung cancer cells (Lim et al. 2017).

Recently, Kim and their team members (Kim et al. 2021) identified the natural products **(Ginsenosides Rk1 and Rg5)** obtained from *Panax ginseng Meyer* that exhibited anticancer activity in A549 lung cancer cells by inhibiting the transforming growth factor-β receptor I (Kim et al. 2021).

Hypaconitine is a natural product obtained from the root of *Aconitum* species possessing a wide range of pharmacological properties. It includes anti-inflammatory, analgesic, and cardiotoxic properties. It falls under the category of diterpenoid alkaloids. Hai-Tao and their research team (2017) reported the antiproliferation properties of hypaconitine in transforming growth factor-β receptor 1-induced epithelial–mesenchymal transition in lung cancer A549 cells (Feng et al. 2017).

IC261 is a synthetic molecule having an indole nucleus. It is a well-known inhibitor of casein kinase. It potentially inhibits the epithelial–mesenchymal transition. In order to know the mechanism involved in the inhibition of epithelial–mesenchymal transition, Kim and Shin studied the effect of IC261 on epithelial–mesenchymal transition using A549 lung cancer cells. IC261 significantly reduces the expression of TGF-β-induced mesenchymal cell markers as well as the capacity of cells to migrate via Smad2/3 phosphorylation in A549 cells (Kim and Shin 2022).

Resveratrol is a phenolic compound, chemically known as *trans*-3,4,5-trihydroxystilbene. It is present in grapes, blueberries, raspberries, mulberries, peanuts, and in many other plants. In 2013, Wang et al. provided evidence that resveratrol suppresses lung cancer invasion and metastasis in vitro by inhibiting transforming growth factor-β receptor I-induced EMT (Wang et al. 2013).

Sanguiin H6 is a polyphenol compound derived from ellagitannin. Sanguiin showed an antiproliferative effect on the growth of lung cancer A549 cells by inhibiting the TGF β receptor. Among the tested concentrations (1, 2.5, 5, 10, 25, 50, 75, and 100 μM), 50 μM and above concentrations displayed an antiproliferative effect (Ko et al. 2015).

Osthol is a coumarin nucleus containing natural products. It is also known as osthole (Sun et al. 2021). Osthol is obtained from *Cnidium monnieri* and *Angelica pubescens*. Feng et al. disclosed the possible mechanism involved in the antiproliferative property of the osthol, TGF-b1-induced EMT, adhesion, migration, and invasion through inactivation of NF-kB-Snail pathways in lung cancer A549 cells (Feng et al. 2017).

9.3 Conclusions

Many IDO inhibitors are under clinical trials at various levels, and most clinical trials involve the combination of IDO inhibitors with other anticancer agents. In the past few decades, many research teams are actively involved in the discovery and development of new and potent IDO inhibitors from natural and synthetic sources. The existing well-known IDO inhibitors (epacadostat, navoximod, isomers of 1-methyltryptophan, and norharmane) serve as substrates and activate the AhR. Hence, identifying the exact pharmacophoric elements of the IDO inhibitors may enable medicinal chemists to discover potent IDO inhibitors with few or negligible adverse effects.

Like IDO inhibitors, TGF-β receptor I inhibitors are discovered to combat a wide range of cancers. The well-known or most studied IDO inhibitors possess either imidazole or pyrazole as a center core moiety. To discover new or potent molecules various approaches, ligand-based, structure-based high-throughput screening and screening of natural products, are employed. To get the synergistic effect, TGF-β receptor I inhibitors are administered along with other classes of anticancer drugs in clinical trials. The recent literature clearly indicates the potential exploitation of natural products for the development of anticancer agents, particularly for the treatment of lung cancer.

References

Adedokun KA, Imodoye SO, Bello IO, Lanihun A-A, Bello IO (2023) Therapeutic potentials of medicinal plants and significance of computational tools in anti-cancer drug discovery. In: Egbuna C, Rudrapal M, Tijjani H (eds) Drug discovery update, phytochemistry, computational tools and databases in drug discovery. Elsevier, Amsterdam, pp 393–455., ISBN 9780323905930. https://doi.org/10.1016/B978-0-323-90593-0.00017-4

Arteaga CL, Hurd SD, Winnier AR, Johnson MD, Fendly BM, Forbes JT (1993) Anti-transforming growth factor (TGF)-beta antibodies inhibit breast cancer cell tumorigenicity and increase mouse spleen natural killer cell activity. Implications for a possible role of tumor cell/host TGF-beta interactions in human breast cancer progression. J Clin Invest 92(6):2569–2576. https://doi.org/10.1172/JCI116871

Avila-Carrasco L, Majano P, Sánchez-Toméro JA, Selgas R, López-Cabrera M, Aguilera A, González Mateo G (2019) Natural plants compounds as modulators of epithelial-to-mesenchymal transition. Front Pharmacol 10:715. https://doi.org/10.3389/fphar.2019.00715

Bagchi M, Patel S, Zafra-Stone S, Bagchi D (2011) Selected herbal supplements and nutraceuticals. In: Gupta RC (ed) Reproductive and developmental toxicology. Academic, Cambridge, MA, pp 385–393. https://doi.org/10.1016/B978-0-12-382032-7.10030-X. ISBN 9780123820327

Beatty GL, O'Dwyer PJ, Clark J, Shi JG, Bowman KJ, Scherle PA, Newton RC, Schaub R, Maleski J, Leopold L, Gajewski TF (2017) First-in-human phase I study of the Oral inhibitor of Indoleamine 2,3-Dioxygenase-1 Epacadostat (INCB024360) in patients with advanced solid malignancies. Clin Cancer Res 23(13):3269–3276. https://doi.org/10.1158/1078-0432.CCR-16-2272

Bhide RS, Cai ZW, Zhang YZ, Qian L, Wei D, Barbosa S, Lombardo LJ, Borzilleri RM, Zheng X, Wu LI, Barrish JC, Kim SH, Leavitt K, Mathur A, Leith L, Chao S, Wautlet B, Mortillo S, Jeyaseelan R Sr, Kukral D, Hunt JT, Kamath A, Fura A, Vyas V, Marathe P, D'Arienzo C, Derbin G, Fargnoli J (2006) Discovery and preclinical studies of (R)-1-(4-(4-fluoro-2-methyl-1H-indol-5-yloxy)-5-methylpyrrolo[2,1-f][1,2,4]triazin-6-yloxy)propan-2-ol

(BMS-540215), an in vivo active potent VEGFR-2 inhibitor. J Med Chem 49(7):2143–2146. https://doi.org/10.1021/jm051106d

Boer J, Young-Sciame R, Lee F, Bowman KJ, Yang X, Shi JG, Nedza FM, Frietze W, Galya L, Combs AP, Yeleswaram S, Diamond S (2016) Roles of UGT, P450, and gut microbiota in the metabolism of Epacadostat in humans. Drug Metab Dispos 44(10):1668–1674. https://doi.org/10.1124/dmd.116.070680

Brandes AA, Carpentier AF, Kesari S, Sepulveda-Sanchez JM, Wheeler HR, Chinot O, Cher L, Steinbach JP, Capper D, Specenier P, Rodon J, Cleverly A, Smith C, Gueorguieva I, Miles C, Guba SC, Desaiah D, Lahn MM, Wick W (2016) A phase II randomized study of galunisertib monotherapy or galunisertib plus lomustine compared with lomustine monotherapy in patients with recurrent glioblastoma. Neuro-Oncology 18(8):1146–1156. https://doi.org/10.1093/neuonc/now009

Brochez L, Chevolet I, Kruse V (2017) The rationale of indoleamine 2,3-dioxygenase inhibition for cancer therapy. Eur J Cancer 76:167–182. https://doi.org/10.1016/j.ejca.2017.01.011

Cabezas R, Avila MF, Torrente D, Gonzalez J, El-Bachá RS, Guedes R, Barreto GE (2015) Natural antioxidants in dementia: an overview. In: Martin CR, Preedy VR (eds) Diet and nutrition in dementia and cognitive decline. Academic, Cambridge, MA, pp 827–836. https://doi.org/10.1016/B978-0-12-407824-6.00076-8. ISBN 9780124078246

Capece L, Arrar M, Roitberg AE, Yeh SR, Marti MA, Estrin DA (2020) Substrate stereo-specificity in tryptophan dioxygenase and indoleamine 2,3-dioxygenase. Proteins 78(14):2961–2972. https://doi.org/10.1002/prot.22819

Cassidy KC, Gueorguieva I, Miles C, Rehmel J, Yi P, Ehlhardt WJ (2018) Disposition and metabolism of [^{14}C]-galunisertib, a TGF-βRI kinase/ALK5 inhibitor, following oral administration in healthy subjects and mechanistic prediction of the effect of itraconazole on galunisertib pharmacokinetics. Xenobiotica 48(4):382–399. https://doi.org/10.1080/00498254.2017.1323137

Chauhan J, Dasgupta M, Luthra T, Awasthi A, Tripathy S, Banerjee A, Paul S, Nag D, Chakrabarti S, Chakrabarti G, Sen S (2018) Design, synthesis and biological evaluation of a novel library of antimitotic C_2-aroyl/arylimino tryptamine derivatives that are also potent inhibitors of indoleamine-2,3-dioxygenase (IDO). Eur J Pharm Sci 124:249–265. https://doi.org/10.1016/j.ejps.2018.08.033

Choi D, Kim CL, Kim JE, Mo JS, Jeong HS (2020) Hesperetin inhibit EMT in TGF-β treated podocyte by regulation of mTOR pathway. Biochem Biophys Res Commun 528(1):154–159. https://doi.org/10.1016/j.bbrc.2020.05.087

DaCosta BS, Major C, Laping NJ, Roberts AB (2004) SB-505124 is a selective inhibitor of transforming growth factor-beta type I receptors ALK4, ALK5, and ALK7. Mol Pharmacol 65(3):744–752. https://doi.org/10.1124/mol.65.3.744

Davar D, Bahary N (2018) Modulating tumor immunology by inhibiting Indoleamine 2,3-dioxygenase (IDO): recent developments and first clinical experiences. Target Oncol 13(2):125–140. https://doi.org/10.1007/s11523-017-0547-9

Du Q, Feng X, Wang Y, Xu X, Zhang Y, Qu X, Li Z, Bian J (2019) Discovery of phosphonamidate IDO1 inhibitors for the treatment of non-small cell lung cancer. Eur J Med Chem 182:111629. https://doi.org/10.1016/j.ejmech.2019.111629

Esatbeyoglu T, Wagner AE, Schini-Kerth VB, Rimbach G (2015) Betanin-a food colorant with biological activity. Mol Nutr Food Res 59(1):36–47. https://doi.org/10.1002/mnfr.201400484

Fan C, Zhang J, Hua W, Dijke P (2019) TGF-β in cancer progression: from tumor suppressor to tumor promotor. In: Boffetta P, Hainaut P (eds) Encyclopedia of cancer (third edition). Academic, Cambridge, MA, pp 455–470. https://doi.org/10.1016/B978-0-12-801238-3.64983-8. ISBN 9780128124857

Fang K, Dong G, Li Y, He S, Wu Y, Wu S, Wang W, Sheng C (2018) Discovery of novel Indoleamine 2,3-dioxygenase 1 (IDO1) and histone deacetylase (HDAC) dual inhibitors. ACS Med Chem Lett 9(4):312–317. https://doi.org/10.1021/acsmedchemlett.7b00487

Feng X, Liao D, Liu D, Ping A, Li Z, Bian J (2020) Development of Indoleamine 2,3-dioxygenase 1 inhibitors for cancer therapy and beyond: a recent perspective. J Med Chem 63(24):15115–15139. https://doi.org/10.1021/acs.jmedchem.0c00925

Feng H, Lu JJ, Wang Y, Pei L, Chen X (2017) Osthole inhibited TGF β-induced epithelial-mesenchymal transition (EMT) by suppressing NF-κB mediated snail activation in lung cancer A549 cells. Cell Adhes Migr 11(5–6):464–475. https://doi.org/10.1080/19336918.2016.1259058

Feng HT, Zhao WW, Lu JJ, Wang YT, Chen XP (2017) Hypaconitine inhibits TGF-β1-induced epithelial-mesenchymal transition and suppresses adhesion, migration, and invasion of lung cancer A549 cells. Chin J Nat Med 15(6):427–435. https://doi.org/10.1016/S1875-5364(17)30064-X

Fu J, Ke X, Tan S, Liu T, Wang S, Ma J, Lu H (2016) The natural compound codonolactone attenuates TGF-β1-mediated epithelial-to-mesenchymal transition and motility of breast cancer cells. Oncol Rep 35(1):117–126. https://doi.org/10.3892/or.2015.4394

Gellibert F, Woolven J, Fouchet MH, Mathews N, Goodland H, Lovegrove V, Laroze A, Nguyen VL, Sautet S, Wang R, Janson C, Smith W, Krysa G, Boullay V, De Gouville AC, Huet S, Hartley D (2004) Identification of 1,5-naphthyridine derivatives as a novel series of potent and selective TGF-beta type I receptor inhibitors. J Med Chem 47(18):4494–4506. https://doi.org/10.1021/jm0400247

Gomes B, Driessens G, Bartlett D, Cai D, Cauwenberghs S, Crosignani S, Dalvie D, Denies S, Dillon CP, Fantin VR, Guo J, Letellier MC, Li W, Maegley K, Marillier R, Miller N, Pirson R, Rabolli V, Ray C, Streiner N, Torti VR, Tsaparikos K, Van den Eynde BJ, Wythes M, Yao LC, Zheng X, Tumang J, Kraus M (2018) Characterization of the selective Indoleamine 2,3-Dioxygenase-1 (IDO1) catalytic inhibitor EOS200271/PF-06840003 supports IDO1 as a critical resistance mechanism to PD-(L)1 blockade therapy. Mol Cancer Ther 17(12):2530–2542. https://doi.org/10.1158/1535-7163.MCT-17-1104

Grygielko ET, Martin WM, Tweed C, Thornton P, Harling J, Brooks DP, Laping NJ (2005) Inhibition of gene markers of fibrosis with a novel inhibitor of transforming growth factor-beta type I receptor kinase in puromycin-induced nephritis. J Pharmacol Exp Ther 313(3):943–951. https://doi.org/10.1124/jpet.104.082099

Haque S, Morris JC (2017) Transforming growth factor-β: a therapeutic target for cancer. Hum Vaccin Immunother 13(8):1741–1750. https://doi.org/10.1080/21645515.2017.1327107

Hatami E, Jaggi M, Chauhan SC, Yallapu MM (2020) Gambogic acid: a shining natural compound to nanomedicine for cancer therapeutics. Biochim Biophys Acta Rev Cancer 1874(1):188381. https://doi.org/10.1016/j.bbcan.2020.188381

Hewlings SJ, Kalman DS (2017) Curcumin: a review of its effects on human health. Foods 6(10):92. https://doi.org/10.3390/foods6100092

Hornyák L, Dobos N, Koncz G, Karányi Z, Páll D, Szabó Z, Halmos G, Székvölgyi L (2018) The role of Indoleamine-2,3-dioxygenase in cancer development, diagnostics, and therapy. Front Immunol 9:151. https://doi.org/10.3389/fimmu.2018.00151

Huang CY, Chung CL, Hu TH, Chen JJ, Liu PF, Chen CL (2021) Recent progress in TGF-β inhibitors for cancer therapy. Biomed Pharmacother 134:111046. https://doi.org/10.1016/j.biopha.2020.111046

Huang Q, Zheng M, Yang S, Kuang C, Yu C, Yang Q (2011) Structure-activity relationship and enzyme kinetic studies on 4-aryl-1H-1,2,3-triazoles as indoleamine 2,3-dioxygenase (IDO) inhibitors. Eur J Med Chem 46(11):5680–5687. https://doi.org/10.1016/j.ejmech.2011.08.044

Jeon HS, Jen J (2010) TGF-beta signaling and the role of inhibitory Smads in non-small cell lung cancer. J Thorac Oncol 5(4):417–419. https://doi.org/10.1097/JTO.0b013e3181ce3afd

Jung SY, Hwang S, Clarke JM, Bauer TM, Keedy VL, Lee H, Park N, Kim SJ, Lee JI (2020) Pharmacokinetic characteristics of vactosertib, a new activin receptor-like kinase 5 inhibitor, in patients with advanced solid tumors in a first-in-human phase 1 study. Investig New Drugs 38(3):812–820. https://doi.org/10.1007/s10637-019-00835-y

Jung KH, LoRusso P, Burris H, Gordon M, Bang YJ, Hellmann MD, Cervantes A, Ochoa de Olza M, Marabelle A, Hodi FS, Ahn MJ, Emens LA, Barlesi F, Hamid O, Calvo E, McDermott D, Soliman H, Rhee I, Lin R, Pourmohamad T, Suchomel J, Tsuhako A, Morrissey K, Mahrus S, Morley R, Pirzkall A, Davis SL (2019) Phase I study of the Indoleamine 2,3-dioxygenase 1 (IDO1) inhibitor Navoximod (GDC-0919) administered with PD-L1 inhibitor (Atezolizumab) in advanced solid tumors. Clin Cancer Res 25(11):3220–3228. https://doi.org/10.1158/1078-0432.CCR-18-2740

Jung SY, Yug JS, Clarke JM, Bauer TM, Keedy VL, Hwang S, Kim SJ, Chung EK, Lee JI (2020) Population pharmacokinetics of vactosertib, a new TGF-β receptor type I inhibitor, in patients with advanced solid tumors. Cancer Chemother Pharmacol 85(1):173–183. https://doi.org/10.1007/s00280-019-03979-z

Katz LH, Li Y, Chen JS, Muñoz NM, Majumdar A, Chen J, Mishra L (2013) Targeting TGF-β signaling in cancer. Expert Opin Ther Targets 17(7):743–760. https://doi.org/10.1517/14728222.2013.782287

Kim H, Choi P, Kim T, Kim Y, Song BG, Park YT, Choi SJ, Yoon CH, Lim WC, Ko H, Ham J (2021) Ginsenosides Rk1 and Rg5 inhibit transforming growth factor-β1-induced epithelial-mesenchymal transition and suppress migration, invasion, anoikis resistance, and development of stem-like features in lung cancer. J Ginseng Res 45(1):134–148. https://doi.org/10.1016/j.jgr.2020.02.005

Kim YW, Kim YK, Kim DK, Sheen YY (2008) Identification of human cytochrome P450 enzymes involved in the metabolism of IN-1130, a novel activin receptor-like kinase-5 (ALK5) inhibitor. Xenobiotica 38(5):451–464. https://doi.org/10.1080/00498250701871121

Kim YW, Kim YK, Lee JY, Chang KT, Lee HJ, Kim DK, Sheen YY (2008) Pharmacokinetics and tissue distribution of 3-((5-(6-methylpyridin-2-yl)-4-(quinoxalin-6-yl)-1H-imidazol-2-yl)methyl)benzamide; a novel ALK5 inhibitor and a potential anti-fibrosis drug. Xenobiotica 38(3):325–339. https://doi.org/10.1080/00498250701781924

Kim J, Lee KW, Lee HJ (2014) Polyphenols suppress and modulate inflammation: possible roles in health and disease. In: Watson RR, Preedy VR, Zibadi S (eds) Polyphenols in human health and disease. Academic, Cambridge, MA, pp 393–408., ISBN 9780123984562. https://doi.org/10.1016/B978-0-12-398456-2.00029-3

Kim BG, Malek E, Choi SH, Ignatz-Hoover JJ, Driscoll JJ (2021) Novel therapies emerging in oncology to target the TGF-β pathway. J Hematol Oncol 14(1):55. https://doi.org/10.1186/s13045-021-01053-x

Kim SJ, Shin MS (2022) IC261 inhibits the epithelial-mesenchymal transition induced by TGF-β in A549 lung cancer cells. Appl Biol Chem 65:21. https://doi.org/10.1186/s13765-022-00690-1

Knox WE, Mehler AH (1950) The conversion of tryptophan to kynurenine in liver. I. The coupled tryptophan peroxidase-oxidase system forming formylkynurenine. J Biol Chem 187(1):419–430

Ko H (2015) (2015) Geraniin inhibits TGF-β1-induced epithelial-mesenchymal transition and suppresses A549 lung cancer migration, invasion and anoikis resistance. Bioorg Med Chem Lett 25(17):3529–3534. https://doi.org/10.1016/j.bmcl.2015.06.093

Ko H, Jeon H, Lee D, Choi HK, Kang KS, Choi KC (2015) Sanguiin H6 suppresses TGF-β induction of the epithelial-mesenchymal transition and inhibits migration and invasion in A549 lung cancer. Bioorg Med Chem Lett 25(23):5508–5513. https://doi.org/10.1016/j.bmcl.2015.10.067

Li Q, Harden JL, Anderson CD, Egilmez NK (2016) Tolerogenic phenotype of IFN-γ-induced IDO+ dendritic cells is maintained via an autocrine IDO-kynurenine/AhR-IDO loop. J Immunol 197(3):962–970. https://doi.org/10.4049/jimmunol.1502615

Li W, Saud SM, Young MR, Colburn NH, Hua B (2015) Cryptotanshinone, a Stat3 inhibitor, suppresses colorectal cancer proliferation and growth in vitro. Mol Cell Biochem 406(1–2):63–73. https://doi.org/10.1007/s11010-015-2424-0

Lim WC, Kim H, Kim YJ, Choi KC, Lee IH, Lee KH, Kim MK, Ko H (2017) Dioscin suppresses TGF-β1-induced epithelial-mesenchymal transition and suppresses A549 lung cancer migration and invasion. Bioorg Med Chem Lett 27(15):3342–3348. https://doi.org/10.1016/j.bmcl.2017.06.014

Liu S, Ren J, Ten Dijke P (2021) Targeting TGFβ signal transduction for cancer therapy. Signal Transduct Target Ther 6(1):8. https://doi.org/10.1038/s41392-020-00436-9

Liu M, Wang X, Wang L, Ma X, Gong Z, Zhang S, Li Y (2018) Targeting the IDO1 pathway in cancer: from bench to bedside. J Hematol Oncol 11(1):100. https://doi.org/10.1186/s13045-018-0644-y

Luo B, Que ZJ, Zhou ZY, Wang Q, Dong CS, Jiang Y, Hu B, Shi H, Jin Y, Liu JW, Li HG, Wang L, Tian JH (2018) Feiji recipe inhibits the growth of lung cancer by modulating T-cell immunity through indoleamine-2,3-dioxygenase pathway in an orthotopic implantation model. J Integr Med 16(4):283–289. https://doi.org/10.1016/j.joim.2018.04.008

Ma S, Suchomel J, Yanez E, Yost E, Liang X, Zhu R, Le H, Siebers N, Joas L, Morley R, Royer-Joo S, Pirzkall A, Salphati L, Ware JA, Morrissey KM (2019) Investigation of the absolute bioavailability and human mass balance of navoximod, a novel IDO1 inhibitor. Br J Clin Pharmacol 85(8):1751–1760. https://doi.org/10.1111/bcp.13961

Ma S, Zhang N, Hou J, Liu S, Wang J, Lu B, Zhu F, Wei P, Hong G, Liu T (2022) Synthesis and discovery of Ligustrazine-heterocycle derivatives as antitumor agents. Front Chem 10:941367. https://doi.org/10.3389/fchem.2022.941367

Massaous J, Hata A (1997) TGF-beta signalling through the Smad pathway. Trends Cell Biol 7(5):187–192. https://doi.org/10.1016/S0962-8924(97)01036-2

Melisi D, Ishiyama S, Sclabas GM, Fleming JB, Xia Q, Tortora G, Abbruzzese JL, Chiao PJ (2008) LY2109761, a novel transforming growth factor beta receptor type I and type II dual inhibitor, as a therapeutic approach to suppressing pancreatic cancer metastasis. Mol Cancer Ther 7(4):829–840. https://doi.org/10.1158/1535-7163.MCT-07-0337

Moon YW, Hajjar J, Hwu P, Naing A (2015) Targeting the indoleamine 2,3-dioxygenase pathway in cancer. J Immunother Cancer 3:51. https://doi.org/10.1186/s40425-015-0094-9

Muller AJ, Sharma MD, Chandler PR, Duhadaway JB, Everhart ME, Johnson BA 3rd, Kahler DJ, Pihkala J, Soler AP, Munn DH, Prendergast GC, Mellor AL (2008) Chronic inflammation that facilitates tumor progression creates local immune suppression by inducing indoleamine 2,3 dioxygenase. Proc Natl Acad Sci U S A 105(44):17073–17078. https://doi.org/10.1073/pnas.0806173105

Munn DH, Sharma MD, Baban B, Harding HP, Zhang Y, Ron D, Mellor AL (2005) GCN2 kinase in T cells mediates proliferative arrest and anergy induction in response to indoleamine 2,3-dioxygenase. Immunity 22(5):633–642. https://doi.org/10.1016/j.immuni.2005.03.013

Naruse T, Aoki M, Fujimoto N, Arase S, Oura H, Ueda Y, Ikeda A (2017) Novel ALK5 inhibitor TP0427736 reduces TGF-β induced growth inhibition in human outer root sheath cells and elongates anagen phase in mouse hair follicles. Pharmacol Rep 69(3):485–491. https://doi.org/10.1016/j.pharep.2017.01.024

Nayak-Kapoor A, Hao Z, Sadek R, Dobbins R, Marshall L, Vahanian NN, Jay Ramsey W, Kennedy E, Mautino MR, Link CJ, Lin RS, Royer-Joo S, Liang X, Salphati L, Morrissey KM, Mahrus S, McCall B, Pirzkall A, Munn DH, Janik JE, Khleif SN (2018) Phase Ia study of the indoleamine 2,3-dioxygenase 1 (IDO1) inhibitor navoximod (GDC-0919) in patients with recurrent advanced solid tumors. J Immunother Cancer 6(1):61. https://doi.org/10.1186/s40425-018-0351-9

Ogunjimi AA, Zeqiraj E, Ceccarelli DF, Sicheri F, Wrana JL, David L (2012) Structural basis for specificity of TGFβ family receptor small molecule inhibitors. Cell Signal 24(2):476–483. https://doi.org/10.1016/j.cellsig.2011.09.027

Pallotta MT, Fallarino F, Matino D, Macchiarulo A, Orabona C (2014) AhR-mediated, non-genomic modulation of IDO1 function. Front Immunol 5:497. https://doi.org/10.3389/fimmu.2014.00497

Prendergast GC, Malachowski WJ, Mondal A, Scherle P, Muller AJ (2018) Indoleamine 2,3-dioxygenase and its therapeutic inhibition in cancer. Int Rev Cell Mol Biol 336:175–203. https://doi.org/10.1016/bs.ircmb.2017.07.004

Reardon DA, Desjardins A, Rixe O, Cloughesy T, Alekar S, Williams JH, Li R, Taylor CT, Lassman AB (2020) A phase 1 study of PF-06840003, an oral indoleamine 2,3-dioxygenase 1 (IDO1) inhibitor in patients with recurrent malignant glioma. Investig New Drugs 38(6):1784–1795. https://doi.org/10.1007/s10637-020-00950-1

Röhrig UF, Awad L, Grosdidier A, Larrieu P, Stroobant V, Colau D, Cerundolo V, Simpson AJ, Vogel P, Van den Eynde BJ, Zoete V, Michielin O (2010) Rational design of indoleamine 2,3-dioxygenase inhibitors. J Med Chem 53(3):1172–1189. https://doi.org/10.1021/jm9014718. PMID: 20055453

Röhrig UF, Reynaud A, Majjigapu SR, Vogel P, Pojer F, Zoete V (2019) Inhibition mechanisms of Indoleamine 2,3-dioxygenase 1 (IDO1). J Med Chem 62(19):8784–8795. https://doi.org/10.1021/acs.jmedchem.9b00942

Shimizu T, Nomiyama S, Hirata F, Hayaishi O (1978) Indoleamine 2,3-dioxygenase. Purification and some properties. J Biol Chem 253(13):4700–4706

Smith JR, Evans KJ, Wright A, Willows RD, Jamie JF, Griffith R (2012) Novel indoleamine 2,3-dioxygenase-1 inhibitors from a multistep in silico screen. Bioorg Med Chem 20(3):1354–1363. https://doi.org/10.1016/j.bmc.2011.10.068

Soliman HH, Minton SE, Han HS, Ismail-Khan R, Neuger A, Khambati F, Noyes D, Lush R, Chiappori AA, Roberts JD, Link C, Vahanian NN, Mautino M, Streicher H, Sullivan DM, Antonia SJ (2016) A phase I study of indoximod in patients with advanced malignancies. Oncotarget 7(16):22928–22938. https://doi.org/10.18632/oncotarget.8216

Sugimoto H, Oda S, Otsuki T, Hino T, Yoshida T, Shiro Y (2006) Crystal structure of human indoleamine 2,3-dioxygenase: catalytic mechanism of O2 incorporation by a heme-containing dioxygenase. Proc Natl Acad Sci U S A 103(8):2611–2616. https://doi.org/10.1073/pnas.0508996103

Sun M, Sun M, Zhang J (2021) Osthole: an overview of its sources, biological activities, and modification development. Med Chem Res 30(10):1767–1794. https://doi.org/10.1007/s00044-021-02775-w

Tabe Y, Shi YX, Zeng Z, Jin L, Shikami M, Hatanaka Y, Miida T, Hsu FJ, Andreeff M, Konopleva M (2013) TGF-β-neutralizing antibody 1D11 enhances Cytarabine-induced apoptosis in AML cells in the bone marrow microenvironment. PLoS One 8(6):e62785. https://doi.org/10.1371/journal.pone.0062785

Tan Y, Liu M, Li M, Chen Y, Ren M (2022) Indoleamine 2, 3-dioxygenase 1 inhibitory compounds from natural sources. Front Pharmacol 13:1046818. https://doi.org/10.3389/fphar.2022.1046818

Tang K, Wu YH, Song Y, Yu B (2021) Indoleamine 2,3-dioxygenase 1 (IDO1) inhibitors in clinical trials for cancer immunotherapy. J Hematol Oncol 14(1):68. https://doi.org/10.1186/s13045-021-01080-8

Tchimene MK, Okunji CO, Iwu MM, Kuete V (2013) 1-monoterpenes and related compounds from the medicinal plants of Africa. In: Kuete V (ed) Medicinal plant research in Africa. Elsevier, Amsterdam, pp 1–32., ISBN 9780124059276. https://doi.org/10.1016/B978-0-12-405927-6.00001-1

Terashima H, Kato M, Ebisawa M, Kobayashi H, Suzuki K, Nezu Y, Sada T (2014) R-268712, an orally active transforming growth factor-β type I receptor inhibitor, prevents glomerular sclerosis in a Thy1 nephritis model. Eur J Pharmacol 734:60–66. https://doi.org/10.1016/j.ejphar.2014.03.045

Tojo M, Hamashima Y, Hanyu A, Kajimoto T, Saitoh M, Miyazono K, Node M, Imamura T (2005) The ALK-5 inhibitor A-83-01 inhibits Smad signaling and epithelial-to-mesenchymal transition by transforming growth factor-beta. Cancer Sci 96(11):791–800. https://doi.org/10.1111/j.1349-7006.2005.00103.x

van den Bulk J, de Miranda NFCC, Ten Dijke P (2021) Therapeutic targeting of TGF-β in cancer: hacking a master switch of immune suppression. Clin Sci (Lond) 135(1):35–52. https://doi.org/10.1042/CS20201236

Wang H, Chen M, Sang X, You X, Wang Y, Paterson IC, Hong W, Yang X (2020) Development of small molecule inhibitors targeting TGF-β ligand and receptor: structures, mechanism, preclinical studies and clinical usage. Eur J Med Chem 191:112154. https://doi.org/10.1016/j.ejmech.2020.112154

Wang K, Ye K, Zhang X, Wang T, Qi Z, Wang Y, Jiang S (2023) Zhang K (2023) dual nicotinamide Phosphoribosyltransferase (NAMPT) and Indoleamine 2,3-dioxygenase 1 (IDO1) inhibitors for the treatment of drug-resistant nonsmall-cell lung cancer. J Med Chem 66(1):1027–1047. https://doi.org/10.1021/acs.jmedchem.2c01954

Wang H, Zhang H, Tang L, Chen H, Wu C, Zhao M, Yang Y, Chen X, Liu G (2013) Resveratrol inhibits TGF-β1-induced epithelial-to-mesenchymal transition and suppresses lung cancer invasion and metastasis. Toxicology 303:139–146. https://doi.org/10.1016/j.tox.2012.09.017

Wei J, Zhu Y, Xu G, Yang F, Guan Z, Wang M, Fang Y (2014) Oxymatrine extracted from Sophora flavescens inhibited cell growth and induced apoptosis in human osteosarcoma MG-63 cells in vitro. Cell Biochem Biophys 70(2):1439–1444. https://doi.org/10.1007/s12013-014-0078-2

Wick A, Desjardins A, Suarez C, Forsyth P, Gueorguieva I, Burkholder T, Cleverly AL, Estrem ST, Wang S, Lahn MM, Guba SC, Capper D, Rodon J (2020) Phase 1b/2a study of galunisertib, a small molecule inhibitor of transforming growth factor-beta receptor I, in combination with standard temozolomide-based radiochemotherapy in patients with newly diagnosed malignant glioma. Investig New Drugs 38(5):1570–1579. https://doi.org/10.1007/s10637-020-00910-9

Wu H, Sun Y, Wong WL, Cui J, Li J, You X, Yap LF, Huang Y, Hong W, Yang X, Paterson IC, Wang H (2020) The development of a novel transforming growth factor-β (TGF-β) inhibitor that disrupts ligand-receptor interactions. Eur J Med Chem 189:112042. https://doi.org/10.1016/j.ejmech.2020.112042

Yang S, Dai W, Wang J, Zhang X, Zheng Y, Bi S, Pang L, Ren T, Yang Y, Sun Y, Zheng Z, Wu S, Kong J (2022) Osthole: an up-to-date review of its anticancer potential and mechanisms of action. Front Pharmacol 13:945627. https://doi.org/10.3389/fphar.2022.945627

Yang S, Li X, Hu F, Li Y, Yang Y, Yan J, Kuang C, Yang Q (2013) Discovery of tryptanthrin derivatives as potent inhibitors of indoleamine 2,3-dioxygenase with therapeutic activity in Lewis lung cancer (LLC) tumor-bearing mice. J Med Chem 56(21):8321–8331. https://doi.org/10.1021/jm401195n

Yang Y, Ye WL, Zhang RN, He XS, Wang JR, Liu YX, Wang Y, Yang XM, Zhang YJ, Gan WJ (2021) The role of TGF-*β* signaling pathways in cancer and its potential as a therapeutic target. Evid Based Complement Alternat Med 2021:6675208. https://doi.org/10.1155/2021/6675208

Yap TA, Vieito M, Baldini C, Sepúlveda-Sánchez JM, Kondo S, Simonelli M, Cosman R, van der Westhuizen A, Atkinson V, Carpentier AF, Löhr M, Redman R, Mason W, Cervantes A, Le Rhun E, Ochsenreither S, Warren L, Zhao Y, Callies S, Estrem ST, Man M, Gandhi L, Avsar E, Melisi D (2021) First-in-human phase I study of a next-generation, Oral, TGFβ receptor 1 inhibitor, LY3200882, in patients with advanced cancer. Clin Cancer Res 27(24):6666–6676. https://doi.org/10.1158/1078-0432.CCR-21-1504

Ye Z, Yue L, Shi J, Shao M, Wu T (2019) Role of IDO and TDO in cancers and related diseases and the therapeutic implications. J Cancer 10(12):2771–2782. https://doi.org/10.7150/jca.31727

Zhang XX, Zuo JQ, Wang YT, Duan HY, Yuan JH, Hu YH (2022) Paeoniflorin in Paeoniaceae: distribution, influencing factors, and biosynthesis. Front Plant Sci 13:980854. https://doi.org/10.3389/fpls.2022.980854

OX40 and CD40 Agonists for the Treatment of Lung Cancer

10

Nitin Verma, Komal Thapa, Neha Kanojia, Parul Sood, Jatin Kumar, Nikita Thakur, and Kamal Dua

10.1 Introduction

Among all malignancies, lung cancer has the greatest fatality rate. Lung cancer accounted for 1.8 million cases worldwide in 2012 or 13% of total cancer cases stated internationally. Lung cancer alone caused 162,510 fatalities in the United States, with 243,820 recent instances being reported. Gender ratio is 2:1, and men 60 years of age and older make up the majority of those diagnosed. According to recent investigations, it is most common amid females in North America and Eastern Asia, as well as in Eastern, Central, and Southern Europe. According to current data, environmental variables including the airborne presence of harmful chemicals like lead and radon are the main contributors to its prevalence (Pardoll 2012). It is also observed that the number of lung cancer cases recorded is rising proportionally as smoking prevalence rises, especially in emerging nations. According to their morphological characteristics, small-cell lung cancer and non-small-cell lung cancer are the two main types of lung cancer. Another classification of non-small-cell lung cancer (NSCLC) includes adenocarcinoma, squamous cells, and large cell carcinoma (Drake et al. 2014). In China, Japan, and Saudi Arabia, it has been noted that women are reported in cases five times more frequently than men are. As per recent research, cigarette components, e-cigarette use, and environmental variables are all contributing to the growth in adenocarcinoma instances. Squamous cell carcinoma was thought to be the most prevalent kind of cancer prior to 1979, and it is currently

N. Verma (✉) · K. Thapa · N. Kanojia · P. Sood · J. Kumar · N. Thakur
Chitkara University, School of Pharmacy, Chitkara University,
Solan, Himachal Pradesh, India
e-mail: nitin.verma@chitkarauniversity.edu.in

K. Dua
Discipline of Pharmacy, Graduate School of Health, University of Technology Sydney,
Sydney, NSW, Australia

S. Bhatt et al. (eds.), *Immunotherapy Against Lung Cancer*,
https://doi.org/10.1007/978-981-99-7141-1_10

the most prevalent type of lung cancer in the Netherlands, Russia, and India (Chen and Flies 2013).

10.1.1 Tumor Microenvironment in Lung Cancer

A new method for treating cancer involves focusing on immune cells expression of costimulatory and co-inhibitory agonists. The concept that may enhance the T-cell function can have beneficial effects on individuals with lung tumor were currently authorized by FDA by the uses of monoclonal CTLA-4 inhibitory molecular antibody (Sharma and Allison 2015). Various other monoclonal Ab therapies that are now under clinical phase have been investigated. Few of these mAbs activate classes of the tumor necrosis factor and superfamily of immune cell surface compounds. This protein having 50 members is expressed by immune cells and is membrane-bound as well as soluble. An ample variety of cellular effects, such as increased formation of cytokines or chemokines as well as differentiation of cell, apoptosis, multiplication and subsistence have been discussed when these proteins are attached by either their agonist antibodies and homologous receptor agonist a (Srivastava et al. 2022; Thakur et al. 2020; Granier et al. 2017). This compound also acts as ideal stimulator for pioneering immunotherapies due to the specific expression of few TNFRSF components on antigen-particular T cells. From ancient times, immunotherapy has been proposed as a valuable therapy for inhibiting tumor growth (Marin-Acevedo et al. 2018). The advancement of mAb that either activates immune-stimulating receptors as well as inhibitory receptors in the previous generations has revealed to improve antitumor immunity in cancer-bearing individuals, causing therapeutic effectiveness. These strategies are based on the concept that cancer-bearing individuals have T lymphocytes in their bodies that are particular for tumor Ags, but their activity is hindered by the tumor microenvironment. Consequently, by improving the prevalence as well as usefulness of antigen-presenting cells and T cells, these immune-modulating Abs help in avoiding this immunological inhibition leading to tumor regression (Workman et al. 2002). Strong associations among the T-cell receptor peptide antigens as well as MHC, the involvement of costimulatory substances produced by APC are important for the perfect stimulation of native T cells (Dholaria et al. 2016). Co-stimulation is an important process for an effective T-cell reaction since the death of activated native T cells or becomes anergic without these costimulatory signals (Anderson et al. 2016).

To best produce effector and memory T cells after an antigen interaction, additional co-stimulatory proteins must be present in addition to OX40 and CD40. The TNFR superfamily includes a number of these costimulatory proteins (He et al. 2016). Formerly believed to be expressed on activated T and B lymphocytes and antigen-presenting cells (APCs), several of these receptors are now understood to promote cell survival and proliferation, differentiation, and maturation as well as provide signals directly to T cells. Numerous research teams have used agonist

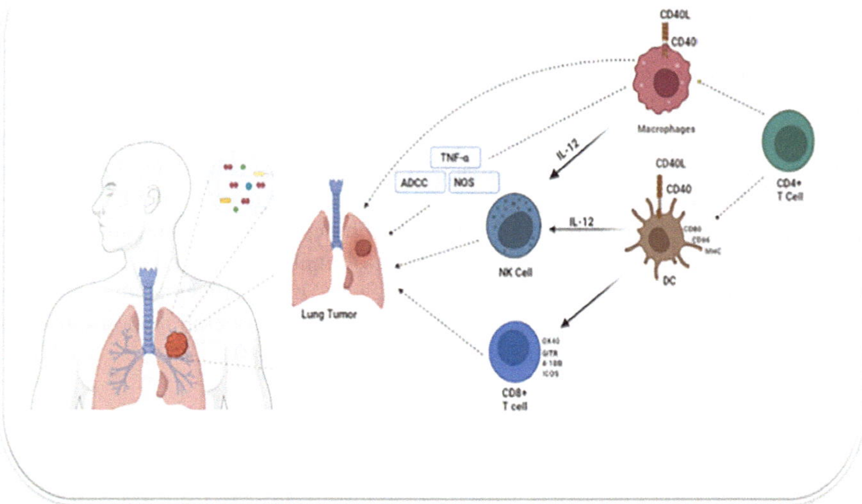

Fig. 10.1 Targeting tumor microenvironment in lung cancer by various receptors

mAbs to target TNFRs aiming to enhance activity of lymphocytes specifically in the functionalization of tumor immunotherapy, since of the diverse T-cell stimulating characteristics of these receptors (Woo et al. 2012). Figure 10.1 shows targeting tumor microenvironment in lung cancer by various receptors.

10.2 Development of Immunotherapy for Lung Cancer

Tumor immunology research will continue to be important for the development of immunotherapy. In 1991, according to the findings of phase-I clinical studies, researchers came to the conclusion that treating NSCLC patients with IL-2 and IFN- was futile. According to a 1993 study, the injection of recombinant IL-2 treatment led to an increase in circulating immune cells that may have anticancer effect (Goldberg and Drake 2011).

The BLP25 liposomal vaccine underwent a phase-I clinical study in 2001, and it was found that patients with lung cancer experienced an immunological response after receiving the vaccination. Further clinical trials of these peptides were required after it was demonstrated in 2006 that patients with NSCLC responded immunogenetically to telomerase peptide vaccination (Andrews et al. 2017). Recent data came to the conclusion that chemotherapy and cytokine-induced killer cells could assist patients recover by reducing their cellular reaction. According to recent research, older patients with a variety of comorbidities benefited most from radio immunotherapy with cetuximab. Haploidentical cytokine-induced killer cells appeared to extend the survival of NSCLC patients, according to studies carried out by Wang and other authors (Brignone et al. 2009).

A clinical trial having an epidermal growth factor vaccination was done in 2016 by Rodriguez et al. and coworkers and revealed the therapeutic potential in the treatment of EGF-dependent NSCLC tumors. An autologous tumor-derived autophagosome vaccine (DRibbles) was the main subject of a clinical trial to access its therapeutic effectiveness, and it was reported that when merging with GM-CSF, the vaccine might activate an immune reaction toward tumor cell (Wang-Gillam et al. 2013). In NSCLC patients with progressive illnesses, Zhao et al. and their coworkers revealed that hindering PD-1 when combined with vitronectin-stimulated cytokine-induced killer cells was effective. Nivolumab has currently been reported as a propitious antibody for individuals with NSCLC by Martin et al. and coworkers (2020). Both Pembrolizumab and docetaxel improved the overall response reaction in individuals with advanced illnesses (Brignone et al. 2010).

10.2.1 Non-small-Cell Lung Cancer Stem Cells

The NSCL cancer's hostility and therapy impedance demonstrated the disorder's heterogeneity and enhanced the probability that stem cells were found. Hindering unknown growth, a trait of undifferentiated/stem cells, is the main obstacle to controlling malignant cells. Additionally, stem cells can also contribute to the dormant/quiescent phase of proliferation when cancer stem cells might hideaway (Nguyen and Ohashi 2015). This ability is one of the reasons behind inherent and acquired treatment resistance. Numerous research studies showed the adaptability of various cancer cells, including NSCLC. According to a review, several investigations found a connection between metastatic invasion and NSCLC stemness. Stem cells with NSCLC displayed poor susceptibility to various antitumor medications. The above-mentioned results demonstrate the importance of stem cell research in germinal cell therapies and prognosis. In order to effectively treat NSCLC, we must therefore concentrate on using stem cells, as these unseen offenders need to be identified (Ascierto et al. 2017; Sakuishi et al. 2013).

10.3 Molecular-Based Targeted Therapies for Lung Cancer

10.3.1 OX40

T cells are essential for coordinating cell-mediated immunity, especially the immune response to malignant cells in tumors, despite the fact that there are numerous subsets with specific responsibilities. T cells are strictly regulated due to their strong cytotoxic potential through its activation process involving multiple steps and interaction of various receptors on their surface (Du et al. 2017). Firstly, T cells require exposure to foreign antigens to recognize them with the help of its T-cell receptor. Antigen-presenting cell (APC) interactions between a variety of T cells and their receptors on the surface and their ligands, made possible by the development of close contact and interaction through an immunological synapse, between the two cells for the exchange of required for T-cell activation, results in costimulatory signal for full T-cell activation (Gorman et al. 2014). One well-known costimulatory receptor is between CD28 on the T cell and CD80/CD86 on the APC. This interaction provides a positive signal that supports T-cell activation. Other co-stimulatory receptors have also been discovered, one of which is a subset that does not express itself by default but is instead increased in response to antigen priming; such receptors are believed to offer additional costimulatory signals, which are essential for sustaining immune response and for creating immunological memory. The OX40 protein is a member of this category (Ebrahim et al. 2014). Around 24–48 hours after antigen exposure, OX40 is expressed on the surface of T cells. OX40 belongs to the tumor necrosis factor, a superfamily of proteins, along with many other co-stimulatory molecules that enhance T-cell activation and co-inhibitory molecules that play role in downregulating and deactivating the T-cell receptors such as CTLA-4 and PD-1 and the TNF family (Fiori et al. 2012).

10.3.1.1 Targeting of OX40 in Lung Cancer

OX40L, which exists on the outermost layers of activated APCs, binds to OX40 to begin the OX40 signaling cascade. When OX40 is activated, it associates with several adaptor proteins, including the TNF receptor-associated factors (TRAFs) such as TRAF2, TRAF3, and TRAF5, and then leads to the activation of nuclear factor kappa B and c-Jun N-terminal kinase in downstream signaling pathways (Ohue et al. 2016). OX40 has no enzymatic activity by itself. T-cell activation, survival, memory formation, and the prevention of T-cell tolerance may cause reduction in T-cell regulation. Any of these activating signals must be present for T cells to operate correctly; otherwise, they fail to multiply, often become inactive (a condition known as T-cell anergy), or even end up dying. This is frequently exploited by cancer cells, which either upregulate or downregulate the expression of costimulatory molecules or co-inhibitory molecules respectively. The antitumor T-cell-mediated immune response is thwarted as a result of the cancer cells' ability to co-opt these pathways (Zhu et al. 2005).

The level of expression of OX40 on T cells within tumor microenvironment has been a subject of investigation in a number of studies. X40 expression on infiltrating T cells is often observed in different types of cancer, indicating that these T cells have undergone priming and activation in response to tumor-associated antigens (Yu et al. 2009). OX40L expression within the tumor is often low, making it unlikely that the T cells will become completely activated. Surprisingly, regulatory T cells that infiltrate tumors and work to inhibit the immune system appear to have the highest expression of OX40. Indeed, monoclonal antibodies targeting the PD-1 receptor or its ligand, PD-L1, have been developed to block the co-inhibitory pathway and enhance antitumor immune responses. This therapeutic strategy, known as immune checkpoint blockade, aims to unleash the immune system's potential by "taking the brakes off" and overcoming the immune evasion mechanisms employed by cancer cells (Zhu et al. 2005; Yu et al. 2009).

10.3.1.2 OX40 Agonist Development

By focusing on costimulatory chemicals, scientists have created a distinct class of medication. Costimulatory agonists have the ability to mimic the actions of ligands by attaching to receptors and starting downstream signaling, ultimately boosting the antitumor immune response. Unlike immune checkpoint inhibitors that target inhibitory pathways (the "brakes"), agonists provide a "go" signal, activating and enhancing T-cell responses against tumors. Since 2006, OX40 agonists have been under development, 5 years before the very first immune-mediated checkpoint inhibitor, ipilimumab (Yervoy), which targets CTLA-4, was approved (Ohue et al. 2016). The initial development of OX40 agonists involved the use of a mouse anti-human monoclonal antibody.

In 30 patients with metastatic cancer, intravenous treatment of the OX40 agonist antibody at 3 distinct doses (0.1 mg/kg, 0.4 mg/kg, or 2 mg/kg) was well tolerated in a phase I clinical trial. The results demonstrated strong immune-stimulating impact and at least one metastatic lesion regression in 30% of total patients. However, the medication did not meet the RECIST (Response Evaluation Criteria in Solid Tumors) standards for an objective response. One factor that contributed to its limited success was the development of anti-mouse antibodies in patients, which restricted repeat dosing of mouse-derived antibody (Yu et al. 2009).

10.3.1.3 Drugs Targeting OX40 and OX40L in Lung Cancers

Agonists of these markers are being investigated in the treatment of various malignancies based on the biological basis and roles of OX40 and its ligand. In several preclinical cancer models developed in mice, including melanoma, glioblastoma multiforme (GBM), breast cancer, colon cancer, renal and prostatic cancer, and lung carcinoma, as well as chemically produced sarcomas, effective treatment responses with OX40 agonists have been seen (Stanietsky et al. 2009; Casado et al. 2009).

Preoperative MEDI6469, an OX40 agonist after administration, was found to be safe in the clinical trial (NCT02274155) and to result in increased activation and generation of T cells within the tumor in 2 weeks after OX40 agonist infusion (Johnston et al. 2015). Another trial revealed that an OX40 agonist Ab enhanced humoral and cellular immunity, displaying antitumor efficacy (Chauvin et al. 2015). A HCC trial with PF-8600 revealed safety and efficacy as well as the persistence of stable illness (17–18 months) in half of the study participants (Lines et al. 2014). The outcomes of animal research, however, have not been adequately duplicated in human studies due to methodologically flawed designs, which is a significant barrier to the success of medication development. Recently, some researchers examined a panel of anti-human OX40 antibodies (anti-hOX40 mAb) and assessed their binding and in vitro activity. The efficiency and mechanism of action of anti-hOX40 mAb were then evaluated in a range of in vivo models, leading to the conclusion that targeting a particular isotype and domain-binding site can affect such antibodies (Le Mercier et al. 2014; Lines et al. 2014). Combining other ICB therapeutic agents enhanced antitumor response synergistically by enhancing immune cell function. However, after stimulation, the production of the costimulatory molecules only lasts a brief while. Repetitive agonistic T-cell activation may result in immunological fatigue, which is another obstacle to this sort of treatment (Picarda et al. 2016). As a result, immunological checkpoints-based therapeutic drugs are essential for the treatment of cancer, and researchers are currently evaluating combinations of medicines that target OX40 in addition to other therapy modalities. However, this combination should be targeted by taking into account the tumor's immunogenicity, the mediators engaged in various routes of immune stimulation, as well as the timing and schedule of the administration of certain drugs in combinatorial tactics (Castellanos et al. 2017). Additionally, effective T-cell agonism and anticancer activity are elicited by targeting certain isotypes with the proper therapeutic design. However, this combination should be targeted by taking into account the tumor's immunogenicity, the mediators engaged in various routes of immune stimulation, as well as the timing and schedule of the administration of certain drugs in combinatorial tactics. Additionally, effective T-cell agonism and anticancer activity are elicited by targeting certain isotypes with the proper therapeutic design (Powderly et al. 2015).

10.3.2 CD40

CD40, a class of the TNF receptor family that stimulated T cells, highly expresses CD154, the agonist ligand. Release of B-cell cytokine release is activated by CD40-CD154 association, resulting in T-cell activation as well as death of cancerous cell (Weidle et al. 2014; Tolcher et al. 2016). Instead of therapeutic potential for synergy with other antitumor remedies and treatments, the application of CD40 agonists has also been related with various toxic effects such as cytokine release disorder, thromboembolic incidences as well as cancer angiogenesis (Kramer et al. 2010; Leone et al. 2015; Zhang 2010; Vijayan et al. 2017). Discovery of ideal drug combinations and the patient compliance associated with it are the various challenges encountered with this specific therapy (Emens et al. 2017; Antonioli et al. 2017).

10.3.2.1 Biological Relevance of CD40/CD40L

A prior review covered the pleiotropic roles that CD40 signaling plays in vivo. Expression of CD40 on monocytes, as well macrophages, DC, and B cells, has an important role to play in immunity (Paulos and June 2010). Having a very high level of flexibility, monocytes are innate immune progenitor cells. Monocyte maturation is largely driven by CD40 signaling, which also promotes the differentiation of monocytes into DC and M1 spectral macrophages (Malissen et al. 2017; Lan et al. 2017; Massague 2008). By stimulating DC, CD40L improves antigen presentation to T cells, which is one of its key roles. By upregulating surface proteins like CD54 and CD86, this process, known as "licensing," improves the contact between DC and T cells, activating the latter (Wendt et al. 2012; Thomas and Massagué 2005).

The CD40L protein also targets B cells. In order to maintain CD40-expressing B cells and to promote the negative selection of autoreactive T cells, a significant interaction between T cells and B cells is necessary in the thymus. Direct contact between B cells and CD4+ T cells causes the T cells to express CD40L, which prevents B cells from going through apoptosis (Padua and Massague 2009; Neuzillet et al. 2015; Smith et al. 2012; Bogdahn et al. 2011; Hwang et al. 2016). Through the activation of PI3K/Akt in this role, CD40L transmits a survival signal that helps activated B cells survive longer and differentiate into plasma cells. The overexpression of anti-apoptotic Bcl-2 family members maintains the homeostatic proliferation and survival of antigen-specific B cells via CD40.8 In fact, deficiencies in antibody class switching and somatic hypermutation in B cells (hyper-IgM syndrome) are linked to abnormalities of the CD40/CD40L system (Gulley et al. 2017; Brandes et al. 2016; Long et al. 2001; Dahlberg et al. 2015; Muntasell et al. 2017; Benson and Caligiuri 2014).

10.3.2.2 Implications for the Development of CD40 Agonists

Agonistic chemicals must have a three-dimensional structure based on the distinct receptor clustering patterns for TNF-R-SF receptors to produce effective downstream signals (Leichner et al. 2016; Schmitt et al. 2017; Bagot et al. 2017). Numerous methods to stimulate CD40 signaling have been investigated because of the crucial part that CD40 has an important function in antitumor immune reaction (Gyori et al. 2017). The latter group can be further broken down into gene therapy techniques and recombinant protein approaches that use CD40L mimics to introduce the CD40L gene into sites required for targeting (Tolcher et al. 2017). Recombinant CD40L and cellular vaccines that overexpressed CD40L were both tried in these initial trials. About 5 years later, the first agonistic antibody studies with CP-870,893 and SGN-40 got underway. Although the early clinical trials produced some positive findings, clinical activity has been constrained for a variety of possible reasons (Liu et al. 2017; Weiskopf 2017; Sikic et al. 2016; Thompson et al. 2017).

10.3.2.3 Bispecific Approaches Targeting CD40

Bispecific CD40/targeting concepts include a variety of methods, including the development of enhanced CAR-T cells (also known as "cellular bispecifics") that express the CAR together with other constituents such as CD40L, antibodies that identify two different epitopes in the trans or cis form, along with bifunctional compounds that associate a targeting domain and a functional domain into a single entity (Willoughby et al. 2017). Tthough, the advancement of bispecific CD40 agonists is difficult because of the doubtful expression of CD40. More research on CD40 bispecifics such as CEA as well as other antigens that target tumors is currently under process (Aspeslagh et al. 2016; Linch et al. 2015; Turner et al. 2001; Curti et al. 2013; Infante et al. 2016; Hamid et al. 2016).

10.3.2.4 Combination Treatment with Other Therapies

Given the overall expression profile and biological activities of CD40, it is worth noting that while investigating the interaction of CD40 agonists with many other treatment options, preclinical studies have explored their potential synergistic effects with various therapeutic modalities (Dempke et al. 2017a). Combining

CD40-targeted therapies with other immunomodulators or checkpoint inhibitors has revolutionized cancer treatment by unleashing the immune system's antitumor activity. Thus, researchers hope to achieve more effective and durable responses in cancer treatment as preclinical studies have shown promising results when CD40-targeted therapies are coupled with chemotherapy or kinase inhibitors (Knee et al. 2016).

One of the mainstays of cancer therapy, radiation (RT) is administered to up to 70% of all cancer patients at some point during their course of treatment. Two of the anticipated outcomes of RT are the release of tumor antigens and the development of a local TME that is pro-inflammatory. As a result, extensive preclinical research studies have proven the use of CD40 agonists with RT to enhance the RT-induced immunization and elicit systemic antitumor effects (Koon et al. 2016; Siu et al. 2017). The ultimate goal of TME regulation is to activate/prime antitumor cytotoxic T cells, which can be facilitated by certain inhibitory checkpoint blocking pathways via PD-1, PD-L1, or CTLA-4 to evade immune surveillance. In non-immunogenic cancer model systems, these medicines have improved the remodeling of the macrophage compartment (Tran et al. 2017). According to a non-controlled Phase I study, there is some indication of clinical benefit in particular when combined with CD40 antibody with checkpoint inhibitors, notably anti-PD-L1 and anti-CTLA-4 antibodies. In preclinical models, several combinations have been documented. Additionally, in mice models of glioma and for other reasons, CD40 ligation has demonstrated potential for therapy when combined with cancer vaccination techniques (Sanmamed et al. 2015). In a mouse B16 melanoma model, it has also increased the effectiveness of adoptive cell transfer therapy. Finally, there are some data that suggest that a combination treatment using CAR-T cells and anti-CD40 agonists may enhance the immune response against tumors in a mouse model having cancer of the pancreas as well as the CD40L-expressing CAR-T cells already stated. These first findings are promising, but bigger, randomized clinical studies are required to fully assess the potential of CD40-targeting combination treatment (Fan et al. 2014; Harvey et al. 2015; Burris et al. 2017; Chester et al. 2016).

10.4 Other Potential Targets

10.4.1 IDO

Tryptophan is broken down by the enzyme indoleamine 2,3-dioxygenase (IDO), converting it to kynurenines. By raising the differentiation and activity of Treg and lowering the quantity and activity of CD8 T cells, kynurenines provide an immunosuppressive environment, which is only exacerbated by the high levels of PD-1/PD-L1 that are concurrently present (Takeda et al. 2010). Numerous tumor cell types, including melanoma, chronic lymphocytic leukemia, ovarian, CRC, and more recently, sarcomas, have been found to have high IDO expression (Tolcher et al. 2016; Segal et al. 2017). Furthermore, high levels of IDO may contribute to drug resistance to chemotherapeutic drugs in addition to correlating with poor outcomes in specific malignancies (Massarelli et al. 2016). IDO inhibitor therapy has also brought up distinct issues, despite their potential to balance the immunosuppressive tumor microenvironment. IFN- γ and other inflammatory chemicals first cause IDO to be produced. As a result, a poor response to anti-IDO drugs may be linked to the absence of inflammation in the tumor microenvironment (Perez-Ruiz et al. 2017). Secondly, healthy tissue also expresses IDO and other comparable enzymes, thus blocking them could have unintended side effects. IDO inhibitors, however, continue to be a major focus of research in immune checkpoint therapy, and several compounds are being tested.

A once-daily, powerful, and selective oral IDO1 inhibitor called BMS-986205 is currently being tested in phase I clinical trial alongside nivolumab (NCT02658890). With the exception of three occurrences of grade 3 hepatitis, dermatitis, and hypophosphatemia, all recorded toxicities have been grades 1–2. There was no effectiveness reported (Denoeud and Moser 2011; van de Ven and Borst 2015).

Phase II clinical trials with indoximod, another IDO inhibitor, are being conducted for melanoma, pancreatic cancer, and castrate-resistant prostate cancer (CRPC) (NCT02073123, NCT02077881, and NCT01560923). In total, 52% of melanoma patients who took indoximod when combined with pembrolizumab, nivolumab, or ipilimumab experienced ORR (Zakharia et al. 2016). Human subject with pancreatic cancer had an ORR of 37% when receiving indoximod, gemcitabine, and nab-paclitaxel at the same time (Michot et al. 2016). The median PFS for metastatic CRPC patients using indoximod rose from 4.1 to 10.3 months when compared to placebo (Owonikoko et al. 2016). Phase I/II clinical trials evaluating epacadostat, an additional oral medication that blocks the IDO pathway, are being conducted to treat various tumors (the trials' NCT numbers are 02327078 and 02178722). The ORR varied from melanoma, which had an ORR of 75%, to CRC, which had an ORR of 4%. It appears safe to use alongside pembrolizumab (Sanborn et al. 2016). Even though no dose-limiting toxicities have been observed in clinical trial, but up to 3% of patients have ceased their medication as a result of adverse events indicating that adverse events experienced by patients are severe enough to require treatment interruption or discontinuation (Vonderheide and Glennie 2013; Dempke et al. 2017b).

10.4.2 TLR

Toll-like receptors (TLRs) are thought to be essential for pathogen detection and immune response regulation. However, they play a far more nuanced part in the onset of cancer. Some TLRs, such as TLR4, can activate Tregs or PD-L1 to speed up the growth of cancer by promoting inflammation in the tumor microenvironment. By recognition of a "danger signal" inside the tumor microenvironment, it alerts the immunity when combined with several malignant cells and activates TLRs, proteins such as TLR7, TLR8, and TLR9 to initiate antitumor response (Cabo et al. 2017). In addition to promoting an immune response against cancer, medications that impact these TLRs pathways induce the death of cancer cells through the induction of autophagy (Moon et al. 2015). When using TLR treatment, there are a few important considerations to make. The nonspecific ability of the compound to stimulate both cytotoxic T cells and immunosuppressive cells within the tumor microenvironment firstly reduces the overall tumoricidal efficacy (Toulmonde et al. 2017; Bilir and Sarisozen 2017). Secondly, it's uncertain which patients and whose couples might benefit most from using these drugs together, having stronger anticancer effects than any single therapy (Siu et al. 2017). It has been established that using these substances in conjunction with other antitumor therapies like radiation and chemotherapy seems to provide more potent anticancer effects than using either therapy alone (Bahary et al. 2016). Sadly, these mixtures may raise the risk of toxicity and immunological responses. In spite of these difficulties, multiple clinical studies are testing various drugs. MEDI9197, a dual TLR7/8 agonist, in combination with these TLR pathways, induces the death of cancer cells through the induction of autophagy (Jha et al. 2017). When using TLR treatment, there are a few important considerations to make. The nonspecific ability of the compound to stimulate the immune cells having both c and immunosuppressive functions within the tumor microenvironment firstly reduces the overall tumoricidal efficacy with durvalumab, and RT is now being studied in the patients being affected with metastatic or locally advanced solid tumors (NCT02556463). According to preliminary research, the agent is typically safe and only has modest side effects. At this time, there are no efficacy statistics available (Hamid et al. 2017; Perez et al. 2017). Patients with advanced solid tumors were administered the TLR9/IL-12 agonist PG545 (pixatimod, pINN) in a phase I clinical trial (NCT02042781). The trial outcome indicated that three out of 23 patients experienced dose-limiting toxicities, while a disease control rate of 38% was observed (Beatty et al. 2017; Lu 2014; Shi et al. 2016). In a recent phase I clinical trial, patients with HCC who were not candidates for surgery were treated with radiation and the potent TLR3 agonist polyinosinic-polycytidylic acid polylysine carboxymethylcellulose (poly-ICLC) (de la Torre et al. 2017). The majority of the drug's side effects, grade I or II, have been demonstrated to be typically safe for intratumoral injection. PFS of 66% at 6 months, 28% at 24 months, and OS of 69% at 1 year, 38% at 2 years were also demonstrated (Dowling and Mansell 2016; Li et al. 2017).

10.4.3 Arginase Inhibitors

The activation and growth of T cells depend on the amino acid arginine. Malignant cells and MDSCs both produce large amounts of arginase, which reduces arginine and causes the emergence of immune-suppressive effects in the tumor microenvironment (Dredge et al. 2017). Combining the arginase inhibitors with other treatment modalities such as with radiation therapy or other immune checkpoint inhibitors is a strategy aimed to synergistically enhance antitumor effect by reducing the immunosuppressive effects within the tumor microenvironment. The inhibition of arginase may directly impact tumor growth beyond to its immunomodulatory effect. Lowering the availability of arginine, a vital nutrient for cancer cell growth and proliferation, can hinder tumor cell metabolism and survival (de la Torre et al. 2017). Finally, because the cancer microenvironment produces arginine at a higher level than plasma, the use of these drugs may have a more tailored and nontoxic effect compared to other types of immunotherapies. Preliminary research investigated the effects of CB-1158, a selective arginase inhibitor when given alone or when given in combination with nivolumab (NCT02903914) in human subject with metastatic solid tumors. Initial findings indicate that CB-1158 demonstrates favorable tolerability, achieves more than 90% arginase inhibition, and causes significant rise in blood plasma arginine level with a rise of up to four times (Tomala and Kovar 2016; Jiang et al. 2016; Su et al. 2015; Diab et al. 2017).

10.4.4 Oncolytic Peptides

The cytotoxic chemotherapeutic peptide LTX-315, which is produced from lactoferrin, penetrates the mitochondrial membrane and causes necrosis without the help of caspase (Su et al. 2015; Diab et al. 2017; Bernatchez et al. 2017; Ananieva 2015; Timosenko et al. 2017). This medication changes the cancer microenvironment in conjunction with anti-CLTA-4 drugs by reducing immunosuppressive cells and raising T lymphocytes (Papadopoulos et al. 2017; Zhou et al. 2016; Sveinbjornsson et al. 2017). Tumor antigen is produced when this medication is given intravenously, increasing TIL activity. This delivery mechanism restricts its applicability to more localized tumors while making it a desirable tactic to lessen systemic toxicity. An additional significant feature of LTX-315 is the notable upregulation of CTLA-4 expression observed in the oncolytic therapy. This demonstrates that this kind of therapy may be particularly helpful when paired with anti-CLTA-4 medications (Yamazaki et al. 2016; Spicer et al. 2017). Clinical trial on phase 1 (NCT01986426) is currently seeking individuals who have metastatic solid tumors, such as breast cancer and melanoma, to participate in evaluating the efficacy of this medication either alone or in combination with pembrolizumab or ipilimumab. Encouraging preliminary results indicate that out of 28 human subjects, two achieved complete remission (CR), eight experienced stable disease (SD), and five showed a reduction in tumor size exceeding 50%. Figure 10.2 depicts mechanisms of various agonists in inhibition of lung cancer (Miotto et al. 2010; Zhang et al. 2016; Sun et al. 2015; Naing et al. 2017).

10.5 Conclusions

The biological characteristics of tumors are the current focus of cancer treatment. The roles of OX40 and OX40L in boosting the immune response are well known. However, while clinical studies have noted translational failure, OX40 and its ligand-targeted therapy have shown promising outcomes in diverse animal tumor models.

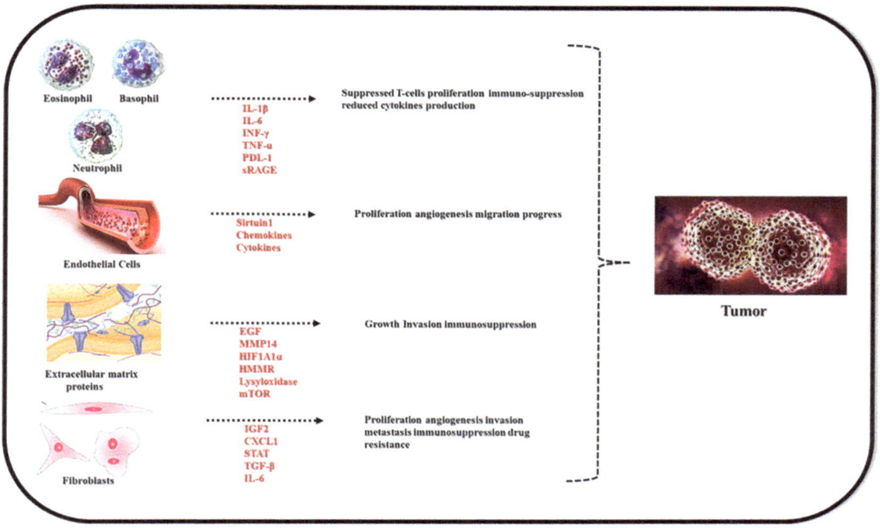

Fig. 10.2 Illustration of mechanism of various agonists in lung cancer

The early clinical findings imply that efficacy of immunotherapy in human patients is constrained. Although the biological basis and fundamental data are inadequate, this also hinders the creation of new drugs and their effectiveness. In the future, understanding the reasoning for developing such treatment drugs and their combinations would help with understanding the expression levels of specific markers or molecules in cancer tissue and blood, with respect to grading and staging for tumor diagnosis and treatment planning. We further recommend that the immunogenicity of various cancers, the burden of tumor mutations, medication design, and the timing of combinatory therapies be examined. By analyzing the expression levels, mutational profiles, and associated biomarkers, clinicians and researchers can gain insights into severity, activity, characteristics of various tumors, selection of appropriate treatment approaches, and monitor treatment response. These factors are important in precision medicine, where treatments are tailored to individual patients by taking into account the specific characteristics of their tumors.

References

Ananieva E (2015) Targeting amino acid metabolism in cancer growth and antitumor immune response. World J Biol Chem 6:281–289

Anderson AC, Joller N, Kuchroo VK (2016) Lag-3, Tim-3, and TIGIT: co-inhibitory receptors with specialized functions in immune regulation. Immunity 44:989–1004

Andrews LP, Marciscano AE, Drake CG, Vignali DAA (2017) LAG3 (CD223) as a cancer immunotherapy target. Immunol Rev 276:80–96

Antonioli L, Novitskiy SV, Sachsenmeier KF et al (2017) Switching off CD73: a way to boost the activity of conventional and targeted antineoplastic therapies. Drug Discov Today 22:1686–1696

Ascierto PA, Melero I, Bhatia S et al (2017) Initial efficacy of anti-lymphocyte activation gene-3 (anti–LAG-3; BMS-986016) in combination with nivolumab(nivo) in pts with melanoma (MEL) previously treated with anti–PD-1/PD-L1 therapy. J Clin Oncol 35:9520–9520

Aspeslagh S, Postel-Vinay S, Rusakiewicz S et al (2016) Rationale for anti-OX40cancer immunotherapy. Eur J Cancer 52:50–66

Bagot M, Porcu P, Ram-Wolff C et al (2017) Phase I study of IPH4102, anti-KIR3DL2 Mab, in relapsed/refractory cutaneous T-cell lymphomas (CTCL): doseescalation safety, biomarker and clinical activity results. Hematol Oncol 35:48–49

Bahary N, Garrido-Laguna I, Cinar P et al (2016) Phase 2 trial of the indoleamine 2,3-dioxygenase pathway (IDO) inhibitor indoximod plus gemcitabine/nabpaclitaxel for the treatment of metastatic pancreas cancer: interim analysis. J Clin Oncol 34:3020–3020

Beatty GL, Dwyer PJ, Clark J et al (2017) First-in-human phase I study of the oral inhibitor of indoleamine 2,3-dioxygenase-1 epacadostat (INCB024360) in patients with advanced solid malignancies. Clin Cancer Res 23:3269

Benson DM, Caligiuri MA (2014) Killer immunoglobulin-like receptors and tumor immunity. Cancer Immunol Res 2:99–104

Bernatchez C, Haymaker CL, Hurwitz ME et al (2017) Effect of a novel IL-2 cytokineimmune agonist (NKTR-214) on proliferating CD8+T cells and PD-1expression on immune cells in the tumor microenvironment in patients with prior checkpoint therapy. J Clin Oncol 35:2545–2545

Bilir C, Sarisozen C (2017) Indoleamine 2,3-dioxygenase (IDO): only an enzyme or a checkpoint controller? J Oncol Sci 3:52–56

Bogdahn U, Hau P, Stockhammer G et al (2011) Targeted therapy for high-grade glioma with the TGF-beta2 inhibitor trabedersen: results of a randomized and controlled phase IIb study. Neuro-Oncology 13:132–142

Brandes AA, Carpentier AF, Kesari S et al (2016) A phase II randomized study of galunisertib monotherapy or galunisertib plus lomustine compared with lomustine monotherapy in patients with recurrent glioblastoma. Neuro Oncol 18:1146–1156

Brignone C, Escudier B, Grygar C et al (2009) A phase I pharmacokinetic and biological correlative study of IMP321, a novel MHC class II agonist, in patients with advanced renal cell carcinoma. Clin Cancer Res 15:6225–6231

Brignone C, Gutierrez M, Mefti F et al (2010) First-line chemoimmunotherapy in metastatic breast carcinoma: combination of paclitaxel and IMP321 (LAG-3Ig) enhances immune responses and antitumor activity. J Transl Med 8:71

Burris HA, Callahan MK, Tolcher AW et al (2017) Phase 1 safety of ICOS agonist antibody JTX-2011 alone and with nivolumab (nivo) in advanced solid tumors; predicted vs observed pharmacokinetics (PK) in ICONIC. J Clin Oncol 35:3033–3033

Cabo M, Offringa R, Zitvogel L et al (2017) Trial watch: immunostimulatory monoclonal antibodies for oncological indications. Onco Targets Ther 6:e1371896

Casado JG, Pawelec G, Morgado S et al (2009) Expression of adhesion molecules and ligands for activating and costimulatory receptors involved in cellmediated cytotoxicity in a large panel of human melanoma cell lines. Cancer Immunol Immunother 58:1517–1526

Castellanos JR, Purvis IJ, Labak CM et al (2017) B7-H3 role in the immune landscape of cancer. Am J Clin Experiment Immunol 6:66–75

Chauvin JM, Pagliano O, Fourcade J et al (2015) TIGIT and PD-1 impair tumor antigen-specific CD8(+) T cells in melanoma patients. J Clin Invest 125:2046–2058

Chen L, Flies DB (2013) Molecular mechanisms of T cell co-stimulation and coinhibition. Nat Rev Immunol 13:227–242

Chester C, Ambulkar S, Kohrt HE (2016) 4-1BB agonism: adding the accelerator to cancer immunotherapy. Cancer Immunol Immunother 65:1243–1248

Curti BD, Kovacsovics-Bankowski M, Morris N et al (2013) OX40 is a potent immune stimulating target in late stage cancer patients. Cancer Res 73:7189–7198

Dahlberg CI, Sarhan D, Chrobok M et al (2015) Natural killer cell-based therapies targeting cancer: possible strategies to gain and sustain anti-tumor activity. Front Immunol 6:605
de la Torre AN, Contractor S, Castaneda I et al (2017) A phase I trial using local regionaltreatment, nonlethal irradiation, intratumoral and systemic polyinosinicpolycytidylic acid polylysine carboxymethylcellulose to treat liver cancer: in search of the abscopal effect. J Hepatocell Carcinoma 4:4
Dempke WCM, Fenchel K, Uciechowski P, Dale SP (2017a) Second- and thirdgeneration drugs for immuno-oncology treatment-the more the better? Eur J Cancer 74:55–72
Dempke WCM, Fenchel K, Uciechowski P, Dale SP (2017b) Second- and third generation drugs for immuno-oncology treatment-the more the better? Eur J Cancer 74:55–72
Denoeud J, Moser M (2011) Role of CD27/CD70 pathway of activation in immunity and tolerance. J Leukoc Biol 89:195–203
Dholaria B, Hammond W, Shreders A, Lou Y (2016) Emerging therapeutic agents for lung cancer. J Hematol Oncol 9:138
Diab A, Tannir NM, Bernatchez C et al (2017) A phase 1/2 study of a novel IL-2 cytokine, NKTR-214, and nivolumab in patients with select locally advanced or metastatic solid tumors. J Clin Oncol 35:e14040–e14040
Dowling JK, Mansell A (2016) Toll-like receptors: the swiss army knife of immunity and vaccine development. Clin Transl Immunol 5:5
Drake CG, Lipson EJ, Brahmer JR (2014) Breathing new life intoimmunotherapy: review of melanoma, lung and kidney cancer. Nat Rev Clin Oncol 11:24–37
Dredge K, Brennan T, Brown MP et al (2017) An open-label, multi-center phase I study of the safety and tolerability of the novel immunomodulatory agent PG545 in subjects with advanced solid tumors. J Clin Oncol 35:3083–3083
Du W, Yang M, Turner A et al (2017) TIM-3 as a target for cancer immunotherapy and mechanisms of action. Int J Mol Sci 18:645
Ebrahim AH, Alalawi Z, Mirandola L et al (2014) Galectins in cancer: carcinogenesis, diagnosis and therapy. Ann Transl Med 2:88
Emens L, Powderly J, Fong L et al (2017) Abstract CT119: CPI-444, an oral adenosine A2a receptor (A2aR) antagonist, demonstrates clinical activity in patients with advanced solid tumors. Cancer Res 77:CT119
Fan XZ, Quezada SA, Sepulveda MA et al (2014) Engagement of the ICOS pathway markedly enhances efficacy of CTLA-4 blockade in cancer immunotherapy. J Exp Med 211:715–725
Fiori V, Magnani M, Cianfriglia M (2012) The expression and modulation of CEACAM1 and tumor cell transformation. Ann Ist Super Sanita 48:161–171
Goldberg MV, Drake CG (2011) LAG-3 in cancer immunotherapy. Curr Top Microbiol Immunol 344:269–278
Gorman JV, Starbeck-Miller G, Pham NL et al (2014) Tim-3 directly enhances CD8 T cell responses to acute listeria monocytogenes infection. J Immunol 192:3133–3142
Granier C, De Guillebon E, Blanc C et al (2017) Mechanisms of action and rationale for the use of checkpoint inhibitors in cancer. ESMO Open 2:2
Gulley JL, Heery CR, Schlom J et al (2017) Preliminary results from a phase 1 trial of M7824 (MSB0011359C), a bifunctional fusion protein targeting PD-L1 and TGF-β, in advanced solid tumors. J Clin Oncol 35:3006–3006
Gyori D, Chessa T, Hawkins PT, Stephens LR (2017) Class (I) phosphoinositide 3- kinases in the tumor microenvironment. Cancers 9:24
Hamid O, Bauer TM, Spira AI et al (2017) Safety of epacadostat 100 mg bid plus pembrolizumab 200 mg Q3W in advanced solid tumors: phase 2 data from ECHO-202/KEYNOTE-037. J Clin Oncol 35:3012–3012
Hamid O, Thompson JA, Diab A et al (2016) First in human (FIH) study of an OX40 agonist monoclonal antibody (mAb) PF-04518600 (PF-8600) in adult patients (pts) with select advanced solid tumors: preliminary safety and pharmacokinetic (PK)/ pharmacodynamic results. J Clin Oncol 34:3079–3079

Harvey C, Elpek K, Duong E et al (2015) Efficacy of anti-ICOS agonist monoclonal antibodies in preclinical tumor models provides a rationale for clinical development as cancer immunotherapeutics. J Immunother Cancer 3:O9
He Y, Rivard CJ, Rozeboom L et al (2016) Lymphocyte-activation gene-3, an important immune checkpoint in cancer. Cancer Sci 107:1193–1197
Hwang L, Ng K, Wang W, Trieu VN (2016) OT-101: an anti-TGF-beta-2 antisense primed tumors to subsequent chemotherapies. J Clin Oncol 34:e15727–e15727
Infante JR, Hansen AR, Pishvaian MJ et al (2016) A phase Ib dose escalation study of the OX40 agonist MOXR0916 and the PD-L1 inhibitor atezolizumab in patients with advanced solid tumors. J Clin Oncol 34:101–101
Jha GG, Gupta S, Tagawa ST et al (2017) A phase II randomized, double-blind study of sipuleucel-T followed by IDO pathway inhibitor, indoximod, or placebo in the treatment of patients with metastatic castration resistant prostate cancer (mCRPC). J Clin Oncol 35:3066–3066
Jiang T, Zhou C, Ren S (2016) Role of IL-2 in cancer immunotherapy. Onco Targets Ther 5:e1163462
Johnston RJ, Yu X, Grogan JL (2015) The checkpoint inhibitor TIGIT limits antitumor and antiviral CD8+ T cell responses. Onco Targets Ther 4:e1036214
Knee DA, Hewes B, Brogdon JL (2016) Rationale for anti-GITR cancer immunotherapy. Eur J Cancer 67:1–10
Koon HB, Shepard DR, Merghoub T et al (2016) First-in-human phase 1 single-dose study of TRX-518, an anti-human glucocorticoid-induced tumor necrosis factor receptor (GITR) monoclonal antibody in adults with advanced solid tumors. J Clin Oncol 34:3017–3017
Kramer K, Kushner BH, Modak S et al (2010) Compartmental intrathecal radioimmunotherapy: results for treatment for metastatic CNS neuroblastoma. J Neuro-Oncol 97:409–418
Lan X, Li S, Gao H et al (2017) Increased BTLA and HVEM in gastric cancer are associated with progression and poor prognosis. Onco Targets Ther 10:919–926
Le Mercier I, Chen W, Lines JL et al (2014) VISTA regulates the development of protective antitumor immunity. Cancer Res 74:1933–1944
Leichner R, Kang H, Haddad R et al (2016) Preliminary efficacy from a phase I/IIstudy of the natural killer cell–targeted antibody lirilumab in combination with nivolumab in squamous cell carcinoma of the head and neck. J Immunother Cancer 4:2051
Leone RD, Lo YC, Powell JD (2015) A2aR antagonists: next generation checkpoint blockade for cancer immunotherapy. Comput Struct Biotechnol J 13:265–272
Li K, Qu S, Chen X et al (2017) Promising targets for cancer immunotherapy: TLRs, RLRs, and STING-mediated innate immune pathways. Int J Mol Sci 18:404
Linch SN, McNamara MJ, Redmond WL (2015) OX40 agonists and combination immunotherapy: putting the pedal to the metal. Front. Oncologia 5:5
Lines JL, Pantazi E, Mak J et al (2014) VISTA is an immune checkpoint molecule forhuman T cells. Cancer Res 74:1924–1932
Lines JL, Sempere LF, Broughton T et al (2014) VISTA is a novel broad-spectrum negative checkpoint regulator for cancer immunotherapy. Cancer Immunol Res 2:510–517
Liu XJ, Kwon H, Li ZH, Fu YX (2017) Is CD47 an innate immune checkpoint for tumor evasion? J Hematol Oncol 10:12
Long EO, Barber DF, Burshtyn DN et al (2001) Inhibition of natural killer cell activation signals by killer cell immunoglobulin-like receptors (CD158). Immunol Rev 181:223–233
Lu H (2014) TLR agonists for cancer immunotherapy: tipping the balance between the immune stimulatory and inhibitory effects. Front Immunol 5:83
Malissen N, Macagno N, Granjeaud S et al (2017) HVEM: a novel cosignaling molecule of major interest in melanoma. J Clin Oncol 35:e14591–e14591
Marin-Acevedo JA, Soyano AE, Dholaria B et al (2018) Cancer immunotherapy beyond immune checkpoint inhibitors. J Hematol Oncol 11:8
Massague J (2008) TGF beta in cancer. Cell 134:215–230
Massarelli E, Segal N, Ribrag V (2016) Clinical safety and efficacy assessment of the CD137 agonist urelumab alone and in combination with nivolumab in patients with hematologic and solid tumor malignancies. J Immunother Cancer 4:O7

Michot J-M, Maerevoet M, Aftimos PG et al (2016) Clinical response observed in a phase I study in T cell lymphoma patients treated with anti-CD70 SIMPLE antibody ARGX-110. J Clin Oncol 34:7556–7556

Miotto D, Lo Cascio N, Stendardo M et al (2010) CD8+ T cells expressing IL-10 areassociated with a favourable prognosis in lung cancer. Lung Cancer 69:355–360

Moon YW, Hajjar J, Hwu P, Naing A (2015) Targeting the indoleamine 2,3- dioxygenase pathway in cancer. J Immunother Cancer 3:51

Muntasell A, Ochoa MC, Cordeiro L et al (2017) Targeting NK-cell checkpoints for cancer immunotherapy. Curr Opin Immunol 45:73–81

Naing A, Wong DJL, Infante JR et al (2017) PEGylated human IL-10 (AM0010) in combination with pembrolizumab in anti-PD1 and CTLA-4 refractory melanoma. J Clin Oncol 35:3084–3084

Neuzillet C, Tijeras-Raballand A, Cohen R et al (2015) Targeting the TGFbeta pathway for cancer therapy. Pharmacol Ther 147:22–31

Nguyen LT, Ohashi PS (2015) Clinical blockade of PD1 and LAG3—potential mechanisms of action. Nat Rev Immunol 15:45–56

Ohue Y, Kurose K, Nishio Y et al (2016) Abstract A101: role of TIM-3/Galectin-9 pathway in lung cancer. Cancer Immunol Res 4:A101–A101

Owonikoko TK, Hussain A, Stadler WM et al (2016) First-in-human multicenter phase I study of BMS-936561 (MDX-1203), an antibody-drug conjugate targeting CD70. Cancer Chemother Pharmacol 77:155–162

Padua D, Massague J (2009) Roles of TGF beta in metastasis. Cell Res 19:89–102

Papadopoulos KP, Tsai FY-C, Bauer TM et al (2017) CX-1158-101: a first-in-human phase 1 study of CB-1158, a small molecule inhibitor of arginase, as monotherapy and in combination with an anti-PD-1 checkpoint inhibitor in patients (pts) with solid tumors. J Clin Oncol 35:3005–3005

Pardoll DM (2012) The blockade of immune checkpoints in cancer immunotherapy. Nat Rev Cancer 12:252–264

Paulos CM, June CH (2010) Putting the brakes on BTLA in T cell-mediated cancer immunotherapy. J Clin Invest 120:76–80

Perez RP, Riese MJ, Lewis KD et al (2017) Epacadostat plus nivolumab in patients with advanced solid tumors: preliminary phase I/II results of ECHO-204. J Clin Oncol 35:3003–3003

Perez-Ruiz E, Etxeberria I, Rodriguez-Ruiz ME, Melero I (2017) Anti-CD137 and PD- 1/PD-L1 antibodies en route toward clinical synergy. Clin Cancer Res 23:5326–5328

Picarda E, Ohaegbulam KC, Zang XX (2016) Molecular pathways: targeting B7-H3 (CD276) for human cancer immunotherapy. Clin Cancer Res 22:3425–3431

Powderly J, Cote G, Flaherty K et al (2015) Interim results of an ongoing phase I, dose escalation study of MGA271 (fc-optimized humanized anti-B7-H3 monoclonal antibody) in patients with refractory B7-H3-expressing neoplasms or neoplasms whose vasculature expresses B7-H3. J Immunother Cancer 3:O8–O8

Sakuishi K, Ngiow SF, Sullivan JM et al (2013) TIM3+FOXP3+ regulatory T cells are tissue-specific promoters of T-cell dysfunction in cancer. Onco Targets Ther 2:e23849

Sanborn RE, Pishvain MJ, Callahan MK et al (2016) Abstract CT023: phase I results from the combination of an immune-activating anti-CD27 antibody (varlilumab) in combination with PD-1 blockade (nivolumab): activation across multiple immune pathways without untoward immune-related adverse events. Cancer Res 76:CT023-CT023

Sanmamed MF, Pastor F, Rodriguez A et al (2015) Agonists of co-stimulation in cancer immunotherapy directed against CD137, OX40, GITR, CD27, CD28,and ICOS. Semin Oncol 42:640–655

Schmitt C, Marie-Cardine A, Bensussan A (2017) Therapeutic antibodies to KIR3DL2 and other target antigens on cutaneous T-cell lymphomas. Front Immunol 8:8

Segal NH, Logan TF, Hodi FS et al (2017) Results from an integrated safety analysis of urelumab, an agonist anti-CD137 monoclonal antibody. Clin Cancer Res 23:1929–1936

Sharma P, Allison JP (2015) The future of immune checkpoint therapy. Science 348:56–61

Shi M, Chen X, Ye K et al (2016) Application potential of toll-like receptors in cancer immunotherapy: systematic review. Medicine 95:e3951

Sikic BI, Narayanan S, Colevas AD et al (2016) A first-in-human, first-in-class phase I trial of the anti-CD47 antibody Hu5F9-G4 in patients with advanced cancers. J Clin Oncol 34:3019–3019

Siu LL, Gelmon K, Chu Q et al (2017) Abstract CT116: BMS-986205, an optimized indoleamine 2,3-dioxygenase 1 (IDO1) inhibitor, is well tolerated with potent pharmacodynamic (PD) activity, alone and in combination with nivolumab (nivo) in advanced cancers in a phase 1/2a trial. Cancer Res 77:CT116

Siu LL, Steeghs N, Meniawy T et al (2017) Preliminary results of a phase I/IIa study of BMS-986156 (glucocorticoid-induced tumor necrosis factor receptor– related gene [GITR] agonist), alone and in combination with nivolumab inmpts with advanced solid tumors. J Clin Oncol 35:104–104

Smith AL, Robin TP, Ford HL (2012) Molecular pathways: targeting the TGF-beta pathway for cancer therapy. Clin Cancer Res 18:4514–4521

Spicer JF, Baurain J-F, Awada A et al (2017) LTX-315, an oncolytic peptide, toconvert immunogenically 'cold' tumors to 'hot' in patients with advanced or metastatic tumours: results from an ongoing phase I study. J Clin Oncol 35:3085–3085

Srivastava S, Dubey AK, Madaan R, Bala R, Gupta Y, Dhiman BS, Kumar S (2022) Emergence of nutrigenomics and dietary components as a complementary therapy in cancer prevention. Environ Sci Pollut Res 29:1–21

Stanietsky N, Simic H, Arapovic J et al (2009) The interaction of TIGIT with PVR and PVRL2 inhibits human NK cell cytotoxicity. Proc Natl Acad Sci U S A 106:17858–17863

Su EW, Moore CJ, Suriano S et al (2015) IL-2Rα mediates temporal regulation of IL-2 signaling and enhances immunotherapy. Sci Transl Med 7:311ra170–311ra170

Sun ZJ, Fourcade J, Pagliano O et al (2015) IL10 and PD-1 cooperate to limit the activity of tumor-specific CD8(+) T cells. Cancer Res 75:1635–1644

Sveinbjornsson B, Camilio KA, Haug BE, Rekdal O (2017) LTX-315: a first-in-class oncolytic peptide that reprograms the tumor microenvironment. Future Med Chem 9:1339–1344

Takeda K, Kojima Y, Uno T et al (2010) Combination therapy of established tumors by antibodies targeting immune activating and suppressing molecules. J Immunol 184:5493–5501

Thakur AK, Chellappan DK, Dua K, Mehta M, Satija S, Singh I (2020) Patented therapeutic drug delivery strategies for targeting pulmonary diseases. Expert Opin Ther Pat 30(5):375–387

Thomas DA, Massagué J (2005) TGF-β directly targets cytotoxic T cell functions during tumor evasion of immune surveillance. Cancer Cell 8:369–380

Thompson JA, Akilov O, Querfeld C et al (2017) A phase 1 dose-escalation trial of intratumoral TTI-621, a novel immune checkpoint inhibitor targeting CD47, in subjects with relapsed or refractory percutaneously-accessible solid tumors and mycosis fungoides. J Clin Oncol 35:TPS3101-TPS3101

Timosenko E, Hadjinicolaou AV, Cerundolo V (2017) Modulation of cancer-specific immune responses by amino acid degrading enzymes. Immunotherapy 9:83–97

Tolcher AW, Alley EW, Chichili G et al (2016) Phase 1, first-in-human, open label, dose escalation ctudy of MGD009, a humanized B7-H3 x CD3 dual-affinity retargeting (DART) protein in patients with B7-H3-expressing neoplasms or B7- H3 expressing tumor vasculature. J Clin Oncol 34:TPS3105-TPS3105

Tolcher A, Hong D, Sullivan R et al (2017) Abstract CT089: IPI-549-01—a phase 1/ 1b, first-in-human study of IPI-549, a PI3K-γ inhibitor, as monotherapy and in combination with nivolumab in patients with advanced solid tumors. Cancer Res 77:CT089-CT089

Tolcher AW, Sznol M, Hu-Lieskovan S et al (2016) Phase Ib study of PF-05082566 in combination with pembrolizumab in patients with advanced solid tumors. J Clin Oncol 34:3002–3002

Tomala J, Kovar M (2016) IL-2/anti-IL-2 mAb immunocomplexes: a renascence of IL-2 in cancer immunotherapy? Onco Targets Ther 5:5

Toulmonde M, Penel N, Adam J et al (2017) Use of pd-1 targeting, macrophage in filtration, and ido pathway activation in sarcomas: a phase 2 clinical trial. JAMA. Oncology 4:93

Tran B, Carvajal RD, Marabelle A et al (2017) Dose escalation results from a first-inhuman, phase 1 study of the glucocorticoid-induced TNF receptor-related protein (GITR) agonist AMG 228 in patients (pts) with advanced solid tumors. J Clin Oncol 35:2521–2521
Turner JG, Rakhmilevich AL, Burdelya L et al (2001) Anti-CD40 antibody induces antitumor and antimetastatic effects: the role of NK cells. J Immunol 166:89–94
van de Ven K, Borst J (2015) Targeting the T-cell co-stimulatory CD27/CD70 pathway in cancer immunotherapy: rationale and potential. Immunotherapy 7:655–667
Vijayan D, Young A, Teng MWL, Smyth MJ (2017) Targeting immunosuppressive adenosine in cancer (vol 17, pg 709, 2017). Nat Rev Cancer 17:724–724
Vonderheide RH, Glennie MJ (2013) Agonistic CD40 antibodies and cancer therapy. Clin Cancer Res 19:1035–1043
Wang-Gillam A, Plambeck-Suess S, Goedegebuure P et al (2013) A phase I study of IMP321 and gemcitabine as the front-line therapy in patients with advanced pancreatic adenocarcinoma. Investig New Drugs 31:707–713
Weidle UH, Kontermann RE, Brinkmann U (2014) Tumor-antigen-binding bispecific antibodies for cancer treatment. Semin Oncol 41:653–660
Weiskopf K (2017) Cancer immunotherapy targeting the CD47/SIRP alpha axis. Eur J Cancer 76:100–109
Wendt MK, Tian MZ, Schiemann WP (2012) Deconstructing the mechanisms and consequences of TGF-beta-induced EMT during cancer progression. Cell Tissue Res 347:85–101
Willoughby J, Griffiths J, Tews I, Cragg MS (2017) OX40: structure and function—what questions remain? Mol Immunol 83:13–22
Woo SR, Turnis ME, Goldberg MV et al (2012) Immune inhibitory molecules LAG-3 and PD-1 synergistically regulate T-cell function to promote tumoral immune escape. Cancer Res 72:917–927
Workman CJ, Dugger KJ, Vignali DA (2002) Cutting edge: molecular analysis of the negative regulatory function of lymphocyte activation gene-3. J Immunol 169:5392–5395
Yamazaki T, Pitt JM, Vétizou M et al (2016) The oncolytic peptide LTX-315 overcomes resistance of cancers to immunotherapy with CTLA4 checkpointblockade. Cell Death Differ 23:1004–1015
Yu X, Harden K, Gonzalez LC et al (2009) The surface protein TIGIT suppresses T cell activation by promoting the generation of mature immunoregulatory dendritic cells. Nat Immunol 10:48–57
Zakharia Y, Drabick JJ, Khleif S et al (2016) Updates on phase 1b/2 trial of the indoleamine 2,3-dioxygenase pathway (IDO) inhibitor indoximod plus checkpoint inhibitors for the treatment of unresectable stage 3 or 4melanoma. J Clin Oncol 34:3075–3075
Zhang B (2010) CD73: a novel target for cancer immunotherapy. Cancer Res 70:6407–6411
Zhang H, Wang Y, Hwang ES, He YW (2016) Interleukin-10: an immune-activating cytokine in cancer immunotherapy. J Clin Oncol 34:3576
Zhou H, Forveille S, Sauvat A et al (2016) The oncolytic peptide LTX-315 triggers immunogenic cell death. Cell Death Dis 7:7
Zhu C, Anderson AC, Schubart A et al (2005) The Tim-3 ligand galectin-9 negatively regulates T helper type 1 immunity. Nat Immunol 6:1245–1252

Exploring the Therapeutic Potential of ICOS and GITR Agonists in Lung Cancer

11

Shiveena Bhatia, Shravani P. Vaidya, Apurva Sagade, Priyamvada Nair, Nikita, and Rajeev Taliyan

11.1 Introduction and Epidemiology

According to the 2023 Statistics by the American Cancer Society, the second most prevalent cancer in both men and women is lung cancer, which includes both small cell and non-small cell lung cancers. It is mainly found to occur in people aged 65 years and above. The disastrous tumour is found to be the primary reason for most of the cancer fatalities in United States claiming lives of one in five of all cancer deaths (American Cancer Society 2023) (https://www.cancer.org/cancer/lung-cancer/about/key-statistics.html). The search for therapeutic options for cancer is now diverting towards the immunotherapy. In addition to being influenced by the characteristics of cancer cells, interaction with the tumour cells also contributes to the progression of cancer (Schiller et al. 1995; Sundar et al. 2014). The immune system is in continuous contact with the tumour cells beginning from the onset towards the progression. Various genetic and epigenetic variations cause cancer cells to express antigens differently as compared to the host cells. Tumour recognition is imperative in order to cause phagocytosis of the tumour cells (Fig. 11.1). The T-lymphocytes are presented with the tumour which triggers their activation followed by killing of the cells. Multiple stimulatory and inhibitory signals modulate this T-cell-mediated immune response. Some of the immune co-stimulatory molecules comprise of OX-40, glucocorticoid-induced tumour necrosis factor receptor (GITR), CD28 and CD137 whereas the co-inhibitory molecules comprise of cytotoxic T-lymphocyte antigen-4 (CTLA-4), programmed death-1 (PD-1),

S. Bhatia · S. P. Vaidya · A. Sagade · P. Nair · Nikita · R. Taliyan (✉)
Neuropsychopharmacology Division, Department of Pharmacy, Birla Institute of Technology and Science-Pilani, Pilani, Rajasthan, India

S. Bhatt et al. (eds.), *Immunotherapy Against Lung Cancer*,
https://doi.org/10.1007/978-981-99-7141-1_11

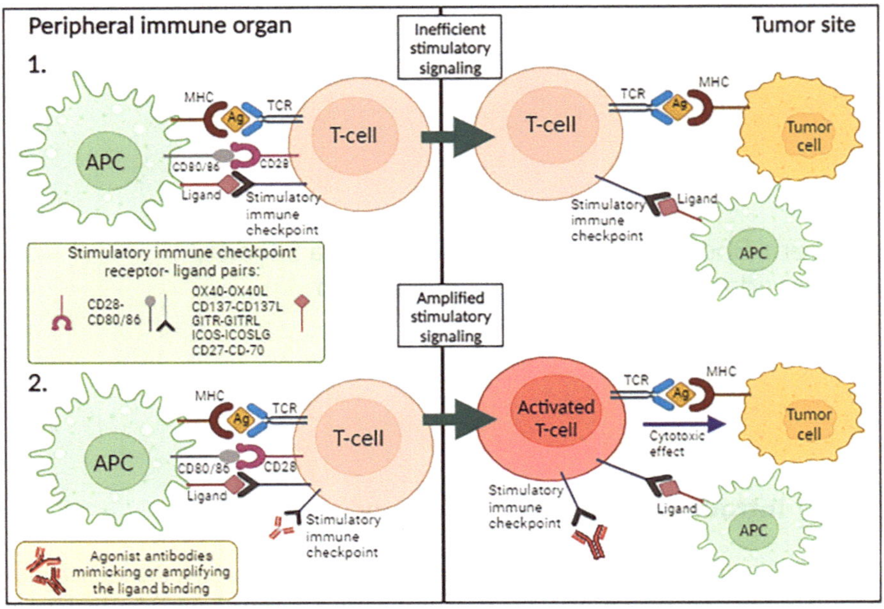

Fig. 11.1 (1) Mechanism of activation of T-cell via interaction with CD28, CD80 or CD86 which results in TCR signalling, further triggering its activation. (2) Agonistic antibodies led to elevation in the effector activity of T-cells by amplification of the binding of ligands to the stimulatory immune checkpoints ultimately leading to expected elimination of cancer cells

lymphocyte-activation gene 3 (LAG3) and T-cell immunoglobulin- and mucin domain-containing molecule 3 (TIM-3) (Fig. 11.2). Under physiological conditions, these immune checkpoints guard against the occurrence of autoimmunity or inflammation. But any alterations in their functioning which can happen in a neoplastic state can induce the development of tumour tolerance and allow tumours to resist immune system intervention (Sundar et al. 2014).

The cancer cells tend to ditch the body's immune system by utilising these checkpoints that keep the immune system under control. These are identified to secrete cytokines like interleukins (IL-10) and transforming growth factor (TGF) or alter their metabolic processes in order to potentially escape being recognised and eliminated by the immune cells (Catalano et al. 2022; Croci et al. 2007; Rabinovich et al. 2007; Wellenstein and de Visser 2018). However, of all the ways to dodge the immune system recognition, the activation of immune checkpoint pathways like cytotoxic T-lymphocyte antigen-4, programmed cell death 1(PD-1) and programmed death ligand (PDL1) is the most effective and most widely explored route. Hence, blocking the CTLA-4 and PD-1/PDL-1 can help restore the healthy immune response against the tumour cells (Pardoll 2012; Seidel et al. 2018). The advent of immune checkpoint inhibitors functions on these principles to aggravate the anticancer action by utilising the body's own immune system.

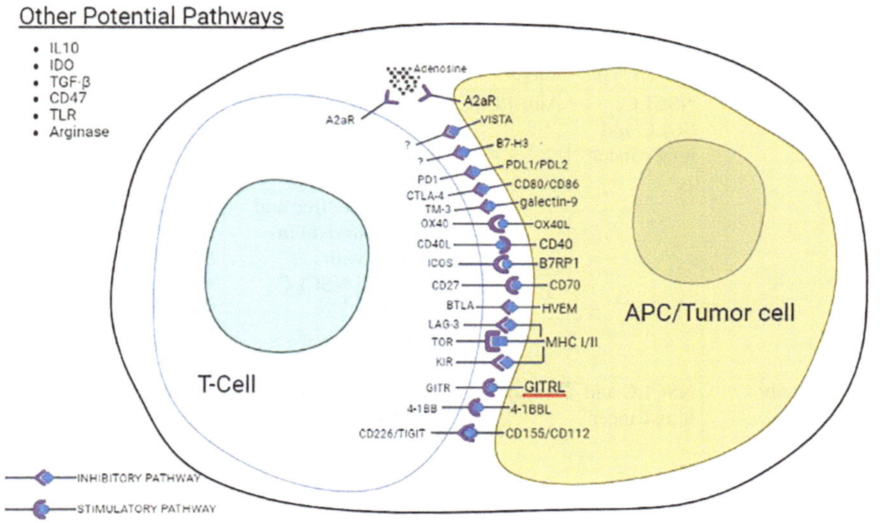

Fig. 11.2 Immune interactions of tumour cells with the T-cells. The figure illustrates various immune co-stimulatory and co-inhibitory molecules

11.2 Promise of Immunotherapy for Lung Cancer

ICIs serve as the primary and the preferred form of treatment for the small cell lung cancer and non-small cell lung cancer with no driver mutation (Singh et al. 2022; Zugazagoitia and Paz-Ares 2022). Currently, approved drugs and trials have targeted CTLA-4 and PD-1/PD-L1. A number of ICIs have been granted approval for the lung cancer therapy so far (Table 11.1).

Many novel immune checkpoints localised on various immune cells like T-cells, B-cells and NK cells like inducible T-cell co-stimulator (ICOS), lymphocyte activation gene 3 (LAG3), T-cell immunoglobulin and mucin-domain containing-3 (TIM-3), B7 homolog 3 protein (B7H3), B-and T-lymphocyte attenuator (BTLA) and V-domain Ig suppressor of T-cell activation (VISTA) have been identified and are currently being researched in various clinical trials (Fig. 11.2). This chapter will focus on two of these novel checkpoint molecules and how these can be targeted to control the progression of lung cancer.

Table 11.1 Monoclonal antibodies being researched for targeting immune checkpoint

Name of the intervention	Cancer type	Target	Results/status	Clinical trial ID
Pembrolizumab	NSCLC, SCLC and lung cancer	Anti-PD-1	Approved by FDA for second-line treatment. It improved progression-free and overall survival in patients with advanced NSCLC and PDL-1 expression	Clinicaltrials.gov ID: NCT02220894, NCT03302234, NCT03134456, NCT02142738, NCT02864394, NCT01905657, NCT02775435, NCT02504372, NCT03066778 and NCT03322540
Nivolumab	NSCLC and lung cancer	Anti-PD-1	First drug to receive accelerated approval by FDA in 2015. Superior response and survival rates as compared to docetaxel	Clinicaltrials.gov ID: NCT02031533, NCT01642004, NCT01673867 and NCT03348904
Ipilimumab	NSCLC	Anti-CTLA-4	Approved in combination with nivolumab for first-line therapy for PD-L1-positive diseases	Clinicaltrials.gov ID: NCT03469960, NCT03351361, NCT02785952 and NCT03302234
Avelumab	NSCLC	Anti-PD-L1	Phase III/phase IV trials going on, results are still awaited	Clinicaltrials.gov ID: NCT02576574 and NCT02395172
Atezolizumab	NSCLC and extensive stage small cell lung cancer	Anti-PD-L1	Approved by FDA for second-line treatment of patients with stages II–III for NSCLC with positive PD-L1	Clinicaltrials.gov ID: NCT02813785, NCT02367794, NCT02008227, NCT02409355, NCT02657434, NCT02367781, NCT02366143, NCT02409342, NCT03191786, NCT03456063 and NCT02763579

(continued)

Table 11.1 (continued)

Name of the intervention	Cancer type	Target	Results/status	Clinical trial ID
Durvalumab	NSCLC and squamous cell lung carcinoma	Anti-PD-L1	The treatment resulted in progression-free survival for patients with positive PD-L1 and not receiving chemotherapy. Approved with or without tremelimumab as first-line therapy	Clinicaltrials.gov ID: NCT02352984, NCT03003962, NCT02453282, NCT02273375, NCT02542293, NCT03164616, NCT02125461, NCT02154490 and NCT02551159
Tremelimumab	Metastatic NSCLC	Anti-CTLA-4	Approved by FDA in combination with durvalumab and chemotherapy. The combination improved the overall survival as compared to the chemotherapy alone	Clinicaltrials.gov ID: NCT03164616
REGN2810 (cemiplimab)	NSCLC	Anti-PD-L1	The monotherapy was found to significantly enhance the overall and progression-free survival in advances NSCLC patients with PD-1	Clinicaltrials.gov ID: NCT03409614 and NCT03088540
IBI308 (sintilimab)	Squamous cell lung carcinoma	Anti-PD-L1	Compared to docetaxel, sintilimab was found to significantly improve overall and progression-free survival	Clinicaltrials.gov ID: NCT03150875
BGB-A317 (tislelizumab)	NSCLC	Anti-PD-L1	It was found to significantly enhance the overall and progression-free survival in advanced NSCLC patients with PD-1	Clinicaltrials.gov ID: NCT03358875
BCD-100	NSCLC	Anti-PD-L1	Phase II/phase III trial still in progress, results awaited	Clinicaltrials.gov ID: NCT03288870

11.3 Inducible T-Cell Co-Stimulatory (ICOS)

ICOS belongs to CD28 receptor family that controls activation of T-lymphocytes and is involved in adaptive immune responses. It is induced in activated T-lymphocytes (Wu et al. 2022). ICOS expression requires T-cell receptor (TCR) and CD28 signalling. Signals from both the TCR and CD28 promote its expression, which is usually minimal. After TCR interaction, ICOS is swiftly induced to transmit co-stimulatory signal. ICOS signalling starts upon interaction with its specific ligand, ICOSL. ICOSL is identified to be present on antigen-presenting cells (APCs) such as dendritic cells (DCs), macrophages and B-cells, as well as other endothelial cells (Amatore et al. 2018). ICOSL would be elevated by TNF-α (tumour necrosis factor-alpha) along with other pro-inflammatory cytokines that plays a crucial co-stimulatory effect in T-cell activation via endothelial cells, particularly for the reactivation of effector T-cells/memory T-cells on the endothelium, thereby facilitating immune cell migration into inflamed tissue (Amatore et al. 2020).

The primary function of ICOS co-stimulation is the formation as well as preservation of germinal centres (GCs) within lymphatic organs and antibody class switching, along with T-cell-dependent B-cell assistance. ICOS is responsible for both T-cell activation and differentiation into T-follicular helper (Tfh) cells, as well as for the movement of CXCR5+ Tfh-cells across the T–B-cell boundary within the follicle (Akiba et al. 2005). ICOS facilitates Tfh-cells to differentiate by activating PI3K, which favours T-cell persistence in motility. Moreover, co-stimulation via ICOS causes the IL-21 production in Tfh, along with expression of CXCR5, that are equally necessary for the conservation and differentiation of T-follicular helper cells and germinal centres, along with B-cell differentiation (Gigoux et al. 2009). Also, ICOS/ICOSL path seems to be essential for survival, development and also proliferation of other CD8+ and CD4+ T-cell subgroups. It increases multiple effector cytokine production, including TNF-α and interleukins (IL-4, IL-5, IL-6, IL-10, IL-21). Amplification of CD8+ T-cell effect by ICOS is presumably one among the major tumour-fighting mechanism pathways promoted by the ICOS/ICOSL cascade (Amatore et al. 2020). It is found to serve two important functions in cancer development. In the first case, it is evident that the co-stimulatory ICOS/ICOSL signal contributes towards the antitumour T-cell reaction whereas on the contrary, ICOS signalling also demonstrates pro-tumoural characteristics that is associated with activation of regulatory T-cell immunity suppressive activity (Amatore et al. 2018). Additionally, it is crucial for functioning and maintenance of regulatory T-cells (Treg), particularly via IL-10 and TGF-α secretion. Tregs, which belong to CD4+ CD25+ T-cell subpopulation, generates forkhead box protein 3 (FoxP3), a transcription factor that dampens immune responses which in turn fosters the evasion of antitumour immunity. These are known to provide immune tolerance in the tumour microenvironment via various routes and mechanisms comprising FAS-L (Fas ligand), CTLA-4, PD-1, perforins or CD39/adenosine, as well as IL-10 secretion, which provides a repressive effect towards dendritic cell functions (Amatore et al. 2018). Tregs were found in the tumour microenvironment of numerous malignancies. ICOS is found to strictly modulate the population of Tregs. In addition, ICOS+ Tregs are more suppressive than their negative counterparts. The ICOS/ICOSL pathway produces Tregs through distinct mechanisms. Th17-to-Treg cell trans-differentiation is one of the examples which is controlled through ICOS that is characterised with the gradual transformation of tumour-induced Th17 lymphocytes into IL-17A-positive Foxp3+ along with IL-17A-negative Foxp3+ T-cells throughout cancer development (Downs-Canner et al. 2017). Invasion of Tregs into the microenvironment of a tumour is typically correlated with a poor prognosis (Amatore et al. 2018). This validates that ICOS/ICOSL pathway serves dual function of being an antitumour agent and pro-tumour-causing agent.

Now addressing lung carcinoma, tumour-infiltrating lymphocytes (TIL) consist of a diverse group of CD4+ helper T-cells, CD8+ cytotoxic T-cells and FOXP3+ regulatory T-cells (Tregs). TIL stimulation is tightly controlled, necessitating antigen recognition in some circumstances of suitable major histocompatibility complex (MHC) molecules as well as binding of CD28, CD40, OX40, GITR, ICOS and other co-stimulatory molecules (Neeve et al. 2019). Expression of ICOS on FoxP3+ Tregs has been demonstrated within the human malignancy. Comparatively Treg tumour-infiltrating lymphocytes (TIL) at the periphery exhibit higher FoxP3 levels and also various additional indicators, such as CTLA-4, ICOS and glucocorticoid-induced TNFR family-related gene, thus increasing the levels of TGF and IL-10 production (Solinas et al. 2020). A recent study suggested correlation between ICOS and prognosis and immune infiltration levels in lung adenocarcinoma. Greater ICOS expression was observed in superior tumour immune microenvironment. ICOS is found to be a potential biomarker and target for therapy linked to immunity and prognosis in lung adenocarcinoma (Wu et al. 2022). ICOS + Tregs isolated from melanoma were found to be more immunosuppressive than ICOS − Tregs and had the capacity to convert CD4+ CD25− T-cells (non-Tregs) into suppressive type 1 regulatory T-cells (Tr1) expressing IL-10 (Solinas et al. 2020).

Immuno-oncology relies on enhancing immune response of the patient against malignancy. T-Lymphocytes have been triggered via interaction of T-cell receptor (TCR) and co-stimulatory and/or co-inhibitory receptors belonging to the B7/CD28 superfamily (Greaves and Gribben 2013). Blocking co-inhibitory receptors, like CTLA (cytotoxic T-lymphocyte-associated molecule)-4 and PD (programmed cell death)-1, is the present primary approach to combating numerous types of malignancy. The simultaneous introduction of anti-PD-1 and anti-CTLA-4 antibodies may promote greater responses than monotherapies, despite numerous and sometimes severe side effects. Thus, a number of preclinical and clinical investigations suggest that co-stimulatory receptor agonists, alone or in combination with co-inhibitory blockers, could enhance response rates. Therefore, a prospective target is inducible T-cell co-stimulator (ICOS), a T-cell enhancing co-stimulatory receptor. ICOS agonist mAbs can enhance the inhibitory checkpoint blocking action (Amatore et al. 2020). ICOS-mediated co-stimulation is weaker as compared with that of other co-stimulatory mechanisms such as CD28-induced co-stimulation, which is due to decreased IL-2 secretion (Amatore et al. 2018).

11.4 Targeting ICOS for Immunotherapy

Due to the predominance of CD4 expression, ICOS seems to be a less effective immunotherapy route than the remaining techniques. However, when used in conjunction with other approaches, particularly in combination with CTLA-4 blockade, it results in a powerful synergistic effect that is ascribed to an increased ICOS expression following anti-CTLA-4 treatment (Pourakbari et al. 2021). Table 11.2 gives an account of various ICOS agonist Abs that are in clinical trials.

Table 11.2 Monoclonal antibodies currently being researched for targeting ICOS

Name of the intervention	Cancer type	Target	Status	Clinical trial
Ipilimumab	NSCLC	CTLA-4 blockade along with ICOS expression on CD4 T-cell	**Approved** showed improved clinical results	Clinicaltrials.gov ID: NCT03469960, NCT03351361, NCT02785952 and NCT03302234
Vopratelimab (JTX-2011)	Advanced solid tumours	CTLA-4 and anti-PD-1	**Approved** exhibited potent antitumour activity with response of both increasing effector T-cell activity and decreasing Treg cells in tumours	Clinicaltrials.gov ID: NCT04319224 and NCT04549025
GSK3359609 BMS-986226	Advanced solid tumours	ICOS + anti-PD-1 mAbs	**Results awaited** Phase I/phase II	Clinicaltrials.gov ID: NCT02723955 and NCT03251924
KY1044 (anti-ICOS Ab)	NSCLC	ICOS + PD-L1 mAbs	**Results awaited** Phase II	Clinicaltrials.gov ID: NCT03829501
INDUCE-1 (feladilimab (ICOS agonist Ab) alone or combined with pembrolizumab	Advanced solid tumours and NSCLC	PD-L1 + ICOS	**Results awaited** Phase II/phase III	Clinicaltrials.gov ID: NCT02723955, NCT05553808 and NCT04128696
Vopratelimab (JTX-2011) in combination with nivolumab	Advanced solid tumour	Anti-CTLA-4 and anti-PD-1	Phase II	Clinicaltrials.gov ID: NCT02904226 and NCT03989362
MEDI-570	Non-Hodgkin lymphomas	IgG1 monoclonal antibody targeting ICOS	Phase I	Clinicaltrials.gov ID: NCT02520791

11.5 Glucocorticoid-Induced TNFR-Related Protein (GTIR) Agonists

Glucocorticoid-induced TNFR-related protein (GITR, TNFRSF18, CD375) (Pourakbari et al. 2021) is a one of the co-stimulators which is constitutively expressed at higher number on regulatory T-(Treg) cells, with further rise in expression on stimulation (Shevach and Stephens 2006). In contrast, CD375 is expressed in minimal levels in CD4+ CD8+ T-cells, and its expression is enhanced upon TCR stimulation within 24–72 h and remains for prolonged period of time on surface of T-cells. Its ligand (GITRL), predominantly expressed on endothelial cells and antigen-presenting cells (APCs) (Tian et al. 2020), upon interaction with GITR, initiates signalling via TNF receptor-associated factors (TRAFs), which is a family of six proteins (Buzzatti et al. 2019). It is complex consisting of a two TRAF-2 and one TRAF-5 proteins, which activates NF-κβ and MAPK pathway, though there are various transduction pathways that are yet to be uncovered. This co-stimulation augments T-cell survival, effector function and proliferation as it upregulates IL-2, IL-2Rα and IFNγ. It also protects T-cells from activation-induced cell death (AICD) and a surge in memory T-cells (Sanmamed et al. 2015). GITR is responsible for suppression of Tregs and creates resistance to inhibition by Tregs (Shevach and Stephens 2006). Hence, we can conclude that Treg cells supresses T-cells, thereby limiting their antitumour activity, while activation of GITR on effector T- cells enhances their effector function by developing resistance to Treg suppression.

GITR came into light when reports of DTA-1 (rat monoclonal immunoglobulin G2a, IgG2a) were published showing that its stimulation by DTA-1 mAb abrogated T regs mediated suppression in vivo and in vitro and induced autoimmunity (Shimizu et al. 2002). This gave an idea that GITR can be targeted in cancer to invade tumour suppressive microenvironment and prevent immune escape of tumour cells. As a result, first phase 1 trial of a fully humanised Fc-dysfunctional monoclonal antibody (mAb), TRX518, was conducted in patients with refractory solid tumour as monotherapy (Zappasodi et al. 2019). Currently, TRX518 is being assessed in two clinical studies or trials against advanced refractory solid tumour, multiple myeloma and other solid tumours (Vence et al. 2019). GITR agonistic antibodies inhibited tumour growth and prolonged survival, and depleted tumour-infiltrating Tregs have been considered as primary mechanism of action (Vence et al. 2019). However, the results so far have illustrated the insufficient efficacy of the monotherapy; consequently, now these are being evaluated as a combination therapy with various anti-PD-1 mAbs.

Seeing its potential in tumour suppression, researchers have started targeting it for the management of lung cancer. Vence et al. (2019) characterised and compared GITR expression in solid tumours, where data suggested that NSCLC, RCC and melanoma should be given priority for anti-GITR therapy development. In the presence of mesenchymal stromal cells (MSC) that express GITRL, GITR-expressing SCLC cell lines induced cell death by increasing the production of an apoptosis-inducing factor (Kopru et al. 2018). In mice with lung cancer, GITR agonistic antibody promoted apoptosis of tumour cells and enhanced the activity of NK cells, T-lymphocytes and APCs, accompanied by a decrease in pro-angiogenic

Table 11.3 Monoclonal antibodies currently being researched for targeting GITR

Name of the intervention	Disease	Target	Phase	Clinical trial ID
BMS-986156 (ipilimumab + nivolumab radiation)	Metastatic lung carcinoma and other diseases (Zhu et al. 2020)	Anti-GITR agonistic mAb	I/II (active)	Clinicaltrials.gov ID: NCT04021043
MEDI1873	NSCLC, head and neck squamous cell carcinoma (HNSCC) and colorectal cancer (CRC) (Balmanoukian et al. 2020)	GITR ligand/IgG1 agonist fusion protein	I (phase I study completed, but further study was terminated due to lack of substantial efficacy)	Clinicaltrials.gov ID: NCT02583165
AMG 228	NSCLC, head and neck squamous cell carcinoma (HNSCC) and colorectal cancer	GITR agonist IgG1 human mAb	I (terminated due to sponsor's decision)	Clinicaltrials.gov ID: NCT02437916

chemokines and an increase in anti-angiogenic chemokines (Zhu et al. 2015). A preclinical analysis of non-small cell lung carcinoma (NSCLC) mouse models indicated that a GITR agonist in combination with radiation therapy and anti-PD-1 produced tumour-free status and significantly enhanced survival in 50% of the mice examined (Schoenhals et al. 2018). A phase I/phase II trial has been initiated to assess the safety and efficacy of agonistic anti-GITR mAb (BMS-986156) in combination with PD-1/CTLA-4 blockade against the metastatic lung cancer and other tumours (Zhu et al. 2020). Table 11.3 gives an account of some of the GITR agonists undergoing clinical trials at present.

11.6 Conclusion and Future Prospects

Impressive findings in the tumour immunotherapy and the treatment of many different types of solid tumours with immune checkpoint blockade have been witnessed over the past decades. The immunological and molecular effects of the PD-1/PD-L1 pathways and CTLA-4 have clearly demonstrated that these checkpoint inhibitors can restore anti-cancer immune activities, especially when the two pathways were coupled. In recent years, however, researches have demonstrated that even in patients administered with immune checkpoint blockade medication, some types of resistance mechanism inevitably arises and considerable proportion of patients have failed to benefit from this regimen (Pourakbari et al. 2021). As the tumour evolves, the tumour cells undergo some genetic changes which make the tumour heterogenous which may result in cells no longer able to present the molecules sensed by the immune cells. As a result, cells that are identified by the immune system get taken care of while the ones that have grown resistant multiply and become more prevalent. In such cases, the patient grows resistant to the prescribed immunotherapy. Hence, combination regimen was implemented to amplify the therapeutic benefits and downregulate the side effects. The timing and order of antibody treatments that target both inhibitory and co-stimulatory receptors must be taken into account if combination therapy is to be successful. Other adjuvant strategies that can be implemented comprise of radiation, immunisation and chemotherapeutics that are proposed to supplement the antitumour action of the stimulatory molecules. However, since these methods are rather new, clinical trials are very limited and still under development. Despite major advancements in cancer therapeutics, this debilitating disease still continues to pose a serious risk to the human life and is one of the most complex and dangerous disorders to cure.

Immunotherapy is not only difficult to deliver and control but also poses a new threat of inducing toxicities. Pulmonary toxicities related to the immune system, for example, pneumonitis, are very common in the trials of lung cancer which involved combining CTLA-4 and PD-1 antibodies (Porcu et al. 2019). Cytokine release syndrome or CRS, an inflammatory response triggered by some drugs and infections, is a common side effect resulting from immuno-modulation, be it suppression or promoting the immune response. CRS has been reported in many cases of antibody-based therapies. While low-grade CRS can be treated with antihistamines and antipyretics, higher-grade CRS may pose a life-threatening situation (Shimabukuro-Vornhagen et al. 2018). Hence, there are chances that ICOS agonists, when introduced in a patient, may result in CRS. Other toxicities related to this type of treatment could be an increase in hepatic enzymes and an accumulation of fluid in the lungs known as pleural effusion (Solinas et al. 2020). And like any immunotherapy method, there is always a risk of triggering autoimmune reactions in the body. And since these methods are still under trial, the long-term effects and risks pertaining to the safety and efficacy of these treatments are yet to be researched in detail.

References

Akiba H, Takeda K, Kojima Y, Usui Y, Harada N, Yamazaki T, Ma J, Tezuka K, Yagita H, Okumura K (2005) The role of ICOS in the CXCR5+ follicular B helper T cell maintenance in vivo. J Immunol 175(4):2340–2348

Amatore F, Gorvel L, Olive D (2018) Inducible co-stimulator (ICOS) as a potential therapeutic target for anti-cancer therapy. Expert Opin Ther Targets 22(4):343–351. https://doi.org/10.1080/14728222.2018.1444753

Amatore F, Gorvel L, Olive D (2020) Role of inducible co-stimulator (ICOS) in cancer immunotherapy. Expert Opin Biol Ther 20(2):141–150

American Cancer Society (2023) About lung cancer what is lung cancer? American Cancer Society, Atlanta, GA, pp 1–15

Balmanoukian AS, Infante JR, Aljumaily R, Naing A, Chintakuntlawar AV, Rizvi NA, Ross HJ, Gordon M, Mallinder PR, Elgeioushi N (2020) Safety and clinical activity of MEDI1873, a novel GITR agonist, in advanced solid tumors. Clin Cancer Res 26(23):6196–6203

Buzzatti G, Dellepiane C, Del Mastro L (2019) New emerging targets in cancer immunotherapy: the role of GITR. ESMO Open 4:e000738

Catalano M, Shabani S, Venturini J, Ottanelli C, Voltolini L, Roviello G (2022) Lung cancer immunotherapy: beyond common immune checkpoints inhibitors. Cancer 14(24):6145. https://doi.org/10.3390/cancers14246145

Croci DO, Zacarías Fluck MF, Rico MJ, Matar P, Rabinovich GA, Scharovsky OG (2007) Dynamic cross-talk between tumor and immune cells in orchestrating the immunosuppressive network at the tumor microenvironment. Cancer Immunol Immunother 56(11):1687–1700. https://doi.org/10.1007/s00262-007-0343-y

Downs-Canner S, Berkey S, Delgoffe GM, Edwards RP, Curiel T, Odunsi K, Bartlett DL, Obermajer N (2017) Suppressive IL-17A+ Foxp3+ and ex-Th17 IL-17AnegFoxp3+ Treg cells are a source of tumour-associated Treg cells. Nat Commun 8(1):14649

Gigoux M, Shang J, Pak Y, Xu M, Choe J, Mak TW, Suh W-K (2009) Inducible costimulator promotes helper T-cell differentiation through phosphoinositide 3-kinase. Proc Natl Acad Sci 106(48):20371–20376

Greaves P, Gribben JG (2013) The role of B7 family molecules in hematologic malignancy. Blood 121(5):734–744

Kopru CZ, Cagnan I, Akar I, Esendagli G, Korkusuz P, Gunel-Ozcan A (2018) Dual effect of glucocorticoid-induced tumor necrosis factor–related receptor ligand carrying mesenchymal stromal cells on small cell lung cancer: a preliminary in vitro study. Cytotherapy 20(7):930–940

Neeve SC, Robinson BW, Fear VS (2019) The role and therapeutic implications of T cells in cancer of the lung. Clin Transl Immunol 8(8):e1076. https://doi.org/10.1002/cti2.1076

Pardoll DM (2012) The blockade of immune checkpoints in cancer immunotherapy. Nat Rev Cancer 12(4):252–264

Porcu M, De Silva P, Solinas C, Battaglia A, Schena M, Scartozzi M, Bron D, Suri JS, Willard-Gallo K, Sangiolo D (2019) Immunotherapy associated pulmonary toxicity: biology behind clinical and radiological features. Cancer 11(3):305

Pourakbari R, Hajizadeh F, Parhizkar F, Aghebati-Maleki A, Mansouri S, Aghebati-Maleki L (2021) Co-stimulatory agonists: an insight into the immunotherapy of cancer. EXCLI J 20:1055

Rabinovich GA, Gabrilovich D, Sotomayor EM (2007) Immunosuppressive strategies that are mediated by tumor cells. Annu Rev Immunol 25(1):267–296. https://doi.org/10.1146/annurev.immunol.25.022106.141609

Sanmamed MF, Pastor F, Rodriguez A, Perez-Gracia JL, Rodriguez-Ruiz ME, Jure-Kunkel M, Melero I (2015) Agonists of co-stimulation in cancer immunotherapy directed against CD137, OX40, GITR, CD27, CD28, and ICOS. Semin Oncol 42(4):640–655

Schiller JH, Morgan-Ihrig C, Levitt ML (1995) Concomitant administration of Interleukin-2 plus tumor necrosis factor in advanced non-small cell lung cancer. Am J Clin Oncol 18(1):47. https://journals.lww.com/amjclinicaloncology/Fulltext/1995/02000/Concomitant_Administration_of_Interleukin_2_Plus.10.aspx

Schoenhals JE, Cushman TR, Barsoumian HB, Li A, Cadena AP, Niknam S, Younes AI, Caetano MDS, Cortez MA, Welsh JW (2018) Anti-glucocorticoid-induced tumor necrosis factor–related protein (GITR) therapy overcomes radiation-induced treg immunosuppression and drives abscopal effects. Front Immunol 9:2170

Seidel JA, Otsuka A, Kabashima K (2018) Anti-PD-1 and anti-CTLA-4 therapies in cancer: mechanisms of action, efficacy, and limitations. Front Oncol 8:86

Shevach EM, Stephens GL (2006) The GITR–GITRL interaction: co-stimulation or contrasuppression of regulatory activity? Nat Rev Immunol 6(8):613–618

Shimabukuro-Vornhagen A, Gödel P, Subklewe M, Stemmler HJ, Schlößer HA, Schlaak M, Kochanek M, Böll B, von Bergwelt-Baildon MS (2018) Cytokine release syndrome. J Immunother Cancer 6(1):56. https://doi.org/10.1186/s40425-018-0343-9

Shimizu J, Yamazaki S, Takahashi T, Ishida Y, Sakaguchi S (2002) Stimulation of CD25+ CD4+ regulatory T cells through GITR breaks immunological self-tolerance. Nat Immunol 3(2):135–142

Singh N, Temin S, Baker S, Blanchard E, Brahmer JR, Celano P, Duma N, Ellis PM, Elkins IB, Haddad RY, Hesketh PJ, Jain D, Johnson DH, Leighl NB, Mamdani H, Masters G, Moffitt PR, Phillips T, Riely GJ, Jaiyesimi IA et al (2022) Therapy for stage IV non–small-cell lung cancer without driver alterations: ASCO living guideline. J Clin Oncol 40(28):3323–3343. https://doi.org/10.1200/JCO.22.00825

Solinas C, Gu-Trantien C, Willard-Gallo K (2020) The rationale behind targeting the ICOS-ICOS ligand costimulatory pathway in cancer immunotherapy. ESMO Open 5(1):e000544

Sundar R, Soong R, Cho B-C, Brahmer JR, Soo RA (2014) Immunotherapy in the treatment of non-small cell lung cancer. Lung Cancer 85(2):101–109. https://doi.org/10.1016/j.lungcan.2014.05.005

Tian J, Zhang B, Rui K, Wang S (2020) The role of GITR/GITRL interaction in autoimmune diseases. Front Immunol 11:588682

Vence L, Bucktrout SL, Fernandez Curbelo I, Blando J, Smith BM, Mahne AE, Lin JC, Park T, Pascua E, Sai T (2019) Characterization and comparison of GITR expression in solid tumors. Clin Cancer Res 25(21):6501–6510

Wellenstein MD, de Visser KE (2018) Cancer-cell-intrinsic mechanisms shaping the tumor immune landscape. Immunity 48(3):399–416. https://doi.org/10.1016/j.immuni.2018.03.004

Wu G, He M, Ren K, Ma H, Xue Q (2022) Inducible co-stimulator ICOS expression correlates with immune cell infiltration and can predict prognosis in lung adenocarcinoma. International Journal of General Medicine 15:3739–3751

Zappasodi R, Sirard C, Li Y, Budhu S, Abu-Akeel M, Liu C, Yang X, Zhong H, Newman W, Qi J (2019) Rational design of anti-GITR-based combination immunotherapy. Nat Med 25(5):759–766

Zhu LX, Davoodi M, Srivastava MK, Kachroo P, Lee JM, St. John M, Harris-White M, Huang M, Strieter RM, Dubinett S (2015) GITR agonist enhances vaccination responses in lung cancer. Onco Targets Ther 4(4):e992237

Zhu H-H, Feng Y, Hu X-S (2020) Emerging immunotherapy targets in lung cancer. Chin Med J (Engl) 133(20):2456–2465. https://doi.org/10.1097/CM9.0000000000001082

Zugazagoitia J, Paz-Ares L (2022) Extensive-stage small-cell lung cancer: first-line and second-line treatment options. J Clin Oncol 40(6):671–680. https://doi.org/10.1200/JCO.21.01881

Vaccines and Oncolytic Virus for the Treatment of Lung Cancer

12

Arghya Kusum Dhar, Narahari N. Palei, and Dilipkumar Reddy Kandula

12.1 Introduction

Lung cancer accounts for around 2.2 million new cancer diagnoses (11.4%) and 1.8 million cancer-related deaths (18.0%) (Sung et al. 2021). Lung cancer can be categorized into two primary categories such as small cell lung cancer (SCLC) and non-small cell lung cancer (NSCLC). The incidence of NSCLC is roughly 15%, while that of SCLC is only 5%. Lung adenocarcinomas account for around 40% of NSCLC cases, while squamous cell carcinomas account for about 25–30%, and giant cell carcinomas account for about 10–15% (Wang et al. 2020; Yuan et al. 2019; Cortés-Jofré et al. 2019). Symptoms of lung cancer are uncommon in its early stages. The vast majority of lung cancer cases are detected at a late stage (stages III and IV). Patients with lung cancer tend to be older (70 years on average at diagnosis), with peak incidence between the ages of 65 and 75. Fifty percent to seventy percent of these patients are detected with stage IV cancer. Rates of survival after 5 years for NSCLC were reported by the International Association for the Study of Lung Cancer (IASLC) to be 36%, 26%, 13%, and 6% for stages IIIA, IIIB, and IV, respectively. This presents a problem for lung cancer treatment, as the elderly often cannot receive harsh therapies due to the age-related loss in the functionality of numerous organs (Cáceres-Lavernia et al. 2021; Losanno and Gridelli 2017). Life expectancy is believed to be lower for people diagnosed with advanced lung cancer compared to those diagnosed at an earlier stage. Thus, it is essential to create

A. K. Dhar (✉)
School of Pharmacy, The Neotia University, Sarisha, West Bengal, India

N. N. Palei
Amity Institute of Pharmacy, Amity University Uttar Pradesh, Lucknow, Uttar Pradesh, India

D. R. Kandula
Institute of Pharmacy, Shri Jagdishprasad Jhabarmal Tibrewala University, Jhunjhunu, Rajasthan, India

S. Bhatt et al. (eds.), *Immunotherapy Against Lung Cancer*,
https://doi.org/10.1007/978-981-99-7141-1_12

screening and early disease detection methods, as well as new cancer therapies for treating tumors at more advanced stages. When diagnosing lung cancer, the stage of the tumor is crucial. Patients with NSCLC at stages I and II are often treated with surgical resection. Adjuvant chemotherapy based on platinum is suggested for stage II tumors following surgical removal. Curative radiation is administered to patients who are not candidates for resection. Radio chemotherapy is given to patients at stage IIIB, while palliative therapies are given to those at stage IV (Cortés-Jofré et al. 2019; Hammerschmidt and Wirtz 2009; Stevens et al. 2020). The use of targeted therapy in the management of NSCLC is expanding in importance. Epidermal growth factor receptor (EGFR), PI3K/AKT/mTOR, RAS-MAPK, and NTRK/ROS1 are just a few of the primary pathways that it aims to disrupt. Several drugs that work by inhibiting these pathways have been developed, and they have improved survival rates and patient's well-being. Drug resistance emerges among tumor cells despite the treatment's promise of pinpointing malignancies (Hammerschmidt and Wirtz 2009; Stevens et al. 2020).

To address the demands for novel drugs to increase survival in lung cancer, new therapeutic approaches for patients with advanced NSCLC must be discovered and developed. Access of NSCLC patients to cutting-edge cancer immunotherapy has ushered in a new era in cancer care (Cortés-Jofré et al. 2019; Schirrmacher 2020), thanks to the rising body of research that has shed light on the relationship between the immune system and cancer cells during the past decade. Immunotherapy uses the body's own defenses against cancer, rather than directly attacking the tumors as do conventional cancer treatments. ICIs and cancer vaccines have been the primary immunotherapeutic techniques studied in NSCLCs. The introduction of ICIs has given patients with advanced or metastatic NSCLC a new therapeutic alternative. It has demonstrated exceptional benefits and significantly improved clinical outcomes in a sample of individuals with NSCLC. Despite of success of ICIs in treating lung cancer, the first-line treatment with ICIs is ineffective for the vast majority of patients with metastatic NSCLC. Second- and third-line treatments had an even lower response rate (20%) than first-line treatments. Clearly, there is still work to be done before the immune response can be fully harnessed and used to improve patient care on a wide scale (van der Hoorn et al. 2021; Badrinath and Yoo 2019). Cancer vaccination attempts to induce robust immune responses against the immunological evasion of tumors and is another immunotherapeutic technique with significant promise to overcome these challenges. Cancer vaccine research has been expanding rapidly and has shown encouraging results. Numerous phase I and phase II clinical trials have confirmed the safety and efficacy of cancer vaccines in NSCLC. Late-stage clinical trials have been conducted during the past decade (Cascone et al. 2021; Jung and Antonia 2018; Nemunaitis et al. 2006), but no favorable data has been revealed. The lack of success of cancer vaccines for treatment of NSCLC can be attributed to a number of causes, including ineffective adjuvants (Nemunaitis et al. 2009), inappropriate antigen targeting (Nemunaitis et al. 2009), tumor-induced immunosuppression (Oliveres et al. 2018), and immunosenescence (Zhang et al. 1996). To overcome these challenges and produce effective vaccine strategies for the therapy of NSCLC, cutting-edge studies in the immunology of tumor and vaccine development are desperately needed.

Recent years have seen the use of oncolytic viruses (OVs) in the therapy of advanced stages of many different cancer types. OVs can be utilized in combination with other immunotherapies like ICIs or cancer vaccines to boost therapeutic anticancer effects because of their ability to preferentially multiply in and destroy tumor cells and then elicit systemic antitumor immune responses. Vaccinia virus (VV) is being investigated as a potential cancer therapy. Many different types of cancer have been demonstrated to respond well to VV-based therapy. Further, research on therapeutic cancer vaccines employing VV as a powerful immunological adjuvant has focused on stimulating robust antitumor immune responses in patients with NSCLC (Nemunaitis et al. 2009; Cuzzubbo et al. 2021; Rodriguez and Sanchez 2013). Therefore, the purpose of this chapter is to review the most up-to-date uses of OVs and vaccines in NSCLC treatment and to speculate on the prospects for these cutting-edge approaches.

12.1.1 Current Lung Cancer Therapy

Common early-stage NSCLC treatments include surgery, chemotherapy, and radiation therapy. However, these methods fail miserably when applied to more severe or persistent cases. Since NSCLC has a high tumor mutational burden (TMB), immunotherapy is the most effective therapeutic approach (Stevens et al. 2020). In particular, high TMB is linked to higher expression of immune-recognizable tumor-specific antigens (neoantigens), which improves the likelihood that the immune system will recognize and eliminate tumor cells, enhancing the response to cancer immunotherapy (Page et al. 2021; Saxena et al. 2021; Fusco et al. 2021). New advances in the treatment of NSCLC have been made possible by applications of immunotherapy, and patients with NSCLC now have better clinical outcomes as a result. The only immunotherapy treatments for NSCLC that have been given the green light so far are ICIs (Stevens et al. 2020). Despite this promising research, only a tiny percentage of patients benefit from ICI therapy for NSCLC (van der Hoorn et al. 2021; Cascone et al. 2021; Jung and Antonia 2018), making current treatment unsatisfactory. There is an urgent clinical need to investigate a new therapeutic modality for NSCLC, the causes of which are still poorly understood.

12.2 Vaccines for Lung Cancer

An emerging immunotherapeutic strategy for the management of NSCLC is cancer vaccination (Shao et al. 2020; Wu et al. 2020). Therapeutic cancer vaccines work by training the immune system to target cancer cells by recognizing their unique tumor antigens (Mellstedt et al. 2011). Thus, cancer vaccinations can induce permanent immunological memory to restrain tumor growth and avoid recurrence with minimal side effects. Because of this, cancer vaccines may be a more secure and efficient therapeutic approach than other drugs currently used to treat cancer (Badrinath and Yoo 2019; Dessureault et al. 2007). Phase III clinical studies are presently underway for several cancer vaccines, and they are all made with the goal of making NSCLC treatment easier than it is now. More research into cancer vaccines could lead to better results for patients with NSCLC.

Cell-based vaccines use dead or living tumor cells to stimulate the immune system of host to prevent disease or infection. This method makes use of allogenic tumor cell lines, autologous tumor cells that have been irradiated, and autologous tumor lysates (Dranoff et al. 1993). The efficiency of whole-cell vaccines was enhanced by the addition of cytokines like interleukin-2 or granulocyte macrophage colony-stimulating factor (GM-CSF) (Disis et al. 1996; Higano et al. 2009).

Peptide vaccines are designed to stimulate an immune response against cancer by mimicking the epitopes of antigen. Immune responses were not strong in early trials using short peptides based on a single antigen. Prior to the introduction of ICI, patients with metastatic melanoma who received the gp100 peptide vaccination in combination with IL-2 had a greater response rate and an extended progression-free survival (PFS) than those who received IL-2 alone (Vinageras et al. 2008). NSCLC research has looked into several peptide–/protein-targeted vaccines. Viral vectors are employed in vaccines to deliver antigens to the host and stimulate an immune response. Plasmid-based DNA vaccines use tumor antigen-encoding genes to elicit an adaptive immune response against cancer cells. Based on the melanoma-associated antigen family A 3 (MAGE-A3), the pVAX1-MAGEA3-sPD1 DNA vaccination is boosted by soluble programmed death-1 (sPD1). Inhibition of tumor growth and immunogenicity in mice were demonstrated with an array of DNA plasmids containing MAGE-A3 and the extracellular motif of murine sPD1 (Addeo et al. 2021).

RNA vaccines have a different method of action than DNA vaccines, which gives them a few advantages. Since RNA does not need to be incorporated into the DNA machinery for expression, its carcinogenic potential is reduced (Miao et al. 2021), and its overall safety in a therapeutic setting is bolstered. New interest in mRNA technology has been prompted by the performance of the SARS-CoV-2 vaccines, and numerous mRNA vaccine platforms are currently being developed for application in the cancer setting (Polack et al. 2020).

Downregulation of major histocompatibility complex class I (MHCI) and abnormalities in antigen-presenting mechanism have been linked to several factors that lead to acquired resistance to immunotherapies, suggesting that ppCT and other signal sequence-derived peptides and their transporter proteins may be useful in the advancement of therapeutic cancer vaccines (Malone et al. 1989). The significant decline in death rates related to SARS-CoV-2 infection can be attributed in large part to the rapid transformation of 30 years of investigation into new mRNA vaccines (Sahin et al. 2020). This has altered our views on the clinical production and application of vaccinations. Applying this understanding to the realm of cancer vaccines is a logical next phase, given the heightened interest in mRNA vaccines for use in cancer in the wake of the pandemic. There is also an ongoing investigation of mRNA vaccines for NSCLC. Sequence-optimized messenger RNAs (mRNAs) encoding various cancer antigens are used in the development of the mRNA-based cancer vaccines CV9201 and CV9202 (Papachristofilou et al. 2019; Sebastian et al. 2019; Lang et al. 2022), which are designed to elicit an adaptive cellular and humoral immune response.

Improvements in the knowledge of the recognition of neoantigens by T-cells and computational techniques for somatic mutation identification and prediction may pave the way for more effective neoantigen-based immunotherapies in the future (Ott et al. 2020). High-affinity immunological T-cell responses can be elicited by personalized cancer vaccinations based on neoantigens of each individual. Patients with NSCLC, bladder cancer, and melanoma participated in a phase Ib trial that paired the anti-PD-1 ICI nivolumab with the neoantigen peptide vaccination NEO-PV-01. It was safe and had a 39% response rate in 18 NSCLC patients (Gridelli et al. 2020).

Multiple types of cancer, including NSCLC, are driven by the KRAS mutation. Highly immunogenic tumor-specific neoantigens are encoded by KRAS mutations (Voena et al. 2015). Although cancer vaccines targeting the KRAS mutation have demonstrated promising preclinical effects, the immunosuppressive tumor microenvironment may restrict their clinical utility. More than one clinical investigation (NCT05202561, NCT05254184, and NCT04117087) is looking into the potential of using combinations of treatments.

Approximately 5–6% of NSCLC cases have an ALK rearrangement. Preclinical experiments conducted by Voena et al. (LUNGevity Found 2022) demonstrated the efficacy of an ALK vaccination comprising a DNA plasmid encoding the intracytoplasmic domain of ALK in generating a tumor-specific cytotoxic response in a mouse model of ALK-rearranged NSCLC (Sankar et al. 2021; Kim et al. 2021).

12.2.1 Mechanism of Action of Lung Cancer Vaccines

Vaccines against cancer have dual potential as cancer preventatives and therapeutics (Roy et al. 2021). Cancer vaccines have the potential to stimulate immune systems to react toward antigens expressed by tumors. Figure 12.1 depicts the mechanism of action of cancer vaccines. Dendritic cells (DCs) and other types of antigen-presenting cells (APCs) are responsible for delivering tumor-associated antigens (TAAs) to the immune system following administration of a cancer vaccine. Following digestion, the TAAs are displayed on the cell surface along with MHC class I and class II molecules. In order to activate CD4+ T helper cells and CD8+ T effector cells, tumor antigens on MHC complexes must bind to receptors on T-cells (TCRs). By releasing IFN-γ, IL-2, and IL-12, CD4+ T helper cells also boost the immune response, which in turn activates CD8+ T-cells and cytotoxic T lymphocytes (CTLs). Antigens on tumor cells are recognized by CTLs, which then trigger apoptosis (cellular immune attack) against tumor cells. In addition, CD4(+) T-cells boost natural killer cell killing and macrophage phagocytosis when activated, and they prime B cells to produce antibodies against a particular antigen via differentiation of plasma cells (a humoral immune response). Tumor antigens are neutralized

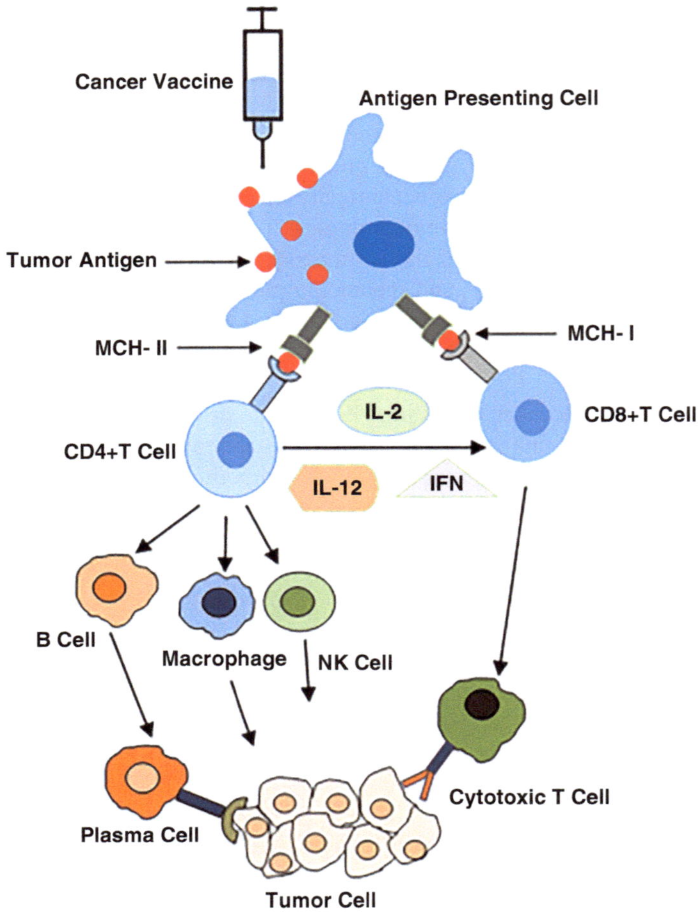

Fig. 12.1 Mechanism of action of lung cancer vaccines (Liu et al. 2018)

when these antibodies attach to them (Jeong and Yoo 2020; Decoster et al. 2012; Giaccone et al. 2015).

12.3 Clinical Studies with Vaccines for the Treatment of Lung Cancer

Many cancer vaccines for the treatment of metastatic NSCLC have shown encouraging outcomes in preliminary clinical studies (Table 12.1) examining their efficacy and safety aspects. Therapeutic cancer vaccines for NSCLC include autologous whole-cell vaccines, protein/peptide vaccines, vector-based vaccines, and vaccines containing DNA.

Table 12.1 Clinical trials of cancer vaccines for the treatment of NSCLC

Name and type of the vaccine	Clinical trial phase	Stage of lung cancer	Outcome	Reference
GVAX, cell-based	I/II	IV	Positive. After procured tumor tissue has been successfully processed into a vaccine, patients are vaccinated against lung cancer with GVAX intradermally (ID) (6–7 injections each immunization) on weeks 1, 3, 5, 7, and 9. In a lack of disease progression or intolerable toxicity, treatment is maintained	Hirschowitz et al. (2011)
Belagenpumatucel-L, cell-based	III	IIIA–B/IV	Negative. The two groups had similar rates of survival. Identical rates of progression-free survival are present	Rodriguez et al. (2016)
1650-G cell-based	II	I–IIB (adjuvant)	Positive	Creelan et al. (2013)
CIMAvax-EGF peptide-based	III	IIIB–IV	Negative. The vaccine group had a median survival time (MST) of 12.43 months compared to the control group's MST of 9.43 months. The mean survival time (MST) was 14.66 months in immunized patients whose baseline EGF concentration was high	Gray et al. (2018) and Grah et al. (2014)
MAGE-A3 peptide-based	III	IB–IIA	Negative. The MAGE-A3 immunotherapeutic was not effective as an adjuvant in improving disease-free survival. The MAGE-A3 immunotherapeutic for non-small cell lung cancer has been halted in its development	Alfonso et al. (2014)
Racotumomab-alum peptide-based	III	IIIA–IV	Positive. Patients who received the vaccine had a median progression-free survival (PFS) of 5.33 months compared to 3.90 months for those who received the placebo	Butts et al. (2014)

(continued)

Table 12.1 (continued)

Name and type of the vaccine	Clinical trial phase	Stage of lung cancer	Outcome	Reference
Tecemotide (L-BLP25), peptide-based	IIB	IIIB/IV	Negative. Despite the immunization increasing survival by 4.4 months, this difference did not reach statistical significance	Ramlau et al. (2008)
The preferentially expressed antigen in melanoma (PRAME), peptide-based	I	IB, II, and IIIA	Negative. No cancer regression was seen during the experiment, despite the presence of anti-PRAME humoral responses	Somaiah et al. (2019)
TG4010, virus-based	II	III/IV	Positive. When compared to the combination of placebo and treatment, TG4010 appears to increase PFS	Donninger et al. (2021)
LV305 virus-based	I	III/IV	Positive	Butts et al. (2005)
Elenagen, DNA vaccines	I/IIA	Advanced solid tumors	The majority of patients had 8 weeks or more of illness stability	Buonaguro and Tagliamonte (2020)

12.4 Development of Therapeutic Vaccines for Lung Cancer: Challenges and Limitations

Therapeutic cancer vaccines attempt to induce a persistent immune memory against tumor cells within the host, resulting in efficient tumor shrinkage with minimal off-target effects (Hollingsworth and Jansen 2019). Despite the fact that therapeutic cancer vaccines show great promise as an adjuvant to ICIs as they are safe and specific and can induce long-term response after generating immunological memory, they have been surprisingly unsuccessful as monotherapy. The focus of current clinical research is on creating therapeutic cancer vaccines that can induce a strong and long-lasting T-cell response to tumor antigens (Hollingsworth and Jansen 2019).

However, a poor immunogenicity, an immunosuppressive tumor microenvironment, a chronic illness problem, and an ineffective lasting memory development are four significant difficulties that therapeutic cancer vaccines must overcome (Vansteenkiste et al. 2016; Hegde and Chen 2020). Effective cancer vaccines face significant challenges, one of the most significant being the difficulties of identifying target tumor antigens that are common to several types of tumors but that are also distinctive to or excessively expressed by tumor cells relative to healthy cells. However, the efficacy of the prospective vaccine is constrained by the elimination of high-affinity T-cells identifying self-antigens during development via the tolerance mechanisms of immune system. Cancer vaccines typically include tumor-associated antigens (TAAs) or non-mutated excessively expressed self-antigens.

Low-affinity T-cell receptors (TCR) on the T-cells stimulated by these vaccines would prevent them from successfully stimulating an anticancer response (Woo et al. 2002). Consequently, other mechanisms are needed.

Despite their immunogenicity, cancer cells can secrete immunosuppressive chemokines, induce MHC antigen loss, and recruit more immunosuppressive cells to the tumor microenvironment (TME) (Thibodeau et al. 2012; Rabinovich et al. 2007). Target antigens, MHC, and co-stimulatory molecules can be downregulated by cancer cells to evade T-cell detection (Thomas and Massagué 2005). Lung cancer cells produce a number of immunosuppressive substances, including TGF-beta, prostaglandin E2, interleukin-10, and cyclooxygenase-2 (Gray et al. 2021; Mardis 2021). These molecules affect dendritic cell processing, presentation, and cytotoxic T lymphocyte effector activity. Advanced methods of antigen screening, immunotherapy administration, and therapeutic combinations have been studied to avoid TME immunosuppression and tumor escape (Quoix et al. 2011).

12.5 Oncolytic Virus for Lung Cancer Therapy

In oncolytic virotherapy (OVT), OVs are used in immunotherapy to specifically target and kill cancer cells without affecting healthy tissue. By replicating only in cancer cells and destroying them, OVs trigger an antitumor immunity reaction throughout the body (Fig. 12.2). Over the past two decades, OVT has shown encouraging results in the cancer therapy. Patients in the later stages of cancer who have not responded to standard treatments like chemotherapy or radiation have benefited greatly from the usage of OVs. Because of their high therapeutic efficacy with relatively low toxicity, OVs are increasingly being used to treat cancer. Several viruses, including vaccinia, coxsackie, adeno, reo, measles, and maraba viruses, are being

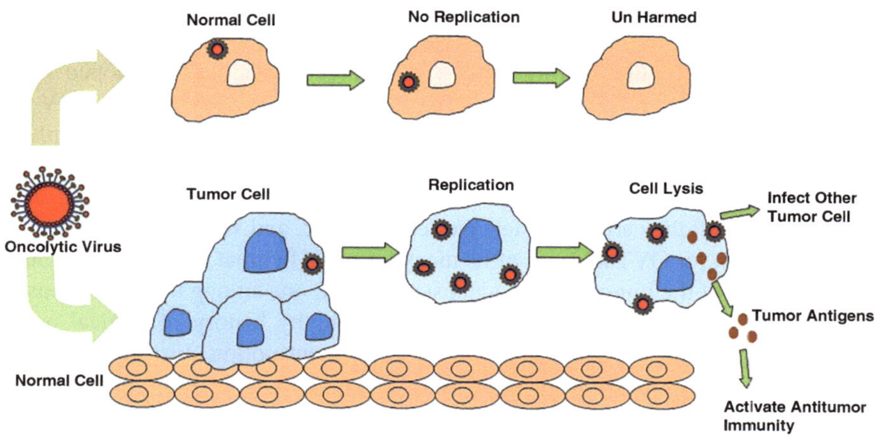

Fig. 12.2 Mechanism of action of OVs

researched for their possible utility in the treatment of various stages of cancer (Thomas et al. 2019; Dash and Patel 2017; Garcia-Carbonero et al. 2017).

12.5.1 Anticancer Mechanism of Oncolytic Virus

The ability of OV to both directly kill cancer cells and stimulate the body's natural defenses against them is making it an increasingly vital component of cancer treatment (Fig. 12.2). OVs activate host antitumor immunity by preferentially infecting and reproducing within tumors, hence disrupting intratumoral immunosuppression and increasing influx of immune mediators into the cancer microenvironment (Zhang et al. 1996; Mondal et al. 2020). Earlier identified as ColoAd1, enadenotucirev is a chimeric adenovirus that targets tumors selectively. Enadenotucirev has been demonstrated to reside in resectable NSCLC, where it stimulates localized strong antitumor immune reaction, including CD8+ T-cell infiltration (Kaufman et al. 2015).

In addition, high-risk populations can be vaccinated with a reprogrammed somatic-derived tumor cell vaccine (VIReST) regime that employs oncolytic adenovirus or vaccinia virus infection to halt tumor progression and kick off tracking the reactions of immune system to tumors over time (Truong and Yoo 2022). Moreover, computers could determine which subunits of a lung cancer-causing oncogenic virus would make the best vaccine candidates; these epitopes hold great therapeutic potential as lung cancer vaccines.

12.5.2 Vaccinia Virus

The vaccinia virus (VV) belongs to the family Chordopoxvirinae, genus *Orthopoxvirus*. The genome of VV is roughly 192 kilobases (kb) long and is made up of two strands of DNA. In mammalian cells, the VV life cycle takes place entirely within the cytoplasm. Throughout its life cycle, VV develops into three distinct viral particles: an intracellular mature virion (IMV), a cell-associated enveloped virion (CEV), and an extracellular enveloped virion (EEV). Most of the time, IMV and EEV are used on building sites. Unlike IMV, which enters cells by fusing with the plasma membrane, EEV is taken into the cells by endocytosis (Badrinath et al. 2016; Yoo et al. 2017a). To date, the characteristics of three major VV strains have been established; they are the Lister, Western Reserve, and Wyeth strains. VV is an attractive agent for OVT because of its many benefits. In great part, VV contributed to the success of the immunization against smallpox, one among the most devastating health issues in human history. VV has a lengthy history of clinical use in humans, suggesting it is a secure oncolytic treatment option. Viruses with a big genome can have substantial amounts of foreign DNA inserted into them without suffering a drastic decrease in their ability to replicate (Yoo et al. 2016). All of the replications takes place inside the cell; therefore there is no danger of insertional mutagenesis. VV employs proteins encoded by the virus itself for replication of

DNA and synthesis of mRNA, allowing it to replicate in many distinct cell types and evade host defenses. In contrast to other OVs, VV can infect a wide variety of host organisms (Badrinath et al. 2016; Parato et al. 2012; Yoo et al. 2017b, 2019). This benefit makes it much simpler to conduct clinical trials using VV after initial studies in animal models. Additionally, the VV has a high tropicity toward tumor cells (Haddad 2017) which is viewed as an advantage over those of other oncolytic viruses. VV platforms have been used to launch numerous cancer treatment experiments. These include using a cancer vaccine to transport antigens linked to tumors and immunoregulatory molecules, using an oncolytic medication that grows preferentially in cancer cells and destroys them and using a virus as a means of delivery for anticancer transgenes (Yoo et al. 2017a; Guo et al. 2019; Kaufman et al. 2016; Shafren et al. 1997; Miyamoto et al. 2012).

12.5.3 Coxsackievirus

Coxsackievirus, a type of non-enveloped, single-stranded RNA enterovirus, belongs to the Picornaviridae family (Janmaat et al. 2006). Infection with the coxsackievirus does not lead to insertional mutagenesis because the virus can multiply in the cytoplasm without a DNA replication step. In addition, its oncolytic and nontoxic properties do not call for intricate genetic engineering (Janmaat et al. 2006). Since some tumors, including multiple myeloma, melanoma, and breast cancer, overexpress ICAM-1 and/or DAF for cell entry (Guo et al. 2005), the coxsackievirus A21 (Cavatak; CVA21) has a usual tropism for cancer cells. Coxsackievirus not only kills tumor cells directly, but it also boosts the immune reaction by encouraging the discharge of damage-associated molecular patterns (DAMPs) like calreticulin (CRT), adenosine triphosphate (ATP), and high-mobility group box 1 protein (HMGB-1) (Deng et al. 2019). The effectiveness of coxsackievirus for previously treated cases of NSCLC is a foremost argument in its favor. Intratumoral administration of coxsackievirus B3 (CVB3) against radiation- and EGFR tyrosine kinase inhibitor gefitinib-resistant A549 lung cancer xenografts has been found to have a significant antitumor effect (Bischoff et al. 1996; Rao et al. 1992).

DAF upregulation by NSCLC cells serves as a defense mechanism against complement-mediated cytotoxicity and as a prime CVB3 target. Preclinical studies showed that CVB3 increased caspase-facilitated apoptosis and consequent oncolysis in NSCLC cells (Deng et al. 2019; Nemunaitis et al. 2000).

12.5.4 Adenovirus

Adenoviruses are non-enveloped, double-stranded DNA viruses, with icosahedral capsids that surround a 35-Kb linear genome (Janmaat et al. 2006). The large genome allows for many man-made upgrades by inserting long DNA sequences. Adenoviruses enter cells and express viral propagation-critical early genes (E1A and E1B) in the nucleus. E1A and E1B block p53 and pRb for cell cycle progression. Adenoviral E1A and E1B proteins directly target host p53 and pRb in normal host cells, causing apoptosis and viral clearance (Schenk et al. 2020; Rudin et al. 2011). ONYX-015 and H101 lack the inactivating region of E1B; therefore they replicate only in cancer cells without active p53. Adenovirus can deliver wild-type p53 gene into mutant p53 tumor cells (Bischoff and Samuel 1989).

12.5.5 Seneca Valley Virus

Seneca valley virus is a picornavirus, a type of non-enveloped RNA virus that prefers SCLC as its host. Intravenous administration is feasible since the virus is resistant to hemagglutination, a mechanism that often leads to early viral clearance and decreased delivery to the tumor site after intravenous administration (Strong et al. 1998). It cannot become part of the host genome because it lacks a DNA phase during replication. Seneca valley virus (SVV-001) was tested on 30 patients with advanced solid tumors, including 6 with SCLC in a phase I trial (Sei et al. 2009). There were no serious adverse effects from taking SVV-001. All patients were proven to have achieved viral clearance, which was found to be linked with the production of antiviral antibodies.

12.5.6 Reovirus

Reoviruses are non-enveloped, double-stranded RNA viruses that target cancer cells with an overactive RAS signaling system. The protein kinase R (PKR) pathway is activated when a reovirus invades a normal healthy cell and begins producing viral RNAs in the cytoplasm. By blocking protein translation, activated PKR stops the virus from replicating and spreading (Li et al. 2020a). RAS-transformed cancer cells, on the other hand, are unable to start the PKR pathway, making them vulnerable to infection and apoptosis (Ahmed et al. 2020). The downside is that it is ineffective against tumor cells without an active RAS pathway. Preclinical evidence suggests that the combination of reovirus with chemotherapy is beneficial for patients with NSCLC (Taunk et al. 2017).

12.6 Combination Therapeutic Strategy for Lung Cancer

Combining oncolytic virotherapy with chemotherapy has recently demonstrated that the use of these two medicines with very different antitumor mechanisms may also lead to synergistic interactions, ultimately resulting in greater therapeutic outcomes. The synergistic effects of oncolytic viruses (OVs) and chemotherapeutic drugs are only now beginning to be understood. However, it is clear that the efficacy of these OV-drug combinations varies substantially depending on the specific OV, the drug(s) chosen, and the type of cancer being treated.

12.6.1 Combination of Oncolytic Virus with Conventional Therapy

Patients with lung cancer who underwent combination therapy with oncolytic viruses had greater objective rates of response than those who had conventional therapy alone, according to a meta-analysis examining the effectiveness and safety of this approach (Li et al. 2013). OV has the potential to help lung cancer patients since it can target lingering tumors and boost an immune system that has been weakened by surgery (Kellish et al. 2019). This may improve postoperative survival by lowering the likelihood of a recurrence or spreading of tumor. Since radiotherapy has revealed remarkable immunoediting action in NSCLC, merging it with OV is an effective approach for treating lung cancer (Fox and Parks 2019). The ability of combination therapy to selectively target and eliminate human NSCLC tumor cells has been demonstrated (Quoix et al. 2016). It was found that when chemotherapeutic agents were combined with oncolytic viruses, the resulting combination exhibited enhanced cytotoxicity and oncolytic effects. Treatment of lung cancer with small-dose cisplatin and the OV and myxoma virus (MYXV) has been shown to increase survival rates (Villalona-Calero et al. 2016). P/V-CPI-5 infection predisposes airway cancer cells to the DNA-destructive effects of chemotherapy, which has proven beneficial in the elimination of these malignant cells (Gomez-Gutierrez et al. 2016). Combining TG4010 (Mva-Muc1-Il2) with conventional chemotherapy is safe and effective for patients with advanced NSCLC (Hofmann et al. 2014). In patients with advanced NSCLC, TG4010 improves the efficacy of treatment (Liu et al. 2009). When used with chemotherapy, TG4010 can lengthen the time between relapses (Zhang et al. 2020). Combining paclitaxel and carboplatin with Pelareorep (Reolysin) was well tolerated, and the addition of reovirus improved the efficacy of chemotherapy (Longo et al. 2019). The combination of temozolomide with oncolytic adenoviruses (OAds) greatly slows the progression of lung cancer (Ribas et al. 2017). Synergistic antitumor activity of cyclophosphamide and GLV-1 h68 was noticed against PC14PE6-RFP lung cancer xenografts (Parakrama et al. 2020). Therapeutic synergism between OBP-301 (Telomelysin) and gemcitabine was observed in human lung tumor xenografts (Jiang et al. 2017).

12.6.2 Combination of Oncolytic Virus with Immunotherapy

ICIs have become routine treatment for various kinds of cancer, including NSCLC due to their potential to prevent cancer-mediated immunosuppression (Masemann et al. 2021). There are a number of interesting immunomodulatory therapeutics, and OV is one among them. These can improve immune system function by modifying the tumor and increasing T-cell permeation. However, immunotherapy based on ICI does not work well for a majority of patients. Within the tumor, it can boost the efficacy of anti-PD-1 immunotherapy by increasing the responsiveness of ICIs (Sun et al. 2020; Zuo et al. 2021a). Inducing cancer cell destruction and stimulating immune-driven tumor cell detection and death, viruses have gained widespread recognition as an immunosensitizer (Zuo et al. 2021b). Potent antitumor immunity is generated through the proliferation of CD8+ T-cells with high specificity for tumor-associated antigens and the activation of tumor-specific lymphocytes when tumor-specific ICIs are combined with the oncolytic adenovirus delta-24-RGDOX, which expresses the immune co-stimulatory factor OX40 ligand (OX40L) (McKenna et al. 2021). Treatment with ICI coupled with infection with less virulent influenza virus (IAV) enhances M1-polarized macrophages in the alveolar cavity and lung invasion by cytotoxic T-cells in NSCLC, suggesting synergistic anticancer and immune-modulating activity of IAV against ICI-resistant lung cancer (Varudkar et al. 2021; Patel et al. 2020). Relapsed lung cancer patients benefit more from a triple therapy approach that combines oVV (oncolytic VV) with either PD-1 or TIM-3 inhibition (Goodwin et al. 2012). The use of oncolytic viruses in conjunction with ICIs that specifically target tumors is a promising approach to treating lung cancer.

The novel genetically engineered oncolytic VV (VV-α-TIGIT) encodes a completely monoclonal antibody against T-cell immunoglobulin and ITIM domain (TIGIT), which considerably raises recruitment and activation of T-cells in the tumor microenvironment (TME) (Xia et al. 2021). VV-scFv-TIGIT is an engineered oncolytic vaccinia virus that promotes strong antitumor immunity (Yang et al. 2015). It encodes a single-chain variable fragment (scFv) that binds to the T-cell immunoglobulin and ITIM domain. Oncolytic viruses producing antibodies against immune checkpoint domains have been found to boost anticancer efficacy by combining the advantages of OV with intratumoral expression of ICIs. The use of OV in combination with therapeutics other than ICIs is beginning to get interest. To effectively treat solid tumors with adoptive cell therapy, one must overcome the immunosuppressive TME. Oncolytic immunotherapy employing modified adenovirus abolishes the TME by infecting tumor cells and adjacent stroma to increase tumor-directed chimeric antigen receptor (CAR)-T-cell activity (Russell and Barber 2018). PM21-NK cells were shown in another investigation to be more effective at killing lung cancer cells infected with the P/V virus (Li et al. 2011). Researchers have employed an endostatin-expressing herpes simplex virus 1 mutant (HSV-Endo) in a mouse model of lung cancer as a potential antiangiogenic therapy. The orthotopic flank model considerably decreased tumor burden and microvessel density (Lu et al. 2020). The oncolytic activity of measles attenuated Edmonston strain (MV-Edm) and its ability to trigger apoptosis in human lung cancer cells A549 and H1299 were both improved by co-incubation with the NF-B signaling pathway inhibitor pS1145 (Tysome et al. 2012). ZD55-TRAIL, an oncolytic adenovirus loaded with the apoptosis-inducing protein TRAIL, displays greater cytotoxicity and causes apoptosis in A549 spheres through the mitochondrial pathway, indicating it has potential for application in lung cancer therapy (Nishio et al. 2014). Combining regular lung cancer treatment with OV is becoming an area of considerable interest.

12.6.3 Other Novel Combinations of Oncolytic Virus

Several cutting-edge avenues are being investigated to boost the effectiveness of OVs. The immunoadjuvant actions of OVs can help stimulate and increase tumor-reactive cytotoxic T-cells (CTLs) when combined with tumor antigen-targeting vaccinations (Suryadevara et al. 2015). Chemotaxis of lymphocyte populations were improved in vitro and in vivo after tumor-bearing animals were vaccinated with type 1 polarized dendritic cells (DC1) and then treated with oncolytic VV expressing CCL5 (vvCCL5; receptors that are found on CTLs produced by DC1) (Wing et al. 2018). Increasing vaccine immunogenicity by pre-infecting with adenovirus and oncolytic vaccinia virus has been supported by several preclinical researches (Cook and Chauhan 2020; Atasheva et al. 2020). Chimeric antigen receptor T-(CAR-T) cell treatment and OVs can work well together. Oncolytic adenovirus expressing RANTES and IL-15 (Ad524) improved CAR-T cell migration and proliferation in a mouse model of neuroblastoma (Patel et al. 2020). Similarly, tumor-bearing mice saw an improvement in OS when treated with a combination of Ad524 and CAR-T cells (Patel et al. 2020; Hu et al. 2018). Bispecific T-cell engagers (BiTEs) are a type of bispecific antibodies characterized by the presence of a CD3-specific antibody on one arm and a tumor-specific antibody on the other (Qiao et al. 2020). In order to boost antitumor activity and survival in several mice cancer models, Wing et al. (Garofalo et al. 2018) engineered an oncolytic adenovirus equipped with an EGFR-targeting BiTE (OAd-BiTE).

12.7 Delivery of Oncolytic Virus

The therapeutic efficacy of OVs is severely hampered by the limited viral dissemination and unfavorable immune modulation in the cancer microenvironment (Hong et al. 2015). This is due to the formation of barriers by the tumor-associated stroma, which prevents the virus from penetrating the tumor and spreading. Intravenous delivery of oncolytic viruses has the disadvantage of making systemic administration more difficult due to antiviral immunity. Researchers have specifically targeted functional regions of the viral capsid to create the adenoviral vector Ad5-3 M. Researchers found that oncolytic viruses replicated in tumor cells, inhibited tumor growth, and were resistant to antiviral immunity in mice with lung cancer (Yurchenko et al. 2018). Excellent anticancer activity and animal survival in an immune-deficient mouse model of non-small cell lung cancer (NSCLC) were demonstrated by VSV-IFN-infected human blood outgrowth endothelial cells (BOECs). Using BOECs infected with A549 xenograft model mice, VSV-IFN was found to protect itself against antibodies and destroy NSCLC cells in vitro (Ye et al. 2018). Mice with an A549 lung tumor responded well to microfluidic oncolytic adenoviral encapsulation as an anticancer treatment in vivo. This was discovered by chance, but it turns out that this method of delivery simultaneously reduces proliferation, boosts oncolysis, and, maybe, immunomodulates cancer (Chai et al. 2014). When oncolytic adenovirus and paclitaxel were administered systemically in EV preparations, transduction rates and infection titers were considerably increased in vitro, and the proliferation of human lung cancer cells in animal xenograft-based models was successfully decreased (Hu et al. 2015). As a vehicle for other therapies, the virus also offers therapeutic promise. Different aerosol delivery technologies in combination with viral vectors and cationic carriers can produce novel, targeted carriers for the therapy of lung cancer (Yaacov et al. 2008).

12.8 Preclinical and Clinical Studies with Oncolytic Virus for the Treatment of Lung Cancer

The precise mechanisms of effect of OVs on lung cancer treatment have been the subject of various preclinical studies. In a preclinical study, the Newcastle disease virus (NDV) destroyed cancer cells without harming healthy ones (Deng et al. 2019). When exposed to NDV, immunogenic cell death with great efficiency was observed (Liu et al. 2020). Recombinant Newcastle disease virus D90 strain (rNDV-GFP) continued to replicate selectively in tumors and caused apoptosis in tumor cells as observed in a study (Liu et al. 2021). Lung cancer spheroids treated with NDV-FMW undergo AKT/mTOR pathway inhibition, caspase-dependent apoptosis, and autophagic disintegration (Chodkowski et al. 2021). Increased rates of viral gene transcription, translation, and offspring virus generation have been linked to NDV-HUJ virus-selective oncolysis (Hu et al. 2018). Coxsackievirus B3 (CVB3) was found to be an effective oncolytic virus for the treatment of lung adenocarcinomas harboring the KRAS mutation (Chaurasiya et al. 2020). Virus with a microRNA modification (miR-CVB3) was able to infect and destroy lung adenocarcinoma cells with the KRAS mutation and SCLC cells with the TP53/RB1 mutation (Qiu et al. 2021; Masemann et al. 2018). The EHV-1 animal virus readily multiplied in the human cancer cell line A549 (Boisgerault et al. 2013). In a study with oncopox-trail, the oncolytic poxviruses that carried the trail gene were more cytotoxic because the TRAIL protein primarily caused apoptosis and prevented necrosis (Zhao et al. 2019). CD8+ T-cell infiltrations of tumors were observed with oncolytic virus CF33-GFP (Song et al. 2021). Tumors infected with herpesvirus 1 in bovines (BoHV-1) had lower protein levels of histone deacetylase (HDAC) because the virus caused DNA damage (Cohen and Kaufman 2004). Upon infection with less pathogenic oncolytic IAV, immunosuppressed tumor-associated lung macrophages in Raf-BxB mice regained their M1-like pro-inflammatory active phenotype (Rochlitz et al. 2003). Oncolysis produced by measles virus (MV) vaccination strains is linked to caspase-3 activation in vivo (Ramlau et al. 2008). The oncolytic myxoma virus (MYXV) has been found to produce growth inhibition and necrosis in tumors due to the infiltration of cytotoxic immune cells (Quoix et al. 2011). Oncolytic adenovirus H101 was found to have significant cytotoxicity, cell lysis, and tumor growth inhibition (Quoix et al. 2016). Targeting the AMPK/mTOR signaling system, the recombinant oncolytic adenovirus Ad-apoptin suppresses glycolysis, migration, and invasion in lung cancer cells (Pandha et al. 2017).

OVs have been subjected to various clinical studies also. Table 12.2 summarizes the progress made in clinical trials of OVs for lung cancer therapy. Tumor-associated MUC1 antigen expression is targeted by the vector-based vaccine TG4010 (MVA-MUC1-IL-2) (Schuler et al. 2001). The viral suspension mostly consists of Ankara virus, a weakened VV modified genetically to express MUC-1 and IL-2. The maximum tolerable dose was found to be 108 PFU per injection in a phase I dose escalation study (Swisher et al. 1999). One of the three patients with metastatic NSCLC in this experiment saw a decrease in numerous tumor sites two months after the final vaccination. Two different schedules of combining TG4010 with first-line chemotherapy were investigated in a randomized, double-blind, placebo-controlled phase IIB multicenter trial involving 65 patients with stage IIIB/stage IV NSCLC (Guerrero et al. 2021).

In treatment group 1, TG4010, cisplatin, and vinorelbine were used. Patients in treatment group 2 were given TG4010 and the treatment from treatment group 1 once their cancer had progressed. Partial responses were seen in 13/37 individuals in group 1 or 35.1%. Because TG4010 was ineffective in group 2, that group was discarded. The first group had a median OS of 12.7 months, but the second group fared better at 14.9 months. Injection site reactions, symptoms resembling the flu, and weariness were the most prevalent adverse effects of TG4010. Patients who responded showed evidence of MUC1-specific cellular immunology in their lymphocytes.

A phase IIb study of TG4010 as first-line therapy in patients with advanced NSCLC and MUC1 expression by immunohistochemistry (IHC) (Aggarwal et al. 2018) was conducted. Patients were given either a combination of cisplatin and gemcitabine (TG4010) or treatment alone. Six-month progression-free survival was higher in the combination group (43.2% vs. 35.1%) than in the chemotherapy-alone group ($p = 0.33$). In addition, there was no statistically noteworthy variation in median survival or time to progression. Phase IIb of a phase IIb/III randomized study including 222 patients with stage IV NSCLC compared the efficacy of TG4010 in combination with standard chemotherapy vs. standard treatment alone (Bradbury et al. 2018). PFS was the primary outcome, and the secondary goal was to verify that a pretreatment level of CD16, CD56, and CD69 triple-positive activated lymphocytes (TrPAL) was an accurate predictor of PFS. The median PFS for TG4010 was 5.9 months, but it was only 5.1 months for placebo (HR 0.74; one-sided p = 0.019). In patients with TrPAL levels below the ULN, the primary goal was achieved, with a hazard ratio (HR) of 0.75 (0.54–1.03) for PFS. There were no serious adverse events associated with the combination treatment. For this reason, TG4010 was evaluated in a phase II trial (NCT03353675) in combination with chemotherapy and nivolumab for PD-L1 50% advanced NSCLC. The main target, overall response rate (ORR) of the experiment, was not met in 2019, therefore ending further research into TG4010.

In a phase Ib STORM study, CVA21 was administered to patients with various types of advanced solid tumors as a monotherapy or in combination therapy with pembrolizumab, with dose increments between cycles (Villalona-Calero et al. 2016). On days 1, 3, and 22, and then once every 3 weeks, six additional infusions

Table 12.2 Clinical trials of oncolytic virus for the treatment of lung cancer (Liu et al. 2018; Wechman et al. 2016)

Oncolytic virus	Description of the trial	Type of trial	Phase
MEM-288 intratumoral injection MEM-288 is a conditionally replicative oncolytic adenovirus vector encoding transgenes for human interferon beta (IFNβ) and a recombinant chimeric form of CD40-ligand (MEM40)	Study of MEM-288 oncolytic virus in solid tumors including non-small cell lung cancer (NSCLC)	Open label	Phase I
Oncolytic adenovirus (ColoAd1)	Study of action mechanisms of ColoAd1	Open label	Phase I
Ad-MAGEA3 MG1-MAGEA3	Treatment of NSCLC with ad-MAGEA3 vaccine and MG1-MAGEA3 oncolytic protein and pembrolizumab	Multi-center and open-label	Phase I Phase II
Oncolytic vaccinia virus (BT-001) Containing genes encoding the 4-E03 human recombinant anti-hCTLA4 antibody and human GM-CSF	Study the effects of BT-001 alone and in conjunction with pembrolizumab on patients with advanced or metastatic solid tumors	Multicenter, open-label, consecutive cohorts	Phase II/phase II
Reovirus serotype 3—Dearing strain (REOLYSIN®) is a naturally occurring, ubiquitous, non-enveloped human reovirus	Combination of REOLYSIN®, paclitaxel, and carboplatin for patients with KRAS- or EGFR-activated non-small cell lung cancer: a phase II study	Open label	Phase II 114 and 115
Herpes simplex virus thymidine kinase (ADV/HSV-tk) expression using an adenovirus as a vector	The purpose of this phase II study was to evaluate the safety and efficacy of window-of-opportunity treatment with stereotactic body radiation therapy (SBRT) and in situ oncolytic virus therapy in patients with metastatic triple-negative breast cancer (TNBC) and metastatic NSCLC prior to administration of pembrolizumab. Treatment ADV/HSV-tk and valacyclovir will constitute in situ oncolytic viral therapy	Open label	Phase II

(continued)

Table 12.2 (continued)

Oncolytic virus	Description of the trial	Type of trial	Phase
CAdVEC	Binary oncolytic adenovirus in combination with human epidermal growth factor receptor 2 (HER2)-specific autologous CAR VST and advanced HER2 positive solid tumors (VISTA)	Open label	Phase I
Recombinant L-IFN adenovirus injection	Safety and efficacy of recombinant oncolytic adenovirus L-IFN injection in relapsed/refractory solid tumors clinical study (YSCH-01)	Single-arm and open label	Early phase I
Oncolytic virus injection (RT-01)	Combining the PD-1 inhibitor nivolumab with an oncolytic virus injection (RT-01) in patients with advanced solid tumors to assess safety and efficacy	Single-arm and open label	Phase I
TBio-6517, engineered oncolytic vaccinia virus	Evaluation of TBio-6517 in individuals with solid tumors, either alone or in combination with pembrolizumab	Nonrandomized open label	Phase I/phase II
Recombinant vaccinia GMCSF, RAC VAC GM-CSF (JX-594)	Safety study of recombinant vaccinia virus to treat refractory solid tumors	Nonrandomized open label	Phase I
Seneca Valley virus, or SVV-001, is a picornavirus that is capable of replication	Seneca Valley virus (SVV-001) safety evaluation in patients with neuroendocrine solid tumors	Nonrandomized open label	Phase I 110
The oncolytic virus HSV1716 is a mutant of herpes simplex virus (HSV) type I that lacks the RL1 gene for the ICP34.5 protein	A phase I/phase IIa study of safety, tolerability, and biological effect involving the intrapleural administration of herpes simplex virus type 1716 (HSV1716), a selectively replication-competent virus, to patients with inoperable malignant pleural mesothelioma	Single group open label	Phase I/phase II
Oncolytic measles virus encoding thyroidal sodium iodide symporter	Intrapleural measle virus therapy in patients with malignant pleural mesothelioma	Single group open label	Phase I

of CVA21 were administered. A maximum of 2 years of pembrolizumab treatment was given to certain patients. The detection of CVA21 viral RNA in tumor tissues demonstrated the efficacy of CVA21 in treating cancer. All patients had generated anti-CVA21 neutralizing antibodies by the 22nd day of the research, indicating that the host had mounted an effective antiviral immune response. One patient got a partial response, whereas the disease remained stable in the other four. In clinical trials, there were no major adverse effects and excellent medication tolerance among patients. In the NSCLC extension cohort, 23% (7/31, 2CR + 5PR) of evaluable patients have had an overall response rate (ORR), while 33% (7/21) of patients without EGFR or ALK mutations have had an ORR. Early immunohistochemistry (IHC) tagging of matched samples from evaluable patients with negative or low baseline expression levels of PD-L1 revealed a 62% increase in PD-L1 + cancer cells by day 15 after the combo treatment. Despite the paucity of mature efficacy data, the average OS for individuals with NSCLC is currently 9.5 months.

Twenty-five patients with unresectable NSCLC participated in an open-label, multicenter phase II study, where they received a total of three cycles of paclitaxel and carboplatin or vinorelbine and cisplatin, in addition to an intra-tumoral injection of 7.5×10^{12} particles of Scheme 58,500 (rAd/p53, day 1 of each cycle) (García-Pardo et al. 2022). Cancers treated with p53 gene therapy and chemotherapy had a similar response rate (52% vs. 48%), as were cancers treated with chemotherapy alone (48%). Survival rates at 1 year were 44% for both therapy groups. Transgenes were expressed in 68% of cancers. There were some moderate side effects from the treatment.

Twenty-eight previously treated patients with refractory NSCLC were given an adenovirus vector encoding wild-type p53 complementary DNA (Ad-p53) in a phase I trial (Truong and Yoo 2022). Ad-p53 was injected intratumorally once a month for up to 6 months using CT-guided percutaneous fine needle injection (23 patients) or bronchoscopy (5 patients). Adenovirus vector DNA was detected in 18 (86%) of 21 patients with assessable posttreatment biopsy specimens using real-time polymerase chain reaction (RT-PCR), while vector-specific p53 mRNA was detected in 12 (46%) of 26 individuals. Apoptosis was detected in 11 of the biopsies performed after therapy. Only 2 patients (8% of the total) had a partial response, whereas 16 (64%) had a stable disease for 2–14 months. All participants tolerated the treatment well. This study confirmed the effectiveness of wild-type p53 transgene expression and demonstrated some anticancer activity in patients with advanced NSCLC.

In patients with progressed NSCLC, first-line chemotherapy has not been found to improve survival when combined with intratumoral adenoviral p53 gene therapy. The OV adenovirus-facilitated generation of herpes simplex virus thymidine kinase (ADV/HSV-tk) was injected intratumorally alongside the PD-1 antibody and SBRT in a phase II study for the treatment of stage IV NSCLC (Dash and Patel 2017). Intratumoral ADV/HSV-tk (51,011 vp) was administered to both immune-oncology (IO)-naive and resistant patients, who thereafter underwent SBRT (30 Gy in five fractions) to the same tumor. Nivolumab or pembrolizumab, two anti-PD-1 drugs, were given for a total of 2 years. In comparison to the IO groups 14.2% ORR and 64.2% clinical benefit rate (CBR), the immunotherapy-naive group saw a 28.5% ORR and 61.9% CBR. The thymidine kinase gene (aglatimagene besadenovec, AdV-tk) and the anti-herpes prodrug valacyclovir are topically administered as part of gene-mediated cytotoxic immunotherapy (GMCI) (Doronin et al. 2009). Patients with malignant pleural effusion have finished a phase I dose escalation trial using GMCI in combination with chemotherapy. Intrapleural administration of 1×10^{12} to 1×10^{13} vector particles of AdV-tk was performed in three separate cohorts. Nineteen patients were included, 14 of whom had malignant mesothelioma, 4 had NSCLC, and 1 had breast cancer. A phase II trial with GMCI in conjunction with conventional ICI for IO-resistant NSCLC is now recruiting, and disease stabilization was achieved in three-fourth of individuals with NSCLC 29 months after treatment (Doronin et al. 2009).

Extensive-stage (ES) SCLC patients who had finished initial course of therapy were enrolled in placebo-controlled, double-blind phase II trials using Seneca Valley virus (NTX-010) (Strong et al. 1998). Within 12 weeks of finishing chemotherapy, 50 patients were randomly assigned to receive either a single dose of NTX-010 or a placebo and were participated in the trial between 2010 and 2013. PFS was the primary indicator of success. The project was terminated early due to futility; NTX-010 and placebo groups had a median PFS of 1.7 months (HR 1.03, $p = 0.92$). Patients whose NTX-010 blood levels were high 1–2 weeks after treatment had a shorter PFS. Flu-like symptoms, diarrhea, and fatigue accounted for 34.6% of all adverse events rated as grade 3 or above.

Patients who have far-advanced or metastatic NSCLC and who had progressed on first-line treatment were administered a strain of reovirus serotype 3 known as pelareorep, produced in the dearing lab (Green et al. 2004), in a phase II randomized trial done by the Canadian Cancer trial group. Depending on histology, patients were randomly randomized to receive either chemotherapy (pemetrexed or docetaxel) or pelareorep (4.5101 TCID50, days 1–3 every 21 days). Success was evaluated mostly using PFS. Between 2012 and 2015, there were a total of 166 registrants. The median PFS for those who had pelareorep (3 months) was not significantly longer than those who received single-agent chemotherapy (2.8 months). There was no correlation between having a KRAS or EGFR mutation and a longer PFS. It increased the risk of neutropenic fever, although it was still tolerable. Reolysin (type 3 dearing reovirus) was studied in a first-line setting in conjunction with paclitaxel and carboplatin for individuals with metastatic or repeated NSCLC that had KRAS mutant or EGFR mutated/amplified (Hill and Carlisle 2019). Thirty-seven individuals were administered Reolysin on days 1–5 of every 21-day cycle. The median PFS was 4 months, the median OS was 12 months, and the ORR was 31%. Although the combination therapy was well tolerated, conclusive evidence about its efficacy was lacking (Hill and Carlisle 2019).

12.9 Development of Oncolytic Virus for Lung Cancer: Challenges and Limitations

There are a number of OVs for thoracic malignancies that can only be given in a tumor infusion, so the challenge of viral delivery remains significant. Although vaccine and reovirus are effective systemic delivery viruses, systemic tumor replication requires doses that are high enough to threaten industrial viability (Mondal et al. 2020). This issue can be addressed in a number of ways, one of which is the use of carrier cells for the selective systemic administration of OVs. In order to maximize the efficacy of adoptive cell transfer, it is possible to improve the bioavailability of OVs by mixing them with carrier systems based on immune cells (Reale et al. 2021). OVs have been delivered from the circulatory system to the site of the tumor via a variety of methods, including nanoparticles, liposomes, polyethylene glycol, and polymeric particles (Doronin et al. 2009; Green et al. 2004). Additionally, magnetic drug targeted systems have shown considerable promise as a carrier system for efficiently transporting viruses to tumor cells (Hill and Carlisle 2019).

Restricted diffusion of OVs within solid tumors is another key drawback. The stroma surrounding tumors acts as a barrier, limiting the spread of oncolytic viruses and, more importantly, limiting the effectiveness of the viral therapy used to treat cancer (Hong et al. 2015). One of the downsides of administering intravenous injections of oncolytic viruses is that antiviral immunity may interfere with systemic delivery. Systemic transmission of free virus to the tumor bed is complicated by preexisting neutralizing antiviral antibodies (Liu et al. 2018). Utilizing different virus serotypes, PEGylating the viral coat, covering the virus with a polymer to block antibodies, and neutralization are all viable options for dealing with this issue (Nemunaitis et al. 2000).

AdUV, which has been shown to more effectively lyse cancer cells, was isolated by repeatedly exposing viral particles from the oncolytic adenovirus wild-type Ad5 dl309 to C-type UV radiation (Wechman et al. 2016). Combining the oncolytic adenovirus Ad-hTERT with interleukin 10 (IL-10) increased antitumor efficacy in lung cancer therapy (Chen et al. 2021a). To be effective, oncolytic viruses must first elicit an immune response within the tumor microenvironment. Metastatic lung tumors are more effectively treated with systemic treatment of the IL-12 expressing NV1042 virus than with the non-cytokine parent NV1023 (Varghese et al. 2006). Antitumor effects can be induced using vaccinia virus IL-23, either secreted or membrane-bound (Chen et al. 2021b). Insufficient targeting of tumor of oncolytic adenoviruses following systemic distribution is another notable drawback of viral treatment for metastatic cancer. To be effective, immunotherapy must simultaneously target cancer cells as well as immune-suppressing stromal cells. Bispecific T-cell engager (BiTE) antibodies have been shown to help oncolytic adenoviruses overcome their "targeted limitation" to activate and steer tumor-penetrating T-cells more effectively (Fajardo et al. 2017). It is possible that tumor cells and immunosuppressive stromal cells could be simultaneously targeted by a designed oncolytic group B adenovirus encoded with BiTEs. BiTE induces activation of T lymphocytes and destruction of fibroblast through binding to fibroblast activation protein (FAP) on cancer-associated fibroblasts (CAFs) and CD3 on T-cells (Freedman et al. 2018). OAd-FBiTE, an oncolytic adenovirus when combined with FAP-targeted bispecific lymphocytes (T-cells), can facilitate viral dissemination and T-cell driven cytotoxicity targeting of tumor stroma by diverting infiltrating lymphocytes to CAFs, which have abnormally high expression of the FAP (De Sostoa et al. 2019). Systemic toxicity can be avoided thanks to PD-L1 BiTE, an oncolytic herpesvirus that triggers an inflammatory response and destroys tumor-promoting cells (Khalique et al. 2021).

Since OVs are living organisms and their growth requires systemic administration, the varying viral dosages reaching the tumor may also account for the inadequate effectiveness with OVs seen thus far with lung cancer (Bommareddy et al. 2018). In order to increase efficacy, which is also dependent on enhanced tumor selectivity, attempts should concentrate on increasing the effective viral load in tumor abrasions (Li et al. 2020b).

12.10 Conclusion

OV represents an attractive current experimental approach to the therapy of human cancers because of its potent anticancer effect on malignant tumors. The challenges of establishing an appropriate viral load at all tumor locations, as well as the lack of effect from OV monotherapy, have stymied the development of OVs for lung cancer. Although early trials combining OVs with chemotherapy showed some success, this was not replicated in larger, randomized studies. It may be worthwhile to investigate the potential for establishing novel OV combinations, particularly with ICIs and other immunotherapeutics, to address the meager results to date. However, further progress in OVs for lung cancer will be contingent on the inclusion of pertinent biomarker investigations in addition to significant outcomes in clinical trials. One possible method to enhance the effectiveness of OV is to employ alternative viral delivery mechanisms. There is an even larger need for the development of a vaccination strategy for both prevention and therapy of lung cancer, one that would halt tumor advancement and generate long-lasting antitumor immune response.

References

Addeo A, Friedlaender A, Giovannetti E, Russo A, de Miguel-Perez D, Arrieta O, Cardona AF, Rolfo C (2021) A new generation of vaccines in the age of immunotherapy. Curr Oncol Rep 23:137

Aggarwal C, Haas AR, Metzger S et al (2018) Phase I study of intrapleural gene-mediated cytotoxic immunotherapy in patients with malignant pleural effusion. Mol Ther 26(5):1198–1205

Ahmed J et al (2020) A new oncolytic Vaccinia virus augments antitumor immune responses to prevent tumor recurrence and metastasis after surgery. J Immunother Cancer 8(1):e000415

Alfonso S, Valdés-Zayas A, Santiesteban ER, Flores YI, Areces F, Hernández M, Viada CE, Mendoza IC, Guerra PP, García E et al (2014) A randomized, multicenter, placebo-controlled clinical trial of racotumomab-alum vaccine as switch maintenance therapy in advanced non-small cell lung cancer patients. Clin Cancer Res 20:3660–3671

Atasheva S et al (2020) Systemic cancer therapy with engineered adenovirus that evades innate immunity. Sci Transl Med 12:571

Badrinath N, Yoo SY (2019) Recent advances in cancer stem cell-targeted immunotherapy. Cancer 11:310

Badrinath N, Heo J, Yoo SY (2016) Viruses as nanomedicine for cancer. Int J Nanomedicine 11:4835

Bischoff JR, Samuel CE (1989) Mechanism of interferon action. Activation of the human P1/eIF-2 alpha protein kinase by individual reovirus s-class mRNAs s1 mRNA is a potent activator relative to s4 mRNA. Virology 172(1):106–115

Bischoff JR, Kirn DH, Williams A, Heise C, Horn S, Muna M, Ng L, Nye JA, Sampson-Johannes A, Fattaey A, McCormick F (1996) An adenovirus mutant that replicates selectively in p53-deficient human tumor cells. Science 274(5286):373–376

Boisgerault N et al (2013) Natural oncolytic activity of live-attenuated measles virus against human lung and colorectal adenocarcinomas. Biomed Res Int 2013:387362

Bommareddy PK, Shettigar M, Kaufman HL (2018) Integrating oncolytic viruses in combination cancer immunotherapy. Nat Rev Immunol 18(8):498–513
Bradbury PA, Morris DG, Nicholas G et al (2018) Canadian cancer trials group (CCTG) IND211: a randomized trial of pelareorep (Reolysin) in patients with previously treated advanced or metastatic non-small cell lung cancer receiving standard salvage therapy. Lung Cancer 120:142–148
Buonaguro L, Tagliamonte M (2020) Selecting target antigens for cancer vaccine development. Vaccine 8:615
Butts C, Murray N, Maksymiuk A, Goss G, Marshall E, Soulières D, Cormier Y, Ellis P, Price A, Sawhney R (2005) Randomized phase IIB trial of BLP25 liposome vaccine in stage IIIB and IV non–small-cell lung cancer. J Clin Oncol 23:6674–6681
Butts C, Socinski MA, Mitchell PL, Thatcher N, Havel L, Krzakowski M, Nawrocki S, Ciuleanu TE, Bosquée L, Trigo JM et al (2014) Tecemotide (L-BLP25) versus placebo after chemoradiotherapy for stage III non-small-cell lung cancer (START): a randomized, double-blind, phase 3 trial. Lancet Oncol 15:59–68
Cáceres-Lavernia HH, Nenínger-Vinageras E, Varona-Rodríguez LM, Olivares-Romero YA, Sánchez-Rojas I, Mazorra-Herrera Z, Basanta-Bergolla D, Duvergel-Calderín D, Torres-Cuevas BL, del Castillo-Carrillo C (2021) Racotumomab in non-Small cell lung cancer as maintenance and second-line treatment. MEDICC Rev 23:21–28
Cascone T, Fradette J, Pradhan M, Gibbons DL (2021) Tumor immunology and immunotherapy of non-Small-cell lung cancer. Cold Spring Harb Perspect Med 12:a037895
Chai Z et al (2014) Oncolytic therapy of a recombinant Newcastle disease virus D90 strain for lung cancer. Virol J 11:84
Chaurasiya S et al (2020) A chimeric poxvirus with J2R (thymidine kinase) deletion shows safety and anti-tumor activity in lung cancer models. Cancer Gene Ther 27(3–4):125–135
Chen D et al (2021a) Combining IL-10 and oncolytic adenovirus demonstrates enhanced antitumor efficacy through CD8(+) T cells. Front Immunol 12:615089
Chen L et al (2021b) Intratumoral expression of interleukin 23 variants using oncolytic vaccinia virus elicit potent antitumor effects on multiple tumor models via tumor microenvironment modulation. Theranostics 11(14):6668–6681
Chodkowski M et al (2021) First report of the oncolytic effect of EHV-1 on the non-small lung cancer—in vitro studies. Pol J Vet Sci 24(4):607–610
Cohen S, Kaufman HL (2004) TG-4010 Transgene. Curr Opin Investig Drugs 5(12):1319–1328
Cook M, Chauhan A (2020) Clinical application of oncolytic viruses: a systematic review. Int J Mol Sci 21:20
Cortés-Jofré M, Uranga R, Pombert AT, Prado MCA, Aguirrechu IC, Pacheco C, Reyes RMO, Chuecas F, Bermejo PIM (2019) Therapeutic vaccines for advanced non-small cell lung cancer. Cochrane Database Syst Rev 2019:CD013377
Creelan BC, Antonia S, Noyes D, Hunter TB, Simon GR, Bepler G, Williams CC, Tanvetyanon T, Haura EB, Schell MJ (2013) Phase II trial of a GM-CSF-producing and CD40L-expressing bystander cell line combined with an allogeneic tumor cell-based vaccine for refractory lung adenocarcinoma. J Immunother 36:442–450
Cuzzubbo S, Mangsbo S, Nagarajan D, Habra K, Pockley AG, McArdle SE (2021) Cancer vaccines: adjuvant potency, importance of age, lifestyle, and treatments. Front Immunol 11:3850
Dash AS, Patel MR (2017) Viroimmunotherapy of thoracic cancers. Biomedicine 5:2
De Sostoa J et al (2019) Targeting the tumor stroma with an oncolytic adenovirus secreting a fibroblast activation protein-targeted bispecific T-cell engager. J Immunother Cancer 7(1):19
Decoster L, Wauters I, Vansteenkiste J (2012) Vaccination therapy for non-small-cell lung cancer: review of agents in phase III development. J Ann Oncol 23:1387–1393
Deng H, Liu H, de Silva T et al (2019) Coxsackievirus type B3 is a potent oncolytic virus against KRAS-mutant lung adenocarcinoma. Mol Ther Oncolytics 14:266–278
Dessureault S, Noyes D, Lee D, Dunn M, Janssen W, Cantor A, Sotomayor E, Messina J, Antonia SJ (2007) A phase-I trial using a universal GM-CSF-producing and CD40L-expressing bystander cell line (GM. CD40L) in the formulation of autologous tumor cell-based vaccines for cancer patients with stage IV disease. Ann Surg Oncol 14:869–884

Disis ML, Bernhard H, Shiota FM, Hand SL, Gralow JR, Huseby ES, Gillis SM, Cheever MA (1996) Granulocyte-macrophage colony-stimulating factor: an effective adjuvant for protein and peptide-based vaccines. Blood 88:202–210
Donninger H, Li C, Eaton JW, Yaddanapudi K (2021) Cancer vaccines: promising therapeutics or an unattainable dream. Vaccine 9:668
Doronin K, Shashkova EV, May SM, Hofherr SE, Barry MA (2009) Chemical modification with high molecular weight polyethylene glycol reduces transduction of hepatocytes and increases efficacy of intravenously delivered oncolytic adenovirus. Hum Gene Ther 20(9):975–988
Dranoff G, Jaffee E, Lazenby A, Golumbek P, Levitsky H, Brose K, Jackson V, Hamada H, Pardoll D, Mulligan RC (1993) Vaccination with irradiated tumor cells engineered to secrete murine granulocyte-macrophage colony-stimulating factor stimulates potent, specific, and long-lasting anti-tumor immunity. Proc Natl Acad Sci U S A 90:3539–3543
Fajardo CA et al (2017) Oncolytic adenoviral delivery of an EGFR-targeting T-cell engager improves antitumor efficacy. Cancer Res 77(8):2052–2063
Fox CR, Parks GD (2019) Histone deacetylase inhibitors enhance cell killing and block interferon-beta synthesis elicited by infection with an oncolytic parainfluenza virus. Viruses 11(5):431
Freedman JD et al (2018) An oncolytic virus expressing a T-cell engager simultaneously targets cancer and immune suppressive stromal cells. Cancer Res 78(24):6852–6865
Fusco MJ, West HJ, Walko CM (2021) Tumor mutation burden and cancer treatment. JAMA Oncol 7:316
Garcia-Carbonero R et al (2017) Phase 1 study of intravenous administration of the chimeric adenovirus enadenotucirev in patients undergoing primary tumor resection. J Immunother Cancer 5(1):71
García-Pardo M, Gorria T, Malenica I, Corgnac S, Teixidó C, Mezquita L (2022) Vaccine therapy in non-small cell lung cancer. Vaccine 10:740
Garofalo M et al (2018) Antitumor effect of oncolytic virus and paclitaxel encapsulated in extracellular vesicles for lung cancer treatment. J Control Release 283:223–234
Giaccone G, Bazhenova LA, Nemunaitis J, Tan M, Juhász E, Ramlau R, Van den Heuvel MM, Lal R, Kloecker GH, Eaton KD et al (2015) A phase III study of belagenpumatucel-L, an allogeneic tumour cell vaccine, as maintenance therapy for non-small cell lung cancer. Eur J Cancer 51:2321–2329
Gomez-Gutierrez JG et al (2016) Combined therapy of oncolytic adenovirus and temozolomide enhances lung cancer virotherapy in vitro and in vivo. Virology 487:249–259
Goodwin JM et al (2012) Angiogenesis inhibition using an oncolytic herpes simplex virus expressing endostatin in a murine lung cancer model. Cancer Invest 30(3):243–250
Grah JJ, Katalinic D, Juretic A, Santek F, Samarzija M (2014) Clinical significance of immunohistochemical expression of cancer/testis tumor-associated antigens (MAGE-A1, MAGE-A3/4, NY-ESO-1) in patients with non-small cell lung cancer. Tumori J 100:60–68
Gray JE, Chiappori A, Williams CC, Tanvetyanon T, Haura EB, Creelan BC, Kim J, Boyle TA, Pinder-Schenck M, Khalil F (2018) A phase I/randomized phase II study of GM. CD40L vaccine in combination with CCL21 in patients with advanced lung adenocarcinoma. Cancer Immunol Immunother 67:1853–1862
Gray J, Rodríguez-Abreu D, Powell SF, Hochmair MJ, Gadgeel S, Esteban E, Felip E, Speranza G, De Angelis F, Dómine M et al (2021) FP13.02 Pembrolizumab + Pemetrexed-platinum vs Pemetrexed-platinum for metastatic NSCLC: 4-year follow-up from KEYNOTE-189. J Thorac Oncol 16:S224
Green NK, Herbert CW, Hale SJ et al (2004) Extended plasma circulation time and decreased toxicity of polymer-coated adenovirus. Gene Ther 11(16):1256–1263
Gridelli C, Ciuleanu T, Domine M, Szczesna A, Bover I, Cobo M, Kentepozidis N, Zarogoulidis K, Kalofonos C, Kazarnowisz A et al (2020) Clinical activity of a htert (vx-001) cancer vaccine as post-chemotherapy maintenance immunotherapy in patients with stage IV non-small cell lung cancer: final results of a randomised phase 2 clinical trial. Br J Cancer 122:1461–1466

Guerrero C, Ensor JE, Sun K et al (2021) Stereotactic body radiation therapy and in situ oncolytic virus therapy followed by immunotherapy in metastatic non-small cell lung cancer. J Clin Oncol 39(15_suppl):9115
Guo WF, Lin RX, Huang J et al (2005) Identification of differentially expressed genes contributing to radio resistance in lung cancer cells using microarray analysis. Radiat Res 164(1):27–35
Guo ZS, Lu B, Guo Z, Giehl E, Feist M, Dai E, Liu W, Storkus WJ, He Y, Liu Z (2019) Vaccinia virus-mediated cancer immunotherapy: cancer vaccines and oncolytics. J Immunother Cancer 7:6
Haddad D (2017) Genetically engineered vaccinia viruses as agents for cancer treatment, imaging, and transgene delivery. Front Oncol 7:96
Hammerschmidt S, Wirtz H (2009) Lung cancer: current diagnosis and treatment. Dtsch Ärzteblatt Int 106:809
Hegde PS, Chen DS (2020) Top 10 challenges in cancer immunotherapy. Immunity 52:17–35
Higano CS, Schellhammer PF, Small EJ, Burch PA, Nemunaitis J, Yuh L, Provost N, Frohlich MW (2009) Integrated data from 2 randomized, double-blind, placebo-controlled, phase 3 trials of active cellular immunotherapy with sipuleucel-T in advanced prostate cancer. Cancer 115:3670–3679
Hill C, Carlisle R (2019) Achieving systemic delivery of oncolytic viruses. Expert Opin Drug Deliv 16(6):607–620
Hirschowitz EA, Mullins A, Prajapati D, Baeker T, Kloecker G, Foody T, Damron K, Love C, Yannelli JR (2011) Pilot study of 1650-G: a simplified cellular vaccine for lung cancer. J Thorac Oncol 6:169–173
Hofmann E, Weibel S, Szalay AA (2014) Combination treatment with oncolytic vaccinia virus and cyclophosphamide results in synergistic antitumor effects in human lung adenocarcinoma bearing mice. J Transl Med 12:197
Hollingsworth RE, Jansen K (2019) Turning the corner on therapeutic cancer vaccines. NPJ Vaccines 4:7
Hong SH et al (2015) Aerosol gene delivery using viral vectors and cationic carriers for in vivo lung cancer therapy. Expert Opin Drug Deliv 12(6):977–991
Hu L et al (2015) Oncolytic Newcastle disease virus triggers cell death of lung cancer spheroids and is enhanced by pharmacological inhibition of autophagy. Am J Cancer Res 5(12):3612–3623
Hu J et al (2018) Trail armed oncolytic poxvirus suppresses lung cancer cell by inducing apoptosis. Acta Biochim Biophys Sin Shanghai 50(10):1018–1027
Janmaat ML, Rodriguez JA, Gallegos-Ruiz M, Kruyt FA, Giaccone G (2006) Enhanced cytotoxicity induced by gefitinib and specific inhibitors of the Ras or phosphatidyl inositol-3 kinase pathways in non-small cell lung cancer cells. Int J Cancer 118(1):209–214
Jeong S-N, Yoo SY (2020) Novel oncolytic virus armed with cancer suicide gene and normal vasculogenic gene for improved anti-tumor activity. Cancer 12:1070
Jiang H et al (2017) Oncolytic adenovirus and tumor-targeting immune modulatory therapy improve autologous cancer vaccination. Cancer Res 77(14):3894–3907
Jung CY, Antonia SJ (2018) Tumor immunology and immune checkpoint inhibitors in non-small cell lung cancer. Tuberc Respir Dis 81:29–41
Kaufman HL, Kohlhapp FJ, Zloza A (2015) Oncolytic viruses: a new class of immunotherapy drugs. Nat Rev Drug Discov 14:642–662
Kaufman HL, Kohlhapp FJ, Zloza A (2016) Oncolytic viruses: a new class of immunotherapy drugs. Nat Rev Drug Discov 15(9):660
Kellish P et al (2019) Oncolytic virotherapy for small-cell lung cancer induces immune infiltration and prolongs survival. J Clin Invest 129(6):2279–2292
Khalique H et al (2021) Oncolytic herpesvirus expressing PD-L1 BiTE for cancer therapy: exploiting tumor immune suppression as an opportunity for targeted immunotherapy. J Immunother Cancer 9(4):e001292
Kim CG, Sang YB, Lee JH, Chon HJ (2021) Combining cancer vaccines with immunotherapy: establishing a new immunological approach. Int J Mol Sci 22:8035

Lang F, Schrörs B, Löwer M, Türeci Ö, Sahin U (2022) Identification of neoantigens for individualized therapeutic cancer vaccines. Nat Rev Drug Discov 21:261–282

Li J, O'Malley M, Urban J et al (2011) Chemokine expression from oncolytic vaccinia virus enhances vaccine therapies of cancer. Mol Ther 19(4):650–657

Li JM et al (2013) MicroRNA-145 regulates oncolytic herpes simplex virus-1 for selective killing of human non-small cell lung cancer cells. Virol J 10:241

Li Y et al (2020a) Oncolytic virus combined with traditional treatment versus traditional treatment alone in patients with cancer: a meta-analysis. Int J Clin Oncol 25(11):1901–1913

Li L, Liu S, Han D, Tang B, Ma J (2020b) Delivery and biosafety of oncolytic virotherapy. Front Oncol 10:475

Liu D et al (2009) Preclinical evaluation of synergistic effect of telomerase-specific oncolytic virotherapy and gemcitabine for human lung cancer. Mol Cancer Ther 8(4):980–987

Liu XQ, Xin HY, Lyu YN et al (2018) Oncolytic herpes simplex virus tumor targeting and neutralization escape by engineering viral envelope glycoproteins. Drug Deliv 25(1):1950–1962

Liu H et al (2020) MicroRNA modification of coxsackievirus B3 decreases its toxicity, while retaining oncolytic potency against lung cancer. Mol Ther Oncolytics 16:207–218

Liu H et al (2021) Erratum: MicroRNA modification of coxsackievirus B3 decreases its toxicity, while retaining oncolytic potency against lung cancer. Mol Ther Oncolytics 20:1–2

Longo V et al (2019) Strategies to improve cancer immune checkpoint inhibitors efficacy, other than abscopal effect: a systematic review. Cancers (Basel) 11(4):539

Losanno T, Gridelli C (2017) Recent advances in targeted advanced lung cancer therapy in the elderly. Expert Rev Anticancer Ther 17:787–797

Lu S, Zhang Z, Du P et al (2020) A virus-infected, reprogrammed somatic cell-derived tumor cell (VIReST) vaccination regime can prevent initiation and progression of pancreatic cancer. Clin Cancer Res 26(2):465–476

LUNGevity Found. First vaccine for treating ALK-positive lung cancer. https://www.lungevity.org/blogs/developing-first-vaccine-for-treating-alk-positive-lung-cancer. Accessed 17 Mar 2022

Malone RW, Felgner PL, Verma IM (1989) Cationic liposome-mediated RNA transfection. Proc Natl Acad Sci U S A 86:6077–6081

Mardis ER (2021) Genomic prediction of neoantigens: Immunogenomics before NGS. Nat Rev Genet 22:550–551

Masemann D et al (2018) Oncolytic influenza virus infection restores immunocompetence of lung tumor-associated alveolar macrophages. Onco Targets Ther 7(5):e1423171

Masemann D et al (2021) Synergistic anti-tumor efficacy of oncolytic influenza viruses and B7-H3 immune- checkpoint inhibitors against IC-resistant lung cancers. Onco Targets Ther 10(1):1885778

McKenna MK et al (2021) Mesenchymal stromal cell delivery of oncolytic immunotherapy improves CAR-T cell antitumor activity. Mol Ther 29(5):1808–1820

Mellstedt H, Vansteenkiste J, Thatcher N (2011) Vaccines for the treatment of non-small cell lung cancer: investigational approaches and clinical experience. Lung Cancer 73:11–17

Miao L, Zhang Y, Huang L (2021) mRNA vaccine for cancer immunotherapy. Mol Cancer 20:41

Miyamoto S, Inoue H, Nakamura T, Yamada M, Sakamoto C, Urata Y, Okazaki T, Marumoto T, Takahashi A, Takayama K, Nakanishi Y, Shimizu H, Tani K (2012) Coxsackievirus B3 is an oncolytic virus with immunostimulatory properties that is active against lung adenocarcinoma. Cancer Res 72(10):2609–2621

Mondal M, Guo J, He P, Zhou D (2020) Recent advances of oncolytic virus in cancer therapy. Hum Vaccin Immunother 16:2389–2402

Nemunaitis J, Swisher SG, Timmons T, Connors D, Mack M, Doerksen L, Weill D, Wait J, Lawrence DD, Kemp BL, Fossella F, Glisson BS, Hong WK, Khuri FR, Kurie JM, Lee JJ, Lee JS, Nguyen DM, Nesbitt JC, Perez-Soler R, Pisters KM, Putnam JB, Richli WR, Shin DM, Walsh GL, Merritt J, Roth J (2000) Adenovirus- mediated p53 gene transfer in sequence with cisplatin to tumors of patients with non-small-cell lung cancer. J Clin Oncol 18(3):609–622

Nemunaitis J, Dillman RO, Schwarzenberger PO, Senzer N, Cunningham C, Cutler J, Tong A, Kumar P, Pappen B, Hamilton C (2006) Phase II study of belagenpumatucel-L, a transforming

growth factor beta-2 antisense gene-modified allogeneic tumor cell vaccine in non-small-cell lung cancer. J Clin Oncol 24:4721–4730
Nemunaitis J, Nemunaitis M, Senzer N, Snitz P, Bedell C, Kumar P, Pappen B, Maples P, Shawler D, Fakhrai H (2009) Phase II trial of Belagenpumatucel-L, a TGF-_2 antisense gene modified allogeneic tumor vaccine in advanced non-small cell lung cancer (NSCLC) patients. Cancer Gene Ther 16:620–624
Nishio N, Diaconu I, Liu H et al (2014) Armed oncolytic virus enhances immune functions of chimeric antigen receptor-modified T cells in solid tumors. Cancer Res 74(18):5195–5205
Oliveres H, Caglevic C, Passiglia F, Taverna S, Smits E, Rolfo C (2018) Vaccine and immune cell therapy in non-small cell lung cancer. J Thorac Dis 10:S1602
Ott PA, Hu-Lieskovan S, Chmielowski B, Govindan R, Naing A, Bhardwaj N, Margolin K, Awad MM, Hellmann MD, Lin JJ et al (2020) A phase Ib trial of personalized Neoantigen therapy plus anti-PD-1 in patients with advanced melanoma, non-small cell lung cancer, or bladder cancer. Cell 183:347–362
Page A, Hubert J, Fusil F, Cosset F-L (2021) Exploiting B cell transfer for cancer therapy: engineered B cells to eradicate tumors. Int J Mol Sci 22:9991
Pandha H, Harrington K, Ralph C et al (2017) Phase 1b KEYNOTE 200 (STORM study): a study of an intravenously delivered oncolytic virus, Coxsackievirus A21 in combination with pembrolizumab in advanced cancer patients [abstract]. Proceedings of the American Association for Cancer Research Annual Meeting 2017; 2017 Apr 1–5; Washington, DC Philadelphia (PA): AACR. Cancer Res 77(13 Suppl):Abstract nr CT115
Papachristofilou A, Hipp MM, Klinkhardt U, Früh M, Sebastian M, Weiss C, Pless M, Cathomas R, Hilbe W, Pall G et al (2019) Phase Ib evaluation of a self-adjuvanted protamine formulated mRNA-based active cancer immunotherapy, BI1361849 (CV9202), combined with local radiation treatment in patients with stage IV non-small cell lung cancer. J Immunother Cancer 7:38
Parakrama R et al (2020) Immune characterization of metastatic colorectal cancer patients post reovirus administration. BMC Cancer 20(1):569
Parato KA, Breitbach CJ, Le Boeuf F, Wang J, Storbeck C, Ilkow C, Diallo JS, Falls T, Burns J, Garcia V, Kanji F, Evgin L, Hu K, Paradis F, Knowles S, Hwang TH, Vanderhyden BC, Auer R, Kirn DH, Bell JC (2012) The oncolytic poxvirus JX-594 selectively replicates in and destroys cancer cells driven by genetic pathways commonly activated in cancers. Mol Ther 20(4):749–758
Patel MR et al (2020) Blood outgrowth endothelial cells as a cellular carrier for oncolytic vesicular stomatitis virus expressing interferon-β in preclinical models of non-small cell lung cancer. Transl Oncol 13(7):100782
Polack FP, Thomas SJ, Kitchin N, Absalon J, Gurtman A, Lockhart S, Perez JL, Marc GP, Moreira ED, Zerbini C et al (2020) Safety and efficacy of the BNT162b2 mRNA Covid-19 vaccine. N Engl J Med 383:2603–2615
Qiao H et al (2020) Tumor localization of oncolytic adenovirus assisted by pHdegradable microgels with JQ1-mediated boosting replication and PD-L1 suppression for enhanced cancer therapy. Biomater Sci 8(9):2472–2480
Qiu W et al (2021) Oncolytic bovine herpesvirus 1 inhibits human lung adenocarcinoma A549 cell proliferation and tumor growth by inducing DNA damage. Int J Mol Sci 22(16):8582
Quoix E, Ramlau R, Westeel V, Papai Z, Madroszyk A, Riviere A, Koralewski P, Breton J-L, Stoelben E, Braun D (2011) Therapeutic vaccination with TG4010 and first-line chemotherapy in advanced non-small-cell lung cancer: a controlled phase 2B trial. Lancet Oncol 12:1125–1133
Quoix E et al (2016) TG4010 immunotherapy and first-line chemotherapy for advanced non-small-cell lung cancer (TIME): results from the phase 2b part of a randomised, double-blind, placebo-controlled, phase 2b/3 trial. Lancet Oncol 17(2):212–223
Rabinovich GA, Gabrilovich D, Sotomayor EM (2007) Immunosuppressive strategies that are mediated by tumor cells. Annu Rev Immunol 25:267–296

Ramlau R, Quoix E, Rolski J, Pless M, Lena H, Lévy E, Krzakowski M, Hess D, Tartour E, Chenard MP et al (2008) A phase II study of Tg4010 (Mva-Muc1-Il2) in association with chemotherapy in patients with stage III/IV non-small cell lung cancer. J Thorac Oncol 3:735–744
Rao L, Debbas M, Sabbatini P, Hockenbery D, Korsmeyer S, White E (1992) The adenovirus E1A proteins induce apoptosis, which is inhibited by the E1B 19-kDa and Bcl-2 proteins. Proc Natl Acad Sci U S A 89(16):7742–7746
Reale A, Calistri A, Altomonte J (2021) Giving oncolytic viruses a free ride: carrier cells for oncolytic virotherapy. Pharmaceutics 13(12):2192
Ribas A et al (2017) Oncolytic virotherapy promotes intratumoral T cell infiltration and improves anti-PD-1 immunotherapy. Cell 170(6):1109–1119
Rochlitz C, Figlin R, Squiban P et al (2003) Phase I immunotherapy with a modified vaccinia virus (MVA) expressing human MUC1 as antigen-specific immunotherapy in patients with MUC1-positive advanced cancer. J Gene Med 5(8):690–699
Rodriguez CP, Sanchez B (2013) Challenges and opportunities for cancer vaccines in the current NSCLC clinical scenario. Curr Top Med Chem 13:2551–2561
Rodriguez PC, Popa X, Martínez O, Mendoza S, Santiesteban E, Crespo T, Amador RM, Fleytas R, Acosta SC, Otero Y et al (2016) A phase III clinical trial of the epidermal growth factor vaccine CIMAvax-EGF as switch maintenance therapy in advanced non–small cell lung cancer patients. Clin Cancer Res 22:3782–3790
Roy D, Geoffroy K, Marguerie M, Khan S, Martin N, Kmiecik J, Bobbala D, Aitken A, de Souza C, Stephenson K (2021) Adjuvant oncolytic virotherapy for personalized anti-cancer vaccination. Nat Commun 12:2626
Rudin CM, Poirier JT, Senzer NN et al (2011) Phase I clinical study of Seneca Valley virus (SVV-001), a replication competent picornavirus, in advanced solid tumors with neuroendocrine features. Clin Cancer Res 17(4):888–895
Russell SJ, Barber GN (2018) Oncolytic viruses as antigen-agnostic cancer vaccines. Cancer Cell 33(4):599–605
Sahin U, Oehm P, Derhovanessian E, Jabulowsky RA, Vormehr M, Gold M, Maurus D, Schwarck-Kokarakis D, Kuhn AN, Omokoko T et al (2020) An RNA vaccine drives immunity in checkpoint-inhibitor-treated melanoma. Nature 585:107–112
Sankar K, Nagrath S, Ramnath N (2021) Immunotherapy for ALK-rearranged non-small cell lung cancer: challenges inform promising approaches. Cancer 13:1476
Saxena M, van der Burg SH, Melief CJ, Bhardwaj N (2021) Therapeutic cancer vaccines. Nat Rev Cancer 21:360–378
Schenk EL, Mandrekar SJ, Dy GK, Aubry MC, Tan AD, Dakhil SR, Sachs BA, Nieva JJ, Bertino E, Lee Hann C, Schild SE, Wadsworth TW, Adjei AA, Molina JR (2020) A randomized double-blind phase II study of the Seneca Valley virus (NTX-010) versus placebo for patients with extensive-stage SCLC (ES SCLC) who were stable or responding after at least four cycles of platinum-based chemotherapy: north central cancer treatment group (Alliance) N0923 study. J Thorac Oncol 15(1):110–119
Schirrmacher V (2020) Cancer vaccines and oncolytic viruses exert profoundly lower side effects in cancer patients than other systemic therapies: a comparative analysis. Biomedicine 8:61
Schuler M, Herrmann R, De Greve JL et al (2001) Adenovirus-mediated wildtype p53 gene transfer in patients receiving chemotherapy for advanced non-small-cell lung cancer: results of a multicenter phase II study. J Clin Oncol 19(6):1750–1758
Sebastian M, Schröder A, Scheel B, Hong HS, Muth A, von Boehmer L, Zippelius A, Mayer F, Reck M, Atanackovic D et al (2019) A phase I/IIa study of the mRNA-based cancer immunotherapy CV9201 in patients with stage IIIB/IV non-small cell lung cancer. Cancer Immunol Immunother 68:799–812
Sei S, Mussio JK, Yang QE et al (2009) Synergistic antitumor activity of oncolytic reovirus and chemotherapeutic agents in non-small cell lung cancer cells. Mol Cancer 8:47
Shafren DR, Dorahy DJ, Ingham RA, Burns GF, Barry RD (1997) Coxsackievirus A21 binds to decay-accelerating factor but requires intercellular adhesion molecule 1 for cell entry. J Virol 71(6):4736–4743

Shao C, Li G, Huang L, Pruitt S, Castellanos E, Frampton G, Carson KR, Snow T, Singal G, Fabrizio D (2020) Prevalence of high tumor mutational burden and association with survival in patients with less common solid tumors. JAMA Netw Open 3:e2025109
Somaiah N, Block MS, Kim JW, Shapiro GI, Do KT, Hwu P, Eder JP, Jones RL, Lu H, Ter Meulen JH et al (2019) First-in-class, first-in-human study evaluating LV305, a dendritic-cell tropic lentiviral vector, in sarcoma and other solid tumors expressing NY-ESO-1. Clin Cancer Res 25:5808–5817
Song G et al (2021) Ad-apoptin inhibits glycolysis, migration and invasion in lung cancer cells targeting AMPK/mTOR signaling pathway. Exp Cell Res 409(2):112926
Stevens D, Ingels J, Van Lint S, Vandekerckhove B, Vermaelen K (2020) Dendritic cell-based immunotherapy in lung cancer. Front Immunol 11:620374
Strong JE, Coffey MC, Tang D et al (1998) The molecular basis of viral oncolysis: usurpation of the Ras signaling pathway by reovirus. EMBO J 17(12):3351–3362
Sun F et al (2020) Dual but not single PD-1 or TIM-3 blockade enhances oncolytic virotherapy in refractory lung cancer. J Immunother Cancer 8(1):e000294
Sung H, Ferlay J, Siegel RL, Laversanne M, Soerjomataram I, Jemal A, Bray F (2021) Global cancer statistics 2020: GLOBOCAN estimates of incidence and mortality worldwide for 36 cancers in 185 countries. CA Cancer J Clin 71:209–249
Suryadevara CM, Gedeon PC, Sanchez-Perez L et al (2015) Are BiTEs the "missing link" in cancer therapy? Onco Targets Ther 4(6):e1008339
Swisher SG, Roth JA, Nemunaitis J et al (1999) Adenovirus-mediated p53 gene transfer in advanced non-small-cell lung cancer. J Natl Cancer Inst 91(9):763–771
Taunk NK et al (2017) Immunotherapy and radiation therapy for operable early stage and locally advanced non-small cell lung cancer. Transl Lung Cancer Res 6(2):178–185
Thibodeau J, Bourgeois-Daigneault MC, Lapointe R (2012) Targeting the MHC class II antigen presentation pathway in cancer immunotherapy. Onco Targets Ther 1:908–916
Thomas DA, Massagué J (2005) TGF-beta directly targets cytotoxic T cell functions during tumor evasion of immune surveillance. Cancer Cell 8:369–380
Thomas S et al (2019) Development of a new fusion-enhanced oncolytic immunotherapy platform based on herpes simplex virus type 1. J Immunother Cancer 7(1):214
Truong CS, Yoo SY (2022) Oncolytic vaccinia virus in lung cancer vaccines. Vaccines (Basel) 10(2):240
Tysome JR, Li X, Wang S et al (2012) A novel therapeutic regimen to eradicate established solid tumors with an effective induction of tumor-specific immunity. Clin Cancer Res 18(24):6679–6689
van der Hoorn IAE, Flórez-Grau G, van den Heuvel MM, de Vries IJM, Piet B (2021) Recent advances and future perspective of DC-based therapy in NSCLC. Front Immunol 12:704776
Vansteenkiste JF, Cho BC, Vanakesa T, De Pas T, Zielinski M, Kim MS, Jassem J, Yoshimura M, Dahabreh J, Nakayama H et al (2016) Efficacy of the MAGE-A3 cancer immunotherapeutic as adjuvant therapy in patients with resected MAGE-A3-positive non-small-cell lung cancer (MAGRIT): a randomized, double-blind, placebo-controlled, phase 3 trial. Lancet Oncol 17:822–835
Varghese S et al (2006) Systemic oncolytic herpes virus therapy of poorly immunogenic prostate cancer metastatic to lung. Clin Cancer Res 12(9):2919–2927
Varudkar N et al (2021) Oncolytic parainfluenza virus combines with NK cells to mediate killing of infected and non-infected lung cancer cells within 3D spheroids: role of type I and type III interferon signaling. J Immunother Cancer 9(6):e002373
Villalona-Calero MA et al (2016) Oncolytic reovirus in combination with chemotherapy in metastatic or recurrent non-small cell lung cancer patients with KRAS-activated tumors. Cancer 122(6):875–883
Vinageras EN, de la Torre A, Rodríguez MO, Ferrer MC, Bravo I, del Pino MM, Abreu DA, Brooks SA, Rives R, del Castillo Carrillo C et al (2008) Phase II randomized controlled trial of an epidermal growth factor vaccine in advanced non–Small-cell lung cancer. J Clin Oncol 26:1452–1458

Voena C, Menotti M, Mastini C, Di Giacomo F, Longo DL, Castella B, Merlo ME, Ambrogio C, Wang Q, Minero VG et al (2015) Efficacy of a cancer vaccine against ALK-rearranged lung tumors. Cancer Immunol Res 3:1333–1343
Wang C, Long Y, Li W, Dai W, Xie S, Liu Y, Zhang Y, Liu M, Tian Y, Li Q (2020) Exploratory study on classification of lung cancer subtypes through a combined K-nearest neighbor classifier in breathomics. Sci Rep 10:5880
Wechman SL et al (2016) Development of an oncolytic adenovirus with enhanced spread ability through repeated UV irradiation and cancer selection. Viruses 8(6):333
Wing A, Fajardo CA, Posey AD Jr et al (2018) Improving CART-cell therapy of solid tumors with oncolytic virus-driven production of a bispecific T-cell engager. Cancer Immunol Res 6(5):605–616
Woo EY, Yeh H, Chu CS, Schlienger K, Carroll RG, Riley JL, Kaiser LR, June CH (2002) Cutting edge: regulatory T cells from lung cancer patients directly inhibit autologous T cell proliferation. J Immunol 168:4272–4276
Wu Y, Xu J, Xu J, Wang Y, Wang L, Lv W, Hu J (2020) The predictive value of tumor mutation burden for immune checkpoint inhibitors therapy in non-small cell lung cancer is affected by patients' age. Biomark Res 8:9
Xia M, Meng G, Dong J (2021) Synergistic effect of NF-κB signaling pathway inhibitor and oncolytic measles virus vaccine strain against lung cancer and underlying mechanisms. Zhongguo Fei Ai Za Zhi 24(4):245–253
Yaacov B et al (2008) Selective oncolytic effect of an attenuated Newcastle disease virus (NDV-HUJ) in lung tumors. Cancer Gene Ther 15(12):795–807
Yang Y et al (2015) Targeting lung cancer stem-like cells with TRAIL gene armed oncolytic adenovirus. J Cell Mol Med 19(5):915–923
Ye T et al (2018) Oncolytic Newcastle disease virus induces autophagy-dependent immunogenic cell death in lung cancer cells. Am J Cancer Res 8(8):1514–1527
Yoo SY, Bang SY, Jeong S-N, Kang DH, Heo J (2016) A cancer-favoring oncolytic vaccinia virus shows enhanced suppression of stem-cell like colon cancer. Oncotarget 7:16479–16489
Yoo SY, Badrinath N, Woo HY, Heo J (2017a) Oncolytic virus-based immunotherapies for hepatocellular carcinoma. Mediators Inflamm 51:98798
Yoo SY, Jeong S-N, Kang DH, Heo J (2017b) Evolutionary cancer-favoring engineered vaccinia virus for metastatic hepatocellular carcinoma. Oncotarget 8:71489–71499
Yoo SY, Badrinath N, Lee HL, Heo J, Kang D-H (2019) A cancer-favoring, engineered vaccinia virus for cholangiocarcinoma. Cancer 11:1667
Yuan M, Huang L-L, Chen J-H, Wu J, Xu Q (2019) The emerging treatment landscape of targeted therapy in non-small-cell lung cancer. Signal Transduct Target Ther 4:61
Yurchenko KS et al (2018) Oncolytic effect of wild-type Newcastle disease virus isolates in cancer cell lines in vitro and in vivo on xenograft model. PloS One 13(4):e0195425
Zhang Z, Lu S, Dunmall LSC, Wang Z, Cheng Z, Zhang Z, Yan W, Chu Y, Gao D, Wang N (1996) Treatment and prevention of lung cancer using a virus-infected reprogrammed somatic cell-derived tumor cell vaccination (VIReST) regime. Front Immunol 2020:11
Zhang L et al (2020) CAR-T immunotherapy and non-small cell lung cancer: bottleneck and dawn. Zhongguo Fei Ai Za Zhi 23(10):916–920
Zhao H et al (2019) Oncolytic adenovirus rAd.DCN inhibits breast tumor growth and lung metastasis in an immune-competent orthotopic xenograft model. Hum Gene Ther 30(2):197–210
Zuo S et al (2021a) Enhanced antitumor efficacy of a novel oncolytic vaccinia virus encoding a fully monoclonal antibody against T-cell immunoglobulin and ITIM domain (TIGIT). EBioMedicine 64:103240
Zuo S et al (2021b) An engineered oncolytic vaccinia virus encoding a single-chain variable fragment against TIGIT induces effective antitumor immunity and synergizes with PD-1 or LAG-3 blockade. J Immunother Cancer 9(12):e002843

Targeting Toll-Like Receptors for the Treatment of Lung Cancer

13

Sarita Rawat, Karuna Dhaundhiyal, Ishwar Singh Dhramshaktu, Md Sadique Hussain, and Gaurav Gupta

13.1 Introduct.ion

Bacterial infections are known to cause 10–20% of cancer cases. HBV (hepatitis B) illnesses for tumours in the liver and HPV illnesses for cervical cancer are the main reasons for disease in many cancers. Lung cancer (LC) is the leading cause of cancer death with only 15% of individuals living longer than 5 years after diagnosis. The histologic subtypes are adenocarcinoma, squamous carcinoma, and large cell carcinoma (also known as NSCLS and SCLCs) (Alexander et al. 2016; Ando et al. 2015). The prognosis is still gloomy despite advancements in treatment. This is primarily due to the fact that it typically develops asymptomatically and is only discovered later. LC identification with low-dose computed tomography (LDCT) has only recently demonstrated to improve survival, and its use is increasing everyday (Alharbi et al. 2021; Allam et al. 2022). There are multiple kinds of LCs, but the

S. Rawat
Amrapali Group of Institute, Haldwani, Nainital, Uttarakhand, India

School of Pharmacy, Suresh Gyan Vihar University, Jaipur, Rajasthan, India

K. Dhaundhiyal
Amrapali Group of Institute, Haldwani, Nainital, Uttarakhand, India

Graphic Era Hill University, Dehradun, Uttarakhand, India

I. S. Dhramshaktu
Dr. Sushila Tiwari Medical College and Hospital, Haldwani, Nainital, Uttarakhand, India

M. S. Hussain
School of Pharmaceutical Sciences, Jaipur National University, Jaipur, Rajasthan, India

G. Gupta (✉)
School of Pharmacy, Suresh Gyan Vihar University, Jaipur, Rajasthan, India

S. Bhatt et al. (eds.), *Immunotherapy Against Lung Cancer*,
https://doi.org/10.1007/978-981-99-7141-1_13

NSCLC subtype causes over 80% of all cases. According to reports, 70% of LC patients receive their diagnosis at a stage three or later, making treatment more challenging. Smoking, air pollution, and ageing are three major risk factors underlying LCs. Since smoking is a well-known primary risk factor for developing LCs, epidemiologic patterns for this disease and its variations quite reflect previous patterns in cigarette smoking. As per the International Institute for Research on Cancer's Globocan 2012 cancer report, there were 1.6 million LC deaths and 1.8 million mortalities globally in 2012, comprising nearly around 19% of all cancer-related casualties (Ashique et al. 2022, 2023). Weight loss, coughing, bloody sputum, and feeling tired all of the time are all symptoms of LC. Oncogene activation, tumour suppressor gene inactivation, and gene changes may all have a role in the development of LC. LC therapeutic effectiveness is currently minimal. As a result, more research into the underlying causes of LC and the development of novel and effective treatments for LC are required (Bahmani et al. 2021; Barnie et al. 2014).

The top epithelium of the respiratory system, such as the nasal cavity, throat, and larynx, is in close contact with a variety of bacteria. In cases of respiratory disease or allergy, epithelial cells' primary response is the production of mucus and antimicrobial substances. TLR signalling either directly or indirectly increases mucin (which is a protein component of mucus) expression. TLRs are a kind of receptor that serves as the human body's initial segment of protection against microbes (Bianchi et al. 2020; Bohnert et al. 2019). TLR agonists have been discovered as promising medicines in tumour immunotherapy because of the role of TLR signalling in carcinogenesis. TLRs recognise structurally conserved microbe-derived compounds. TLRs stimulate downstream signalling pathways that coordinate inflammatory responses upon binding to cognate ligands. Recent research showed that the signalling through TLRs, newly identified receptor molecules recognising different pathogens execute a significant part in triggering the growth of anti-tumour immunity. TLR agonists' powerful immune-stimulatory capabilities hold considerable promise for the advancement of active immunotherapy against tumours. Several TLR agonists have been shown in mice and humans to have anticancer influence against existing cancer/cancerous cell lines (North and Christiani 2013; O'Keeffe and Patel 2008; Pallis and Syrigos 2013).

TLRs function as receptors that identify both damage-associated and pathogen-associated molecular patterns (DAMPs and PAMPs). TLR receptors promote immune responses against a variety of invading pathogens by detecting PAMP-specific receptors, which are highly conserved and synthesised by potentially harmful microorganisms involving viruses, parasites, fungi, and bacteria. These PAMPs and DAMPs interact to discriminate between self- and non-self-threat signals. TLRs recognise a wide range of microbial ligands, including bacterial and viral nucleic acids, flagellins, LPS peptidoglycans, lipopeptides, lipoteichoic acids, and so on (Chow et al. 2014, 2015). The ligands bind to certain TLRs, activating a cascade mechanism involved in cell proliferation, cell differentiation, cellular homeostasis, and inducing inflammatory cytokines such as interferons (IFNs), interleukins (IL2, IL6, IL8, IL12, IL16), and TNF-α to eliminate microbes. TLRs are independent membrane-spanning glycoproteins of type I with an extracellular and intracellular domain. While the outer section includes motifs with leucine-rich repeats, the inner section encompasses a highly conserved area designated to as the Toll/interleukin (IL)-1 receptor (TIR). There are 10 functioning TLRs in humans and 12 in mice. TLR1, TLR2, TLR4, TLR5, and TLR6 are located on the outer cell membrane and detect bacterial PAMPs, whereas TLR3, TLR7, TLR8, and TLR9 as well as TLR11 are located in endosomes or lysosomes and detect viral PAMPs. TLRs, including TLR4, may also recognise similar DAMPs (Conti et al. 2013; Droemann et al. 2005). TLRs are classified into two types based on their cellular location: TLR1, TLR2, TLR4, TLR5, TLR6, and TLR10 are cell surface receptors that are principally responsible for recognising bacterial membrane molecular characteristics; TLR3, TLR7, TLR8, and TLR9 are intracellular receptors that are primarily linked to the detection of nucleic acid produced from microbes. TLR3 is found on both the luminal and basal sides of the lower respiratory tract, while TLR1, TLR2, and TLR6 are found on the basolateral side. TLR6 is prevalent, while TLR2, TLR3, TLR4, TLR5, TLR7, TLR9, and TLR10 are found in less levels on both the cell surface and intracellular compartments (Elton et al. 2013; Freire et al. 2022).

TLRs have received a lot of attention due to their probable role in connecting inflammation and LCs; nevertheless, knowledge of their precise functions in LC cells, along with the underlying processes, is still insufficient. TLRs are predominantly expressed on both native lung cells and invading cells of myeloid and lymphoid origin. TLR1, TLR2, TLR3, TLR4, TLR5, TLR6, and TLR9 are all observed to be overexpressed in airway epithelial cells. Unusually, LCs have higher levels of TLR2, TLR4, TLR7/TLR8, and TLR9 expressions than "normal" lung tissue. Recent studies indicate that TLRs are important for the expression of innate immunity (Gergen et al. 2020; Giblin and Midwood 2015). Many immune cells, such as plasmacytoid dendritic cells (DCs), monocytes, and B lymphocytes, as well as epithelial and respiratory cells from humans, express these receptors at low levels (Bhat et al. 2022, 2023). Inflammation can be harmful to the body and has been connected to the growth of cancer as a major physiological response to injury and health problems. TLRs can identify compounds produced from microorganisms that have a similar structure. TLRs control inflammatory responses by stimulating various signalling pathways once they connect to related stimuli. In the mid-nineteenth century, William Coley discovered the role of TLRs in cancer and found that frequent microbial toxicity doses (later known as LPS-Coley's toxin) could be an effective anti-tumour adjuvant therapy. After that, there have been several research on TLR agonists and its potential tumour-fighting effectiveness (Fig. 13.1) (Chan et al. 2020, 2021a).

The lung immunological microenvironment is controlled by TLRs, which promote the advancement and growth of LCs as shown in Fig. 13.1. The prevalence of chronic lung inflammation with behaviour like Th2 (type 2 Helper cells) can promote the multiplication of "transformed" cells that are not identified by the immunity. Th2- and T-reg (regulatory T-cells)-mediated immunity leads to tumour progression while Th1 (type 1 Helper cells) and T cytotoxic (Tc) immune system develops tumour regression (Chan et al. 2021b, 2022).

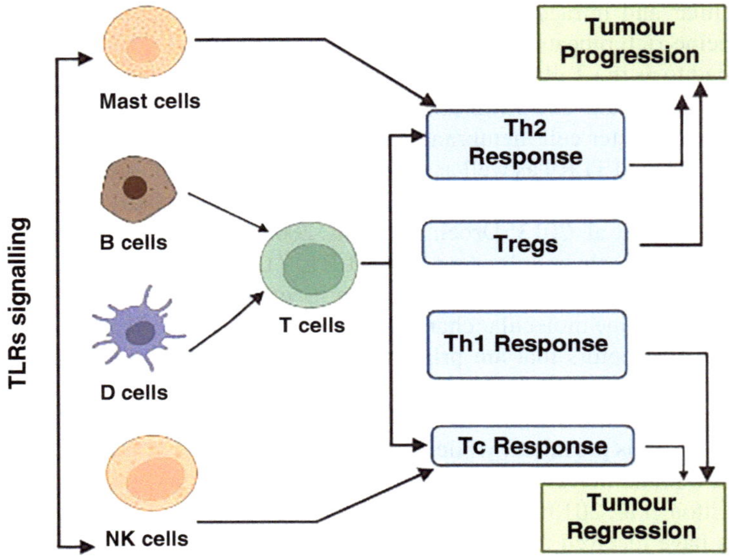

Fig. 13.1 Activation of antigen-presenting cells

13.2 Function of Toll-Like Receptor in Lung Cancer

The initial first line of defence against foreign pathogens is innate immunity, and it is mediated by pathogen recognition molecules known as TLRs. TLRs can also sense endogenous "danger" signals, inducing cytokine synthesis and adaptive immune system activation. At present, infection and long-term inflammation cause approximately 18% of tumour cases, and those with long-term inflammatory diseases are more likely to acquire cancer. TLRs in cancer cells or the tumour's microenvironment may encourage cancer development via several mechanisms like pro-inflammatory, prosurvival, proliferative, and immunosuppressive. TLR expression in LC tissues and their interactions have recently become a focus of research (Gergen et al. 2020; Giblin and Midwood 2015). Airway epithelial cells express TLR1–TLR6 and TLR9. TLRs are found mostly on the cell membrane or in the cytoplasm of LC cells. TLRs are predominantly expressed on both native lung cells and invading cells of myeloid and lymphoid origin. TLR5 was found to be primarily expressed on the membrane of LC cells, while TLR4, TLR8, and TLR9 were found to be primarily expressed in the cells' cytoplasm and TLR7 was found to be primarily expressed surrounding the nucleus. Airway epithelial cells have TLR1–TLR9, and TLRs are predominantly located on the cell membrane or in the cytoplasm of malignant lung cells. For example, TLR5 was discovered to be primarily manifested on the surface of LC cells (Gowing et al. 2019; Henriques et al. 2018). TLR4, TLR8, and TLR9 were generally present in the cells' cytoplasm, whereas TLR7 was mostly found close to the nucleus. TLRs are linked to the development of LC cells. Cancer cells have an unlimited growth capacity as well as anti-apoptotic pathways. TLRs may enhance LC cell proliferation by sending proliferative or anti-apoptotic signals. TLR4 is one of the most well-studied TLRs linked to LC cell proliferation. TLR stimulation on the two cell forms can help in the entry of immunostimulant or tolerogenic cells inside the lungs, in which they contribute to the cancer-causing mechanism (Chellappan et al. 2022a, b). TLR stimulation on epitheliums encourages the synthesis of chemokines like CXCL-8 (IL-8), an effective neutrophil chemo attractant, as well as the expulsion of growth elements like VEGF that leases blood vessels to inflamed and harmed breathing epithelium (Li et al. 2022; Loizidou and Lim 2021; Lovly 2022). TLR stimulation of innate resistant cells, such as APCs (i.e. DCs), can also improve the adaptive immune system via the following processes: (1) antigen preparation and presentation, (2) upregulation of co-stimulatory substances including CD80/CD86, and (3) control of T regulatory cell (Treg) action via cytokine generation such as IL-6 (Table 13.1) (Chellappan et al. 2020; Chin et al. 2020).

There are two types of lung DCs: conventional and plasmacytoid (pDCs). Throughout the formation of LCs, DCs have a key TLR-dependent reaction that connects both the adaptive and innate immunity. TLR2 and TLR4 trigger Th1- or Th2-like proliferative immune reactions in lung-derived DCs that are typically inactive in a lack of TLRs. LC microenvironments are assumed to be Th2-like, which means pro-tumours, with undeveloped DCs and TLR7, TLR8, and TLR9, are all highly active on pDCs. The role of IL-6 in LCs should be treated with care, despite the fact that IL6 observes to play a pro-tumoural part in cancer by encouraging multiplication, survival, angiogenesis, metastasis, and immunoevasion, an entirely novel role in causing anti-tumour immunity (Clarence et al. 2022; Gupta et al. 2018a). Upon recognising pathogens, TLRs on immune cells activate signalling pathways that lead to the release of chemokines and cytokines, so setting off both adaptive and innate immune responses. The agonists of the TLR are currently being investigated in preclinical and clinical trials to control anticancer immunity, and their activity on immune cells has been frequently used to elicit an anti-tumour immune reaction (Hirsh et al. 2011; Hsu et al. 2017).

Table 13.1 Toll-like receptor function in lung cancer

TLRs	Main cell type involved (anti-cancer activity)	Anti-cancer activity
TLR2	Mast cell	TLR2 stimulation on mast cells reversed their pro-tumour function
TLR3	NSCLCs	Leads to apoptosis Reactivate innate local reactions
TLR4	NSCLC dendritic cell	NSCLC is hindered by regulation
TLR5	NSCLCs	Increases anti-cancer activity
TLR7/8	Dendritic cell and Nk cell	Increases DC and NK cell stimulation
TLR7	NSCLCs	Angiogenesis is inhibited.
TLR9	PBMC human primary	CpG-ODN-stimulating TLR9 results in anti-tumour activity

LC lung cancer; *NSCLCs* non-small cell LCs, *NK* natural killer

TLR5 has been stated to have an anti-tumoural impact because of its function in the immune response via the regulation of DC that may eliminate cancer cells. TLRs, on the other hand, appear to have both functions in either encouraging or inhibiting tumour growth depending on the type of malignancy; for instance, TLR7/TLR8 has been shown to have anti-tumour effects due to their role in DCs and natural killer (NK) cell stimulation. NK cells are innate immune system actuators that eliminate cancerous cells (Jones and Baldwin 2018; Jonna and Subramaniam 2019). They are activated by DCs and cause cell damage by using the independent MyD88 pathway. Mast cells are a different kind of innate immune cell that involves carcinomas and are considered to be pro-tumour by promoting cancer angiogenesis. Cytotoxic T-cells are the most adaptable cellular effectors in cancer regression, and cancer regression depends on the MyD88-dependent signalling pathway, which regulates MHC-I expression (Fig. 13.2) (Gupta et al. 2018b; Kaur et al. 2022).

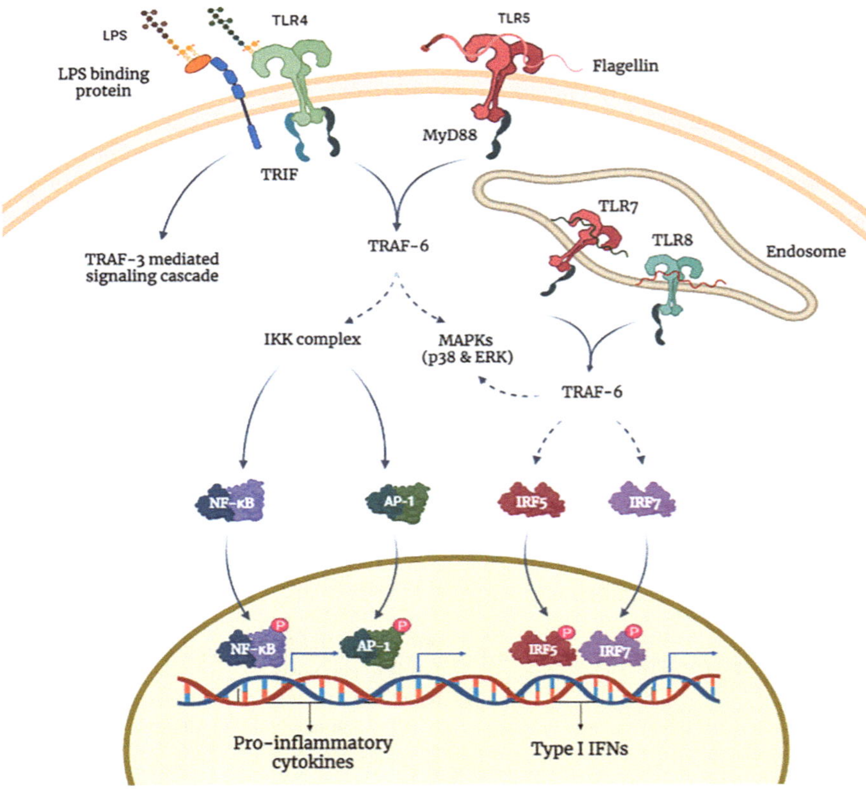

Fig. 13.2 The TLR4, TLR5, TLR7, and TLR8 signalling cascade, which plays a significant part in the innate immunity induction of the inflammatory response

13.3 Toll-Like Receptors and Their Ligands

TLRs are transmembrane proteins of type I, characterised by three primary domains: an outer domain containing leucine-rich repeats responsible for facilitating the binding of PAMPs, a transmembrane domain with lipophilic properties, and inner TIR domains located intracellularly, which engage with downstream adaptor proteins. Based on sequence homology, vertebrate TLRs are divided into six groups. TLR1, TLR2, TLR6, TLR10, TLR4, TLR5, TLR7, TLR11, TLR12, and TLR13 are the receptors. They are further categorised based on where they are located. TLR1, TLR2, TLR4, TLR5, TLR6, and TLR10 are found on the cellular surface, while TLR3, TLR7, TLR8, TLR9, TLR11, TLR12, and TLR13 are intracellularly expressed (Izadparast et al. 2022; Jiang et al. 2014). TLR3 has been discovered in human astrocytes at both the intracellular and plasma membrane levels, which is unusual. Each TLR molecule is unique in terms of molecular and structural biology, coreceptor(s), and capacities. TLRs have the potential to be ligand-drug targets in infectious and autoimmune diseases, cancer, and other inflammatory diseases and disorders. TLRs are expressed in a range of cell types, including immunological and non-immune cells, according to growing data. TLR2, TLR3, TLR4, and TLR8 are primarily expressed by macrophages and myeloid DC, whereas TLR7 and TLR9 are preferentially expressed by plasmacytoid dendritic cells or natural interferon-producing cells (IPC). TLRs are located in endosomes and lysosomes, as well as on the plasma membrane. TLRs on bacterial cell surfaces are able to detect flagellin (TLR5), bacterial lipoproteins (TLR2/TLR1 and TLR2/TLR6), and the lipopolysaccharide of Gram-negative bacteria (TLR4) (Kang et al. 2020; Ke et al. 2015). On the other hand, endosomal TLRs are specifically capable of detecting nucleic acids such as double-stranded DNA (TLR9), double-stranded RNA (TLR3), and single-stranded RNA (TLR7) (Table 13.2) (Lee et al. 2021; Mohgan et al. 2022). TLR2, TLR3, TLR4, and TLR8 are typically expressed by macrophages and myeloid DC, whereas TLR7 and TLR9 are primarily expressed by plasmacytoid dendritic cells (also known as IPC).

Table 13.2 Toll-like receptors and their ligands in lung cancer

Toll-like receptors (TLRs)	Ligand
TLR2	Peptidoglycan, lipoprotein, lipoteichoic acid, and lipoarabinomannan
TLR3	Double-stranded ribonucleic acid (dsRNA)
TLR4	Lipopolysaccharides
TLR5	Flagellin
TLR6	Diacyl lipopeptides
TLR7	ssRNA and imidazoquinolines
TLR8	ssRNA and imidazoquinolines (only in humans)
TLR9	CpG DNA

ssRNA single-stranded RNA

13.3.1 Toll-Like Receptor 2 (TLR2)

Both Gram-positive bacteria (peptidoglycan and lipoteichoic acid) and Gram-negative bacteria (lipoproteins from *Borrelia burgdorferi*, *Mycoplasma fermentans*, and *Treponema pallidum*) may be recognised by TLR2. *Mycobacterial lipoarabinomannan*, *Trypanosoma cruzi* glycosylphosphatidylinositol anchoring, *Staphylococcus epidermis* phenol-soluble modulin, fungal zymosan, and *Treponema maltophilum* glycolipids are all detected. It has been shown that TLR2 heterodimerises with its co-receptors, TLR1 and TLR6. Such combinations provide a broader range of ligand recognitions (Hoy et al. 2019; Jain and Roy-Chowdhuri 2021). TLR2:TLR6 complexes have been confirmed to stimulate immune responses, while TLR2:TLR1 complexes have been shown to suppress T-cell immunity. TLR2 and TLR6 complexes have been linked to enhanced LC development. TLR1 and TLR2 complexity has been discovered as an intriguing prospective biomarker for LC and m-MDSC proliferation. TLR1 and TLR2 are intimately related to LCs, and increased levels of proteins can act as valuable biological indicators in recognising LC growth or development (Pradhan et al. 2019; Prasher et al. 2021). TLR2 is active initially in the development of LCs, and it relates to increased survival and clinical transformation. TLR2 inhibits the progression of early LC by activating cell intrinsic cell cycle arrest mechanism and the proinflammatory senescence-associated secretory phenotype (SASP). The SASP regulates anti-tumour responses that extend beyond individual cells, such as the immune monitoring of precancerous cells. Deleting TLR2 diminishes the recruitment of myeloid cells to LCs. TLR2 agonist treatment inhibits LC growth, which suggests its potential therapeutic target. Early-stage NSCLC requires surgical removal for cure. Nonetheless, the prevalence of postpartum bacterial pneumonia persists elevated, perhaps increasing the likelihood of metastasis. TLRs, which recognise microbial molecules on the outermost layer of different cell types in the lung, regulate the inflammatory response; yet limited has been discovered regarding how host TLRs enhance NSCLC metastasis. TLR2 recognises the elements of Gram-positive bacterial cell walls and triggers innate immunity (Khan et al. 2021; Ko et al. 2018; Li et al. 2015).

13.3.2 Toll-Like Receptor 3 (TLR3)

TLR3 differs from other TLRs in that it does not possess a specific proline residue in its cytoplasmic region, unlike proline 712 in the Tlr4 gene. TLR3, like TLR2, is a pro- or anti-tumour receptor. TLRs are also present on epithelial cells, encompassing several histotypes of cancerous cells. TLR3 stimulation on cancerous cells has been demonstrated to induce apoptosis in a variety of tumour histotypes, mostly by an extrinsic pathway. TLR3 recognises tumoural exosomal RNA in lung epithelial cells, which is essential for neutrophil recruitment and the development of a lung metastatic microenvironment. TLR3 has also been demonstrated to identify double-stranded RNA from LC cells, which activates the endothelium SLIT2 gene and promotes metastatic growth (Hamann et al. 2018; Hashemi et al. 2017). TLR3 activation by the most important tumoural exosomal ribonucleic acid causes chemokine release in lung epithelial cells, and there is an immediate link between TLR3 impairment and decreased LC progression. TLR3 has been tested by using vitro model in NSCLCs to kill cancer cells, stimulate lung DCs, and trigger favourable immune responses (Sharma et al. 2021, 2023). TLRs have a role in tumour cell growth regulation, yet each TLR's individual role and effect on cancer inhibition or acceleration are complicated. However, only a small number of studies have looked at TLR3 activation's prognostic effects on tumour cells independently of immune cells. Patients with hepatocellular carcinoma (HCC) who have TLR3 expression in their tumour parenchyma and immune cells invading the tumour have a better chance of survival. Tumoural TLR3 expression, on the other hand, is strongly linked to poor overall survival in patients with resectable gastric tumours, as shown by immunohistochemistry (IHC). Lung microenvironment may always be conducive to TLR3 activation due to the persistent presence of exogenous TLR3 ligands. Inflammatory immune microenvironment may shift towards a tumour-supportive microenvironment after TLR3 activation on immune cells (Li et al. 2019; Lin et al. 2017). TLR3 expression on immune systems affecting the tumour stroma may contribute to the maintenance of inactive immune surroundings because of the known strong connection between TLR3-s and PD-1 on immune cells; TLR3-s' interaction with its ligand PD-L1 on tumour cells minimises functional communication that hinders the body's defences from harming tumour cells (Long et al. 2018).

13.3.3 Toll-Like Receptor 4 (TLR4)

TLR4 was discovered to be the first human Toll analogue, and it has been discovered that it is expressed not only on immune cells but additionally on various kinds of malignancy cells. TLR4 expression in lung endothelial cells is essential for neutrophil recruitment and capillary sequestration. TLR4 is one of the most carefully analysed TLRs, with numerous artificial agonists now being used as adjuvants in vaccines towards immunogenic targets. TLR4 is found in higher concentrations in LC tissue than in non-LC tissue. TLR4 has been confirmed to contribute to LC cells in refusing the immune response by generating immunosuppressive cytokines such as TGF-b, VEGF, and IL-8 and boosting resistance to proapoptotic proteins such as tumour necrosis factor-alpha (Ernster 1996; Evans 2013; Fortenbaugh 1998; Ge et al. 2020; Giaccone and Smit 2005; Gilliland and Samet 1994). TLR2 and TLR4 have been associated with a greater likelihood of numerous cancer types, and TLR4 is linked in the identification of a number of ligands as well as lipopolysaccharide. Lipopolysaccharide (LPS) is a key element of Gram-negative bacteria's outer surface and has strong immunoregulatory activity. TLR4 may have anti-cancer effects on non-small lung cells, with calreticulin (CALR) acting as an antigen, and activating the CALR-TLR4-MyD88 confirmation pathway enhances DC migration and development, which is a critical stage in cancer regression (Sharma et al. 2019; Shrivastava et al. 2021). TLR4 has a crucial function in eliminating bacteria in both *Pseudomonas pneumonia* and *Klebsiella pneumonia*. This process is facilitated by GM-CSF, a versatile growth factor that protects the alveolar epithelium. TLR4 also plays a significant role in orchestrating macrophage inflammatory reactions to hyaluronan fragments during lung damage induced by bleomycin (Long et al. 2018; Lu et al. 2019).

13.3.4 Toll-Like Receptor 5 (TLR5)

TLR5 is clearly manifested on the basolateral edge of intestinal epithelial cells but not on the anterior edge, and it plays a crucial role in microbial detection at the mucosal membrane. TLR5 is mainly linked to anti-tumour actions in LCs, with a small amount of pro-tumour activity in other forms of malignancies. After flagellin therapy, TLR5 signalling increases in NSCLC cells, which may regulate invasion, migration, and proliferation, indicating a link between TLR5 identifying new bacterium flagella and the lung. Flagellin, which activates TLR5, which has been discovered to have a crucial part in activating macrophages in injured or diseased pulmonary tissue, is thought to provide shielding from the host's immune response (Shukla et al. 2022a, b).

13.3.5 Toll-Like Receptor 6 (TLR6)

TLR6 has not been demonstrated to play an important part in LCs, even though it has been discovered to effectively connect with TLR2 in the identical manner as TLR1. TLR6's entrance into macrophage cell lines decreased TNF generation in reactions to peptidoglycan but not in reaction to bacterial lipopeptides, which are both tracked by TLR2 (Tew et al. 2020; Wadhwa et al. 2020).

13.3.6 Toll-Like Receptor 7 (TLR7)

TLR7 has been linked to the immunological response to antiviral medications. The immunological responses caused by imidazoquinoline are caused via TLR7. TLR7 is found in the endosomal membrane and cannot be generated from single-strand RNA. TLR7 is greatly expressed in NSCLC cells and plays a role in treatment of drug resistance. TLR7 activation has been reported to increase cell survival, chemoresistance, and inflammation in primary LC cells (Aberle and Brown 2008; Abolfathi et al. 2021). The development of new blood vessels, which feed energy to tumours, is directly linked to tumour growth. It was shown that TLR7 hinders LC vascularisation. The Toll-like receptor 7 (TLR7) is a member of the large family of immune receptors known as "sensors" that respond to signals sent by pathogens and damaged cells. New blood vasculature creation in non-small cell LC is inhibited by TLR7 because it stimulates the production of chemicals with inhibitory effects. Specialist pro-resolving mediators (SPMs) are molecules synthesised from omega-3 and omega-6 fatty acids that are being studied as new therapeutic targets and approaches for LC (Manegold et al. 2008, 2012). In the context of influenza infection, TLR7 is also crucial. They are produced by pDCs and boost cell-specific immune responses by inducing IFN through the transcription factor MyD88. B-Cell isotype shift, mediated by MyD88 and IPS-1, is also seen during influenza infection. Recent research has found that combining R848 (resiquimod, an antiviral imidazoquinoline derivative) with chemotherapy or nanoparticles has therapeutic benefits in LC. R848 was initially delivered intravenously because TLR7 was shown to be significantly expressed in TiLs (tumour-infiltrating lymphocytes). R848 injections directly into cancer masses, on the other hand, inhibited spontaneous tumour formation. Because TLR7 is abundantly expressed in TiLs, R848 encapsulated in nanoparticles or combined with TiL-targeting medicines may be worth exploring further in the future (Markman et al. 2013; Martín-Medina et al. 2022; Murata 2008).

13.3.7 Toll-Like Receptor 8 (TLR8)

TLR8 and TLR7 genes are very similar and are both found on the human X chromosome. TLR8 has been found to detect TLR7 ligands imidazoquinolines and single-stranded RNA. TLR7 and TLR8 are structurally identical and can recognise viral ssRNA; the differences between them may be seen in their attachment regions, which have different characteristics (Ernster 1996; Evans 2013; Fortenbaugh 1998). TLR8 is not found in pDCs or B cells but is common in myeloid cells, and when synthetic inhibitors like resiquimod (R848) are used, TLR8 may be considered a more developed target pathway. R848 specifically increases innate and adaptive immunity in the host by engaging and boosting DCs, NKs, and T-cells despite decreasing TME regulatory T-cells. TLR8 is extensively expressed in primary NSCLC cells and contributes to drug resistance (Abu Rous et al. 2023; Avasarala and Rickman 2022).

13.3.8 Toll-Like Receptor 9 (TLR9)

TLR9 is found in a variety of immune and non-immunological cells. The expulsion of components of cells including DNA, nucleotides, and proteins inside normal physiological regions induces a favourable inflammatory reaction and preserves cellular waste disposal balance. The activation of mtDNA and TLR9 throughout pathological cellular damage and stress signals serves as a warning indicator for the onset of autoimmune and inflammatory diseases. TLR9 is necessary for bacterial and viral DNA recognition of the CpG pattern; TLR9, like TLR7, plays a role in the onset of autoimmune disorders and exhibits activity in LCs at both the messenger RNA and protein sites. TLR9 is known to encourage metastasis, and there is proof that the agonist CpG ODN encourages and improves cancer growth and proliferation (Collins et al. 2007; de Sousa and Carvalho 2018). TLR9 had been demonstrated to be predominant in B-lymphocytes, monocytes, plasmacytoid cells, and DCs, with minimal levels in human airway cells. TLR9 has been identified in a broad spectrum of human LC cell lines and tissues. TLR9 and mitochondrial DNA (mtDNA) expression are lower in NSCLC patients who have not metastasis compared to those who have metastasis; consequently, TLR9 and mtDNA may act as possible indicators for the establishment and spread of LCs (Bade et al. 2020; Cheung and Juan 2017). In a mouse model of LC, the activation of TLR9 by mononuclear cells was discovered to be linked to a negative prognosis. Furthermore, the expression of TLR9 was connected to an angiogenic phenotype in a subset of patients with early-stage NSCLC. The angiogenic phenotype, influenced by TLR9, seems to contribute to the initial stages of cancer advancement (Persano et al. 2017; Pfirschke et al. 2016; Pu et al. 2021).

13.4 Conclusion

TLRs are the highly significant receptors for regulating the effects of innate immunity. It has an enormous effect on triggering an immune response against several pathogens and different disease stages, including the development of malignancies. TLRs belong to a family of glycoprotein receptors that are classified as type I transmembrane proteins. They possess ligand recognition domains at their N-terminus, transmembrane domains, and C-terminal signalling domains located intracellularly. TLRs are essential components of innate immunity and are expressed not only in immune cells but also in tumour cells. TLR activation results in both pro- and anti-tumour actions. TLR activation is necessary for the host's defence against foreign pathogens, and TLR agonists could be used as immune adjuvants in tumour or combination immunotherapy. Many tumours are often triggered by inflammation, where TLRs play very important roles. TLR activation can also affect the development, spread, and treatment of cancer by modifying the inflammatory environment. TLRs play a broad spectrum of activities in the advancement of LCs. The functions of a single factor are likely to differ within cells and tissue components. To verify the involvement of TLRs in signalling cascade regulation underlying LC development, a cell culture procedure should be carried out. Due to the opposing pro- and anti-tumour effects of TLRs, the therapeutic value of this approach has yet to be limited. The molecular origins of these cellular responses are yet unknown; however, it appears that the conflicting effects of these receptors remain microenvironment specific. However, inappropriate TLR activation in tumour cells may promote abnormal cytokine profiles associated with immune tolerance, tumour growth, and tumour microenvironment proliferation. At the present time, therapeutic targeting of TLRs in malignancies with multiple TLR agonists has been enormously potential in clinical and advanced preclinical studies. TLR agonist clinical development necessitates rigorous agent screening and evaluation since stimulation of TLRs in tumour cells has been demonstrated to promote tumour development and metastasis. TLRs acting as sensors on LC cells may increase cell proliferation, vascular development, and aggressiveness and affect the behaviour of CSCs (cancer stem cells), though further research is needed to identify this. Novel TLR-targeting drugs might help in preventing the progression of LC. TLR agonists have been recognised or are undergoing clinical studies as cancer therapeutic alternatives. Bacillus Calmette-Guérin (BCG), a TLR2 and TLR4 agonists, is now authorised for the therapy of superficial bladder carcinoma. TLRs are a historically preserved family of pattern-recognising receptors (PRRs). More research is needed to understand TLRs' diverse actions on cell types associated with LCs. Although LC has long been associated with late-stage detection and limited options for therapy, the previous decade has witnessed positive outcomes with LC screening in high-risk populations and significant advancement in systemic treatments for cellular subgroups of individuals with advanced tumours. New molecular targets are discovered on a regular basis, resulting in the development of new drugs. Future combination therapy, such as the use of targeted medications or immunotherapies, could be an additional curative option for specific subgroups of people with NSCLC.

References

Aberle DR, Brown K (2008) Lung cancer screening with CT. Clin Chest Med 29:1–14. v

Abolfathi H, Sheikhpour M, Shahraeini SS, Khatami S, Nojoumi SA (2021) Studies in lung cancer cytokine proteomics: a review. Expert Rev Proteomics 18:49–64

Abu Rous F, Singhi EK, Sridhar A, Faisal MS, Desai A (2023) Lung cancer treatment advances in 2022. Cancer Invest 41:12–24

Alexander CM, Xiong KN, Velmurugan K, Xiong J, Osgood RS, Bauer AK (2016) Differential innate immune cell signatures and effects regulated by toll-like receptor 4 during murine lung tumor promotion. Exp Lung Res 42:154–173

Alharbi KS, Fuloria NK, Fuloria S, Rahman SB, Al-Malki WH, Javed Shaikh MA, Thangavelu L, Singh SK, Allam VSRR, Jha NK, Chellappan DK, Dua K, Gupta G (2021) Nuclear factor-kappa B and its role in inflammatory lung disease. Chem Biol Interact 345:109568

Allam V, Chellappan DK, Jha NK, Shastri MD, Gupta G, Shukla SD, Singh SK, Sunkara K, Chitranshi N, Gupta V, Wich PR, MacLoughlin R, Oliver BGG, Wernersson S, Pejler G, Dua K (2022) Treatment of chronic airway diseases using nutraceuticals: mechanistic insight. Crit Rev Food Sci Nutr 62:7576–7590

Ando T, Ito H, Arioka Y, Ogiso H, Seishima M (2015) Combination therapy with α-galactosylceramide and a toll-like receptor agonist exerts an augmented suppressive effect on lung tumor metastasis in a mouse model. Oncol Rep 33:826–832

Ashique S, De Rubis G, Sirohi E, Mishra N, Rihan M, Garg A, Reyes RJ, Manandhar B, Bhatt S, Jha NK, Singh TG, Gupta G, Singh SK, Chellappan DK, Paudel KR, Hansbro PM, Oliver BG, Dua K (2022) Short chain fatty acids: fundamental mediators of the gut-lung axis and their involvement in pulmonary diseases. Chem Biol Interact 368:110231

Ashique S, Gupta K, Gupta G, Mishra N, Singh SK, Wadhwa S, Gulati M, Dureja H, Zacconi F, Oliver BG, Paudel KR, Hansbro PM, Chellappan DK, Dua K (2023) Vitamin D-A prominent immunomodulator to prevent COVID-19 infection. Int J Rheum Dis 26:13–30

Avasarala SK, Rickman OB (2022) Endobronchial therapies for diagnosis, staging, and treatment of lung cancer. Surg Clin North Am 102:393–412

Bade BC, Dela Cruz CS, Cancer L (2020) Epidemiology, etiology, and prevention. Clin Chest Med 41(2020):1–24

Bahmani B, Gong H, Luk BT, Haushalter KJ, DeTeresa E, Previti M, Zhou J, Gao W, Bui JD, Zhang L, Fang RH, Zhang J (2021) Intratumoral immunotherapy using platelet-cloaked nanoparticles enhances antitumor immunity in solid tumors. Nat Commun 12:1999

Barnie PA, Zhang P, Lu P, Chen X, Su Z, Wang S, Xu H (2014) CpG-oligodeoxynucleotides suppress the proliferation of A549 lung adenocarcinoma cells via toll-like receptor 9 signaling and upregulation of runt-related transcription factor 3 expression. Biomed Rep 2:374–377

Bhat AA, Gupta G, Alharbi KS, Afzal O, Altamimi ASA, Almalki WH, Kazmi I, Al-Abbasi FA, Alzarea SI, Chellappan DK, Singh SK, MacLoughlin R, Oliver BG, Dua K (2022) Polysaccharide-based nanomedicines targeting lung cancer. Pharmaceutics 14:2788

Bhat AA, Thapa R, Goyal A, Subramaniyan V, Kumar D, Gupta S, Singh SK, Dua K, Gupta G (2023) Curcumin-based nanoformulations as an emerging therapeutic strategy for inflammatory lung diseases. Future Med Chem 15:583–586

Bianchi F, Alexiadis S, Camisaschi C, Truini M, Centonze G, Milione M, Balsari A, Tagliabue E, Sfondrini L (2020) TLR3 expression induces apoptosis in human non-small-cell lung Cancer. Int J Mol Sci 21:1440

Bohnert KR, Goli P, Roy A, Sharma AK, Xiong G, Gallot YS, Kumar A (2019) The toll-like receptor/MyD88/XBP1 signaling axis mediates skeletal muscle wasting during cancer cachexia. Mol Cell Biol 39:e00184

Chan Y, Ng SW, Mehta M, Gupta G, Chellappan DK, Dua K (2020) Sugar-based nanoparticles for respiratory diseases: a new paradigm in the nanoworld. Future Med Chem 12:1887–1890

Chan Y, Mehta M, Paudel KR, Madheswaran T, Panneerselvam J, Gupta G, Su QP, Hansbro PM, MacLoughlin R, Dua K, Chellappan DK (2021a) Versatility of liquid crystalline nanoparticles in inflammatory lung diseases. Nanomedicine (Lond) 16:1545–1548

Chan Y, Prasher P, Löbenberg R, Gupta G, Singh SK, Oliver BG, Chellappan DK, Dua K (2021b) Applications and practice of advanced drug delivery systems for targeting toll-like receptors in pulmonary diseases. Nanomedicine (Lond) 16:783–786

Chan Y, Singh SK, Gulati M, Wadhwa S, Prasher P, Kumar D, Kumar AP, Gupta G, Kuppusamy G, Haghi M, George Oliver BG, Adams J, Chellappan DK, Dua K (2022) Advances and applications of monoolein as a novel nanomaterial in mitigating chronic lung diseases. J Drug Deliv Sci Technol 74:103541

Chellappan DK, Yee LW, Xuan KY, Kunalan K, Rou LC, Jean LS, Ying LY, Wie LX, Chellian J, Mehta M, Satija S, Singh SK, Gulati M, Dureja H, Da Silva MW, Tambuwala MM, Gupta G, Paudel KR, Wadhwa R, Hansbro PM, Dua K (2020) Targeting neutrophils using novel drug delivery systems in chronic respiratory diseases. Drug Dev Res 81:419–436

Chellappan DK, Paudel KR, Tan NW, Cheong KS, Khoo SSQ, Seow SM, Chellian J, Candasamy M, Patel VK, Arora P, Singh PK, Singh SK, Gupta G, Oliver BG, Hansbro PM, Dua K (2022a) Targeting the mitochondria in chronic respiratory diseases. Mitochondrion 67:15–37

Chellappan DK, Prasher P, Saravanan V, Vern Yee VS, Wen Chi WC, Wong JW, Wong JK, Wong JT, Wan W, Chellian J, Molugulu N, Prabu SL, Ibrahim R, Darmarajan T, Candasamy M, Singh PK, Mishra V, Shastri MD, Zacconi FC, Chakraborty A, Mehta M, Gupta PK, Dureja H, Gulati M, Singh SK, Gupta G, Jha NK, George Oliver BG, Dua K (2022b) Protein and peptide delivery to lungs by using advanced targeted drug delivery. Chem Biol Interact 351:109706

Cheung CHY, Juan HF (2017) Quantitative proteomics in lung cancer. J Biomed Sci 24:37

Chin LH, Hon CM, Chellappan DK, Chellian J, Madheswaran T, Zeeshan F, Awasthi R, Aljabali AA, Tambuwala MM, Dureja H, Negi P, Kapoor DN, Goyal R, Paudel KR, Satija S, Gupta G, Hsu A, Wark P, Mehta M, Wadhwa R, Hansbro PM, Dua K (2020) Molecular mechanisms of action of naringenin in chronic airway diseases. Eur J Pharmacol 879:173139

Chow A, Zhou W, Liu L, Fong MY, Champer J, Van Haute D, Chin AR, Ren X, Gugiu BG, Meng Z, Huang W, Ngo V, Kortylewski M, Wang SE (2014) Macrophage immunomodulation by breast cancer-derived exosomes requires toll-like receptor 2-mediated activation of NF-κB. Sci Rep 4:5750

Chow SC, Gowing SD, Cools-Lartigue JJ, Chen CB, Berube J, Yoon HW, Chan CH, Rousseau MC, Bourdeau F, Giannias B, Roussel L, Qureshi ST, Rousseau S, Ferri LE (2015) Gram negative bacteria increase non-small cell lung cancer metastasis via toll-like receptor 4 activation and mitogen-activated protein kinase phosphorylation. Int J Cancer 136:1341–1350

Clarence DD, Paudel KR, Manandhar B, Singh SK, Devkota HP, Panneerselvam J, Gupta V, Chitranshi N, Verma N, Saad S, Gupta G, Hansbro PM, Oliver BG, Madheswaran T, Dua K, Chellappan DK (2022) Unravelling the therapeutic potential of nano-delivered functional foods in chronic respiratory diseases. Nutrients 14:3828

Collins LG, Haines C, Perkel R, Enck RE (2007) Lung cancer: diagnosis and management. Am Fam Physician 75:56–63
Conti L, Lanzardo S, Arigoni M, Antonazzo R, Radaelli E, Cantarella D, Calogero RA, Cavallo F (2013) The noninflammatory role of high mobility group box 1/toll-like receptor 2 axis in the self-renewal of mammary cancer stem cells. FASEB J 27:4731–4744
de Sousa VML, Carvalho L (2018) Heterogeneity in lung cancer. Pathobiology 85:96–107
Droemann D, Albrecht D, Gerdes J, Ulmer AJ, Branscheid D, Vollmer E, Dalhoff K, Zabel P, Goldmann T (2005) Human lung cancer cells express functionally active toll-like receptor 9. Respir Res 6:1
Elton TS, Selemon H, Elton SM, Parinandi NL (2013) Regulation of the MIR155 host gene in physiological and pathological processes. Gene 532:1–12
Ernster VL (1996) Female lung cancer. Annu Rev Public Health 17:97–114
Evans M (2013) Lung cancer: needs assessment, treatment and therapies. Br J Nurs 22:S15–S16. s18, s20–12
Fortenbaugh C (1998) Lung cancer. Nurs Spectr 8:12–14
Freire T, Landeira M, Giacomini C, Festari MF, Pittini Á, Cardozo V, Brosque A, Monin L, da Costa V, Faral-Tello P, Robello C, Osinaga E (2022) Trypanosoma cruzi-derived molecules induce anti-tumour protection by favouring both innate and adaptive immune responses. Int J Mol Sci 23:15032
Ge X, Zhang Z, Zhi X, Wang J (2020) Research progress of circular RNA in lung cancer. Zhongguo fei ai za zhi (Chin J Lung Cancer) 23:1095–1100
Gergen AK, Kohtz PD, Halpern AL, Li A, Meng X, Reece TB, Fullerton DA, Weyant MJ (2020) Activation of toll-like receptor 2 promotes proliferation of human lung adenocarcinoma cells. Anticancer Res 40:5361–5369
Giaccone G, Smit E (2005) Lung cancer. Cancer Chemother Biol Response Modif 22:413–442
Giblin SP, Midwood KS (2015) Tenascin-C: form versus function. Cell Adh Migr 9:48–82
Gilliland FD, Samet JM (1994) Lung cancer. Cancer Surv 19-20:175–195
Gowing SD, Chow SC, Cools-Lartigue JJ, Chen CB, Najmeh S, Goodwin-Wilson M, Jiang HY, Bourdeau F, Beauchamp A, Angers I, Giannias B, Spicer JD, Rousseau S, Qureshi ST, Ferri LE (2019) Gram-negative pneumonia augments non-small cell lung Cancer metastasis through host toll-like receptor 4 activation. J Thorac Oncol 14:2097–2108
Gupta G, Chellappan DK, de Jesus Andreoli T, Pinto PM, Hansbro M, Bebawy KD (2018a) Tumor suppressor role of miR-503. Panminerva Med 60:17–24
Gupta G, de Jesus Andreoli T, Pinto DK, Chellappan A, Mishra H, Malipeddi KD (2018b) A clinical update on metformin and lung cancer in diabetic patients. Panminerva Med 60:70–75
Hamann HA, Ver Hoeve ES, Carter-Harris L, Studts JL, Ostroff JS (2018) Multilevel opportunities to address lung cancer stigma across the cancer control continuum. J Thorac Oncol 13:1062–1075
Hashemi ZS, Khalili S, Forouzandeh Moghadam M, Sadroddiny E (2017) Lung cancer and miRNAs: a possible remedy for anti-metastatic, therapeutic and diagnostic applications. Expert Rev Respir Med 11:147–157
Henriques F, Lopes MA, Franco FO, Knobl P, Santos KB, Bueno LL, Correa VA, Bedard AH, Guilherme A, Birbrair A, Peres SB, Farmer SR, Batista ML Jr (2018) Toll-like receptor-4 disruption suppresses adipose tissue remodeling and increases survival in cancer cachexia syndrome. Sci Rep 8:18024
Hirsh V, Paz-Ares L, Boyer M, Rosell R, Middleton G, Eberhardt WE, Szczesna A, Reiterer P, Saleh M, Arrieta O, Bajetta E, Webb RT, Raats J, Benner RJ, Fowst C, Meech SJ, Readett D, Schiller JH (2011) Randomized phase III trial of paclitaxel/carboplatin with or without PF-3512676 (toll-like receptor 9 agonist) as first-line treatment for advanced non-small-cell lung cancer. J Clin Oncol 29:2667–2674
Hoy H, Lynch T, Beck M (2019) Surgical treatment of lung cancer. Crit Care Nurs Clin North Am 31:303–313

Hsu HY, Lin TY, Lu MK, Leng PJ, Tsao SM, Wu YC (2017) Fucoidan induces toll-like receptor 4-regulated reactive oxygen species and promotes endoplasmic reticulum stress-mediated apoptosis in lung cancer. Sci Rep 7:44990

Izadparast F, Riahi-Zajani B, Yarmohammadi F, Hayes AW, Karimi G (2022) Protective effect of berberine against LPS-induced injury in the intestine: a review. Cell Cycle 21:2365–2378

Jain D, Roy-Chowdhuri S (2021) Advances in cytology of lung cancer. Semin Diagn Pathol 38:109–115

Jiang DS, Wang YW, Jiang J, Li SM, Liang SZ, Fang HY (2014) MicroRNA-26a involved in toll-like receptor 9-mediated lung cancer growth and migration. Int J Mol Med 34:307–312

Jones GS, Baldwin DR (2018) Recent advances in the management of lung cancer. Clin Med (Lond) 18:s41–s46

Jonna S, Subramaniam DS (2019) Molecular diagnostics and targeted therapies in non-small cell lung cancer (NSCLC): an update. Discov Med 27:167–170

Kang X, Li P, Zhang C, Zhao Y, Hu H, Wen G (2020) The TLR4/ERK/PD-L1 axis may contribute to NSCLC initiation. Int J Oncol 57:456–465

Kaur J, Gulati M, Corrie L, Awasthi A, Jha NK, Chellappan DK, Gupta G, MacLoughlin R, Oliver BG, Dua K, Singh SK (2022) Role of nucleic acid-based polymeric micelles in treating lung diseases. Nanomedicine (Lond) 17:1951–1960

Ke X, Wu M, Lou J, Zhang S, Huang P, Sun R, Huang L, Xie E, Wang F, Gu B (2015) Activation of Toll-like receptors signaling in non-small cell lung cancer cell line induced by tumor-associated macrophages. Chin J Cancer Res (Chung-kuo yen cheng yen chiu) 27:181–189

Khan S, Shafiei MS, Longoria C, Schoggins JW, Savani RC, Zaki H (2021) SARS-CoV-2 spike protein induces inflammation via TLR2-dependent activation of the NF-κB pathway. Elife 10:e68563

Ko EC, Raben D, Formenti SC (2018) The integration of radiotherapy with immunotherapy for the treatment of non-small cell lung cancer. Clin Cancer Res 24:5792–5806

Lee LY, Hew GSY, Mehta M, Shukla SD, Satija S, Khurana N, Anand K, Dureja H, Singh SK, Mishra V, Singh PK, Gulati M, Prasher P, Aljabali AAA, Tambuwala MM, Thangavelu L, Panneerselvam J, Gupta G, Zacconi FC, Shastri M, Jha NK, Xenaki D, MacLoughlin R, Oliver BG, Chellappan DK, Dua K (2021) Targeting eosinophils in respiratory diseases: biological axis, emerging therapeutics and treatment modalities. Life Sci 267:118973

Li W, Xiao J, Zhou X, Xu M, Hu C, Xu X, Lu Y, Liu C, Xue S, Nie L, Zhang H, Li Z, Zhang Y, Ji F, Hui L, Tao W, Wei B, Wang H (2015) STK4 regulates TLR pathways and protects against chronic inflammation-related hepatocellular carcinoma. J Clin Invest 125:4239–4254

Li Y, Zhou D, Ren Y, Zhang Z, Guo X, Ma M, Xue Z, Lv J, Liu H, Xi Q, Jia L, Zhang L, Liu Y, Zhang Q, Yan J, Da Y, Gao F, Yue J, Yao Z, Zhang R (2019) Mir223 restrains autophagy and promotes CNS inflammation by targeting ATG16L1. Autophagy 15:478–492

Li Y, Wu X, Yang P, Jiang G, Luo Y (2022) Machine learning for lung cancer diagnosis, treatment, and prognosis. Genomics Proteomics Bioinformatics 20:850–866

Lin CH, Lin HH, Kuo CY, Kao SH (2017) Aeroallergen Der p 2 promotes motility of human non-small cell lung cancer cells via toll-like receptor-mediated up-regulation of urokinase-type plasminogen activator and integrin/focal adhesion kinase signaling. Oncotarget 8:11316–11328

Loizidou A, Lim E (2021) Is small cell lung cancer a surgical disease at the present time? Thorac Surg Clin 31:317–321

Long T, Liu Z, Shang J, Zhou X, Yu S, Tian H, Bao Y (2018) Polygonatum sibiricum polysaccharides play anti-cancer effect through TLR4-MAPK/NF-κB signaling pathways. Int J Biol Macromol 111:813–821

Lovly CM (2022) Expanding horizons for treatment of early-stage lung cancer. N Engl J Med 386:2050–2051

Lu Y, Qiu Y, Chen P, Chang H, Guo L, Zhang F, Ma L, Zhang C, Zheng X, Xiao J, Zhong R, Han L, Xu X, Zhang Y, Li D, Zhong G, Boyton R, Huang Y, He Y, Hu R, Wei B, Wang H (2019) ER-localized Hrd1 ubiquitinates and inactivates Usp15 to promote TLR4-induced inflammation during bacterial infection. Nat Microbiol 4:2331–2346

Manegold C, Gravenor D, Woytowitz D, Mezger J, Hirsh V, Albert G, Al-Adhami M, Readett D, Krieg AM, Leichman CG (2008) Randomized phase II trial of a toll-like receptor 9 agonist oligodeoxynucleotide, PF-3512676, in combination with first-line taxane plus platinum chemotherapy for advanced-stage non-small-cell lung cancer. J Clin Oncol 26:3979–3986

Manegold C, van Zandwijk N, Szczesna A, Zatloukal P, Au JSK, Blasinska-Morawiec M, Serwatowski P, Krzakowski M, Jassem J, Tan EH, Benner RJ, Ingrosso A, Meech SJ, Readett D, Thatcher N (2012) A phase III randomized study of gemcitabine and cisplatin with or without PF-3512676 (TLR9 agonist) as first-line treatment of advanced non-small-cell lung cancer. Ann Oncol 23:72–77

Markman JL, Rekechenetskiy A, Holler E, Ljubimova JY (2013) Nanomedicine therapeutic approaches to overcome cancer drug resistance. Adv Drug Deliv Rev 65:1866–1879

Martín-Medina A, Cerón-Pisa N, Martinez-Font E, Shafiek H, Obrador-Hevia A, Sauleda J, Iglesias A (2022) TLR/WNT: a novel relationship in immunomodulation of lung cancer. Int J Mol Sci 23:6539

Mohgan R, Candasamy M, Mayuren J, Singh SK, Gupta G, Dua K, Chellappan DK (2022) Emerging paradigms in bioengineering the lungs. Bioengineering (Basel) 9:195

Murata M (2008) Activation of toll-like receptor 2 by a novel preparation of cell wall skeleton from *Mycobacterium bovis* BCG Tokyo (SMP-105) sufficiently enhances immune responses against tumors. Cancer Sci 99:1435–1440

North CM, Christiani DC (2013) Women and lung cancer: what is new? Semin Thorac Cardiovasc Surg 25:87–94

O'Keeffe P, Patel J (2008) Women and lung cancer. Semin Oncol Nurs 24:3–8

Pallis AG, Syrigos KN (2013) Lung cancer in never smokers: disease characteristics and risk factors. Crit Rev Oncol Hematol 88:494–503

Persano S, Guevara ML, Li Z, Mai J, Ferrari M, Pompa PP, Shen H (2017) Lipopolyplex potentiates anti-tumor immunity of mRNA-based vaccination. Biomaterials 125:81–89

Pfirschke C, Engblom C, Rickelt S, Cortez-Retamozo V, Garris C, Pucci F, Yamazaki T, Poirier-Colame V, Newton A, Redouane Y, Lin YJ, Wojtkiewicz G, Iwamoto Y, Mino-Kenudson M, Huynh TG, Hynes RO, Freeman GJ, Kroemer G, Zitvogel L, Weissleder R, Pittet MJ (2016) Immunogenic chemotherapy sensitizes tumors to checkpoint blockade therapy. Immunity 44:343–354

Pradhan R, Singhvi G, Dubey SK, Gupta G, Dua K (2019) MAPK pathway: a potential target for the treatment of non-small-cell lung carcinoma. Future Med Chem 11:793–795

Prasher P, Sharma M, Chellappan DK, Gupta G, Jha NK, Singh SK, MacLoughlin R, Pinto TJA, Löbenberg R, Dua K (2021) Advanced drug delivery systems targeting NF-κB in respiratory diseases. Future Med Chem 13:1087–1090

Pu R, Pu M, Huang H, Cui Y (2021) MicroRNA 144 inhibits cell migration and invasion and regulates inflammatory cytokine secretion through targeting toll like receptor 2 in non-small cell lung cancer. Arch Med Sci 17:1028–1037

Sharma P, Mehta M, Dhanjal DS, Kaur S, Gupta G, Singh H, Thangavelu L, Rajeshkumar S, Tambuwala M, Bakshi HA, Chellappan DK, Dua K, Satija S (2019) Emerging trends in the novel drug delivery approaches for the treatment of lung cancer. Chem Biol Interact 309:108720

Sharma A, Kumar D, Dahiya K, Hawthorne S, Jha SK, Jha NK, Nand P, Girgis S, Raj S, Srivastava R, Goswami VK, Gregoriou Y, El-Zahaby SA, Ojha S, Dureja H, Gupta G, Singh S, Chellappan DK, Dua K (2021) Advances in pulmonary drug delivery targeting microbial biofilms in respiratory diseases. Nanomedicine (Lond) 16:1905–1923

Sharma A, Shambhwani D, Pandey S, Singh J, Lalhlenmawia H, Kumarasamy M, Singh SK, Chellappan DK, Gupta G, Prasher P, Dua K, Kumar D (2023) Advances in lung cancer treatment using nanomedicines. ACS Omega 8:10–41

Shrivastava G, Aljabali AA, Shahcheraghi SH, Lotfi M, Shastri MD, Shukla SD, Chellappan DK, Jha NK, Anand K, Dureja H, Pabari RM, Mishra V, Almutary AG, Alnuqaydan AM, Charbe N, Prasher P, Negi P, Goyal R, Dua K, Gupta G, Serrano-Aroca Á, Bahar B, Barh D, Panda PK, Takayama K, Lundstorm K, McCarron P, Bakshi H, Tambuwala MM (2021) Targeting LIN28: a new hope in prostate cancer theranostics. Future Oncol 17:3873–3880

Shukla MK, Dubey A, Pandey S, Singh SK, Gupta G, Prasher P, Chellappan DK, Oliver BG, Kumar D, Dua K (2022a) Managing apoptosis in lung diseases using nano-assisted drug delivery system. Curr Pharm Des 28:3202–3211

Shukla SD, Shastri MD, Vanka SK, Jha NK, Dureja H, Gupta G, Chellappan DK, Oliver BG, Dua K, Walters EH (2022b) Targeting intercellular adhesion molecule-1 (ICAM-1) to reduce rhinovirus-induced acute exacerbations in chronic respiratory diseases. Inflammopharmacology 30:725–735

Tew XN, Xin Lau NJ, Chellappan DK, Madheswaran T, Zeeshan F, Tambuwala MM, Aljabali AA, Balusamy SR, Perumalsamy H, Gupta G, Oliver BG, Hsu A, Wark P, Reddy K, Wadhwa R, Hansbro PM, Dua K (2020) Immunological axis of berberine in managing inflammation underlying chronic respiratory inflammatory diseases. Chem Biol Interact 317:108947

Wadhwa R, Paudel KR, Mehta M, Shukla SD, Sunkara K, Prasher P, Panth N, Goyal R, Chellappan DK, Gupta G, Hansbro PM, Aljabali AAA, Tambuwala MM, Dua K (2020) Beyond the obvious: smoking and respiratory infection implications on Alzheimer's disease. CNS Neurol Disord Drug Targets 19:698–708

14 Current and Future Perspectives of Combining Chemotherapy and Stereotactic Body Radiation Therapy with Immunotherapy in the Treatment of Lung Cancer

Abhishek Krishna, Elroy Saldanha, Vijay Marakala, Paul Simon, Thomas George, Raymond Anthony, Pankaj Prabhakar, Princy Louis Palatty, and Manjeshwar Shrinath Baliga

A. Krishna
Department of Radiation Oncology, Kasturba Medical College, Mangalore, Karnataka, India

E. Saldanha · R. Anthony
Department of Oncosurgery, Father Muller Medical College, Kankanady, Mangalore, Karnataka, India

V. Marakala
Department of Basic Biomedical Sciences, College of Medicine, University of Bisha, Bisha, Saudi Arabia

P. Simon
Department of Radiation Oncology, P.D.Hinduja Hospital and Medical Research Centre, Mahim, Mumbai, Maharashtra, India

T. George
Internal Medicine, Coney Island Hospital, Brooklyn, NY, USA

P. Prabhakar
Department of Pharmacology, Indira Gandhi Institute of Medical Sciences (IGIMS), Sheikhpura, Patna, Bihar, India

P. L. Palatty
Department of Pharmacology, Amrita Institute of Medical Sciences, Amrita Vishwa Vidyapeetham, Kochi, Kerala, India

M. S. Baliga (✉)
Research Unit, Mangalore Institute of Oncology, Pumpwell, Mangalore, Karnataka, India

S. Bhatt et al. (eds.), *Immunotherapy Against Lung Cancer*, https://doi.org/10.1007/978-981-99-7141-1_14

14.1 Introduction

Worldwide, carcinoma lung is the second most prevalent cancer with annual incidence of approximately 2,206,771 cases (Song et al. 2021). Lung cancer kills the most people each year, and global differences, medical facilities, and socioeconomic variables affect its care. Lung cancer accounted for 11.4% of 19.3 million cases in 2020 and 1.8 million fatalities (Song et al. 2021). In India, incidences of new cases are high and the cumulative risk for developing lung cancer is 0.60 (Deshpand et al. 2022). According to the findings of the GLOBOCAN 2018 study, it is the fourth highest cause of cancer overall (5.9% of cases), across all age groups and genders. In addition, lung cancer was the cause of death for 63,475 people (8.1% of all cancer-related fatalities), making it the third greatest cause of cancer-related mortality (Deshpand et al. 2022). Lung cancer kills most people, and impoverished countries have a 15% 5-year survival rate, three times lower than industrialized countries. Late detection and unaffordability for most people are the major contributing factors towards the same.

Smoking tobacco causes 85% of lung cancer cases, while non-smokers contribute 10–15%. These situations are often caused by genetics and air contaminants such as air pollution, radon gas, asbestos, and second-hand smoke. Lung cancer in never-smokers is more common in women than males worldwide, and burning biomass (wood, charcoal, crop wastes, or dung) or coal is a major cause. In addition to inhaling environmental tobacco/second-hand smoke, it also depends on time of tobacco exposure, and age, especially in the younger population, has been connected to lung cancer.

Lung cancer arises from the bronchus (bronchioles) or alveolus and is generally categorized into non-small cell lung carcinoma (NSCLC) and small cell lung carcinoma. NSCLC accounts for 80% of those diagnosed, while SCLC accounts for 20%. LUAD, LUSC, and LCC are NSCLC subtypes, while SCLC is a neuroendocrine tumour. SCLC is aggressive pathologically and usually treated non-surgically, but NSCCs require surgery and adjuvant therapy. Metastatic NSCLC and SCLC patients survive 5 years at 4%. India has 29% stage III NSCLC. Locally advanced cancers with variable disease extension and lymph node involvement are difficult to treat.

14.2 Lung Cancer Treatment Modality

Radiation, surgery, or chemotherapy can be administered alone or combination for the treatment of lung cancers. 1.5%–5.3% of early-stage lung cancer patients have surgery. All lung cancer therapies include radiation therapy, which is appropriate for older patients who cannot undergo surgery. In many of the locally advanced lung cancer treatment begins with concurrent, or sequential, with radiation therapy as the sole modality.

Third, chemotherapy can treat NSCLC before or after surgery. Neoadjuvant therapy decreases the tumour burden before surgery, while adjuvant therapy cures the disease. Radiation and chemotherapy reduce tumour size but are harmful.

Chemotherapy helps patients but costs families. Cancer drugs and treatment devour most Indians' lifetime wages. Over 90% of Indians lack health insurance, and this leads to financial burden to the family.

14.2.1 Role of Surgery in Lung Cancer

Surgery is recommended in the early stages and thoracic surgeons perform surgical staging and evaluates for the possibility of resection. According on the stage of the disease and the size of the tumour, four distinct types of surgical procedures are used to treat lung cancer. Cancerous lung tissue and some adjacent healthy tissue are removed during a wedge resection. The term "segmental resection" is used to describe the removal of numerous sections of the lungs all at once. A lobectomy is a surgical surgery in which one of the lung's five lobes is removed. The surgical removal of both lungs is known as a pneumonectomy (Fig. 14.1).

As a prerequisite, CT/PET/CT staging should be done 60 days before surgery, and resection is the optimal local treatment for medically operable disease in patients considering curative local therapy. A multidisciplinary review with a radiation oncologist is indicated for high-risk or borderline operable patients considering SABR. Before starting non-emergency treatment, it is important to determine the treatment plan and imaging studies. Thoracic surgeons should actively engage in lung cancer multidisciplinary meetings. Smokers should receive counselling and encouragement to quit, but they should not be denied surgery.

Most NSCLC patients require pulmonary resection. Anatomically adequate and margin-negative lung-sparing anatomic resection (lobectomy) along with mediastinal lymphadenectomy is recommended over pneumonectomy. T3 and T4 local extension cancers necessitate en bloc excision of the affected component with negative margins. If R_0 resection is doubtful, then a second opinion from a high-volume specialty centres or combination of other modalities like neoadjuvant chemotherapy or radiotherapy has to be considered. To establish local recurrence risk, surgical pathology must be correlated with apparent close or positive margins.

Lung cancer resections should accompany mediastinal lymph node sampling or dissection with three N2 stations along with N1 and N2 node resection. Stage IIIA (N2) patients undergoing resection require formal ipsilateral mediastinal lymph node dissection. Complete resection is achieved through R_0 resection of the lung margin along with systematic node dissection and sampling of highest tumour-free mediastinal node. R_+ margin, positive lymph nodes, or pleural/pericardial effusions indicate incomplete resection. Surgery for pathologically N_2 confirmed disease is controversial. Surgery is based on relevant imaging modality or plan for appropriate diagnostic mediastinoscopy/bronchoscopic-guided biopsy when there is possibility of N_2-positive disease. Mediastinal nodal illness affects prognosis and treatment decisions; hence radiologic and invasive staging should be done before starting treatment. VATS patients with N_2 disease may have induction therapy before surgery. Mediastinal dissection must encompass sampling of the contralateral lymph nodes and subcarinal station. EBUS (endobronchial ultrasound) along with EUS (endoscopic ultrasound) can be coupled with mediastinoscopy for minimally invasive pathologic mediastinal staging. Before considering the surgical option, it is

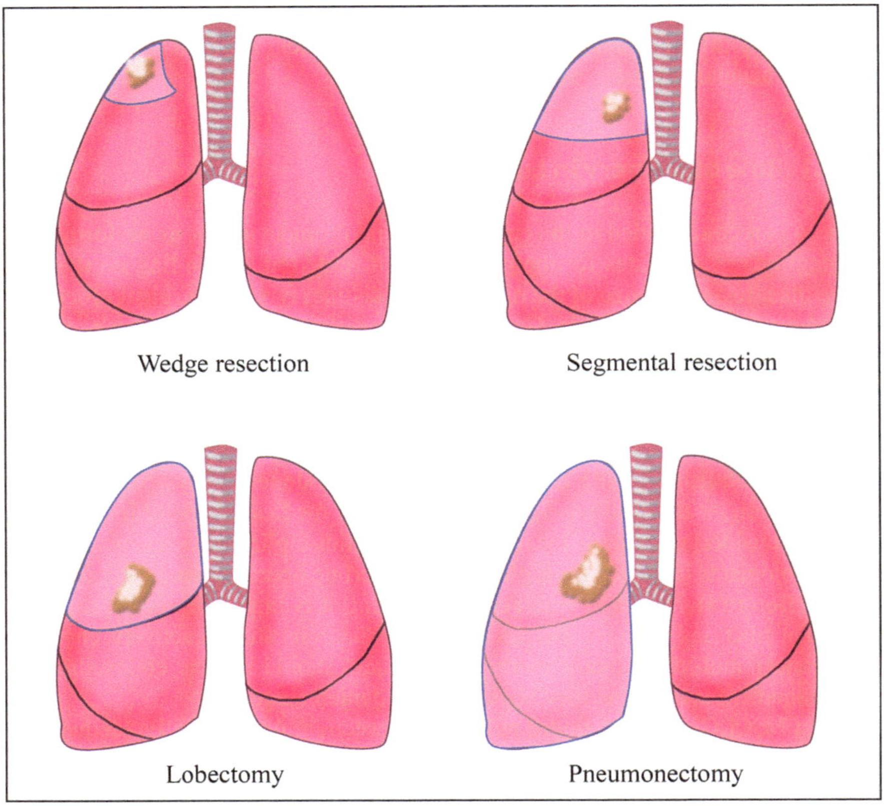

Fig. 14.1 Different types of surgeries done in cancer depending on the extent and place of the tumour in the lung

vital to map the nodal stations affected and confirm involvement of the contralateral lymph node.

14.2.2 Chemotherapy for Lung Cancer

Currently, platinum-based chemotherapy along with taxanes (paclitaxel and docetaxel), gemcitabine, and vinca alkaloids (vinorelbine) works best for NSCLC (Huang et al. 2017a). As first-line lung cancer treatment, current guidelines recommend cisplatin or carboplatin plus pemetrexed, gemcitabine, a taxane (paclitaxel, docetaxel), or vinorelbine. Cisplatin doublets outperformed carboplatin-based chemotherapy in meta-analyses (Hotta et al. 2004; Ardizzoni et al. 2007). Bevacizumab, a monoclonal VEGF antibody, was licensed in late 2006 as a first-line therapy for NSCLC along with paclitaxel and carboplatin (Cohen et al. 2007; Sandler et al. 2006). Most cancer cells die when cisplatin forms intra- and inter-strand DNA adducts (Cohen and Lippard 2001). Paclitaxel and docetaxel bind to tubulin and in turn disrupt mitotic spindle, the "building block" of microtubules, at the metaphase and phase junction of mitosis. Microtubules form, transport, secrete, and transmit neurotransmitters (Gligorov and Lotz 2004). Oral gefitinib is effective against NSCLC acts by targeting the epidermal growth factor receptor (Anderson et al. 2001). In EGFR-overexpressing cells, gefitinib-IRESSA suppresses ER-negative cell proliferation (Anderson et al. 2001).

14.2.3 Immunotherapy for Lung Cancer

The immune system kills most cancer cells daily. "Cancer-immunity cycles have seven phases: (1) Release of cancer cell neoantigens which are captured by dendritic cells followed by (2) cancer cell antigen presentation to MHCs, (3) T cell activation (priming phase), (4) migration, (5) infiltration, (6) cancer cell recognition, and (7) attack and eradication of cancer cells (effector phase)" (Chen and Mellman 2013; Onoi et al. 2020). Low immunogenicity cancer cells without cancer neoantigens may bypass this immune response and survive longer (equilibrium phase) (Chen and Mellman 2013; Schreiber et al. 2011). Mutations in cancer cells, the production of Tregs and immunosuppressive cells like MDSCs (myeloid suppressor cells), and the overexpression of the immune checkpoint markers like PD-L1 promote uncontrolled proliferative tumour growth (escape phase) (Chen and Mellman 2013; Schreiber et al. 2011). Thus, some of the cancer cells reach the escape phase and multiply wildly to evade immunological response. ICIs (immune checkpoint inhibitors) prevent cancer cell immunosuppression. Unlike cytocidal anticancer medications, which disrupt the cell cycle, and molecularly targeted therapies, which bind to gene mutation sites and decrease proliferative signals, ICIs combat cancer through host autoimmune processes. Anti-PD-1/PD-L1 antibodies cure lung and other cancers. PD-L1 determines lung cancer treatment. Anti-PD-1/PD-L1 antibodies may detect microsatellite instability in gastric, triple-negative breast, and colorectal cancer.

In 2011, the FDA approved ipilimumab for advanced cases of malignant melanoma, which is an anticytotoxic T-lymphocyte antigen 4 antibody (CTLA-4). In 2015, it approved the combination of ipilimumab with nivolumab. Sunitinib was previously used in renal cell carcinoma and NSCLC; currently combination of nivolumab + ipilimumab outperformed effects of sunitinib (Motzer et al. 2018; Carbone et al. 2017). Ipilimumab and nivolumab combo therapy may improve survival rates. This review analyses the commonly acknowledged processes of ICIs in vivo; however many sections are questionable. Anti-PD-1/PD-L1 antibodies influence cancer immunity's effector phase as effector T cells kill cancerous cells. However, PD-L1 on cancer cells binds to PD-1 on effector T cells, limiting their attack. T cells attack when anti-PD-1/PD-L1 antibodies inhibit this link. Thus, these antibodies may hinder cancer immunity priming (Hui et al. 2017; Onoi et al. 2020).

Anti-CTLA-4 antibodies activate dendritic cells and T cells during priming. T cell activation requires TCRs, the MHC1-cancer antigen complex acts on dendritic cells, and CD28 and B7 (CD80/86) act on T cells and dendritic cells, respectively (Sansom 2000). CTLA-4 binds B7 better than T cell CD28. Thus, enhanced CTLA-4 remains connected to B7 and blocks the costimulatory signal, suppressing T cell activation (Rowshanravan et al. 2018). Anti-CTLA-4 antibodies stimulate T cells and combat cancer via binding CD28-B7 (Malas et al. 2014). Cancer-induced CTLA-4 on Treg surfaces binds to dendritic cell B7 to suppress T cell activation. Thus, anti-CTLA-4 antibodies may attack tumours by binding and killing Tregs.

14.2.4 Radiation Therapy for Lung Cancer

RT can be definitive/consolidative or palliative at all stages of lung cancer. All patients with early-stage disease that is inoperable, not consenting for surgery, or is a high-risk surgical candidate, stage III NSCLC, and stage IV disease may benefit from local radiation therapy and should consider radiation oncology as part of a multidisciplinary evaluation.

CT images in the RT treatment position with proper immobilisation are optimal for simulation. In individuals with central tumours or nodal illness, IV contrast with or without oral contrast improves target/organ delineation whenever possible. Intense enhancement may require density masking or a pre-contrast scan because IV contrast can impair tissue heterogeneity correction estimates. For patients with IV CT contrast contraindications and substantial atelectasis, PET/CT increases targeting accuracy. PET/CT RT planning prevented fruitless radical RT, reduced recurrences, and improved overall survival. NSCLC can advance rapidly; hence PET/CT should be done in the treatment position within 4 weeks.

Inoperable node-positive stage II and stage III NSCLC patients should receive concurrent chemo- and radiotherapy (RT). Supportive care prevents RT interruptions and dose decreases for controllable acute toxicities. RT alone or sequential chemotherapy/RT is appropriate for patients who cannot tolerate concurrent therapy. If concomitant chemotherapy is not tolerated, sequential or RT-only accelerated RT regimens may be effective. Resectable stage IIIA NSCLC patients can choose preoperative systemic therapy and postoperative RT or preoperative concurrent chemotherapy/RT, especially for superior sulcus tumours. If the patient does not undergo surgery, the RT must be planned to continue to a final dose. The appropriate timing of RT in trimodality therapy is debatable, so preoperative or postoperative with chemotherapy and resectability should be determined before starting the treatment. Stage III NSCLC patients should visit a multidisciplinary team before surgery. Two randomized studies found no overall survival advantage of postoperative RT in patients with clinical stage I/stage II upstaged surgically to N2 with totally resected disease. However, locoregional control was greatly improved. PORT may be considered for selected high-risk N2 disease patients with extracapsular extension, multi-station involvement, inadequate lymph node dissection/sampling, and/or refusal or intolerance of adjuvant systemic therapy. Intensity-modulated RT or proton treatment reduces lung and cardiac toxicity. Involved field irradiation without elective nodal irradiation allows tumour dose escalation and reduces the chance of isolated nodal relapse, especially in PET-/CT-staged patients.

Definitive RT doses are usually 60–70 Gy in 2 Gy per fraction. Dose escalation improves survival in sequential chemotherapy/RT, non-randomized RT alone, and concurrent chemotherapy/RT comparisons. While appropriate RT dosage intensification is still debated, dose more than 74 Gy is not recommended for frequent use. Accelerated fractionation RT treatments enhanced survival in a meta-analysis, while RTOG 1106 found that PET-based customized dose intensification may improve local control but not overall survival.

14.3 Limitations of Conventional RT in Lung Cancers

Regardless of the histology, stage, or primary modality used to treat (chemotherapy, radiation therapy, surgery, or combinations of these), disease recurrence is likely to be the leading cause of mortality in patients with lung cancer. Failure might be local, regional, or distant (brain, liver, bone). Eighty-five percent of locally advanced NSCLC patients relapse after chemoradiotherapy. It was believed that following definitive EBRT, RT would either surpass tissue tolerances or could only be administered for palliation, since patients would not live long enough to experience long-lasting impacts. Both lung cancers respond well to radiation, although normal tissue damage prevents local control in many patients. For curative thoracic high-dose radiation, 3DCRT (three-dimensional conformal radiation therapy) or IMRT (intensity-modulated radiation therapy) is the standard. The fields are then conformed to the target (malignancy involving the lung and lymph nodes and perhaps microscopic illness), delivering the prescribed dose while taking into account the typical tissue tolerances of the surrounding tissues with typical dose ranging from 60 to 66 Gy in 30 to 33 fractions.

Higher radiation doses improve local control in dose-escalation trials and very hypo-fractionated stereotactic body radiotherapy procedures. Chest tissue sensitivities prevent significant radiation doses for most people. Target definition, mobility, and low radiation dosage causing harm to lung tissue can occur with IMRT for lung cancers. Even a fractionated dose of 20–25 Gy can harm the lungs. Radiation lung injury severity and clinical manifestation depend largely on volume. Although 20 Gy given equally to both lungs can be fatal, if it is confined to a very tiny amount, it might not be apparent. The lung often receives a larger dosage of radiation, followed by the liver (5–10 Gy) or none at all. Patients may have temporary moderate radiation pneumonitis (2–6 months following therapy), severe, or deadly pneumonitis depending on dose volume, lung reserve, radiobiological variables, and concurrent therapy. Thus, volumetric parameters like V20 (the fraction of lung volume receiving 20 Gy or more), the mean lung dose, and lower doses (e.g. 05 [lung volume getting 5 Gy or more] and V10 [lung volume getting 1013 Gy or more]) are the strongest predictors of radiotherapy-induced lung damage. Unless it uses appropriate dosages with a low risk of clinically severe irradiation pneumonitis, "radical" radiation will not remove most tumours.

Lungs are the most radiation-sensitive organ in the thorax. Heart, oesophagus, and spinal cord restrict lung cancer radiotherapy dosages. To provide centrally located cancers higher doses, cord-sparing procedures expose more lung capacity to radiation. For tumours located in the vertebral body or proximal rib at the intravertebral foramen, 3DCRT cannot safely implement programmes with a large dosage reduction. Acute radiation damage, which can be evident with even modest doses and gets exacerbated as more tissue receive high doses, can cause severe morbidity (pain, thirst, and weight loss) and thus typically prevents dose escalation. The critical dosage threshold for the oesophagus is lower than that for the spinal cord. When radiotherapy and chemotherapy are utilized to treat mediastinal tumour mass, significant amounts of oesophageal tissue might get exposed. Inhalation spreads tumours, complicating lung cancer treatment. Without on-board imaging, conventional radiation requires a big margin. The lung is covered by the primary tumour, lymph nodes, and target volume, limiting the dose to 60–66 Gy. Smokers almost always have preexisting lung diseases such as COPD (chronic obstructive pulmonary disease), interstitial lung disease, TB, and others, which limits safe dosage escalation because many of them are hazardous at 50 Gy.

14.4 SBRT and Its Use in Lung Cancer

SBRT focuses on delivering a high radiation dosage to limited and well-defined areas in a single dose or a few fractions (Potters et al. 2004). The cutting-edge therapy requires precision, accuracy, and reproducibility. Using stereotactic lesion localisation or image guidance, target identification, margin reduction, and dose delivery require manoeuvres to prevent target volume movement. Immobilising patients and delivering of radiation should be precise, and early SBRT trials show promising local tumour reduction and manageable late effects (Garau 2017).

SBRT has shown excellent clinical control in numerous clinical trials. The radiobiological mechanisms of SBRT and SRS (stereotactic radiosurgery) are still uncertain, but in conventional fractionated radiation therapy, DNA double-strand break-induced chromosomal abnormalities contribute to the destruction of cancer cells. SBRT and SRS influence cancers beyond DNA damage by damaging tumour microenvironment cells and inflicting indirect effects (Song et al. 2021; Garau 2017). This is confirmed by the findings of Park et al., who identified a wide range of characteristics in radiation-induced vascular changes including blood vessel size, shape, and density in animal and human malignancies (Park et al. 2012). They discovered that exposure to radiation at doses greater than 10 Gy in a single fraction or 20–60 Gy in a small number of fractions results in severe vascular damage, which kills tumour cells inadvertently because of the abrupt drop in blood perfusion that causes the tumour to become oedematous. Acid sphingomyelinase-mediated ceramide formation may induce endothelial cell death after high radiation exposure (Fuks and Kolesnick 2005). There is insufficient evidence to conclude that this phenomenon plays a crucial role in how high-dose radiation affects all cancers, albeit it may vary depending on tumour type, location, total radiation dose, and fraction size. The research is divided on whether indirect cell death by devascularisation occurs and how to represent it because the LQ model does not take it into consideration (Fuks and Kolesnick 2005).

Recent studies reveal that radiation may actually stimulate the immune system in some radiotherapy patients. Radiation induces immunogenic cell death (ICD) (Moding et al. 2015; Kroemer et al. 2013). Dying cancer cells release DAMPs (damage-associated molecular patterns), which stimulate the absorption of tumour-derived antigens by dendritic cells and their presentation of these antigens, thereby defining an ICD. Dendritic cells must cross present tumour-derived antigens to lymph node T cells to initiate the typical antitumour T cell response. Interferon I, which is required for the recruitment and activation of dendritic cells, is also secreted in response to radiation. Tumour type, fraction size, genetic alterations, immunogenicity, and radiation dose determine tumour cell death.

SBRT generates chemokines and endothelial vascular adhesion molecules that allow CD8+ T cell extravasation into tumours, increasing effector T cell trafficking and homing to malignancies. Radiation activates MHC I molecules and death receptors, helping cytotoxic CD8+ T lymphocytes to detect tumour cells. Thus, radiation releases cancer cell neoantigens into the immune system, allowing effector T cells to circulate, detect, and destroy tumour cells. Radiation has immunostimulatory effects, but its immunosuppressive or microenvironmental effects counteract them (Garau 2017; Song et al. 2021).

Radiation therapy may have unintended effects (Formenti and Demaria 2009). The abscopal effect—also known as out-of-field or distant bystander effects—describes a tumour response inside the same organism that occurs away from the irradiation volume (Mole 1953). Radiation-induced abscopal impact is rare and likely underreported (Siva et al. 2015). Cytokines or immune system activation may generate the abscopal effect (Kaminski et al. 2005). The tumour-specific abscopal action, immune-mediated in experimental animals, and radiation-induced distant tumour suppression require T cells (Demaria et al. 2004). Tumour cells are immune-resistant (Hanahan and Weiberg 2011). Malignant tumours grow when neoplastic cells develop immune surveillance evasion and/or immune system effector cell attack limitation mechanisms (Dunn et al. 2004). Immunological mechanisms are constantly alert for transformed cells. Thus, immunotherapy again targets antitumour immunity, tumour immune evasion, and pharmacological countermeasures.

14.5 Combination Therapy: Rationale and Evidence

Local lung cancer radiotherapy (RT) has worked for decades, and exposure to ionising radiation damages DNA, killing cells (Lauber et al. 2012). Damage to the DNA that is caused by radiation can be divided into four categories: base damage, single-strand breaks, complicated double-strand breaks, and direct ionisation or free oxygen radical-induced DNA crosslinks (Olive 1998). Normal cells can repair radiation-damaged DNA. Radiation stress kills cancer cells, which have little repair capacity and cause tumour shrink (Lauber et al. 2012).

There have been advancements made in VMAT (volumetric modulated arc therapy), tomotherapy, stereotactic radiosurgery (SRS), and SBRT. The tumour microenvironment (TME) immune response may be increased by SBRT, which targets a tiny target with high radiation doses. SBRT is beneficial for treating cancers of the lung, liver, and prostate. In comparison to normal RT, it features a reduced number of fractions, increased doses, and improved targeting. These advantages resulted in an improvement in tumour control as well as toxicity and outcomes. Both the immunological function and the systemic effects of RT are improved by SBRT. Increased tumour control and maybe abscopal effects can be achieved by the use of SBRT, which increases tumour-associated antigens and immune cell activation.

SBRT induces pro-inflammatory cytokines, effector cell infiltration, and tumour immunogenicity. Lung cancer irradiation enhances MHC-I expression; later immune effector cells like dendritic cells or CD8+ T lymphocytes are also presented with antigens by MHC-I (Reits et al. 2006; Sridharan and Schoenfeld 2015; Zeng et al. 2019). Irradiation increases CD8+ T cell-dependent lung cancer tumour cell PD-L1 expression (Dovedi et al. 2017). SBRT increases NSCLC NKG2D ligands, which interact with NKG2D receptors on NK, NKT, and T cells to kill tumour cells (Kim et al. 2006). SBRT impacts T cell priming and DC activation in melanoma mice (Burnette et al. 2011).

Thoracic irradiation increases lung inflammatory cytokines such as TNF, IL-1α, and IL-6 in vitro, which may contribute to the abscopal tumour response outside the radiation area (Burnette et al. 2011). DCs and macrophages may identify RT-generated tumour-derived antigens, including neoantigens. Radiation-induced immunogenic cell death (ICD) needs calreticulin, HMGB1, and ATP (Golden et al. 2014). Importantly, pro-inflammatory cytokines, radiation-induced TME alterations, and angiogenesis attract activated CD8+ T cells (Mondini et al. 2015), which facilitate local and distant immunological effects of RT (Chakravarty et al. 1999).

Chemotherapy boosts tumour immunogenicity and immunity (Zheng et al. 2017; Gameiro et al. 2012). Most systemic lung cancer treatments include pemetrexed, vinorelbine, etoposide, platinum compounds (cisplatin/carboplatin), and paclitaxel. Immunoregulatory function may fight cancer despite bone marrow suppression (Zheng et al. 2017). Conventional chemotherapy boosts tumour immunity by increasing tumour antigenicity, ICD, effector T cell, and immune suppressive pathway responsiveness. Platinum compound is one the most studied anticancer drugs to treat lung cancer. Platinum compounds like cisplatin release tumour antigens and DAMP in the TME (Table 14.1), upregulate MHC class I expression, recruit and proliferate effector cells, upregulate cytotoxic effectors, and downregulate the immune-suppressive microenvironment (Gameiro et al. 2012).

Preclinical studies show that platinum-based chemotherapy synergises with irradiation and radio-sensitisation, making it a promising multimodal treatment

(Boeckman et al. 2005). Golden et al. observed that breast cancer irradiation dose dependently generates ICD, which platinum compounds can augment in vitro (Golden et al. 2014). Etoposide inhibits DNA topoisomerase II, breaking DNA and killing cells (Davou et al. 2019). Etoposide targets S and G2 cells. Myelosuppression makes etoposide immunosuppressive, but its immunomodulatory effect is uncertain. Johnson et al. found that etoposide indirectly promotes apoptosis of activated cells in vitro. These data confirm Ferraro's (2000) questioning of etoposide's role in immune checkpoint inhibition-based therapy.

Vinorelbine breaks spindles and stops tubulin polymerisation, responsible for microtubule formation during cell division. Vinorelbine with platinum-based treatment may boost lung cancer cell immunogenicity. Cisplatin/vinorelbine increased MHC class I expression in H1703 and A549 lung cancer cell lines (Gameiro et al. 2012). Pemetrexed blocks folate metabolism. It is mainly used for non-squamous NSCLC. Pemetrexed induced ICD in colorectal cancer mice (Schaer et al. 2019). Pemetrexed boosts T cell activation, infiltration, and innate immune pathways, making a viable radiation and immunotherapy combined.

Paclitaxel, unlike other tubulin-binding chemotherapeutics, stimulates microtubule assembly and prevents their dissociation, inhibiting mitosis, cell cycle progression, and tumour growth. Paclitaxel upregulates mitotic Aurora kinase A (AURKA) and its cofactor targeting protein for xenopus kinesin-like protein 2 (TPX2), causing radiosensitisation, according to Orth et al. (2018). Paclitaxel kills tumour cells, releases tumour antigens, and may promote antigen-presenting cell phagocytosis. Paclitaxel decreases Tregs and enhances IL-10 and dendritic cell-mediated antigen presentation (Zhu and Chen 2019).

Radiotherapy and chemotherapy are known to alter immune function (Demaria et al. 2004; Golden et al. 2014; Formenti et al. 2018). Preclinical research suggests that radiotherapy and chemotherapy induce ICD, modify tumour immunogenicity, and release pro-inflammatory cytokines to promote immune-mediated anticancer effects. Immune checkpoint inhibitors are used alone and in combination (Formenti et al. 2018; Reck et al. 2016; Krummel and Allison 1995). Ipilimumab, tremelimumab, nivolumab, pembrolizumab, sintilimab, atezolizumab, and durvalumab target CTLA-4, PD-1, and PD-L1. CTLA-4 inhibition works in melanoma and is being explored in NSCLC (Formenti et al. 2018). CTLA-4 mechanism is unknown but assumed to suppress activated T cells (Krummel and Allison 1995). CTLA-4 decreases signal by attaching a phosphatase on the TCR (T cell receptor) (Lee et al. 1998). Metastatic NSCLC's full and durable abscopal response supported ipilimumab irradiation. RT with CTLA-4 inhibition produced systemic antitumour T cells in 21 chemo-refractory metastatic NSCLC patients (Formenti et al. 2018). Neither chemotherapy nor anti-CTLA-4 antibodies worked.

PD-1/PD-L1 pathway suppression is the most researched metastatic NSCLC immunotherapy (Reck et al. 2016; Rizvi et al. 2016). PD-1 inhibits tumour and TME-specific T cell activation. PDL2 and PD-1 bind. PD-L1 on tumour cells and PD1 on tumour-infiltrating CD8+ T cells reduce cytotoxic T cell activity, protecting

Table 14.1 Details of clinical trial where cytotoxic drugs and immunotherapy are combined

Trial	Phase	Patients	Study design	Treatment	Response rate	Survival
KEYNOTE 189 (Gandhi et al. 2018)	III	616	Non-squamous NSCLC, any PD-L1	Pembrolizumab carboplatin pemetrexed vs. carboplatin pemetrexed	Response rate was 47.6% in the pembrolizumab-combination group and 18.9% in the chemotherapy arm	OS at 12 months 69.2% in chemoimmunotherapy arm vs. 49.4% in chemotherapy arm Hazard ratio for death, 0.49; 95% CI, 0.38–0.64 Median progression-free survival was 8.8 months in the pembrolizumab-combination group and 4.9 months in chemotherapy arm
KEYNOTE 047 (Paz Ares et al.)	III	559	Untreated metastatic, squamous NSCLC	Pembrolizumab or placebo; all the patients also received carboplatin and either paclitaxel or albumin-bound paclitaxel for the first four cycles	57.9% (95% CI, 51.9 to 63.8) in the pembrolizumab-combination group and 38.4% (95% CI, 32.7–44.4) in the placebo-combination group	Median OS 13.2 months vs. 11.3 months Median PFS 6.4 months vs. 4.8 months
Impower 150 (Socinski et al. 2018)	III	356	Non-squamous, any PD-L1	Atezolizumab bevacizumab carboplatin paclitaxel vs. bevacizumab carboplatin paclitaxel	Objective response was 63.5% in the ABCP group and 48.0% in the BCP group	The median progression-free survival was longer in the ABCP group than in the BCP group (8.3 months vs. 6.8 months Median overall survival (19.2 months vs. 14.7 months)
Impower 130 (Cappuzzo et al. 2018)	III	724	Non-squamous, any PD-L1	Atezolizumab carboplatin nab-paclitaxel vs. carboplatin nab-paclitaxel	Atezolizumab plus chemotherapy group 49.2%, vs. 31.9% in chemotherapy-alone group	Median OS: 18·6 months in the atezolizumab plus chemotherapy group and 13.9 months in the chemotherapy group Median PFS 7 months vs. 5.5 months

Trial	Phase	Patients	Study design	Treatment	Response rate	Survival
Impower131 (Jotte et al.)	III	1021	Squamous, any PD-L1	Atezolizumab + carboplatin + paclitaxel vs. atezolizumab +carboplatin + nab-paclitaxel vs. carboplatin + nab-paclitaxel	Chemoimmunotherapy arm 59.4% vs. immunotherapy arm 51.3%	PFS 6.3 months vs. 5.6 months OS 14.2 months vs. 13.5 months
Impower 132 (Papadimitrakopoulou et al.)	III	578	Non-squamous, any PD-L1	Atezolizumab in combination with cisplatin or carboplatin plus pemetrexed (APP) vs. cisplatin or carboplatin plus pemetrexed (PP)	Chemoimmunotherapy arm 47% vs. 32% in chemotherapy arm	Median PFS 7.6 vs. 5.2 months Median OS 18.1 months vs. 13.6 months

tumour cells from immunological attack. Blocking the interaction between PD-L1 and PD-1 using antibodies against both of these proteins results in an increase in antitumour CD8+ T cell responses. According to Zou (2016), anti-PD-1/PD-L1 therapy raises the level of PD-L1 expression in tumour cells. Because PD-L1 suppression benefitted tumours that did not have PD-L1, its predictive value has been called into question. There is a need for improved biological and imaging prognostic indicators for host immune cells and PD-L1 expression. RNA sequencing results showed that tumours had lower levels of PD-L1 gene expression than the noncancerous lung tissue that was around the tumour (Reynders et al. 2018). Peripheral blood mononuclear cells expressed PD-1/PDL1 (Boffa et al. 2017). Before and after therapy, tumour and peripheral blood PD-L1 expression can change significantly (Daly et al. 2015). Immunotherapy and combo treatments require immune response monitoring.

ICD correlation studies predict tumour response and treatment. Following concurrent CRT, the prognosis of patients with locally advanced NSCLC was reported to be impacted by tumour cell PD-L1 expression. These PD-L1-positive individuals had a shorter progression-free survival (PFS), which may be evaluated by measuring PD-L1 expression in circulating tumour cells (CTCs) prior to radio- or chemoradiotherapy in NSCLC (Wang et al. 2018). More than 5% of the CTCs in these patients were positive for the PD-L1 protein. In a study carried out by Gennen and colleagues, the researcher found that these patients had a lower rate of overall survival (Gennen et al. 2020). According to Dovedi (2017), mice given fractionated RT had lower levels of antitumour immunity and higher levels of PD-L1 expression in their tumour cells. Depending on the level of PD-L1 expression, RT combined with PD-1/PD-L1 inhibition may either boost systemic immunity or suppress immunological checkpoints more effectively. According to Dovedi (2017), inhibiting RT and PD-L1 in vivo led to a reduction in the growth of tumours in many malignancies. Synergistic anticancer effects can be achieved through the use of radiotherapy, immunotherapy, chemotherapy, and PD-1/PD-L1 suppression (Demaria et al. 2004; Zheng et al. 2017; Boeckman et al. 2005; Liu et al. 2018; Wang et al. 2018). ICD mechanisms enable all three therapies: radiotherapy, chemotherapy, and immunotherapy. Mechanistic data significantly supports lung cancer RT with PD-1/PD-L1 inhibition and chemotherapy. Nevertheless, research is required into the interaction of radiotherapy, chemotherapy, and immunotherapy so that the results can be effectively applied to clinical studies and practice.

14.5.1 SBRT + Immunotherapy

SBRT has the potential to improve the efficacy of immunotherapy by reducing the size of the tumour. Only 38% of pembrolizumab responders showed a radiological clinical response, whereas 74% showed an immunologic response in their peripheral blood, as reported by Huang et al. (2017b). According to Wherry, tumours shrink because T lymphocytes are depleted in response to tumour inhibitory signals. SBRT can reduce tumour burden and re-energize T cells in patients with limited or oligometastatic disease, allowing the T cells to detect and eliminate micrometastatic illness. Radiation enhances the immune-provoking properties of cell surfaces. Foreign peptides presented by MHC class I can be recognized by T lymphocytes. Sharabi et al. (2015a, b) argues that this is how tumours evade the immune system (Table 14.2).

Radiation dose-dependently increases MHC class I expression, and mice receiving combined radiation and immunotherapy had a longer tumour response than single therapy alone (Reits et al. 2006). Radiation upregulates antigen-presenting proteins calreticulin and HMGB1. Radiation may help immunotherapy find tumour antigens. Radiation can stimulate the body's innate immune response. When activated T cells express FAS ligand, a death receptor, the process of apoptosis is initiated. According to Chakraborty et al. (2004), a single dose of radiation consisting of 8 Gy led to an increase in tumour cell FAS that lasted for 11 days, as well as an increase in T cell infiltration and mortality. After radiation-induced NKG2D expression, natural killer cells go on the attack against tumour cells (Kim et al. 2006). Therefore, a halo effect occurs when tumour cells that have been prepared for apoptosis following radiation are overcome by an immunological response from activated immune cells that are located nearby. Radiation has two different effects. Long-term exposure to substantial volumes of fractionated radiation can lower the number of lymphocytes in all body sites for up to a year (Campian et al. 2013; Grossman et al. 2015). Lymphocytes are radiosensitive, killing 50% after 2 Gy and 10% after 0.5 Gy (Nakamura et al. 1990).

Patients with locally advanced lung cancer were more likely to experience lymphopenia and death after receiving doses to the lungs and heart, according to 2006 research by Contreas. By reducing the amount of blood that receives daily low to intermediate doses of radiation, hypofractionation or SBRT can help prevent iatrogenic immunosuppression (Yovino et al. 2013). Radiation upregulates PD-L1 expression on cell surfaces (Crocenzi et al. 2016), which inhibits the immunogenic cell death essential for effective regional control. When used in conjunction with checkpoint inhibitors, hypofractionated radiation decreases the infiltration of tumour suppressor cells following radiation therapy (Deng et al. 2014). Dendritic cells in the lymph nodes around the tumour get activated and start making additional T cells when the tumour is irradiated (Brix et al. 2017). Checkpoint inhibitors are more immunomodulatory than interleukin-2 and immune cell infusions; thus research is needed to determine their role.

SBRT could boost antitumour immunity and immunomodulation (Sharabi et al. 2015a, b). Hypofractionated radiation raises MHC-1, ICAM-1, and Fas dose-dependently between 1 and 20 Gy (Reits et al. 2006). Tumours downregulate immunogenic cell surface signals to avoid immunology. SBRT upregulates these markers

Table 14.2 Details of clinical trial where SBRT and immunotherapy are combined

Trial	Phase	Number of patients	Trial design	Treatment details	Response	Survival
PEMBRO RT (Theelen et al. 2019)	II	76	Advanced NSCLC randomized to pembrolizumab alone or SBRT followed by pembrolizumab	SBRT 8Gy x 3 fractions	12 weeks ORR: 18% in pembrolizumab-alone arm 36% in pembrolizumab + SBRT	Medial PFS 1.9 months in pembrolizumab alone vs. 6.6 months pembrolizumab + SBRT
MDACC (Welsh et al. 2020)	I/II	100	NSCLC <4 metastasis randomized to pembrolizumab alone or pembrolizumab + RT	SBRT 50 Gy on 4 fractions/ RT 45Gy in 15 fractions	ORR 25% in pembrolizumab-alone arm vs. 22% in the pembrolizumab/RT arm and 38% in pembrolizumab/SBRT arm	Median PFS 5.1 months in pembrolizumab alone arm vs. 9.1 months in pembrolizumab/RT arm
Reynders et al. (2015)	Case series	23	Analysis of SBRT and Abscopal effects in 23 case reports, 1 retrospective, and 13 pre-clinical studies	Various fractionation schedules	Time to documented abscopal response ranged between less than 1 and 24 months, with a median reported time of 5 months	Median PFS 13 months (3–39 months)
Bestvina et al. (2021)	I	37	Metastatic NSCLC randomized to concurrent (SBRT with immunotherapy) or sequential (SBRT followed by immunotherapy) immunotherapy used-ipilimumab, nivolumab	30 Gy in three fractions for osseous, spinal, or paraspinal metastases; 45 Gy in three fractions for peripheral lung, liver, abdominal, and pelvis metastases; 50 Gy in five fractions for central lung and mediastinal/cervical or axillary lymph nodes	Overall best response was as follows: 5.4% (2 of 37) complete response, 40.5% (15 of 37) partial response, 16.2% (6 of 37) stable disease, and 37.8% (14 of 37) progressive disease No difference in response rate and toxicities in sequential/concurrent SBRT	Median progression-free survival was 5.8 months (95% confidence interval: 3.6–11.4 months), ith median follow-up of 17.0 months. Median overall survival was not reached

Table 14.2 (continued)

Trial	Phase	Number of patients	Trial design	Treatment details	Response	Survival
Pakkala et al. (2020)	II	18	Patients with relapsed lung cancer and ≤ 2 previous lines of therapy were randomized to (1) arm A: Durvalumab (D)/ tremelimumab (T) without SBRT or (2) arm B: SBRT to one selected tumour site (9 Gy × 3 fractions) followed by D/T	Durvalumab (D) 1500 mg/ tremelimumab (T) 75 mg SBRT (9 Gy × 3 fractions)	ORR was 0% in arm A 28.6% in arm B	Median PFS—2.1 months in arm A, 3.3 months in ARM B Median overall survival (OS) was 2.8 months in arm A and 5.7 months in arm B ($p = 0.3772$)
Schoenfeld et al. (2022)	II	90	Durvalumab plus tremelimumab alone or with low-dose or with SBRT (24 Gy total delivered over three 8-Gy fractions during the first cycle only), one week after initial durvalumab–tremelimumab administration	Durvalumab: 1500 mg, q4w, for up to 13 cycles Tremelimumab: 75 mg, q4w, for up to 4 cycles Low-dose RT—0.5 Gy delivered twice per day, repeated for 2 days during each of the first four cycles of therapy SBRT—24 Gy total delivered over three 8 Gy fractions during the first cycle only administration	No differences in overall response rates 11.3% (durvalumab-tremelimumab-alone group), 7.7% (low-dose radiotherapy group), and 11.5% (SBRT group)	Median PFS—4 months in SBRT + immunotherapy arm and 3.3 months in immunotherapy only arm

(continued)

Table 14.2 (continued)

Trial	Phase	Number of patients	Trial design	Treatment details	Response	Survival
Mattes et al. (2021)	II	35	CPI immunotherapy alone ($n = 19$) or in combination with four-cycle doublet carboplatin/pemetrexed chemotherapy ($n = 16$) and 3–5 fractions SBRT to a single extracranial target lesion between cycles 1 and 2 of the systemic therapy		Systemic ORR was 53%, and the disease control rate was 73.5% Immunotherapy-alone monotherapy and PD-L1 0–49% had an observed ORR of 20.0% Immunotherapy alone and PD-L1 50–100% had an observed ORR of 64.3% chemotherapy with immunotherapy 53.3%	Fifteen patients (44%) underwent a subsequent course of RT while on immunotherapy; 12 of these patients (80%) continued to develop PD, but 3 patients (20%) experienced progression-free intervals of 12, 16, and 10 months

to assist the immune system respond to abnormal cell changes, increasing anticancer effects (Sharabi et al. 2015a, b).

Preclinical studies suggest that high radiation doses can lead to immunogenic cell death (ICD) through increasing intracellular stress and, more specifically, ROS (reactive oxygen species)-mediated DNA damage (Rapoport and Anderson 2019; Golden et al. 2012; Golden and Apetoh 2015). The ability of ICD to create and display DCs and cross-prime CTLs has been demonstrated to require calreticulin, HMGB1, and ATP. Weichselbaum et al. (2017) states that hypofractionated SBRT exposes and secretes sufficient tumour-associated antigens (TAAs) and damaged dsDNA. In order to transmit signals that activate the immune system, DCs feed on these chemicals. Deng et al. (2014) states that IFN-I production is triggered by cytoplasmic dsDNA through the cGAS-STING pathway.

SBRT produces immunosuppression and immunomodulation and may considerably increase TGFβ (transforming growth factor beta) (Sharabi et al. 2015a, b). TGFβ cannot generate Treg CD4+ T cells, inhibiting radiation-induced antitumour immune response. PD-L1-PD-1 binding promotes immunosuppression and radiation resistance. SDF-1, CSF-1, and C-X-C chemokine receptor type 4 activation in irradiated malignancies boosted TAM infiltration (Spiotto et al. 2016; Xu et al. 2013). TAMs suppress antitumour immunity, encouraging tumour growth, invasion, and metastasis (Ruffell et al. 2014). Radiotherapy, chemotherapy, and immunotherapy preclinical trials are sparse. Radio-chemotherapy-immunotherapy interaction needs research (Boeckman et al. 2005; Liu et al. 2018; Wang et al. 2018).

14.5.2 Immunotherapy and SBRT Trials

Chemotherapy and RT dominates lung cancer treatment. SABR treats oligometastatic disease safely and effectively. This non-invasive local therapy conservatively delivers a high radiation dosage (eight fractions with 5 Gy/fraction) to tumour sites (Bassanelli et al. 2022; Lehrer et al. 2021). Consolidative SABR can be given to stage IV oligometastatic sites (1–3 metastases) (Gomez et al. 2019; Iyengar et al. 2018). RT stimulates DNA-damaging cytotoxic signaling pathways that destroy cancer cells (Qiao et al. 2018; Chen et al. 2020a). Radiation-immune system cross-talk overcomes immunotherapy resistance (Sharabi et al. 2015a, b). Radiation and ICPi (immune checkpoint inhibitors) improve local and distant tumour care in numerous studies (Theelen et al. 2019). Patients with advanced NSCLC who participated in the phase II trial PEMBRO-RT were randomly randomized to receive either pembrolizumab on its own or SBRT (three treatments totalling 8 Gy) to a single tumour location (Theelen et al. 2019). At 12 weeks, the ORR for pembrolizumab was 18%, while the radiation treatment had a 36% success rate. Pembrolizumab alone resulted in a PFS of 1.9 months, while radiation therapy resulted in 6.6 months. The median OS was 7.6 months, compared to 15.9 months.

Only the PD-L1-negative subgroup saw improvement from the SBRT treatment (Table 14.3).

The MDACC (University of Texas MD Anderson Cancer Center) phase I/phase II trial randomly allocated patients with NSCLC who had fewer than four RT-sensitive lung or liver metastases and at least one non-contiguous lesion to receive pembrolizumab with or without RT (Welsh et al. 2020). Stereotactic body irradiation (50 Gy in four fractions) or conventional hypofractionated radiation therapy (45 Gy in 15 fractions) was used to treat lesions, depending on their clinical viability. Median progression-free survival (PFS) was 5.1 months with pembrolizumab alone and 9.1 months when combined with radiotherapy. The objective response rate (ORR) for immune-RT was 22%, whereas the ORR for pembrolizumab was 25%. Pembrolizumab + SBRT showed 38% ORR in non-contiguous lesions and 10% in hypofractionated RT in unirradiated lesions (Theelen et al. 2021).

SBRT and hypofractionated RT impact ALC (absolute lymphocyte count) and immunology (Chen et al. 2020b). Traditional RT reduced ALC more than SBRT (Chen et al. 2020c). SBRT demonstrated better abscopal effects on nonirradiated metastatic lesions than hypofractionated (Dewan et al. 2009). Patients with NSCLC who had RT before pembrolizumab fared better in terms of progression-free survival (PFS, 4.4 months vs. 2.1 months) and overall survival (10.7 months vs. 5.3 months) in the KEYNOTE-001 trial (Shaverdian et al. 2017). Median overall survival (OS) for patients with advanced solid tumours treated with multisite SBRT at 30–50 Gy followed by at least one round of pembrolizumab within 7 days was 9.6 months, ORR was 13.2, and PFS was 3.1 months (Luke et al. 2018). A recent meta-analysis concluded that RT 90 days before to ICPi is safe for a variety of malignancies (Anscher et al. 2022). The pneumonia rate in the RT 90 days group was 6.8%, whereas the rate in the non-RT group was 3.8% (grades 3–4 in 1.9% vs. 1.1%).

In addition to the localisation, there has been increased research on radiation therapy and metastatic immunotherapy. Results from the phase I KEYNOTE-001 pembrolizumab trial demonstrated that 43% of radiation-treated patients had improved progression-free survival and overall survival compared to the control group (Shaverdian et al. 2017). In terms of PD-L1, radiation had no effect (71% vs. 80%). Treatments included 91% extracranial radiation, 74% palliative care, and 29% SBRT. Pembrolizumab was initiated in the radiation group 26 months later than in the control group (17 months vs. 9 months). Another study looked at the difference in outcomes between patients who underwent thoracic radiotherapy and those who did not treat 164 people with metastatic NSCLC with PD-1/PD-L1 inhibitors (Hwang 2018). Most patients began using checkpoint inhibitors 8.6 months after finishing radiation therapy (median 60 Gy, range, 44–79.1 Gy). Despite having fewer patients with good adenocarcinoma (49% vs. 75%) and fewer patients with a targetable mutation (4% vs. 16%), the thoracic radiation group had better OS. The results of a Chinese retrospective study showed that SBRT combined with adoptive immunotherapy enhanced survival rates for patients with advanced cancer (Wang et al. 2013). The overall response rate (RECIST partial or complete response) was

Table 14.3 Details of ongoing clinical trials

Trial	Phase	Trial details	Median FU (months)	Median PFS (months)	Median OS (months)
PACIFIC-1	III	cCRT → durvalumab vs. placebo	25.2	17.2	
PACIFIC-2	III	cCRT + durvalumab → durvalumab vs. cCRT + placebo →	NR	NR	NR
PACIFIC-5	III	cCRT→ durvalumab fixed dose	NR	NR	NR
PACIFIC-6	II	sCRT → durvalumab	NR	NR	NR
COAST	II	cCRT → durvalumab vs. cCRT → durvalumab + oleclumab vs. cCRT → durvalumab + monalizumab	NR	NR	NR
HCRN LUN 14–179	II	cCRT → pembrolizumab	16.4	15.4	NR
RUTGERS	I	cCRT → pembrolizumab and cCRT + pembrolizumab → pembrolizumab	16	18.7	29.4
CONSIST	III	cCRT → dintilimab vs. cCRT alone	NR	NR	NR
POSEIDON	III	Durvalumab + tremelimumab with chemotherapy or durvalumab with chemotherapy or chemotherapy alone	NR	NR	NR
CHECKMATE 568	III	Nivolumab in combination with ipilimumab (part 1); nivolumab plus ipilimumab in combination with chemotherapy (part 2) as first-line therapy in stage IV non-small cell lung cancer	NR	NR	NR
CheckMate 9LA	III	A study of nivolumab and ipilimumab combined with chemotherapy compared to chemotherapy alone in first-line NSCLC	NR	NR	NR
Impower 110	III	A study of atezolizumab (MPDL3280A) compared with a platinum agent (cisplatin or carboplatin) + (pemetrexed or gemcitabine) in participants with stage IV non-squamous or squamous non-small cell lung cancer (NSCLC)	NR	NR	N

(continued)

Table 14.3 (continued)

Trial	Phase	Trial details	Median FU (months)	Median PFS (months)	Median OS (months)
KEYNOTE-715-05/ ECHO-306-05	II	Pembrolizumab plus epacadostat with platinum-based chemotherapy vs. pembrolizumab plus platinum-based chemotherapy plus placebo in metastatic non-small cell lung cancer	NR	NR	NR

increased from 60.2% to 66.8% after the re-injection of interferon-activated monocytes following SBRT (Wang et al. 2013).

14.5.3 Chemotherapy + Immunotherapy

Platinum-based chemotherapy prevents immunological recognition of the disease by encouraging immunogenic cell death (ICD), increasing the expression of tumour neoantigens, and altering the immunosuppressive milieu of the tumour (Kroemer et al. 2013). It is postulated that DCs receive cues to eliminate dead cells and secrete activating and maturing substances via changes in the ICD membrane. These DCs then present tumour antigens to T cells, leading to the development of tumour-targeting effector cells (Kroemer et al. 2013). Several studies, including those by Liu (2010), Tseng (2008), and Suzuki (2005), show that chemotherapy stimulates the growth of antigen-presenting cells and leads to a greater infiltration of CD81 T cells. Preclinical research showed that the activity of effector T cells was amplified by chemotherapy. Pfirschke (2016) found that treatment with oxaliplatin and cyclophosphamide increased CD81 T cell infiltration and hence facilitated immunological recognition of the tumour microenvironment. Lesterhuis et al. (2011) reports that platinum drugs can suppress the T cell inhibitor PD-L2 in human tumour cells and dendritic cells. This led to an uptick in tumour detection and antigen-specific proliferation of T cells. Platinum-based chemotherapy, as stated by Ramakrishnan et al. (2010), promotes the granzyme-B-mediated death of tumour cells by T lymphocytes. Eleven platinum-based medications improve cytotoxic T cell and major histocompatibility complex class I (MHC-I) performance by increasing HLA1 gene complex expression. Several preliminary studies suggest that combining immunotherapy with platinum-based chemotherapy may improve clinical outcomes.

14.5.4 Immunotherapy + Chemotherapy Trials

Three metastatic non-squamous NSCLC trials (KEYNOTE-189, IMpower150, and IMpower130) found that anti-PD-1/PD-L1 antibodies increased overall survival (OS) (Judd and Borghaei 2020). Patients with non-squamous NSCLC who lacked sensitising EGFR (epidermal growth factor receptor) or ALK (anaplastic lymphoma kinase) mutations were randomized to receive either a platinum and pemetrexed doublet and 200 mg pembrolizumab or placebo in the phase III trial known as KEYNOTE-189 (Gandhi et al. 2018; Gadgeel et al. 2019). This regimen of three drugs was administered in four cycles, each lasting 3 weeks, and was followed by maintenance treatment with pemetrexed and pembrolizumab or a placebo. Both primary and secondary outcomes (PFS and OS) benefited from the presence of an objective central review committee (Gadgeel et al. 2019). Median overall survival (OS) was 22.0 months for pembrolizumab and 10.7 months in the most recent 18.7-month follow-up analysis. Overall survival (OS) was prolonged by immunotherapy and chemotherapy regardless of tumour proportion score (TPS) (Gadgeel et al. 2019). Patients treated with pembrolizumab in combination had a 47.6% response rate compared to placebo's 18.9% and 50% of placebo patients converted to pembrolizumab when their disease progressed. There were more AEs (adverse events) in the pembrolizumab group (67.2%) than in the placebo group (65.8%). More people stopped taking the pembrolizumab combination because of adverse events (28% vs. 15%).

Patients receiving platinum-based combination chemotherapy were more likely to experience anaemia (16.3% vs. 15.3%) and neutropenia (15.8% vs. 11.9%) than those receiving pembrolizumab alone. To no one's surprise, the pembrolizumab combination group saw a higher incidence of immune-related adverse events (irAEs; 22.7% vs. 11.9%) than the placebo combination group. The pembrolizumab combination group saw a higher incidence of hypothyroidism and pneumonitis among irAEs. The most prevalent serious adverse events (irAEs) in the pembrolizumab-combination arm were pneumonia (2.7%) and severe skin reactions (2.0%). Three people who were given the pembrolizumab combo died from pneumonia. Pembrolizumab monotherapy and chemotherapy both produced no irAEs in KEYNOTE-024.

Patients with metastatic non-squamous non-small cell lung cancer (NSCLC) were studied in the randomized phase III trial IMpower130, which compared a platinum doublet backbone of carboplatin and nab-paclitaxel with and without atezolizumab (ACnP against CnP) (Cappuzzo et al. 2018). The experimental arm continued to receive atezolizumab, whereas the control arm continued to use switch. ITT-WT median PFS and OS were both enhanced by atezolizumab. Except for those with EGFR/ALK mutations in liver metastases, all PD-L1 subgroups showed an increase in PFS and benefit. ORR was 49.2% for ACnP and 31.9% for CnP. A phase III experiment called IMpower150 compared ACP and BCP to ACP, bevacizumab, carboplatin, and paclitaxel (ABCP) (Socinski et al. 2018). After carboplatin and paclitaxel, atezolizumab or bevacizumab was administered. In terms of overall survival, ABCP was superior to BCP in WT (8.3 vs. 6.8 months). All ITT (intention-to-treat) patients had longer PFS if they had EGFR/ALK mutations, low or negative PD-L1 expression, or liver metastases. WT median OS was greater for ABCP (at 19.2 months) than for BCP (14.7 months). BCP triumphed over ACP. The WT ORR for ABCP was 63.5%, but for BCP, it was only 48.5%. Patients receiving ABCP had a 3.7% success rate compared to BCP's 1.2%.

Results also suggest that both IMpower130 (PFS, 7.0 months; ACnP vs. CnP) and IM power 150 (PFS, 8.3 months; ABCP vs. BCP) benefited from immunotherapy (Cappuzzo et al. 2018). Bevacizumab increased IMpower150's PFS and overall response rate. The median OS for IMpower130 (18.6 vs. 13.9 months with ACNP vs. CnP) was comparable to that of IMpower150 (19.2 vs. 14.7 months with ABCP vs. BCP). In the IMpower150 trial, the four-drug ABCP combination had 58.5% AEs of grade 3 or higher, while the BCP group only had 50.0%. There was a higher death rate due to the treatment (2.8% vs. 2.3%). Deaths were not caused by irAEs despite having more AEs with ABCP (77.4% grade 1) (Cappuzzo et al. 2018). Compared to BCP, more people with ABCP experienced rashes, hepatitis, and hypothyroidism.

Patients with wild type (WT) tumours benefited more with immunotherapy than those treated with second-line TKIs (tyrosine kinase inhibitors) (Herbst et al. 2016; Borghaei et al. 2015; Fehrenbacher et al. 2016). Sensitising mutations in EGFR or ALK were seen in cancer cells. Regardless of PD-L1 expression, immunotherapy performed worse than chemotherapy in patients with EGFR or ALK mutations (Peters et al. 2017; Haratani et al. 2017). This is a result of developments in first-line immunotherapy and TKIs. Similar tumour changes were associated with a progression of illness or intolerable side effects following treatment with at least one approved TKI in the ongoing IM power 150 study. Platinum doublet plus atezolizumab plus bevacizumab was given to ITT patients. Both chemotherapy and blocking VEGF have immunosuppressive effects. The success of immunotherapy has a positive effect on patient survival.

14.6 Safety

Immunotherapy may worsen SBRT side effects. Radiation toxicity occurs when the immune system inflames healthy tissues. Dose, duration, treatment area size, and tumour proximity to healthy tissues determine radiation damage. Toxins include IRAEs. Mild to severe IRAEs harm the skin, gastrointestinal tract, liver, and lungs. Immunotherapy and SBRT may cause IRAEs. Immunotherapy may flare tumours. Before the immune system kills cancer cells, tumour flares grow and inflame. SBRT and immunotherapy can cause tumour flare, discomfort, and other symptoms. Immunotherapy efficacy may decrease with SBRT. Radiation inhibits immune cells, preventing them from recognising and killing cancer cells. SBRT immunotherapy may not work. SBRT and immunotherapy may cause secondary cancer. Radiation damages DNA, causing cancer. Immunotherapy may cause secondary cancers.

SBRT and chemotherapy combined with immunotherapy may improve clinical success, but the regimen may increase patient toxicity, limiting its clinical use. On the other hand, patients diagnosed with NSCLC were able to tolerate the combination treatment with levels of adverse effects that were deemed to be tolerable, as was observed in the KEYNOTE 001 and PACIFIC studies (Shaverdian et al. 2017; Antonia et al. 2017). According to the findings of the secondary analysis of the KEYNOTE-001 study (Shaverdian et al. 2017), individuals who underwent previous thoracic irradiation exhibited a statistically significant difference in treatment-related pulmonary toxicities but not in high-grade ones. In the phase III PACIFIC study, immune-related adverse events (irAEs) of grade 3, the most common of which was pneumonitis, were comparable between the durvalumab and placebo arms (Antonia et al. 2017).

Immune system stress may increase these adverse effects, and the combination of chemotherapy with immunotherapy can increase the toxicity. Immunotherapy activates the immune system, enhancing chemotherapy's side effects. Depending on the cancer, treatment, and patient, chemotherapy and immunotherapy can cause side effects. This treatment may require side effect assistance (Rocco et al. 2019). In the research that has been done, it has been found that gastrointestinal, dermatologic, tiredness, and endocrine toxicities are the most prevalent types of irAEs. On the other hand, musculoskeletal, ocular, pulmonary, renal, and haematological toxicities are quite uncommon (Wang et al. 2017; De Velasco et al. 2017). According to the STIC (Society of Thoracic Surgeons Invasive Cardiac Professionals) and ASCO (American Society of Clinical Oncology) toxicity management instructions (Puzanov et al. 2017), corticosteroids can be used to address these adverse effects, and the withholding of ICI (immune checkpoint inhibitors) is only required in extremely exceptional circumstances.

14.7 Future Directions

Lung cancer treatment has progressed in the previous decade, thanks to the discovery of mutations in oncogenic drivers and the development of immunotherapeutics. In addition to this, combining radiation and immunotherapy has also shown promise in the control of lung malignancies. Hypofractionated doses of 10–12 Gy have been recommended based on preclinical research, and patients with stage III non-small cell lung cancer who underwent definitive chemoradiation saw an improvement in PFS after receiving adjuvant immunotherapy. The possible reason is that immunotherapy, which previously only worked in metastatic tumours with high PD-L1 expression, may be enhanced by radiation treatment. Immunotherapy following SBRT is necessary for NSCLC in the early stage, and reducing tumour load improves immunotherapy response in the development of non-metastatic NSCLC SBRT. It is expected that nivolumab, pembrolizumab, and atezolizumab, three chemoimmunotherapies, may replace platinum-based chemotherapies within 5 years for patients with advanced non-squamous or squamous NSCLC who do not have active autoimmune disorders or positive genetic biomarkers. Concurrent CRT with maintenance PD-1/PD-L1 inhibition is a safe and effective multimodal therapy for patients with inoperable stage III NSCLC.

References

Anderson NG, Ahmad T, Chan K, Dobson R, Bundred NJ (2001) ZD1839 (Iressa), a novel epidermal growth factor receptor (EGFR) tyrosine kinase inhibitor, potently inhibits the growth of EGFR-positive cancer cell lines with or without erbB2 overexpression. Int J Cancer 94:774–782

Anscher MS, Arora S, Weinstock C, Amatya A, Bandaru P, Tang C, Girvin AT, Fiero MH, Tang S, Lubitz R, Amiri- Kordestani L, Theoret MR, Pazdur R, Beaver JA (2022) Association of radiation therapy with risk of adverse events in patients receiving immunotherapy: a pooled analysis

of trials in the US Food and Drug Administration database. JAMA Oncol 8(2):232–240. https://doi.org/10.1001/jamaoncol.2021.6439
Antonia SJ, Villegas A, Daniel D et al (2017) Durvalumab after chemoradiotherapy in stage III non-small-cell lung cancer. N Engl J Med 377:1919–1929
Ardizzoni A, Boni L, Tiseo M, Fossella FV, Schiller JH, Paesmans M et al (2007) Cisplatin- versus carboplatin-based chemotherapy in first-line treatment of advanced non-small-cell lung cancer: an individual patient data meta-analysis. J Natl Cancer Inst 99:847–857
Bassanelli M, Ramella S, Zeuli M, Ceribelli A (2022) Radiotherapy and immunotherapy: the power of the teamwork for the treatment of NSCLC. Anticancer Res 42(5):2241–2247
Boeckman HJ, Trego KS, Turchi JJ (2005) Cisplatin sensitizes cancer cells to ionizing radiation via inhibition of nonhomologous end joining. Mol Cancer Res 3:277–285
Boffa DJ, Graf RP, Salazar MC, Hoag J, Lu D, Krupa R et al (2017) Cellular expression of PD-L1 in the peripheral blood of lung cancer patients is associated with worse survival. Cancer Epidemiol Prev Biomark 26:1139–1145
Borghaei H, Paz-Ares L, Horn L et al (2015) Nivolumab versus docetaxel in advanced nonsquamous nonsmall-cell lung cancer. N Engl J Med 373(17):1627–1639
Brix N, Tiefenthaller A, Anders H et al (2017) Abscopal, immunological effects of radiotherapy: narrowing the gap between clinical and preclinical experiences. Immunol Rev 280:249–279
Burnette BC, Liang H, Lee Y, Chlewicki L, Khodarev NN, Weichselbaum RR et al (2011) The efficacy of radiotherapy relies upon induction of type I interferon–dependent innate and adaptive immunity. Cancer Res 71:2488–2496
Campian JL, Ye X, Brock M et al (2013) Treatment-related lymphopenia in patients with stage III non-small-cell lung cancer. Cancer Invest 31:183–188
Cappuzzo F, McCleod M, Hussein M et al (2018) IMpower130: progression-free survival (PFS) and safety analysis from a randomised phase III study of carboplatin 1 nab-paclitaxel (CnP) with or without atezolizumab (atezo) as first-line (1L) therapy in advanced non-squamous NSCLC. Ann Oncol 29(suppl_8):VIII742. [Abstract nr LBA53]
Carbone DP, Reck M, Paz-Ares L, Creelan B, Horn L, Steins M, Felip E, Heuvel MMVD, Ciuleanu T-E, Badin F et al (2017) First-line Nivolumab in stage IV or recurrent non–small-cell lung cancer. N Engl J Med 376:2415–2426
Chakraborty M, Abrams SI, Coleman CN et al (2004) External beam radiation of tumors alters phenotype of tumor cells to render them susceptible to vaccine-mediated T-cell killing. Cancer Res 64:4328–4337
Chakravarty PK, Alfieri A, Thomas EK, Beri V, Tanaka KE, Vikram B et al (1999) Flt3- ligand administration after radiation therapy prolongs survival in a murine model of metastatic lung cancer. Cancer Res 59:6028–6032
Chen D, Mellman I (2013) Oncology meets immunology: the cancer-immunity cycle. Immunity 39:1–10
Chen D, Patel RR, Verma V, Ramapriyan R, Barsoumian HB, Cortez MA, Welsh JW (2020a) Interaction between lymphopenia, radiotherapy technique, dosimetry, and survival outcomes in lung cancer patients receiving combined immunotherapy and radiotherapy. Radiother Oncol 150:114–120. https://doi.org/10.1016/j.radonc.2020.05.051
Chen D, Verma V, Patel RR, Barsoumian HB, Cortez MA, Welsh JW (2020b) Absolute lymphocyte count predicts abscopal responses and outcomes in patients receiving combined immunotherapy and radiation therapy: analysis of 3 phase 1/2 trials. Int J Radiat Oncol Biol Phys 108(1):196–203. https://doi.org/10.1016/j.ijrobp.2020.01.032
Chen Y, Gao M, Huang Z, Yu J, Meng X (2020c) SBRT combined with PD-1/PD-L1 inhibitors in NSCLC treatment: a focus on the mechanisms, advances, and future challenges. J Hematol Oncol 13(1):105. https://doi.org/10.1186/s13045-020-00940-z
Cohen SM, Lippard SJ (2001) Cisplatin: from DNA damage to cancer chemotherapy. Prog Nucleic Acid Res Mol Biol 67:93–130
Cohen MH, Gootenberg J, Keegan P, Pazdur R (2007) FDA drug approval summary: bevacizumab (Avastin) plus carboplatin and paclitaxel as first-line treatment of advanced/metastatic recurrent nonsquamous non-small cell lung cancer. Oncologist 12:713–718

Crocenzi T, Cottam B, Newell P et al (2016) A hypofractionated radiation regimen avoids the lymphopenia associated with neoadjuvant chemoradiation therapy of borderline resectable and locally advanced pancreatic adenocarcinoma. J Immunother Cancer 4:45

Daly ME, Monjazeb AM, Kelly K (2015) Clinical trials integrating immunotherapy and radiation for non–small-cell lung cancer. J Thorac Oncol 10:1685–1693

Davou GI, Chuwang NJ, Essien UC, Choji TPP, Echeonwu BC, Lugos MD (2019) Cytotoxicity analysis of etoposide and cisplatin on cell lines from human lung cancer and normal human lung. Int Res J Med Sci 7(2):40–47

De Velasco G, Je Y, Bossé D et al (2017) Comprehensive meta-analysis of key immune-related adverse events from CTLA-4 and PD-1/PD-L1 inhibitors in cancer patients. Cancer Immunol Res 5(4):312–318

Demaria S, Ng B, Devitt ML, Babb JS, Kawashima N, Liebes L et al (2004) Ionizing radiation inhibition of distant untreated tumors (abscopal effect) is immune mediated. Int J Radiat Oncol Biol Phys 58:862–870

Deng L, Liang H, Burnette B et al (2014) Irradiation and anti-PD-L1 treatment synergistically promote antitumor immunity in mice. J Clin Invest 124:687–695

Deshpand R, Chandra M, Rauthan A (2022) Evolving trends in lung cancer: epidemiology, diagnosis, and management. Indian J Cancer 59(Supplement):S90–S105. https://doi.org/10.4103/ijc.IJC_52_21

Dewan MZ, Galloway AE, Kawashima N, Dewyngaert JK, Babb JS, Formenti SC, Demaria S (2009) Fractionated but not single-dose radiotherapy induces an immune-mediated abscopal effect when combined with anti-CTLA-4 antibody. Clin Cancer Res 15(17):5379–5388. https://doi.org/10.1158/1078-0432.CCR-09-0265

Dovedi SJ, Cheadle EJ, Popple AL, Poon E, Morrow M, Stewart R et al (2017) Fractionated radiation therapy stimulates antitumor immunity mediated by both resident and infiltrating polyclonal T-cell populations when combined with PD-1 blockade. Clin Cancer Res 23:5514–5526

Dunn GP, Old LJ, Schreiber RD (2004) The three Es of cancer immunoediting. Annu Rev Immunol 22:329–360

Fehrenbacher L, Spira A, Ballinger M et al (2016) Atezolizumab versus docetaxel for patients with previously treated non-small-cell lung cancer (POPLAR): a multicentre, open-label, phase 2 randomised controlled trial. Lancet 387(10030):1837–1846

Ferraro C, Quemeneur L, Fournel S, Prigent A, Revillard J, Bonnefoy-Berard N (2000) The topoisomerase inhibitors camptothecin and etoposide induce a CD95-independent apoptosis of activated peripheral lymphocytes. Cell Death Differ 7:197–206

Formenti SC, Demaria S (2009) Systemic effects of local radiotherapy. Lancet Oncol 10(7):718–726

Formenti SC, Demaria S (2012) Radiation therapy to convert the tumor into an in situ vaccine. Int J Radiat Oncol Biol Phys 84(4):879–880

Formenti SC, Rudqvist N-P, Golden E, Cooper B, Wennerberg E, Lhuillier C et al (2018) Radiotherapy induces responses of lung cancer to CTLA-4 blockade. Nat Med 24:1845–1851

Fuks Z, Kolesnick R (2005) Engaging the vascular component of the tumor response. Cancer Cell 8(2):89–91

Gadgeel SM, Garassino MC, Esteban E et al (2019) KEYNOTE-189: updated OS and progression after the next line of therapy (PFS2) with pembrolizumab(pembro) plus chemo with pemetrexed and platinum placebo plus chemo for metastatic nonsquamous NSCLC. J Clin Oncol 37(15_suppl):9013

Gameiro SR, Caballero JA, Hodge JW (2012) Defining the molecular signature of chemotherapy-mediated lung tumor phenotype modulation and increased susceptibility to T-cell killing. Cancer Biother Radiopharm 27:23–35

Gandhi L, Rodrıguez-Abreu D, Gadgeel S et al (2018) Pembrolizumab plus chemotherapy in metastatic non-small-cell lung cancer. N Engl J Med 378(22):2078–2092

Garau MM (2017) Radiobiology of stereotactic body radiation therapy (SBRT). Rep Pract Oncol Radiother 22(2):86–95

Gennen K, Käsmann L, Taugner J, Eze C, Karin M, Roengvoraphoj O et al (2020) Prognostic value of PD-L1 expression on tumor cells combined with CD8+ TIL density in patients with locally advanced non-small cell lung cancer treated with concurrent chemoradiotherapy. Radiat Oncol 15:5

Gligorov J, Lotz JP (2004) Preclinical pharmacology of the taxanes: implications of the differences. Oncologist 9:3–8

Golden EB, Apetoh L (2015) Radiotherapy and immunogenic cell death. Semin Radiat Oncol 25(1):11–17

Golden EB, Pellicciotta I, Demaria S, Barcellos-Hoff MH, Formenti SC (2012) The convergence of radiation and immunogenic cell death signaling pathways. Front Oncol 2:88

Golden EB, Frances D, Pellicciotta I, Demaria S, Helen Barcellos-Hoff M, Formenti SC (2014) Radiation fosters dose-dependent and chemotherapy-induced immunogenic cell death. Onco Targets Ther 3:e28518

Gomez DR, Tang C, Zhang J, Blumenschein GR Jr, Hernandez M, Lee JJ, Ye R, Palma DA, Louie AV, Camidge DR, Doebele RC, Skoulidis F, Gaspar LE, Welsh JW, Gibbons DL, Karam JA, Kavanagh BD, Tsao AS, Sepesi B, Swisher SG, Heymach JV (2019) Local consolidative therapy vs. maintenance therapy or observation for patients with oligometastatic non-small-cell lung cancer: long-term results of a multi-institutional, phase II, randomized study. J Clin Oncol 37(18):1558–1565. https://doi.org/10.1200/JCO.19.00201

Grossman S, Ellsworth S, Campian J et al (2015) Survival in patients with severe lymphopenia following treatment with radiation and chemotherapy for newly diagnosed solid tumors. J Natl Compr Canc Netw 13:1225–1231

Hanahan D, Weiberg RA (2011) Hallmarks of cancer: the next generation. Cell 144(5):646–674

Haratani K, Hayashi H, Tanaka T et al (2017) Tumor immune microenvironment and nivolumab efficacy in EGFR mutation-positive non-small-cell lung cancer based on T790M status after disease progression during EGFR-TKI treatment. Ann Oncol 28(7):1532–1539

Herbst RS, Baas P, Kim DW et al (2016) Pembrolizumab versus docetaxel for previously treated, PD-L1-positive, advanced non-small-cell lung cancer (KEYNOTE-010): a randomised controlled trial. Lancet 387(10027):1540–1550

Hotta K, Matsuo K, Ueoka H, Kiura K, Tabata M, Tanimoto M (2004) Meta-analysis of randomized clinical trials comparing cisplatin to carboplatin in patients with advanced non-small-cell lung cancer. J Clin Oncol 22:3852–3859

Huang AC, Postow MA, Orlowski RJ et al (2017a) T-cell invigoration to tumour burden ratio associated with anti- PD-1 response. Nature 545:60–65

Huang CY, Ju DT, Chang CF, Reddy PM, Velmurugan BK (2017b) A review on the effects of current chemotherapy drugs and natural agents in treating non–small cell lung cancer. Biomedicine 7(4):23

Hui E, Cheung J, Zhu J, Su X, Taylor MJ, Wallweber HA, Sasmal DK, Huang J, Kim JM, Mellman I et al (2017) T cell costimulatory receptor CD28 is a primary target for PD-1–mediated inhibition. Science 355:1428–1433

Iyengar P, Wardak Z, Gerber DE, Tumati V, Ahn C, Hughes RS, Dowell JE, Cheedella N, Nedzi L, Westover KD, Pulipparacharuvil S, Choy H, Timmerman RD (2018) Consolidative radiotherapy for limited metastatic non-small-cell lung cancer: a phase 2 randomized clinical trial. JAMA Oncol 4(1):e173501. https://doi.org/10.1001/jamaoncol.2017.3501

Judd J, Borghaei H (2020) Combining immunotherapy and chemotherapy for non–small cell lung cancer. Thorac Surg Clin 30(2):199–206

Kaminski JM, Shinohara E, Summers JB et al (2005) The controversial abscopal effect. Cancer Treat Rev 31(3):159–172

Kim JY, Son YO, Park SW et al (2006) Increase of NKG2D ligands and sensitivity to NK cell-mediated cytotoxicity of tumor cells by heat shock and ionizing radiation. Exp Mol Med 38:474–484

Kroemer G, Galluzzi L, Kepp O et al (2013) Immunogenic cell death in cancer therapy. Annu Rev Immunol 31:51–72

Krummel MF, Allison JP (1995) CD28 and CTLA-4 have opposing effects on the response of T cells to stimulation. J Exp Med 182:459–465

Lauber K, Ernst A, Orth M, Herrmann M, Belka C (2012) Dying cell clearance and its impact on the outcome of tumor radiotherapy. Front Oncol 2:116

Lee K-M, Chuang E, Griffin M, Khattri R, Hong DK, Zhang W et al (1998) Molecular basis of T cell inactivation by CTLA-4. Science 282:2263–2266

Lehrer EJ, Singh R, Wang M, Chinchilli VM, Trifiletti DM, Ost P, Siva S, Meng MB, Tchelebi L, Zaorsky NG (2021) Safety and survival rates associated with ablative stereotactic radiotherapy for patients with oligometastatic cancer: a systematic review and meta-analysis. JAMA Oncol 7(1):92–106. https://doi.org/10.1001/jamaoncol.2020.6146

Lesterhuis WJ, Punt CJ, Hato SV et al (2011) Platinum based drugs disrupt STAT6-mediated suppression of immune responses against cancer in humans and mice. J Clin Invest 121(8):3100–3108

Liu WM, Fowler DW, Smith P et al (2010) Pre-treatment with chemotherapy can enhance the antigenicity and immunogenicity of tumours by promoting adaptive immune responses. Br J Cancer 102(1):115–123

Liu Y, Dong Y, Kong L, Shi F, Zhu H, Yu J (2018) Abscopal effect of radiotherapy combined with immune checkpoint inhibitors. J Hematol Oncol 11:104. https://doi.org/10.1186/s13045-018-0647-8

Luke JJ, Lemons JM, Karrison TG, Pitroda SP, Melotek JM, Zha Y, Al-Hallaq HA, Arina A, Khodarev NN, Janisch L, Chang P, Patel JD, Fleming GF, Moroney J, Sharma MR, White JR, Ratain MJ, Gajewski TF, Weichselbaum RR, Chmura SJ (2018) Safety and clinical activity of pembrolizumab and multisite stereotactic body radiotherapy in patients with advanced solid tumors. J Clin Oncol 36(16):1611–1618

Malas S, Harrasser M, Lacy KE, Karagiannis SN (2014) Antibody therapies for melanoma: new and emerging opportunities to activate immunity (review). Oncol Rep 32:875–886

Moding EJ, Castle KD, Perez BA et al (2015) Tumor cells, but not endothelial cells, mediate eradication of primary sarcomas by stereotactic body radiation therapy. Sci Transl Med 7:278ra34

Mole R (1953) Whole body irradiation—radiobiology or medicine? Br J Radiol 26:234–241

Mondini M, Nizard M, Tran T, Mauge L, Loi M, Clémenson C et al (2015) Synergy of radiotherapy and a cancer vaccine for the treatment of HPV-associated head and neck cancer. Mol Cancer Ther 14:1336–1345

Motzer RJ, Tannir NM, McDermott DF, Frontera OA, Melichar B, Choueiri TK, Plimack ER, Barthelemy P, Porta C, George S et al (2018) Nivolumab plus Ipilimumab versus Sunitinib in advanced renal-cell carcinoma. N Engl J Med 378:1277–1290

Nakamura N, Kusunoki Y, Akiyama M (1990) Radiosensitivity of CD4 or CD8 positive human T-lymphocytes by an in vitro colony formation assay. Radiat Res 123:224–227

Olive PL (1998) The role of DNA single-and double-strand breaks in cell killing by ionizing radiation. Radiat Res 150:S42–S51

Onoi K, Chihara Y, Uchino J, Shimamoto T, Morimoto Y, Iwasaku M, Kaneko Y, Yamada T, Takayama K (2020) Immune checkpoint inhibitors for lung cancer treatment: a review. J Clin Med 9(5):1362

Orth M, Unger K, Schoetz U, Belka C, Lauber K (2018) Taxane-mediated radiosensitization derives from chromosomal missegregation on tripolar mitotic spindles orchestrated by AURKA and TPX2. Oncogene 37:52–62

Park HJ, Griffin RJ, Hui S et al (2012) Radiation-induced vascular damage in tumors: implications of vascular damage in ablative hypofractionated radiotherapy (SBRT and SRS). Radiat Res 177(3):311–327

Peters S, Gettinger S, Johnson ML et al (2017) Phase II trial of atezolizumab as first-line or subsequent therapy for patients with programmed death-ligand1-selected advanced non-small-cell lung cancer (BIRCH). J Clin Oncol 35(24):2781–2789

Pfirschke C, Engblom C, Rickelt S et al (2016) Immunogenic chemotherapy sensitizes tumors to checkpoint blockade therapy. Immunity 44(2):343–354

Potters L, Steinberg M, Rose C et al (2004) American Society for Therapeutic Radiology and Oncology and American College of Radiology. Practice guideline for the performance of stereotactic body radiation therapy. Int J Radiat Oncol Biol Phys 60(4):1026–1032

Puzanov I, Diab A, Abdallah K et al (2017) Managing toxicities associated with immune checkpoint inhibitors: consensus recommendations from the Society for Immunotherapy of Cancer (SITC) toxicity management working group. J Immunother Cancer 5(1):95

Qiao M, Jiang T, Ren S, Zhou C (2018) Combination strategies on the basis of immune checkpoint inhibitors in non-small-cell lung cancer: where do we stand? Clin Lung Cancer 19(1):1–11. https://doi.org/10.1016/j.cllc.2017.06.005

Ramakrishnan R, Assudani D, Nagaraj S et al (2010) Chemotherapy enhances tumor cell susceptibility to CTL-mediated killing during cancer immunotherapy in mice. J Clin Invest 120(4):1111–1124
Rapoport BL, Anderson R (2019) Realizing the clinical potential of immunogenic cell death in cancer chemotherapy and radiotherapy. Int J Mol Sci 20:959
Reck M, Rodríguez-Abreu D, Robinson AG, Hui R, Csőszi T, Fülöp A et al (2016) Pembrolizumab versus chemotherapy for PD-L1-positive non-small-cell lung cancer. N Engl J Med 375:1823
Reits EA, Hodge JW, Herberts CA, Groothuis TA, Chakraborty M, Wansley EK et al (2006) Radiation modulates the peptide repertoire, enhances MHC class I expression, and induces successful antitumor immunotherapy. J Exp Med 203:1259–1271
Reynders K, Wauters E, Moisse M, Decaluwé H, De Leyn P, Peeters S et al (2018) RNA-sequencing in non-small cell lung cancer shows gene downregulation of therapeutic targets in tumor tissue compared to non-malignant lung tissue. Radiat Oncol 13:131
Rizvi NA, Hellmann MD, Brahmer JR, Juergens RA, Borghaei H, Gettinger S et al (2016) Nivolumab in combination with platinum-based doublet chemotherapy for first-line treatment of advanced non–small-cell lung cancer. J Clin Oncol 34:2969
Rocco D, Della Gravara L, Battiloro C, Gridelli C (2019) The role of combination chemo-immunotherapy in advanced non-small cell lung cancer. Expert Rev Anticancer Ther 19(7):561–568
Rowshanravan B, Halliday N, Sansom D (2018) CTLA-4: a moving target in immunotherapy. Blood 131:58–67
Ruffell B, Chang-Strachan D, Chan V et al (2014) Macrophage IL-10 blocks CD8+ T cell-dependent responses to chemotherapy by suppressing IL-12 expression in intratumoral dendritic cells. Cancer Cell 26(5):623–637
Sandler A, Gray R, Perry MC, Brahmer J, Schiller JH, Dowlati A et al (2006) Paclitaxel-carboplatin alone or with bevacizumab for nonsmall-cell lung cancer. N Engl J Med 355:2542–2550
Sansom D (2000) CD28, CTLA-4 and their ligands: who does what and to whom? Immunology 101:169–177
Schaer DA, Geeganage S, Amaladas N, Lu ZH, Rasmussen ER, Sonyi A et al (2019) The folate pathway inhibitor pemetrexed pleiotropically enhances effects of cancer immunotherapy. Clin Cancer Res 25:7175–7188
Schreiber RD, Old LJ, Smyth MJ (2011) Cancer immunoediting: integrating immunity's roles in cancer suppression and promotion. Science 331:1565–1570
Sharabi AB, Lim M, DeWeese TL, Drake CG (2015a) Radiation and checkpoint blockade immunotherapy: radiosensitisation and potential mechanisms of synergy. Lancet Oncol 16(13):e498–e509. https://doi.org/10.1016/S1470-2045(15)00007-8
Sharabi AB, Nirschl CJ, Kochel CM et al (2015b) Stereotactic radiation therapy augments antigen-specific PD-1-mediated antitumor immune responses via cross-presentation of tumor antigen. Cancer Immunol Res 3:345
Shaverdian N, Lisberg AE, Bornazyan K, Veruttipong D, Goldman JW, Formenti SC, Garon EB, Lee P (2017) Previous radiotherapy and the clinical activity and toxicity of pembrolizumab in the treatment of non-small-cell lung cancer: a secondary analysis of the KEYNOTE-001 phase 1 trial. Lancet Oncol 18(7):895–903. https://doi.org/10.1016/S1470-2045(17)30380-7
Siva S, MacManus MP, Martin RF, Martin OA (2015) Abscopal effects of radiation therapy: a clinical review for the radiobiologist. Cancer Lett 356(1):82–90
Socinski MA, Jotte RM, Cappuzzo F et al (2018) Atezolizumabfor first-line treatment of metastatic nonsquamous NSCLC. N Engl J Med 378(24):2288–2301
Song CW, Glatstein E, Marks LB, Emami B, Grimm J, Sperduto PW, Kim MS, Hui S, Dusenbery KE, Cho LC (2021) Biological principles of stereotactic body radiation therapy (SBRT) and stereotactic radiation surgery (SRS): indirect cell death. Int J Radiat Oncol Biol Phys 110(1):21–34
Spiotto M, Fu YX, Weichselbaum RR (2016) The intersection of radiotherapy and immunotherapy: mechanisms and clinical implications. Sci Immunol 1(3):EAAG1266
Sridharan V, Schoenfeld JD (2015) Immune effects of targeted radiation therapy for cancer. Discov Med 19:219–228

Suzuki E, Kapoor V, Jassar AS et al (2005) Gemcitabine selectively eliminates splenic gr-11/ CD11b1 myeloid suppressor cells in tumor-bearing animals and enhances antitumor immune activity. Clin Cancer Res 11(18):6713–6721

Theelen WSME, Peulen HMU, Lalezari F, van der Noort V, de Vries JF, Aerts JGJV, Dumoulin DW, Bahce I, Niemeijer AN, de Langen AJ, Monkhorst K, Baas P (2019) Effect of pembrolizumab after stereotactic body radiotherapy vs pembrolizumab alone on tumor response in patients with advanced non-small cell lung cancer: results of the PEMBRO-RT phase 2 randomized clinical trial. JAMA Oncol 5(9):1276–1282. https://doi.org/10.1001/jamaoncol.2019.1478

Theelen WSME, Chen D, Verma V, Hobbs BP, Peulen HMU, Aerts JGJV, Bahce I, Niemeijer ALN, Chang JY, de Groot PM, Nguyen QN, Comeaux NI, Simon GR, Skoulidis F, Lin SH, He K, Patel R, Heymach J, Baas P, Welsh JW (2021) Pembrolizumab with or without radiotherapy for metastatic non-small-cell lung cancer: a pooled analysis of two randomised trials. Lancet Respir Med 9(5):467–475. https://doi.org/10.1016/S2213-2600(20)30391-X

Tseng CW, Hung CF, Alvarez RD et al (2008) Pretreatment with cisplatin enhances E7-specific CD81 T-cell mediated antitumor immunity induced by DNA vaccination. Clin Cancer Res 14(10):3185–3192

Wang YS, Yang G, Wang YY et al (2013) Early efficacy of stereotactic body radiation therapy combined with adoptive immunotherapy for advanced malignancies. Mol Clin Oncol 1:925–929

Wang PF, Chen Y, Song SY et al (2017) Immune-related adverse events associated with anti-PD-1/ PD-L1 treatment for malignancies: a meta-analysis. Front Pharmacol 8:730

Wang W, Green M, Liu JR, Lawrence TS, Zou W (2018) CD8+ T cells in immunotherapy, radiotherapy, and chemotherapy. In: Oncoimmunology. Springer International Publishing AG, Dordrecht, pp 23–39

Weichselbaum RR, Liang H, Deng L, Fu YX (2017) Radiotherapy and immunotherapy: a beneficial liaison? Nat Rev Clin Oncol 14(6):365–379

Welsh J, Menon H, Chen D, Verma V, Tang C, Altan M, Hess K, de Groot P, Nguyen QN, Varghese R, Comeaux NI, Simon G, Skoulidis F, Chang JY, Papdimitrakopoulou V, Lin SH, Heymach JV (2020) Pembrolizumab with or without radiation therapy for metastatic non-small cell lung cancer: a randomized phase I/II trial. J Immunother Cancer 8(2):e001001. PMID: 33051340; PMCID: PMC7555111. https://doi.org/10.1136/jitc-2020-001001

Xu J, Escamilla J, Mok S et al (2013) CSF1R signaling blockade stanches tumor-infiltrating myeloid cells and improves the efficacy of radiotherapy in prostate cancer. Cancer Res 73:2782

Yovino S, Kleinberg L, Grossman SA et al (2013) The etiology of treatment-related lymphopenia in patients with malignant gliomas: modelling radiation dose to circulating lymphocytes explains clinical observations and suggests methods of modifying the impact of radiation on immune cells. Cancer Invest 31:140–144

Zeng H, Zhang W, Gong Y, Xie C (2019) Radiotherapy activates autophagy to increase CD8+ T cell infiltration by modulating major histocompatibility complex class-I expression in non-small cell lung cancer. J Int Med Res 47:3818–3830

Zheng H, Zeltsman M, Zauderer MG, Eguchi T, Vaghjiani RG, Adusumilli PS (2017) Chemotherapy-induced immunomodulation in non-small-cell lung cancer: a rationale for combination chemoimmunotherapy. Immunotherapy 9:913–927

Zhu L, Chen L (2019) Progress in research on paclitaxel and tumor immunotherapy. Cell Mol Biol Lett 24:40

Zou W, Wolchok JD, Chen L (2016) PD-L1 (B7-H1) and PD-1 pathway blockade for cancer therapy: mechanisms, response biomarkers, and combinations. Sci Transl Med 8(328):328rv4. PMID: 26936508; PMCID: PMC4859220. https://doi.org/10.1126/scitranslmed.aad7118

Lung Cancer Therapy: Synergistic Potential of PD-1/PD-L1 and CTLA-4 Inhibitors

15

Kangkan Sharma, Khyati Saini, Pranali Chimaniya, Sibashankar Sahu, Debasis Gantayat, Rajeev Sharma, Shvetank Bhatt, and Satish Shilpi

15.1 Introduction

According to the World Health Organization, lung cancer is known as the second highest diagnosis (11.4%) and the leading cause of death (18%) among all forms of cancer in 2020 (WHO 2020). The 5-year survival rate of the cancer patients across the world was 19% during 2010–2014. Only few countries like Japan (33%), Israel (27%), and Republic of Korea (25%) had higher survival rate (Allemani et al. 2018). The prime reason for low survival rate is late-stage diagnosis, lack of awareness, socioeconomic condition, environmental contamination, and metastatic and intratumoral heterogeneity nature of the tumor (Gss et al. 2014; Van der Heyden et al. 2009; Walters et al. 2013; Zhang et al. 2014).

The common etiological factors for this lung cancer development are smoking of tobacco (which causes 80% of the cases in the USA and other countries), occupational exposure to asbestos (5–10% globally), cannabis or marijuana smoking (4% in the USA at 2002–2014), radon exposure (10% in the Western world), air pollution, group 1 carcinogen arsenic exposure, inflammation and cellular damage during respiratory infection, chronic obstructive pulmonary disease-related inflammation and scar, and family lung cancer history (Alberg et al. 2013; Devesa

K. Sharma · K. Saini · S. Sahu · D. Gantayat · S. Shilpi (✉)
School of Pharmaceuticals and Population Health Informatics, FOP, DIT University, Dehradun, Uttarakhand, India

P. Chimaniya
Ravishankar College of Pharmacy, Bhanpur Square, Bhopal, Madhya Pradesh, India

R. Sharma
Amity Institute of Pharmacy, Amity University Madhya Pradesh, Gwalior, India

S. Bhatt
School of Health Sciences and Technology, Dr. Vishwanath Karad MIT World Peace University, Pune, Maharashtra, India

S. Bhatt et al. (eds.), *Immunotherapy Against Lung Cancer*,
https://doi.org/10.1007/978-981-99-7141-1_15

et al. 2005; Hasin 2018; Krewski et al. 2006; Bade and Dela Cruz 2020; Liu et al. 2012; Brenner et al. 2011; Caramori et al. 2011; Matakidou et al. 2005). Other increased risk factors for this cancer are systemic sclerosis patients, smoker breast cancer survivors, HIV infection patients with idiopathic pulmonary fibrosis, certain fibrotic pneumoconiosis patients, and lung cancer survivors. The abovementioned etiological factorial agents have free radicals, reactive oxygen species, and reactive electrophiles. Depending upon the dose, dimension, bio-durability, and surface reactivity, reactions can modify certain nucleotides in DNA with nitrogen and oxygen atom lesions to distort the basic base pairing arrangement leading to incorrect nucleotide incorporation during replication (Coluzzi et al. 2019; Lodish et al. 2000; Liu et al. 2013; Gout 2012; Yang et al. 2010; Klebe et al. 2019; Kou et al. 2020). Cell repair mechanism can repair the abduct DNA damage. But the escape portions change the coding of the DNA. Repeated exposure to etiological factors which are instruments to a series of genomic changes like variations of copy number (CNVs), insertions/deletions (INDELs), and single-nucleotide variants (SNVs), in exomes in autosomal chromosome, leads to permanent change in the sequence and that start to from the primary tumor followed by metastasis via circulating tumor cells (Weir et al. 2007; Davies et al. 2002; Ni et al. 2013). These genomic mutations affect synthesis of protein and disrupt the cell cycle progression to promote carcinogenesis. The study of circulatory tumor cells for metastatic cancer and genomics of the tumor cells for the noninvasive types helps in diagnosis and prognosis purposes. Circulating tumor cell analysis is helpful for the prediction of disease progression, survivability of patients, and personalized therapy as cell-free DNA fragments are found in peripheral blood (Weir et al. 2007; Davies et al. 2002; Ni et al. 2013; Cristofanilli et al. 2004; Krebs et al. 2011; Magbanua et al. 2012). Lung cancer occurs through either one or a combination of the etiological factors that lead to mutations in proto-oncogenes and tumor suppressor genes, DNA repair gene dysfunction, apoptotic mechanism erosion, limitless telomere replication, sustained angiogenesis, increment of invasion and metastasis, and escape from immunity (Seto et al. 2010; Dalmay and Edwards 2006; Hassanpour and Dehghani 2017; Lazebnik 2010; Macé et al. 2018).

Histologically, lung cancer is classified into non-small-cell lung cancer (NSCLC, 85%) and small cell lung cancer (SCLC, 13%) (Landesman-Milo et al. 2015). NSCLC is divided into three types: squamous-cell-carcinoma (25–30%), large-cell-carcinoma (5–10%), and lung adenocarcinoma (40%) (Travis et al. 1995, 2011; Zappa and Mousa 2016). In 2015, the WHO modified the lung cancer classification based on immunohistochemistry, genetic studies for personalized treatment strategies, and small biopsy and cytologic samples (Zappa and Mousa 2016; Travis et al. 2015; Bychkov 2023). This new classification objective is to overcome the drug resistance, intracellular accumulation, metastasis, invasion, side effects, and toxicity and develop a more effective personalized novel treatment regime (Kim 2016). The current treatment regime depends upon the stage of progression of cancer, the health of the patients, and the affordability during the time of diagnosis. Though the advancement of the treatment regime impacted the treatment profile, late-stage diagnosis (metastasis stage) creates a burden (Gss et al. 2014; Van der Heyden et al.

2009; Walters et al. 2013). Out of the different therapies, chemotherapy and radiotherapy are the preferred therapies after surgery. As a result of its disadvantages such as peripheral neuropathy, numbness, tingling, pain, lymphedema, nausea, hair loss, neutropenia, vomiting, memory/thinking problems, deep vein thrombosis, skin color, nail change, multidrug resistance, and the inability to treat metastasis and invasion, other treatment regimens are becoming increasingly important. Pathway-blocking agents and immunotherapy are two of them; even WHO classification shows this. The emphasis on immunotherapy, or immune oncology, is increasing for the treatment because of its precise targets for the cancer cells, its ability to dynamically adapt immunity to reevaluate and relaunch new attacks to control tumor growth, and its immune system memory to target to eliminate the cancer-like cells and type of cells. Depending upon the disease progression stage, the different treatments are impended in single or combinational therapy (Nurgali et al. 2018; Mansoori et al. 2017).

As the tumor microenvironment hinders the trafficking of CD8+ cells, even the immune system cannot inhibit the tumor (Zhou et al. 2020; Rodrigo et al. 2012; Tashkin and Ferguson 2013; Tammela et al. 2008; Goel et al. 2012). Regulatory T-cell (Treg) limitation, regulation of Axl, Mertk receptor (TAM) regulation, Tyro3 regulation, and inhibition of myeloid-derived suppressor cells (MDSC) are a few methods for overcoming the immune system. TAM overexpression increases cell survival and decreases apoptotic signaling. Again TAM downstreaming promotes metastasis via migration and invasion. Due to the polarization of macrophage M1 to M2, TAM has an immunosuppressive effect. M2 releases immune-suppressive cytokines. M2 blocking agents and M1 reprogramming agents can regulate this immunity suppression. Small molecule tyrosine inhibitors and TAM receptor-targeted ligands can use to regulate it (Gadiyar et al. 2020; Phuengkham et al. 2019; Zanganeh et al. 2016; Mulens-Arias et al. 2015). Treg cell regulates T-cell immune response to maintain cell homeostasis. But in the TME, Treg cells decrease the entry of T-cells. Again, cytotoxic-T-lymphocyte-associated-protein-4-(CTLA-4) antibodies remove the Treg and that can enhance the T-cell's functions (Li et al. 2021). MDSC induces immune suppression by inhibiting T-cell, NK cell, and macrophage functions. Targeting and inhibiting phosphatidylinositol 3-kinase (PI3K)δ, PD-L1 or CTLA-4, and multi-kinase MDSC can control the disease progression (Groth et al. 2019; Mi et al. 2020).

In different studies, researchers found that almost 32.6% of NSCLC cases have increased PD-L1 expression and it acts as a biomarker. Antibodies that are monoclonal directed against PD-L1 can stop its interaction with the PD-1 receptor in the body and can enhance the overall survival (Pawelczyk et al. 2019). Further, researchers have found that low PD-L1-expressed NSCLC overall survival is higher than the higher PD-L1 expression NSCLC. Recently, USFDA had approved two anti-PD-L1 antibodies named nivolumab and pembrolizumab. This approval helps to overcome ineffectiveness of therapies along with probable autoimmune side effect evaluation. But the main challenge in PD-L1 detection is the lack of standardized clinical results in different studies. Further, in chemotherapy or targeted drug delivery therapy, induced patient's PD-L1 expression changes. As reported in the comparison data, protein positivity for PD-L1 was more prevalent than mRNA positivity for PD-L1. Perhaps different thresholds for positivity are responsible for the difference. Immunotherapy may be beneficial to patients who are not identified by immunohistochemistry but may benefit from mRNA in situ hybridization (Yu et al. 2016).

Several lymphomas have genetic changes at the PD-1 gene locus 9p24.1, but lung cancer has yet to explore. Further, several studies concluded that anti-PD-L1 immunotherapy effectiveness depends on neoantigen and mutagen burdens. As with-PD-L1, PD-L2 is also a transmembrane protein-encoded-by the programmed cell death 1 ligand 2 gene ligand for the PD-1 T-cell receptor. PD-L2 plays an important role as a clinical marker in the tumor microenvironment to mediate immunosuppression as has been reported. In a study of KRAS-mutated NSCLC, researchers found that 47% of patients' PD-L2 expression was detected when they used monoclonal anti-PD-L2 (Yu et al. 2016).

In addition to PD-L1/PD-1 inhibitor responses, biomarkers that evaluate other immune checkpoints may also be used to predict the responses. CTLA-4/B7 checkpoint ligand may inhibit innate immunity and cause a patient to not respond to PD-L1/PD-1 inhibitors. In immunotherapy, CTLA-4/B7 ligand checkpoint inhibitors interfere with the connection of the CTLA-4-receptor on T-cells and the B7 ligand on-DCs. After that, the B7 ligand will attach to the CD28 receptor and activate the-immune system's-response (Yu et al. 2016). Early in an immune response, CTLA-4 stimulates the proliferation of T-cells, mainly in lymph nodes, whereas PD-1 inhibits the-proliferation-of T-cell afterward, primarily in peripheral tissues (Buchbinder and Desai 2016).

15.2 T-Cell Activation Pathways

15.2.1 CTLA-4 Pathway

Stimulatory signals are required to activate T-cells. With the help of co-stimulatory signals, the receptor T-cell (TCR) binds to major histocompatibility complexes (MHC) to activate T-cells. For the-T-cell to signal, B7-1(.CD-80) or B7-2.(CD86) molecules on the antigen-presenting cell (APC) need to bind to CD28 molecules on the antigen-presenting cell (APC). T-cells produce growth cytokines like'interleukin-2 (IL-2), increase-energy metabolism, and upregulate genes associated for cell survival when CD28:B7-1/2 binding is adequate. It increases survival of T-cells, proliferation, and differentiation (Masteller et al. 2000; Schneider et al. 2006; Linsley et al. 1996). CTLA-4, the homolog of CD28, has a much higher affinity for-B7; however, CTLA-4 does not stimulate B7, and the competitive binding can block the co-stimulatory-signal of the CD28:B7-binding. T-cell energy activation depends upon the binding ratio of-CD28:B7 against the CTLA-4:B7. Few studies report that CTLA-4:B7 binding can produce an inhibitory signal to counteract the stimulatory effect of CD28:B7 binding. This inhibitory mechanism of intracellular compartmental component CTLA-4 decreases the interaction with antigen-presenting cells. The upregulation of the intracellular compartmental component

CTLA-4 occurs through the stimulatory signals from T-cell receptor and CD28:B7 binding. An inhibitory signal through CTLA-4:B7 inhibits the IL-2 production and progression of the-cell cycle, which prevents activation of the full T-cell. Again, CTLA-4 also controls peripheral tolerance by maintaining regulatory T-cells (Treg) for controlling T-cells. Further, it was found from a study on animal model that deficiency of CTLA-4, impaired the functioning of regulatory T-cell. The mechanism that controls effector T-cells by Treg is the downregulation of B7 ligands on the APCs (Buchbinder and Desai 2016; Krummel and Allison 1996; Piccirillo and Shevach 2004; Takahashi et al. 2000; Wing et al. 2008a; Dijk et al. 2019) (Fig. 15.1).

According to a clinical update by the US patent office, researchers have found that anti-CTLA-4 antibodies antagonize CTLA-4 to control the T-cell functions for controlling immunity (Dijk et al. 2019). In another study, researchers have found that pembrolizumab, as a monotherapy, enhances disease regression with minimal toxicity (Arbeit and Ragan 2019).

15.2.2 PD-L1 Pathway

PD-1 inhibits immune response and promotes self-tolerance by-T-cell activation, antigen-specific T-cell-apoptosis, and regulatory T-cell apoptosis-inhibition. The costimulatory receptor of the B7/CD28 family PD-1 regulates T-cells by binding to its ligands (PD-L1 and PD-L2). It leads to the inhibition of proliferation, existence of T-cells, necrosis of factor-a, interferon-G, and production of IL-2. Early blocking of TCR signal, leads to decreased T-cell activation. Generally, PD-1 is responsible to prevent the TCR signaling by preventing phosphorylation of TCR signaling intermediates. T-cells can exhibit PD-1 with the assistance of a substantial amount of stimulation or a decline in CD4+ T-cell frequency. Infection and tumor control become less efficient as a result of T-cell malfunction (Bennett et al. 2003; Wherry 2011; Cuillerot et al. 2020). Researchers recently discovered that signaling

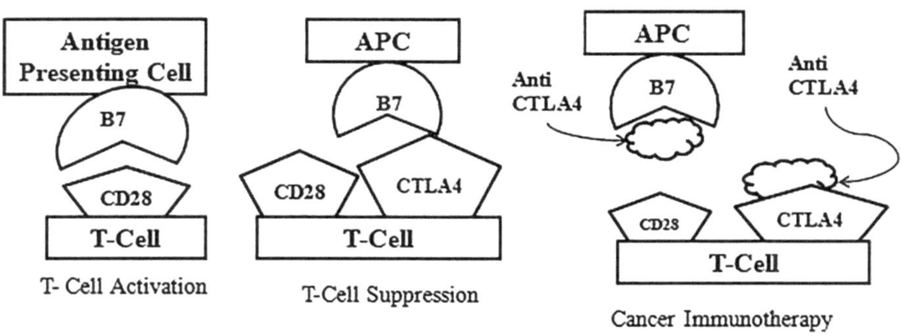

Fig. 15.1 Schematic drawing of the molecular mechanism of checkpoint blockade by therapeutic antibodies. T-cells are activation by the interaction between B7 ligands of antigen-presenting cell (APC) and CD28 on T-cells. CTLA-4 suppresses T-cell activation by competitive binding to B7. Therapeutic antibodies against CTLA-4 block the CTLA-4/B7 interaction

pathways play a significant part in tumorigenesis by modulating the PD-1/PD-L1 axis. PI3K/AKT, MAPK, NF-B, MAPK, Hedgehog, WNT, and JAK-STAT are the signaling pathways (Gowrishankar et al. 2015). In reaction to extracellular signals, the intracellular signal transduction pathway named PI3K/Akt stimulates metabolism, proliferation, cell survival, growth, and angiogenesis via phosphorylating an assortment of downstream substrates on serine and threonine. When PI3K/AKT is activated, CD8-T-cells consume more nutrition and produce more energy. Again mTOR pathway regulates the biological effects of immune cell stimulation. AKT/PI3K activation can result in the expression of PD-L1 by increasing extrinsic signaling or decreasing the negative regulator's expression. One of the negative regulators is PTEN. PTEN inhibition increases PI3K/AKT activation and the PD-L1 expression. In GIT stromal malignancies, PD-1/PD-L1 inhibition restored worn-out CD8+ T-cells through PI3K/Akt/mTOR activity (Zhao et al. 2019).

Mitogen-activated protein kinase is one of the serine/threonine protein kinases that directly influence proliferation, differentiation, invasion, metastasis, and death through phosphorylation activation activity. External stimuli initiate transmitting signals. MAPK subdivisions that are important include c-Jun N-terminal (JNK), MAPK14, ERK MAPK, and RAS/Raf1/MEK/ERK. The proto-oncogene RAS also sends out signals that promote proliferation and growth. In lung adenocarcinomas, inhibition of MAPK functioning, reduced the production of mRNA CD274 and protein PDL1 as well as it induced membrane up-regulation in epidermal growth factor pathway (Stutvoet et al. 2019; Pradhan et al. 2019). Anti-PD-L1 antibodies decreased p-P38 and p-ERK in Hodgkin-Lymphoma cell lines. A MAPK pathway component, MEK1/2, can also significantly prevent PD-L1 expression in renal cell carcinoma (Jalali et al. 2019). The JAK/STAT pathway regulates different extracellular factors like cytokines, interferon, hormones, growth factors, and related molecules to control gene expression (Groner and von Manstein 2017). Recently, in lung adenocarcinoma, the gene-associated IL4I1 through the JAK/STAT-pathway induces PD-L1-expression (Zhu et al. 2023). Additionally, FGFR2 signaling activated the JAK/STAT3 signaling pathway, resulting in increased PD-L1 expression. Overexpression with FGFR2 increases PD-L1 expression and exacerbated tumors in colorectal cancer xenograft models. JAK inhibitors can counteract this impact by inhibiting the JAK/STAT3 pathway (Li et al. 2019). WNT signaling pathways begin with proteins that pass signals into cells via cell surface receptors to govern physiological activities like migration, growth, and differentiation during the process of development and homeostasis. The deregulation of WNT signaling promotes malignant transformation, progression, and treatment resistance. In addition, the abnormal signals of WNT can disrupt immune monitoring in cancer, thereby promoting immune escape and preventing the immune therapies from working, including immune checkpoint inhibitors (Galluzzi et al. 2019; Azbazdar et al. 2021). Investigators recently discovered that thwarting the Wnt/β-catenin signal boosts the curative effect of anti-PD-1 therapy by preventing tumor growth and migratory and encouraging immune infiltration in glioblastoma cells (Zhang et al. 2021) (Fig. 15.2).

A key transcription factor in the inflammation process and immune system function is NF-κB. The NF-κB family has five DNA-binding proteins to form different

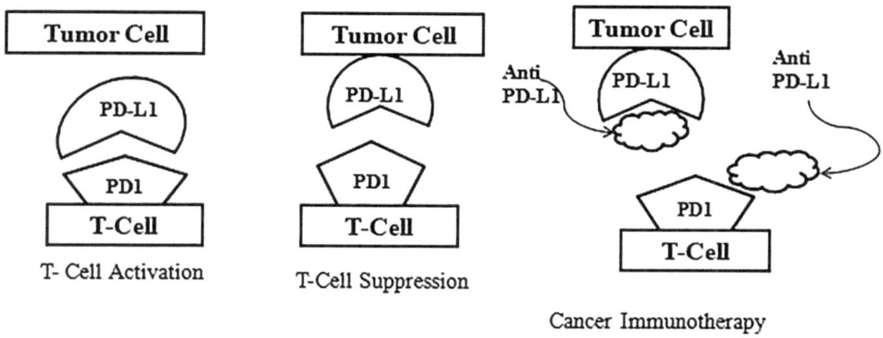

Fig. 15.2 Schematic drawing of the molecular mechanism of T-cell activation, suppression, and antibody drugs for cancer immunotherapy bound to PD-1 or PD-L1, blocking the PD-1/PD-L1 interaction

homodimers and heterodimers. These proteins regulate cell proliferation by controlling adaptive as well as innate immune responses, apoptosis mechanism, invasion and migration of cells, genetic and epigenetic alteration, and cancer stem cell formation. Activation of NF-κB induces immunosuppression via the lipopolysaccharide and tumor necrosis factor. NF-κB regulates lymphocyte functions of T-cells and B cells (Han et al. 2020; Taniguchi and Karin 2018). Yet again, NF-κB can trigger PD-L1 transcription by binding to its promoter and subsequently regulate PD-L1 posttranscriptionally through indirect pathways. Often, tumors are dysregulated in these processes, which promote tissue healing and homeostasis when stressed. Oncogenes, stress, and cytokines trigger inflammation, and chemotherapeutic medications comprise a few of the cues that trigger PD-L1 to be elevated in cancer cells. It is feasible that PD-L1 participates in the remodeling of tissues as revealed by the epithelial/mesenchymal transformation and PD-L1 expression spurred on by a signaling system in epithelial malignancies. By expressing PD-L1, tumor-infiltrating myeloid cell populations may contribute to the immune-suppressive features of the tumor environment (Cha et al. 2019; Bi et al. 2016; Zhou et al. 2021). The caffeic acid phenethyl ester NF-kB modulator suppresses the excitation of PD-L1 by LMP1. Furthermore, INF-induced PD-L1 expression undergoes regulation by NF-kB. The NF-kB inhibitor inhibited IFN-induced PD-L1 expression, whereas MAPK, PI3K, and STAT3 inhibitors had no impact (Bi et al. 2016). According to a study, PD-1 inhibitors engage in conjunction with low-dose carboplatin to rewire the tumor immune milieu via the STING-triggering pathway (Zhou et al. 2021). The hedgehog pathway is essential during embryonic development. It has physiological consequences through influencing the proportion of the activator and repressor versions of the transcription factors involved in gliomas (Skoda et al. 2018). In a study, researchers have found that in gastric cancer, hedgehog activation stimulates PD-L1 expression and tumor cell proliferation (Chakrabarti et al. 2018). Recently, in a clinical update, researchers have found that Avelumab selectively binds to PD-L1 and competitively blocks PD-1 and targets tumor cells better than anti-PD-L1 antibodies that target T-cells with a lower risk of autoimmune-related safety (Cuillerot et al. 2020).

15.3 T-Cell Receptors

15.3.1 Cytotoxic T-Lymphocyte-Associated Antigen-4

CTLA-4 (CD152) receptor appears on the surface of activated T-cell lymphocytes. It was found in 1987 (Chakrabarti et al. 2018) by Brunet et al. using evaluation of mouse in cytolytic T-cell-generated cDNA libraries.

CTLA-4 expression arises from normal T-cell activation, while regulatory T-cells (Tregs) frequently express CTLA4 since they possess a greater amount of FoxP3, a forkhead gene transcription factor that is known to regulate CTLA-4 expression (Brunet et al. 1987; Perkins et al. 1996; Alegre et al. 1996). CTLA-4 acts mainly by competing for B7 ligands (B7-1/CD80 and B7-2/CD86) on antigen-presenting cells (APCs) with CD28 receptors. Crucial subsequent stimulation cue for T-cells is transmitted by the attachment of the CD28 receptor on T-cells to the B7 ligand on APCs during stimulation of T-cells. However, CTLA-4 receptors surpass CD28 receptors for B7 ligand interaction because they have a greater affinity and lesser surface density for doing so. T-cell anergy would result from a lack of an additional stimulation signal in the existence of CTLA-4 receptors. Furthermore, it has been demonstrated that B7 ligands are sequestered by CTLA-4 receptors from the exterior of APCs, significantly reducing the amount of ligands there (Pardoll 2012).

15.3.1.1 Cancer and Cytotoxic CTLA-4

Numerous investigations into antibodies that inhibit CTLA-4 and thus boost the body's immune system toward cancer cells have been concluded. Ipilimumab (ant-iCTLA-4) clinical trial data served as the foundation for the FDA's 2011 acceptance of the medicine for the treatment of individuals with advanced melanoma. The CTLA-4 molecule, a part of the immunological synapse, is attracted via the T-cell effector barrier from the cytoplasm (Antonia et al. 2016b). There are two phases to the stimulation of cytotoxic T-lymphocytes. When the TCR detects the antigen through histocompatibility complexes (MHC of either class I or II) on the outermost layer of the APC, it produces the first signal, which increases the receptivity of the CD4 and CD8 recipients to the antigen. The interaction of co-stimulating CD80/CD86 proteins (B7-1 and B7-2) on the surface of APC with the CD28 proteins on the outer layer of T-cells, resulting in lymphocyte stimulation and sorting, is the second signal necessary for synaptogenesis. When it involves sticking to ligands on the surface of APC cells, CTLA-4 outperforms CD28 because it is more selective for B7 family molecules than CD28, inhibiting CD28 from coming into touch with CD80/86. Because CTLA-4 binds to CD80-B7-1 and CD86-B7-2 on APCs, which sets off a hindering reaction and immunosuppression, the T-lymphocyte accordance is impeded, T-lymphocyte growth declines, Treg lymphocyte exertion is hampered, and cytokine production declines (Wei et al. 2018; Zhao et al. 2018; Rowshanravan et al. 2018; Schadendorf et al. 2015; Ribas et al. 2013; Wojtukiewicz et al. 2021; Sanmamed and Chen 2014). High levels of CTLA-4 expression also result in the functional conversion of T helper cells to regulatory T-lymphocytes that have important immunosuppressive characteristics. CTLA-4 impacts the immune dysfunction found in individuals with cancer. Anti-CTLA-4 antibodies (ipilimumab, tremelimumab) prevent CTLA-4 and lead to T-cell activation, suppression, and recurrence in Fig. 15.1. The goal of antibody therapy is to unblock an immune system response that has been suppressed and activate T-lymphocytes, which are found in the lymph nodes, which leads to a successful immune response and the elimination of malignant cells (Rowshanravan et al. 2018). The way that CTLA-4 inhibitors work varies a little. They make the T-cells to actively search out and destroy cancerous cells. A CTLA-4-specific antibody called ipilimumab is clinically used in immunotherapy to treat cancer but has significant autoimmune side effects. The efficiency and toxicity of CTLA-4-targeting antibodies can potentially be separated using the techniques described in a current paper by Du et al. in *Cell Research* (Wing et al. 2008b). To treat cancer patients, immune checkpoint inhibitors (ICIs) (anti-CTLA-4, anti-PD-1, and anti-PD-L1), a combination of anti-PD-1/PD-L1 with anti-CTLA-4, and anti-ICI (anti-CTLA-4, anti-PD-1, anti-PD-L1) are utilized. This offers an innovative form of immunotherapy for treatment of cancer and has unquestionably been a major development in the area of malignancy in new years. Patients with a variety of cancers now have much better treatment outcomes and prognoses because of ICIs. It is expected that as ICI use grows, carers may run into more challenges trying to manage the negative side effects of taking these medications. PD-1, anti-PD-L1, and a combination of anti-PD-1/PD-L1 with anti-CTLA-4 have unquestionably proven to be significant improvements in the area of cancer treatment in current years. ICIs have significantly improved the prognosis and treatment outcomes for patients with many types of malignancies. With the increased use of ICIs, it is anticipated that carers would encounter additional difficulties, specifically managing the negative side effects brought on by the use of these medications (Pol and Kroemer 2018). Anti-CTLA-4 agents (ipilimumab, tremelimumab) serve as a paradigm of activation of T-cells, suppression, and resurrection. Two signals are necessary for T-cell activation: the first is the binding of MCH with TCR, and the second is the cooperation of CD28 with the T-cell and B7 (CD 80, CD 86) in the APC. After the activation of T-cells, CTLA-4 is pushed to the membrane of the plasma where it serves as an inhibitor of the activation of T-cells. T-cell reactivation is caused by the binding of the anti-CTLA-4 antibody to CTLA-4. The acronyms APC, TCR, CTLA-4, and MHC stand for antigen-presenting cell, T-cell receptor, and major histocompatibility complex, respectively.

15.3.1.2 Anti-CTLA-4 Agents in Anticancer Therapy

15.3.1.2.1 Ipilimumab

The initial ICI was evaluated on cancer patients and shown to have potential as anti-CTLA-4. Ipilimumab was one of the initial antibodies to be approved by the FDA and to be regularly used in healthcare settings with cancer patients. It has been demonstrated that a monoclonal anti-CTLA-4 (IgG1) antibody that is entirely mammalian improves long-term survival in patients with advanced cutaneous melanoma (Wei et al. 2018). Prior to this, there was a strong focus on a significant increase in OS despite a small number of objective reactions to treatment (about 10% of patients) with a relatively small percentage of individuals (20–25%) who witnessed long-term benefits. Additionally, it was revealed that ipilimumab therapy had a peculiar spectrum of adverse effects, notably cutaneous and gastrointestinal problems. Since the introduction of anti-CTLA-4 medicine, the significance of patients obtaining complete medical treatment has been emphasized (Ribas et al. 2013).

15.3.1.2.2 Tremelimumab

Tremelimumab research has not yet yielded good results, in contrast to ipilimumab, which would discourage its broad usage in monotherapy (Schadendorf et al. 2015). In the studies that have been publicized thus far, individuals with HCC who were receiving treatment with tremelimumab and nivolumab experienced rates of response of 15% and 30%, respectively. Tremelimumab and durvalumab combined for therapy are currently being studied, albeit (Ribas et al. 2013; Wojtukiewicz et al. 2021).

15.3.1.2.3 Durvalumab and Tremelimumab

Numerous studies have been executed to assess the efficacy of anti-PD-1/PD-L1 and anti-CTLA-4 antibodies for the treatment of lung tumors. In the initial phases of the 1b research, five oncology organizations in the USA analyzed the safety and efficacy of mixing durvalumab (anti-PD-L1) and tremelimumab (anti-CTLA-4) administration for individuals with advanced squamous or non-squamous NSCLC. The research study observed clinical activity in both PD-L1-positive and PD-L1-negative tumors, with 23% of patients having investigator-determined verified ORR (Wojtukiewicz et al. 2021).

15.3.1.2.4 Nivolumab and Ipilimumab

In a phase 1 trial, nivolumab and ipilimumab were examined for both safety and effectiveness as initial treatments for NSCLC. The two administration schedules for the combination that were assessed in the experiment were nivolumab every 2 weeks along with ipilimumab once every 12 weeks and nivolumab for every 2 weeks plus ipilimumab at a period of 6 weeks. Patients who acquired ipilimumab every 12 weeks exhibited a slightly greater confirmed ORR (47% vs. 38%, respectively) at the time of reporting than in individuals undergoing ipilimumab each 6 weeks (Ready et al. 2019). An open-label stage 3 trial started among individuals with cancer at stage 4 or recurring NSCLC who did not earlier receive chemotherapy treatment. The combination of nivolumab and ipilimumab administration was shown ORR of 45.3%, a disease-free survival rate of 42.6%, and a median PFS of 7.2 months in individuals who had a significant malignant mutational frequency (ten alterations per megabase). In the clinical trial, the group receiving nivolumab alone was found a poor significant result in the comparison of simultaneous administration of nivolumab + ipilimumab for the management of disease in the patients with a malignant mutational strain. Alone nivolumab was shown at least ten alterations per megabase and PD-L1 expression of at least 1%, the median PFS (4.1 months) was assessed while in case of nivolumab + ipilimumab in combination it was found tandem PFS (7.1 months) (Hellmann et al. 2017). When compared to the chemotherapy category, the nivolumab plus ipilimumab combination group had a significantly reduced risk of developing an illness or death. The safety and efficacy of nivolumab plus "low-dose" ipilimumab as first-line therapy for advanced NSCLC were investigated in subsequent open-label stage 2 examinations and the relationship between efficacy and the expression of PD-L1 and cancer mutational frequencies. The research suggested a threshold of ten alterations per megabase for tumor mutational burden and observed that the ORR increased in individuals with cancer mutational complexities, including at least ten different kinds per megabase, irrespective of PD-L1 expression (48% in PD-L1 1% cohort and 47% in PD-L1 1% group).

15.3.1.2.5 Nivolumab Plus Ipilimumab

In addition to progressive NSCLC, patients with metastatic SCLC were given a combination of nivolumab and ipilimumab. Individuals who recovered after at least one prior platinum-containing treatment were given nivolumab along with ipilimumab or nivolumab alone in a multicenter stage 1/stage 2 study. At the stage of evaluation, patients who received both nivolumab and ipilimumab had a higher ORR (23% vs. 10%) and a longer survival (7.7 vs. 4.4 months for the median OS and 43% vs. 33% for the 1-year OS rate) than those getting nivolumab alone. This adds to the evidence for the benefits of combining CTLA-4 antagonists and PD-1 inhibitors (Hellmann et al. 2018).

15.4 PD-L1 Inhibitors

PD-L1 is a co-inhibitory molecule that inhibits the adaptive and innate immune system against cancer. It is primarily located on hematopoietic cell surfaces such as dendric cells, T-cells, B cells, and non-hematopoietic cells and macrophages like astrocytes, vascular endothelial cells, and keratinocytes. It mainly presents on the surface of T-lymphocytes whose primary function is to secrete cytokine and possess antigens. PD-L1 also known as CD289 and B7H1 is a transmembrane glycoprotein carrying amino acids with 290 in number along with IgC and Ig on the cellular surface (Sanmamed and Chen 2014). It is a ligand of PD-1, which embeds 288 amino acids along with a membrane-permeating domain and cytoplasmic tail having two tyrosine base (ITIM and ITSM that are immunoreceptor-based inhibitory and switching motifs) (Neel et al. 2003). PD-1 has high levels of expression in tumor T-lymphocytes. The transcription of PD-1 on tumor cells is governed by certain factors such as interferon regulatory factor 9 (IRF9), forkhead box protein (FOX), and nuclear factor of activated T-cells (NFAT), whereas the conserved upstream regulatory regions-B (CR-B) and conserved upstream regulatory regions-C (CR-C) are support the PD-1 gene expression. Instead of binding c-FOS (a proto-oncogene whose expression causes a multiple stimuli such as development factors and tumor promotors) to the COR-C region, they connect to the sites of the COR-B region and boost PD-1 expression when the T-cell receptor activated is stimulated by the detection of antigens in innocent T-cells. Chronic infections and cancer cell leakage can also contribute to the expression of PD-1 by various mechanisms such as promotor demethylation and upregulations of c-FOS (Han et al. 2020). Initially, it was considered that the PD-L1 on macrophages functions similarly to the PD-L1 on T-cells, which blocks the T-cell response. Various studies were conducted on the parts of PD-L1 on macrophages, and it is found that their function is more complex. According to Singhal et al., PD-L1 acts as a kind of barrier on macrophages rather than preventing the T-cell response (Singhal et al. 2019). The PD-L1 inhibitors' mechanism of action includes the following:

1. Improvement in T-cell function
2. T-cell proliferation stimulation
3. Promotion of cytokine secretion
4. Modulation of tumor microenvironment

15.4.1 Enhancement of T-Cell Activity

Increasing the number of T-cells is frequently more important in case of achieving the required immunogenicity against any particular autoimmune disorder. The enhancement of T-cell function in the case of inhibiting PD-L1 receptors can be done by a bispecific antibody mechanism. This particular bispecific mechanism can be achieved by an antibody called LY3434172. LY3434172 is a special type of antibody that can act in both cases of PD1 and PDL1; that is why it is named as the bispecific mechanism. Some research also states that the bispecific antibody frequently activates the T-cell and further diminishes the effect of cancer cells in vitro rather than the parent antibody which is present inside the body and only capable of killing some significant cancerous protein. In this way, the enhancement of T-cells can be done by a bispecific type of antibody which further helps in the inhibition of the PDL1 receptor (Kotanides et al. 2020).

15.4.2 Induction of T-Cell Proliferation

T-cell proliferation is inhibited by PD-L1 and PDL-2 interactions with PD-1. As a consequence, T-cells cannot be multiplied because of the production of a molecule called L2 (L2 downmodulate cytokine production and cell proliferation). This inhibition can be overcome by CD28 co-stimulation through the induction of interleukin-2 productions. But the overcome is later dominated by the PD-1 lane. CD8+ kind of T-cells is more sensitive to the interaction of PD: PD1 than CD4+ types, as they can produce interleukin-2 (Carter et al. 2002).

15.4.3 Promotion of Cytokine Secretion

Cytokine plays a significant role in regulating adaptive and immune immunity, which can be suppressed via PD-L1. By inhibiting PD-L1, we can restore cytokine formation and reactivate the immune system's function (Han et al. 2020). Various cytokine promoters can be used which are able to bind to certain specific receptors of the targeted area and induce the secretion of cytokine (Corwin 2000).

15.4.4 Modulation of Tumor Microenvironment

By modifying various factors of the cancer microenvironment, we can control the outcome of PD-L1. The tumor microenvironment generally contains vasculature, an extracellular matrix along with a molecular network that holds and regulates various functions (Jiang et al. 2019). PD-L1 expression can be influenced by a variety of factors in the surrounding microenvironment, such as cytokines, exomes, and hypoxia. We can harmonize the microenvironment by adjusting various factors and controlling various secretions that can control the microenvironment (Jiang et al. 2019).

15.5 Synergistically Combinational Approach of CTLA-4 and PD-1 Pathway Inhibitors in Cancer

In general, there are some parallels and few alterations between CTLA-4 and PD-1. Both routes are expressed by TCR signaling to stimulate T-cells and are supporters of the B7 receptor. Additionally, both regulate the intracellular T-cell signaling proteins and the decline in T-cell survival, proliferation, glucose metabolism, and cytokine production. However, the primary variations between the two methods are specifically in lymphoid tissues; a CTLA-4 receptor restricts T-cell responses initially in an immune response, whereas PD-1 receptors restrict immune responses afterward, mostly in peripheral organs. Antigen-presenting cells express both CTLA-4 and PD-1 ligands. Non-immune cells, including tumor cells, are able to produce PD-1 ligands. More T-cell signaling pathways are impacted by a PD-1 engagement than a CTLA-4 engagement. Although PD-1's impact on regulatory T-cells is uncertain, CTLA-4 has an impact on how they operate (Buchbinder and Desai 2016; Masteller et al. 2000; Schneider et al. 2006; Linsley et al. 1996; Krummel and Allison 1996; Piccirillo and Shevach 2004; Takahashi et al. 2000; Wing et al. 2008a; Dijk et al. 2019; Arbeit and Ragan 2019; Bennett et al. 2003; Wherry 2011; Cuillerot et al. 2020). Seven PD-1 and PD-L1 checkpoint inhibitors, as well as CTLA-4 immunotherapy for various cancers, have received approval from various regulatory bodies. A few more inhibitors are still in the advanced stages of development. Although these medications had acceptable safety profiles and improved durable response rates when used as monotherapy, only 50% of the patients saw success. Researchers discovered that nivolumab (anti-PD-1) and combining ipilimumab (anti-CTLA-4) improve response rates to CTLA-4 and inhibitors of PD-1 in patients with advanced melanoma. Compared with a single therapy, patient's survival rate climbed to 58% with these two inhibitors.

15.6 Conclusion

The advanced growth and progression of cancer cells challenge researchers to develop and invent new technology and strategies for its treatment. There are so many pathways explored by researchers which are directly and indirectly related to the growth of the cancer cells. Adaptation of daily bad routine of the societies and environmental factors like pollution is also a big challenge to overcome. Many new drugs and strategies are invented day by day, but above factors may affect their treatment potential which should be consider during strategies' development. Multidrug resistance (MDR) and advanced type of lung cancer may fail all the developed strategies, and it required further advancement in the treatment strategies. Pathways like PD-1 and CTLA-4 inhibition are some pathways to activate T-cell. There are so many PD-1 and CTLA-4 inhibitors that have been developed which can induce the T-cell activation. T-cell activation is beneficial to retard the growth of lung cancer types. Monoclonal antibodies' based targeting alongwith PD-1 and CTLA-4 inhibitors were found significant response on tumor cell growth regression due to T-cell activation.

References

Alberg AJ, Brock MV, Ford JG, Samet JM, Spivack SD (2013) Epidemiology of lung cancer: diagnosis and management of lung cancer, 3rd ed: American College of Chest Physicians evidence-based clinical practice guidelines. Chest 143(5 Suppl):e1S–e29S. https://doi.org/10.1378/chest.12-2345

Alegre ML, Noel PJ, Eisfelder BJ, Chuang E, Clark MR, Reiner SL et al (1996) Regulation of surface and intracellular expression of CTLA4 on mouse T cells. J Immunol 157(11):4762–4770

Allemani C, Matsuda T, Di Carlo V, Harewood R, Matz M, Nikšić M, Bonaventure A, Valkov M, Johnson CJ, Estève J et al (2018) Global surveillance of trends in cancer survival 2000–14 (CONCORD-3): analysis of individual records for 37 513 025 patients diagnosed with one of 18 cancers from 322 population-based registries in 71 countries. Lancet (London, England) 391(10125):1023–1075. https://doi.org/10.1016/S0140-6736(17)33326-3

Antonia SJ, Lopez-Martin JA, Bendell J, Ott PA, Taylor M, Eder JP et al (2016b) Nivolumab alone and nivolumab plus ipilimumab in recurrent small-cell lung cancer (CheckMate 032): a multicentre, open-label, phase 1/2 trial. Lancet Oncol 17(7):883–895

Arbeit RD Ragan PM (2019) Methods for treating cancer. JP2019502741A, 31 Jan 2019

Azbazdar Y, Karabicici M, Erdal E, Ozhan G (2021) Regulation of Wnt signaling pathways at the plasma membrane and their misregulation in cancer. Front Cell Dev Biol 9:631623. https://doi.org/10.3389/fcell.2021.631623

Bade BC, Dela Cruz CS (2020) Lung cancer 2020: epidemiology, etiology, and prevention. Clin Chest Med 41(1):1–24. https://doi.org/10.1016/j.ccm.2019.10.001

Bennett F, Luxenberg D, Ling V et al (2003) Program death-1 engagement upon TCR activation has distinct effects on costimulation and cytokine-driven proliferation: attenuation of ICOS, IL-4, and IL-21, but not CD28, IL-7, and IL-15 responses. J Immunol 170:711–718

Bi XW, Wang H, Zhang WW, Wang JH, Liu WJ, Xia ZJ, Huang HQ, Jiang WQ, Zhang YJ, Wang L (2016) PD-L1 is upregulated by EBV-driven LMP1 through NF-κB pathway and correlates with poor prognosis in natural killer/T-cell lymphoma. J Hematol Oncol 9(1):109. https://doi.org/10.1186/s13045-016-0341-7

Brenner DR, McLaughlin JR, Hung RJ (2011) Previous lung diseases and lung cancer risk: a systematic review and meta-analysis. PLoS One 6(3):e17479. https://doi.org/10.1371/journal.pone.0017479

Brunet JF, Denizot F, Luciani MF, Roux-Dosseto M, Suzan M, Mattei MG et al (1987) A new member of the immunoglobulin superfamily—CTLA-4. Nature 328(6127):267–270

Buchbinder EI, Desai A (2016) CTLA-4 and PD-1 pathways. Am J Clin Oncol 39(1):98–106. https://doi.org/10.1097/coc.0000000000000239

Bychkov A. WHO classification. PathologyOutlines.com website. https://www.pathologyoutlines.com/topic/lungtumorWHO.html. Accessed 3 Apr 2023

Caramori G, Adcock IM, Casolari P, Ito K, Jazrawi E, Tsaprouni L, Villetti G, Civelli M, Carnini C, Chung KF et al (2011) Unbalanced oxidant-induced DNA damage and repair in COPD: a link towards lung cancer. Thorax 66(6):521–527. https://doi.org/10.1136/thx.2010.156448

Carter L, Fouser LA, Jussif J, Fitz L, Deng B, Wood CR, Collins M, Honjo T, Freeman GJ, Carreno BM (2002) PD-1:PD-L inhibitory pathway affects both CD4(+) and CD8(+) T cells and is overcome by IL-2. Eur J Immunol 32(3):634–643. https://doi.org/10.1002/1521-4141(200203)32:3<634::AID-IMMU634>3.0.CO;2-9. PMID: 11857337

Cha JH, Chan LC, Li CW, Hsu JL, Hung MC (2019) Mechanisms controlling PD-L1 expression in cancer. Mol Cell 76(3):359–370. https://doi.org/10.1016/j.molcel.2019.09.030

Chakrabarti J, Holokai L, Syu L, Steele NG, Chang J, Wang J, Ahmed S, Dlugosz A, Zavros Y (2018) Hedgehog signaling induces PD-L1 expression and tumor cell proliferation in gastric cancer. Oncotarget 9(100):37439–37457. https://doi.org/10.18632/oncotarget.26473

Coluzzi E, Leone S, Sgura A (2019) Oxidative stress induces telomere dysfunction and senescence by replication fork arrest. Cells 8(1):19. https://doi.org/10.3390/cells8010019

Corwin EJ (2000) Understanding cytokines. Part I: physiology and mechanism of action. Biol Res Nurs 2(1):30–40. https://doi.org/10.1177/109980040000200104. PMID: 11232509

Cristofanilli M, Budd GT, Ellis MJ, Stopeck A, Matera J, Miller MC, Reuben JM, Doyle GV, Allard WJ, Terstappen LW, Hayes DF (2004) Circulating tumor cells, disease progression, and survival in metastatic breast cancer. N Engl J Med 351(8):781–791. https://doi.org/10.1056/NEJMoa040766

Cuillerot J-M, Heydebreck AV, Yuan G (2020) Pd-1/pd-l1 inhibitors for the treatment of cancer. US20200362040A1, 19 Nov 2020

Dalmay T, Edwards DR (2006) MicroRNAs and the hallmarks of cancer. Oncogene 25(46):6170–6175. https://doi.org/10.1038/sj.onc.1209911

Davies H, Bignell GR, Cox C, Stephens P, Edkins S, Clegg S, Teague J, Woffendin H, Garnett MJ, Bottomley W et al (2002) Mutations of the BRAF gene in human cancer. Nature 417(6892):949–954. https://doi.org/10.1038/nature00766

Devesa SS, Bray F, Vizcaino AP, Parkin DM (2005) International lung cancer trends by histologic type: male: female differences diminishing and adenocarcinoma rates rising. Int J Cancer 117:294–299. https://doi.org/10.1002/ijc.21183

Dijk MV, Mundt CA, Ritter G, Schaer D, Wolchok JD, Merghoub T, Savitsky DA, Wilson NS (2019) Anti-ctla-4 antibodies and methods of use thereof. US20190135919A1, 9 May 2019

Gadiyar V, Patel G, Davra V (2020) Immunological role of TAM receptors in the cancer microenvironment. Int Rev Cell Mol Biol 357:57–79. https://doi.org/10.1016/bs.ircmb.2020.09.011

Galluzzi L, Spranger S, Fuchs E, López-Soto A (2019) WNT signaling in cancer immunosurveillance. Trends Cell Biol 29(1):44–65. https://doi.org/10.1016/j.tcb.2018.08.005

Goel S, Wong AH, Jain RK (2012) Vascular normalization as a therapeutic strategy for malignant and nonmalignant disease. Cold Spring Harb Perspect Med 2(3):a006486. https://doi.org/10.1101/cshperspect.a006486

Gout T (2012) Role of ATP binding and hydrolysis in the gating of the cystic fibrosis transmembrane conductance regulator. Ann Thorac Med 7(3):115–121. https://doi.org/10.4103/1817-1737.98842

Gowrishankar K, Gunatilake D, Gallagher SJ, Tiffen J, Rizos H, Hersey P (2015) Inducible but not constitutive expression of PD-L1 in human melanoma cells is dependent on activation of NF-κB. PLoS One 10(4):e0123410. https://doi.org/10.1371/journal.pone.0123410

Groner B, von Manstein V (2017) Jak Stat signaling and cancer: opportunities, benefits and side effects of targeted inhibition. Mol Cell Endocrinol 451:1–14. https://doi.org/10.1016/j.mce.2017.05.033

Groth C, Hu X, Weber R, Fleming V, Altevogt P, Utikal J, Umansky V (2019) Immunosuppression mediated by myeloid-derived suppressor cells (MDSCs) during tumour progression. Br J Cancer 120(1):16–25. https://doi.org/10.1038/s41416-018-0333-1

Gss PE, Strasser-Weippl K, Lee-Bychkovsky BL, Fan LLJ, Chavarri-Guerra Y, Liedke PER, Pramesh CS, Badovinac-Crnjevic T, Sheikine Y, Chen Z, Qiao Y-L, Shao Z et al (2014) Challenges to effective cancer control in China, India, and Russia. Lancet Oncol 15(5):489–538. https://doi.org/10.1016/S1470-2045(14)70029-4

Han Y, Liu D, Li L (2020) PD-1/PD-L1 pathway: current researches in cancer. Am J Cancer Res 10(3):727–742. PMID: 32266087; PMCID: PMC7136921

Hasin DS (2018) US epidemiology of cannabis use and associated problems. Neuropsychopharmacology 43(1):195–212. https://doi.org/10.1038/npp.2017.198

Hassanpour SH, Dehghani MA (2017) Review of cancer from perspective of molecular. J Cancer Res Pract 4(4):127–129. https://doi.org/10.1016/j.jcrpr.2017.07.001

Hellmann MD, Rizvi NA, Goldman JW, Gettinger SN, Borghaei H, Brahmer JR et al (2017) Nivolumab plus ipilimumab as first-line treatment for advanced nonsmall-cell lung cancer (CheckMate 012): results of an open-label, phase 1, multicohort study. Lancet Oncol 18(1):31–41

Hellmann MD, Ciuleanu TE, Pluzanski A, Lee JS, Otterson GA, AudigierValette C et al (2018) Nivolumab plus ipilimumab in lung cancer with a high tumor mutational burden. N Engl J Med 378(22):2093–2104

Jalali S, Price-Troska T, Bothun C, Villasboas J, Kim HJ, Yang ZZ, Novak AJ, Dong H, Ansell SM (2019) Reverse signaling via PD-L1 supports malignant cell growth and survival in classical Hodgkin lymphoma. Blood Cancer J 9(3):22. https://doi.org/10.1038/s41408-019-0185-9

Jiang X, Wang J, Deng X, Xiong F, Ge J, Xiang B, Wu X, Ma J, Zhou M, Li X, Li Y, Li G, Xiong W, Guo C, Zeng Z (2019) Role of the tumor microenvironment in PD-L1/PD-1-mediated tumor immune escape. Mol Cancer 18(1):10. https://doi.org/10.1186/s12943-018-0928-4. PMID: 30646912; PMCID: PMC6332843

Kim ES (2016) Chemotherapy resistance in lung cancer. Adv Exp Med Biol 893:189–209. https://doi.org/10.1007/978-3-319-24223-1_10

Klebe S, Leigh J, Henderson DW, Nurminen M (2019) Asbestos, smoking and lung cancer: an update. Int J Environ Res Public Health 17(1):258. https://doi.org/10.3390/ijerph17010258

Kotanides H, Li Y, Malabunga M, Carpenito C, Eastman SW, Shen Y, Wang G, Inigo I, Surguladze D, Pennello AL, Persaud K, Hindi S, Topper M, Chen X, Zhang Y, Bulaon DK, Bailey T, Lao Y, Han B, Torgerson S, Chin D, Sonyi A, Haidar JN, Novosiadly RD, Moxham CM, Plowman GD, Ludwig DL, Kalos M (2020) Bispecific targeting of PD-1 and PD-L1 enhances T-cell activation and antitumor immunity. Cancer Immunol Res 8(10):1300–1310. https://doi.org/10.1158/2326-6066.CIR-20-0304. Epub 2020 Jul 27. PMID: 32873605

Kou F, Wu L, Ren X, Yang L (2020) Chromosome abnormalities: new insights into their clinical significance in cancer. Mol Ther Oncolytics 17:562–570. https://doi.org/10.1016/j.omto.2020.05.010

Krebs MG, Sloane R, Priest L, Lancashire L, Hou JM, Greystoke A, Ward TH, Ferraldeschi R, Hughes A, Clack G et al (2011) Evaluation and prognostic significance of circulating tumor cells in patients with non-small-cell lung cancer. J Clin Oncol 29(12):1556–1563. https://doi.org/10.1200/JCO.2010.28.7045

Krewski D, Lubin JH, Zielinski JM, Alavanja M, Catalan VS, Field RW, Klotz JB, Létourneau EG, Lynch CF, Lyon JL et al (2006) A combined analysis of North American case-control studies of residential radon and lung cancer. J Toxicol Environ Health A 69(7):533–597. https://doi.org/10.1080/15287390500260945

Krummel MF, Allison JP (1996) CTLA-4 engagement inhibits IL-2 accumulation and cell cycle progression upon activation of resting T cells. J Exp Med 183:2533–2540

Landesman-Milo D, Ramishetti S, Peer D (2015) Nanomedicine as an emerging platform for metastatic lung cancer therapy. Cancer Metastasis Rev 34(2):291–301. https://doi.org/10.1007/s10555-015-9554-4

Lazebnik Y (2010) What are the hallmarks of cancer? Nat Rev Cancer 10(4):232–233. https://doi.org/10.1038/nrc2827

Li P, Huang T, Zou Q, Liu D, Wang Y, Tan X, Wei Y, Qiu H (2019) FGFR2 promotes expression of PD-L1 in colorectal cancer via the JAK/STAT3 signaling pathway. J Immunol (Baltimore, Md.: 1950) 202(10):3065–3075. https://doi.org/10.4049/jimmunol.1801199

Li H, Zhou L, Zhou J et al (2021) Underlying mechanisms and drug intervention strategies for the tumour microenvironment. J Exp Clin Cancer Res 40:97. https://doi.org/10.1186/s13046-021-01893-y

Linsley PS, Bradshaw J, Greene J et al (1996) Intracellular trafficking of CTLA-4 and focal localization towards sites of TCR engagement. Immunity 4:535–543

Liu P, He K, Li Y, Wu Q, Yang P, Wang D (2012) Exposure to mercury causes formation of male-specific structural deficits by inducing oxidative damage in nematodes. Ecotoxicol Environ Saf 79:90–100. https://doi.org/10.1016/j.ecoenv.2011.12.007

Liu G, Cheresh P, Kamp DW (2013) Molecular basis of asbestos-induced lung disease. Annu Rev Pathol 8:161–187. https://doi.org/10.1146/annurev-pathol-020712-163942

Lodish H, Berk A, Zipursky SL et al (2000) Molecular cell biology, 4th edn. W. H. Freeman, New York. Section 12.4, DNA Damage and Repair and Their Role in Carcinogenesis. https://www.ncbi.nlm.nih.gov/books/NBK21554/

Macé A, Kutalik Z, Valsesia A (2018) Copy number variation. Methods Mol Biol (Clifton, NJ) 1793:231–258. https://doi.org/10.1007/978-1-4939-7868-7_14

Magbanua MJ, Sosa EV, Scott JH, Simko J, Collins C, Pinkel D, Ryan CJ, Park JW (2012) Isolation and genomic analysis of circulating tumor cells from castration resistant metastatic prostate cancer. BMC Cancer 12:78. https://doi.org/10.1186/1471-2407-12-78

Mansoori B, Mohammadi A, Davudian S, Shirjang S, Baradaran B (2017) The different mechanisms of cancer drug resistance: a brief review. Adv Pharm Bull 7(3):339–348. https://doi.org/10.15171/apb.2017.041

Masteller EL, Chuang E, Mullen AC et al (2000) Structural analysis of CTLA-4 function in vivo. J Immunol 164:5319–5327

Matakidou A, Eisen T, Houlston RS (2005) Systematic review of the relationship between family history and lung cancer risk. Br J Cancer 93(7):825–833. https://doi.org/10.1038/sj.bjc.6602769

Mi Y, Guo N, Luan J, Cheng J, Hu Z, Jiang P, Jin W, Gao X (2020) The emerging role of myeloid-derived suppressor cells in the glioma immune suppressive microenvironment. Front Immunol 11:737. https://doi.org/10.3389/fimmu.2020.00737

Mulens-Arias V, Rojas JM, Pérez-Yagüe S, Morales MP, Barber DF (2015) Polyethylenimine-coated SPIONs trigger macrophage activation through TLR-4 signaling and ROS production and modulate podosome dynamics. Biomaterials 52:494–506. https://doi.org/10.1016/j.biomaterials.2015.02.068

Neel BG, Gu H, Pao L (2003) The 'Shp'ing news: SH2 domain-containing tyrosine phosphatases in cell signaling. Trends Biochem Sci 28:284–293

Ni X, Zhuo M, Su Z, Duan J, Gao Y, Wang Z, Zong C, Bai H, Chapman AR, Zhao J et al (2013) Reproducible copy number variation patterns among single circulating tumor cells of lung cancer patients. Proc Natl Acad Sci U S A 110(52):21083–21088. https://doi.org/10.1073/pnas.1320659110

Nurgali K, Jagoe RT, Abalo R (2018) Editorial: adverse effects of cancer chemotherapy: anything new to improve tolerance and reduce sequelae? Front Pharmacol 9:245. https://doi.org/10.3389/fphar.2018.00245
Pardoll DM (2012) The blockade of immune checkpoints in cancer immunotherapy. Nat Rev Cancer 12(4):252–264
Pawelczyk K, Piotrowska A, Ciesielska U, Jablonska K, Gletzel-Plucinska N, Grzegrzolka J, Podhorska-Okolow M, Dziegiel P, Nowinska K (2019) Role of PD-L1 expression in non-small cell lung cancer and their prognostic significance according to clinicopathological factors and diagnostic markers. Int J Mol Sci 20(4):824. https://doi.org/10.3390/ijms20040824
Perkins D, Wang Z, Donovan C, He H, Mark D, Guan G et al (1996) Regulation of CTLA-4 expression during T cell activation. J Immunol 156(11):4154–4159
Phuengkham H, Ren L, Shin IW, Lim YT (2019) Nanoengineered immune niches for reprogramming the immunosuppressive tumor microenvironment and enhancing cancer immunotherapy. Adv Mater (Deerfield Beach, FL) 31(34):e1803322. https://doi.org/10.1002/adma.201803322
Piccirillo CA, Shevach EM (2004) Naturally-occurring CD4 + CD25 + immunoregulatory T cells: central players in the arena of peripheral tolerance. Semin Immunol 16:81–88
Pol J, Kroemer G (2018) RESEARCH HIGHLIGHT Anti-CTLA-4 immunotherapy: uncoupling toxicity and efficacy. Cell Res 28:501–502. https://doi.org/10.1038/s41422-018-0031-9
Pradhan R, Singhvi G, Dubey SK, Gupta G, Dua K (2019) MAPK pathway: a potential target for the treatment of non-small-cell lung carcinoma. Future Med Chem 11(8):793–795. https://doi.org/10.4155/fmc-2018-0468
Ready N, Hellmann MD, Awad MM, Otterson GA, Gutierrez M, Gainor JF et al (2019) First-line nivolumab plus ipilimumab in advanced non-small-cell lung cancer (CheckMate 568): outcomes by programmed death ligand 1 and tumor mutational burden as biomarkers. J Clin Oncol 37(12):992–1000
Ribas A, Kefford R, Marshall MA, Punt CJ, Haanen JB, Marmol M et al (2013) Phase III randomized clinical trial comparing tremelimumab with standard-of-care chemotherapy in patients with advanced melanoma. J Clin Oncol 31(5):616–622. https://doi.org/10.1200/jco.2012.44.6112
Rodrigo GJ, Plaza V, Castro-Rodríguez JA (2012) Comparison of three combined pharmacological approaches with tiotropium monotherapy in stable moderate to severe COPD: a systematic review. Pulm Pharmacol Ther 25(1):40–47. https://doi.org/10.1016/j.pupt.2011.10.006
Rowshanravan B, Halliday N, Sansom DM (2018) CTLA-4: a moving target in immunotherapy. Blood 131(1):58–67. https://doi.org/10.1182/blood-2017-06-741033
Sanmamed MF, Chen L (2014) Inducible expression of B7-H1 (PD-L1) and its selective role in tumor site immune modulation. Cancer J 20:256–261
Schadendorf D, Hodi FS, Robert C, Weber JS, Margolin K, Hamid O, Patt D, Chen TT, Berman DM, Wolchok JD (2015) Pooled analysis of long-term survival data from phase II and phase III trials of ipilimumab in unresectable or metastatic melanoma. J Clin Oncol 33(17):1889–1894. https://doi.org/10.1200/jco.2014.56.2736
Schneider H, Downey J, Smith A et al (2006) Reversal of the TCR stop signal by CTLA-4. Science 313:1972–1975
Seto M, Honma K, Nakagawa M (2010) Diversity of genome profiles in malignant lymphoma. Cancer Sci 101(3):573–578. https://doi.org/10.1111/j.1349-7006.2009.01452.x
Singhal S, Stadanlick J, Annunziata MJ et al (2019) Human tumor-associated monocytes/macrophages and their regulation of T cell responses in early-stage lung cancer. Sci Transl Med 11(479):eaat1500
Skoda AM, Simovic D, Karin V, Kardum V, Vranic S, Serman L (2018) The role of the Hedgehog signaling pathway in cancer: a comprehensive review. Bosn J Basic Med Sci 18(1):8–20. https://doi.org/10.17305/bjbms.2018.2756
Stutvoet TS, Kol A, de Vries EG, de Bruyn M, Fehrmann RS, Terwisscha van Scheltinga AG, de Jong S (2019) MAPK pathway activity plays a key role in PD-L1 expression of lung adenocarcinoma cells. J Pathol 249(1):52–64. https://doi.org/10.1002/path.5280

Takahashi T, Tagami T, Yamazaki S et al (2000) Immunologic self-tolerance maintained by CD25(+) CD4(+) regulatory T cells constitutively expressing cytotoxic T lymphocyte-associated antigen 4. J Exp Med 192:303–309

Tammela T, Zarkada G, Wallgard E, Murtomäki A, Suchting S, Wirzenius M, Waltari M, Hellström M, Schomber T, Peltonen R et al (2008) Blocking VEGFR-3 suppresses angiogenic sprouting and vascular network formation. Nature 454(7204):656–660. https://doi.org/10.1038/nature07083

Taniguchi K, Karin M (2018) NF-κB, inflammation, immunity and cancer: coming of age. Nat Rev Immunol 18:309–324. https://doi.org/10.1038/nri.2017.142

Tashkin DP, Ferguson GT (2013) Combination bronchodilator therapy in the management of chronic obstructive pulmonary disease. Respir Res 14(1):49. https://doi.org/10.1186/1465-9921-14-49

Travis WD, Travis LB, Devesa SS (1995) Lung cancer. Cancer 75(1 Suppl):191–202

Travis WD, Brambilla E, Noguchi M, Nicholson AG, Geisinger KR, Yatabe Y, Beer DG, Powell CA, Riely GJ, Van Schil PE, Garg K (2011) International association for the study of lung cancer/American thoracic society/European respiratory society international multidisciplinary classification of lung adenocarcinoma. J Thorac Oncol 6(2):244–285. https://doi.org/10.1097/JTO.0b013e318206a221

Travis WD, Brambilla E, Nicholson AG, Yatabe Y, Austin JHM, Beasley MB, Chirieac LR, Dacic S, Duhig E, Flieder DB, Geisinger K, WHO Panel (2015) The 2015 World Health Organization classification of lung tumors: impact of genetic, clinical and radiologic advances since the 2004 classification. J Thorac Oncol 10(9):1243–1260. https://doi.org/10.1097/JTO.0000000000000630

Van der Heyden JHA, Schaap MM, Kunst AE, Esnaola S, Borrell C, Cox B, Leinsalu M, Stirbu I, Kalediene R, Deboosere P, Mackenbach JP, Van Oyen H (2009) Socioeconomic inequalities in lung cancer mortality in 16 European populations. Lung Cancer 63(3):322–330. https://doi.org/10.1016/j.lungcan.2008.06.006

Walters S, Maringe C, Coleman MP, Peake MD, Butler J, Young N, Bergström S, Hanna L, Jakobsen E, Kölbeck K et al (2013) Lung cancer survival and stage at diagnosis in Australia, Canada, Denmark, Norway, Sweden and the UK: a population-based study, 2004-2007. Thorax 68(6):551–564. https://doi.org/10.1136/thoraxjnl-2012-202297

Wei SC, Duffy CR, Allison JP (2018) Fundamental mechanisms of immune checkpoint blockade therapy. Cancer Discov 8(9):1069–1086. https://doi.org/10.1158/2159-8290.cd-18-0367

Weir BA, Woo MS, Getz G, Perner S, Ding L, Beroukhim R, Lin WM, Province MA, Kraja A, Johnson LA et al (2007) Characterizing the cancer genome in lung adenocarcinoma. Nature 450(7171):893–898. https://doi.org/10.1038/nature06358

Wherry EJ (2011) T cell exhaustion. Nat Immunol 12:492–499

WHO global report on trends in prevalence of tobacco smoking 2000–2025, 2nd edn. WHO. https://apps.who.int/iris/handle/10665/272694. Accessed 2 Dec 2020

Wing K, Onishi Y, Prieto-Martin P et al (2008a) CTLA-4 control over Foxp3 + regulatory T cell function. Science 322:271–275

Wing K, Onishi Y, Prieto-Martin P, Yamaguchi T, Miyara M, Fehervari Z et al (2008b) CTLA-4 control over Foxp3+ regulatory T cell function. Science 322(5899):271–275

Wojtukiewicz MZ, Rek MM, Karpowicz K, Górska M, Polityńska B, Wojtukiewicz AM, Moniuszko M, Radziwon P, Tucker SC, Honn KV (2021) Inhibitors of immune checkpoints—PD-1, PD-L1, CTLA-4—new opportunities for cancer patients and a new challenge for internists and general practitioners. Cancer Metastasis Rev 40:949–982. https://doi.org/10.1007/s10555-021-09976-0

Yang H, Rivera Z, Jube S, Nasu M, Bertino P, Goparaju C, Franzoso G, Lotze MT, Krausz T, Pass HI, Bianchi ME, Carbone M (2010) Programmed necrosis induced by asbestos in human mesothelial cells causes high-mobility group box 1 protein release and resultant inflammation. Proc Natl Acad Sci U S A 107(28):12611–12616. https://doi.org/10.1073/pnas.1006542107

Yu H, Boyle TA, Zhou C, Rimm DL, Hirsch FR (2016) PD-L1 expression in lung cancer. J Thorac Oncol 11(7):964–975. https://doi.org/10.1016/j.jtho.2016.04.014

Zanganeh S, Hutter G, Spitler R, Lenkov O, Mahmoudi M, Shaw A, Pajarinen JS, Nejadnik H, Goodman S et al (2016) Iron oxide nanoparticles inhibit tumour growth by inducing pro-inflammatory macrophage polarization in tumour tissues. Nat Nanotechnol 11(11):986–994. https://doi.org/10.1038/nnano.2016.168

Zappa C, Mousa SA (2016) Non-small cell lung cancer: current treatment and future advances. Transl Lung Cancer Res 5(3):288–300. https://doi.org/10.21037/tlcr.2016.06.07

Zhang J, Fujimoto J, Zhang J, Wedge DC, Song X, Zhang J, Seth S, Chow CW, Cao Y, Gumbs C, Gold KA et al (2014) Intratumor heterogeneity in localized lung adenocarcinomas delineated by multiregion sequencing. Science (New York, NY) 346(6206):256–259. https://doi.org/10.1126/science.1256930

Zhang H, Bi Y, Wei Y, Liu J, Kuerban K, Ye L (2021) Blocking Wnt/β-catenin signal amplifies Anti-PD-1 therapeutic efficacy by inhibiting tumor growth, migration, and promoting immune infiltration in glioblastomas. Mol Cancer Ther 20(7):1305–1315. https://doi.org/10.1158/1535-7163.MCT-20-0825

Zhao Y, Yang W, Huang Y, Cui R, Li X, Li B (2018) Evolving roles for targeting CTLA-4 in cancer immunotherapy. Cell Physiol Biochem 47(2):721–734. https://doi.org/10.1159/000490025

Zhao R, Song Y, Wang Y, Huang Y, Li Z, Cui Y, Yi M, Xia L, Zhuang W, Wu X, Zhou Y (2019) PD-1/PD-L1 blockade rescue exhausted CD8+ T cells in gastrointestinal stromal tumours via the PI3K/Akt/mTOR signalling pathway. Cell Prolif 52(3):e12571. https://doi.org/10.1111/cpr.12571

Zhou Y, Chen X, Cao J, Gao H (2020) Overcoming the biological barriers in the tumor microenvironment for improving drug delivery and efficacy. J Mater Chem B 8(31):6765–6781. https://doi.org/10.1039/d0tb00649a

Zhou L, Xu Q, Huang L, Jin J, Zuo X, Zhang Q, Ye L, Zhu S, Zhan P, Ren J, Lv T, Song Y (2021) Low-dose carboplatin reprograms tumor immune microenvironment through STING signaling pathway and synergizes with PD-1 inhibitors in lung cancer. Cancer Lett 500:163–171. https://doi.org/10.1016/j.canlet.2020.11.049

Zhu J, Li Y, Lv X (2023) IL4I1 enhances PD-L1 expression through JAK/STAT signaling pathway in lung adenocarcinoma. Immunogenetics 75:17–25. https://doi.org/10.1007/s00251-022-01275-4

16 Synergistic Potential of Antigen-Specific Vaccines and Immunomodulatory Agents for Lung Cancer Treatment

Suresh Krishna Venkataramanan, Nithya Shree Raman, Karthika Rangasamy, Sree Gayathri Ganapathy, Pavithra Vimala Arulrajan, Shibi Muralidar, Gayathri Gopal, and Senthil Visaga Ambi

16.1 Introduction

Lung cancer is a one of the most fatal types of cancer which has been associated with thousands of deaths in the global population. With a very low survival rate, lung cancer-associated deaths are majorly attributed to their late diagnosis in advance stages. The most common subtype of lung cancer, non-small cell lung cancer (NSCLC), accounts for 85% of lung cancer cases, and it is less responsive to existing treatment strategies such as chemotherapies, radiotherapies, and surgical treatments. According to a survey conducted in 2012, 1,800,000 new instances of lung cancer were recorded; 1,600,000 of these cases resulted in fatalities, making the mortality rate for lung cancer as 87% in a single year. It is the second most frequent factor in both men's and women's cancer-related fatalities (Altaf et al. 2022).

Thus, patients with lung cancer must be diagnosed early and intervened in their early stage. Increasing knowledge and exploration on the molecular biology and

S. K. Venkataramanan · N. S. Raman · K. Rangasamy · S. G. Ganapathy · P. V. Arulrajan · S. Muralidar
Biopharmaceutical Research Lab, Anusandhan Kendra-1, School of Chemical and Biotechnology, SASTRA Deemed-to-be-University, Thanjavur, Tamil Nadu, India

G. Gopal · S. V. Ambi (✉)
Biopharmaceutical Research Lab, Anusandhan Kendra-1, School of Chemical and Biotechnology, SASTRA Deemed-to-be-University, Thanjavur, Tamil Nadu, India

Department of Bioengineering, School of Chemical and Biotechnology, SASTRA Deemed-to-be-University, Thanjavur, Tamil Nadu, India
e-mail: senthilvisagaambi@scbt.sastra.edu

S. Bhatt et al. (eds.), *Immunotherapy Against Lung Cancer*,
https://doi.org/10.1007/978-981-99-7141-1_16

pathways associated with lung cancer in the recent decades have radically provided insightful management strategies against lung cancer. Recent advances in immunotherapy and immunomodulatory approaches targeting lung cancer have significantly contributed to improved outcomes in the diseased population. Further, combinatorial treatment strategies are extensively explored to enhance the anticancer immunity that could play a major role in combating the disease progression (Matsushita and Kawaguchi 2018; Altaf et al. 2022). In this line, apart from immunomodulatory and immunotherapy, therapeutic cancer vaccines are a novel intriguing aspect that are recently explored in cancer research. With increasing evidential knowledge on tumor-associated antigens, native immune response and novel antigen delivery technologies have enabled enhanced vaccine design. The ultimate goal of these therapeutic vaccines is to establish a persisting anti-tumor memory and induction of tumor regression with less or no adverse reactions. Tumor-induced immunoresistance and immunosuppression are still a major challenge to overcome in this approach (Saxena et al. 2021).

In this chapter, we summarized the different types of lung cancer vaccines and their effect on host immune response. This chapter also briefly speaks about the existing pros and cons of these vaccines and their clinical efficacy. Apart from conventional treatment options such as chemotherapy, radiotherapy, and surgical treatment, this chapter discusses about the existing immunomodulators and their efficacy in treating lung cancer. Also, we have focused on emerging immunomodulatory therapeutic agents that are currently being developed to tackle lung cancer. Finally, this chapter has discussed the synergistic ability of combining vaccines and immunomodulators in lung cancer. This chapter would provide a roadmap to its reader on existing cancer vaccines, emerging immunomodulatory agents, and the effect of combinatorial treatment (vaccines and immunomodulatory agents) in treating lung cancer patients.

16.2 Cancer Vaccine

The idea behind cancer vaccine is same as any other vaccine which prepares the host immune system by activating an immune response against a specific antigen which might be later useful in mounting a heightened immune response against the same antigen in its next onset. Cancer vaccine can be a therapeutic vaccine to treat existing cancer patients or preventive vaccines that can prevent any future occurrence of tumors. The main parameters determining the success of a vaccine are the antigens used and the adjuvant accompanying it. The cardinal goal of any therapeutic cancer vaccine might be activating the adaptive immune response by targeting the antigen to an effective antigen-presenting cell (dendritic cell) (Pardoll 1998).

16.2.1 Whole Tumor Cell Vaccine

One of the very first cancer vaccines analyzed used the whole tumor cell as an antigen which contains the cancer neoantigens as well as the antigens expressed by normal cells. The tumor cells may be obtained from existing cancer patient and then injected into the patients in vitro (autologous) or from established cancer cell line (allogeneic) (Tagliamonte et al. 2014). A clinical trial (Neller et al. 2008) was conducted on patients possessing different types of cancers to compare the results between tumor cell vaccine and tumor antigen-specific vaccine. The results of the study showed that compared to tumor-specific antigen, whole tumor cell vaccine showed better clinical response in the cancer patients since tumor cell may contain different array of tumor antigens that have a higher efficacy of activating the T-cell responses when compared to the single identified tumor antigen as in the latter case (Chiang et al. 2010). Generally, the release of some inflammatory cytokines or danger signals such as heat shock proteins and uric acid induces the expression of co-stimulatory molecule on the surface of the antigen-presenting cell (APC) such as B7. This interaction is vital for the activation the T-cell responses, and failure of any such action will lead to immune tolerance. In order to evade this immune tolerance, the vaccine will contain excess tumor cells that are undergoing necrosis which release danger signals that can be picked up, processed, and presented by the dendritic cell (Ward et al. 2002). Killing of tumor cells is necessary because the tumor cells secrete TGF-β (transforming growth factor beta) and IL-10 (interleukin-10) that can suppress the immune system and impair dendritic cell (DC) maturation. Similar to necrotic tumor cells, apoptotic cells can also be used in cancer vaccines after irradiation by UV rays. Apoptosis is normally immunologically silent since the antigen will be expressed endogenously, but the irradiation causes the calreticulin to move onto the surface of the apoptotic tumor cell from its endoplasmic reticulum which can be detected by the dendritic cells and initiate cytotoxic T-cell responses. Other than this, the extracellular vesicles known as exosomes secreted by the stressed tumor cells are also shown to induce immunogenicity (Chiang et al. 2010). In a clinical trial, autologous tumor vaccine Belagenpumatucel-L that has TGF-β2 antisense plasmid can improve the survival of individuals with non-small cell lung cancer (NSCLC) since the immunosuppressive TGF-β2 levels can be reduced at the site of vaccination (Brahmer 2013).

16.2.2 Tumor-Specific Antigen Vaccine

Rather than using the whole cell, specific antigens expressed by the tumor cell can be used in the vaccine along with the adjuvant. Tumor antigens are subdivided as tumor-associated antigens (TAA) and tumor-specific antigens (TSA). The former is found in both tumor cells and normal cells whereas the TSA are found only in cancer cells. TAA can be further classified based on whether they are expressed exclusively on a single tumor type (unique) or expressed broadly over a range of tumor cell types (shared). TAA are either expressed only on cancer cells wherein their expressions in a normal cell are silenced (cancer testis) or overexpressed on cancer cells when compared to normal cells. TAA can also be antigens expressed on the tissue from which the tumor originated (Tagliamonte et al. 2014). Melanoma-associated antigen-A3 is an antigen that is expressed only by tumor cells predominantly on melanoma cells but also in some of the NSCLC (Brahmer 2013). The antigenic epitopes may be formulated in the vaccines as either peptides or nucleic acids encoding them. Multipeptides are more effective in eliciting immune response than the single peptide vaccines because the antigen-presenting cells may sometimes fail to uptake/recognize a single epitope (Hu et al. 2018). Tumor antigens that arise due to point mutations are more specific and hence are capable of eliciting a greater extent of immune response than other tumor antigens (Jäger et al. 2001). Even though identifying an optimal tumor antigen is the major step in the process, antigen to which the immune system responds may also change from the selected specific antigen to another antigen during the next wave of the immune response in a process called epitope or determinant spreading. This process in which the target changes to a more potent epitope on same or different antigen that can induce the T-cells to suppress the tumor cells more efficiently (Butterfield 2015). Tumor neoantigens that arise due to mutations on the tumor cells which are not expressed on normal cells are also considered as an effective candidate since they can evade central tolerance. Studies have shown that neoantigen activates preferably helper T-cells over cytotoxic T-cell and it is also shown that the patients who respond positively to the neoantigen vaccine also respond well to anti-PD1 (programmed cell death protein-1) treatment indicating a clear synergy between the cancer vaccine and immunomodulatory agents (Saxena et al. 2021). Clinical trials have shown clear connections between the neoantigen load and their respective cytotoxic T-cell activity on patients with lung cancer (Hu et al. 2018).

16.2.3 Host Immune Response

Despite their types, all cancer vaccines work on same goal of presenting the tumor antigen to the dendritic cells that can ultimately activate the T-cells to infiltrate into the tumor microenvironment and repress the tumor cells. Once the antigen is detected by the dendritic cells, it is processed by either cytosolic or vacuolar pathway and gets translocated to the MHC (major histocompatibility complex) molecule before moving to the secondary lymphoid organs where the immune cells to which the antigen can be presented will be surplus in number. The interaction between the MHC molecule presenting the processed antigen and the receptors on T-cells activates both $CD4^+$ and $CD8^+$ T-cells which then relocate toward the tumor microenvironment to kill the tumor cells. Though the $CD4^+$ T-cells do not have direct tumor killing effect, it is shown that they can greatly amplify the $CD8^+$ T-cells to do the same (Saxena et al. 2021). $CD8^+$ T-cells specific to the tumor antigen are produced when they interact with antigen-loaded DCs and get stimulated by T_{h1} cytokines, whereas on the other hand, the interaction between the DC with MHC class II antigen and B cells in the presence of T_{h2} cytokines leads to tumor antigen-specific antibodies (Hirshowitz et al. 2006). T_{reg} cells which are known to have immunosuppressive effect on the cytotoxic T-cells and the T helper cells are found in higher number when compared to other T-cell subsets in the tumor microenvironment of the lung cancer patients (Brahmer 2013). Hence the suppression of the T_{reg} cells may provide an ideal environment for lung cancer treatment. Interestingly, a glycoprotein CD47 known as the integrin-associated protein is overexpressed on the tumor cells when compared to normal cells. This protein can protect the tumor cells from the macrophage detection, and hence anti-CD47 agents are also studied whether they can expose the tumor cells to the host immune system (Wu et al. 2021).

16.2.4 Pros and Cons of Cancer Vaccines

Both types of cancer vaccines have their own advantages as well as disadvantages and their appropriate usage depends on the application and the constraints present. The primary shortcoming of preparing the tumor antigen specific vaccine is that identifying the optimal antigen is difficult whereas the whole tumor cell vaccine bypasses this step by containing a relevant array of antigen rather than single antigen but suffers from the fact that the variables to be accounted for are more and hence the analysis of their immune response is difficult. Also enough tumor specimen must be present for the production of autologous whole tumor cell vaccine (Offringa et al. 2000). Since the whole tumor cell contain many antigens that are also expressed by normal cells, this may result in immune tolerance which is not the case in tumor specific antigen (Tagliamonte et al. 2014). In addition to possessing the threat of generating autoimmunity, tumor-associated antigen generates weaker immune response when compared to tumor-specific antigen. In neoantigen vaccines, the number of epitopes to be included in the vaccine should be determined precisely to avoid the long production time and also to improve the clinical efficacy of the vaccine (Saxena et al. 2021). The adjuvants used along with the vaccine are also known to have potential side effects (Liu 2014).

16.3 Immune Modulators

Immune modulation is now the most effective cancer therapy approach, the most significant area of study in clinical and translational cancer research, and likely our best, most realistic chance for curing pulmonary neoplasms and other malignancies in the near future. The function of the immunomodulatory agents is to eliminate tumor cell defenses, activate the strength of the immune system, and then utilize it to eradicate cancer cells. With few to no side effects on healthy organs, efficient immunotherapeutic medicines use the immune system's capabilities to target cancer cells. Furthermore, immune system manipulation is believed to be persistent due to the fact that it encompasses immunologic memory in addition to high specificity and reliability (Wang et al. 2022).

16.3.1 Role in Lung Cancer

Lung cancer patients now have a promising new therapeutic option generally referred to as immunotherapy. The immune system of the body can be circumvented by cancer cells, allowing them to spread unabated. Immunomodulators can help stimulate the immune system, improving its capacity to identify and eliminate cancer cells.

Immunotherapy is a method that has been proven to be successful in treating some kinds of lung cancer. They either trigger the immune system's defense against cancer cells or they block the immune system-inhibiting proteins made by cancer cells.

Checkpoint inhibitors, a class of immunomodulators used for diagnosing lung cancer, inhibit cancer cells from expressing the proteins that can evade the immune system. Immune checkpoint proteins like PD-1 and programmed cell death protein ligand-1 (PD-L1) are important in downregulating the immune response, and monoclonal antibodies like pembrolizumab and nivolumab target these proteins (Altaf et al. 2022). By inhibiting these proteins from functioning, these antibodies can raise immune system against cancer cells. Immunomodulatory antibodies against PD-L1/CD274 and cytotoxic T-cell-associated antigen 4 (CTLA-4/CD152) have been clinically used in lung cancer patients (Aerts and Hegmans 2013). Immunomodulatory drugs stimulate the activation and clonal differentiation of T-cells by phosphorylating CD28, which consequently activates both helper and cytotoxic T-cells (Matsushita and Kawaguchi 2018).

Lung cancer growth and spread are also influenced by an assortment of signaling pathways that involve the phosphoinositide 3 kinase (PI3K)/protein kinase B (AKT)/(mechanistic target of rapamycin) mTOR pathway, the Wnt signaling pathway, and the Notch pathway. The development and spread of lung cancer can be facilitated by the deregulation of several pathways, which control cellular proliferation, differentiation, and mortality. Main mutations found in NSCLC and SCLC that promote cell growth and division are Kirsten rat sarcoma (KRAS), anaplastic lymphoma kinase (ALK), ROS1 rearrangements, mutations in epidermal growth factor receptor (EGFR) (Maemondo et al. 2010), TP53, and RB1 (Camidge et al. 2012).

The treatment of lung cancer is frequently used with other medications to improve patient results. Particularly when used in conjunction with other treatments like chemotherapy and radiation therapy, immunomodulators have shown potential as a lung cancer treatment. In people with advanced NSCLC, for instance, combinatorial treatment of pembrolizumab and chemotherapy increased overall survival, nivolumab and ipilimumab have been used in conjunction (Altaf et al. 2022). Certain forms of lung cancer, notably NSCLC, have been proven to respond well to immunomodulators.

16.3.2 Immune Checkpoint Molecules

The adaptive immune response relies on two signals provided by APCs typically a dendritic cell, for the naive T-cell activation. The T-cell receptor and a class I or class II antigenic peptide of the MHC generate the first signal. The next signal is a costimulatory signal that is mediated between CD28 present on the T-cell surface and B7 molecule on the APCs. Both signals cause T-cells to become activated and to multiply clonally. Once the T-cell has been activated, it starts expressing CTLA-4 which is a homologue of CD28 and a member of immunoglobulin superfamily (Tomasini et al. 2012). When compared to CD28, CTLA-4 is mostly found in intracellular vesicles.

CTLA-4 competes with CD28 receptor for binding to B7 molecules on APCs. Both CTLA-4 and CD28 have similar structures and can bind to CD80 and CD86 of B7 family. However, while CD28 binding to B7 molecules produces a stimulatory signal that promotes T-cell activation and proliferation, CTLA-4 binding to B7 molecules transmits an inhibitory signal that suppresses T-cell activation and proliferation. Therefore, the equilibrium between the blocking and stimulatory signals delivered by CTLA-4 and CD28 is critical for regulating the strength and duration of T-cell responses in the immune system (Wang et al. 2022).

PD-1 is a protein primarily found on activated T-cells and has three domains. PD-1 binds with its counterparts PD-L1 and PD-L2 through its IgV domain (immunoglobulin variable domain) and sends a signal to inhibit T-cell activation when activated. This is important in preventing excessive immune activation and tissue damage. However, overexpression of PD-1 can led to immune suppression and contribute to cancer or chronic infections. Therefore, blocking PD-1 or its ligands has become an important strategy in immunotherapy (Wang et al. 2022). Increased PD-1 expression is correlated to cytotoxic T-cell malfunction and decreased immunological response in NSCLC. These proteins may also promote tumor growth by releasing matrix metalloproteinases and triggering angiogenesis (Dasanu et al. 2012).

Moreover, this signaling pathway can be utilized to control the magnitude and severity of the immune response, as well as by cancer cells to escape detection by the immune system. The immune system has built-in inhibitory mechanisms to maintain self-tolerance, which tumor cells use to evade detection by the immune system. In order to sustain themselves, tumor cells overexpress the receptors and inhibitory ligands which govern T-cell effector functions. After the blocking of these immunological checkpoints, antigen-specific T-cell responses have come to its original state. When it comes to immune checkpoint inhibitors (ICI)s, the PD-1 and CTLA-4 have undergone significant research and have proven to be promising therapeutic targets (Wang et al. 2022).

16.3.3 Monoclonal Antibody

The inhibition of immune checkpoints is a highly developing area of study for boosting the immune response against cancer cells. Many monoclonal antibodies are directed against the immune checkpoint molecules and generates anti-tumor response by enhancing the T-cell activation. Among all the various immune checkpoint inhibitors, ipilimumab works against the surface protein known as CTLA-4, which blocks T-cell activation. It is fully humanized IgG1 antibody with a molecular weight of around 148 kDa (Wang et al. 2022). Ipilimumab overcomes ligand competition by binding to CTLA-4 and interacting with the recognition site of CTLA-4:CD28, increasing T-cell recognition of tumor antigens and the subsequent activation of the immune response against tumor (Pinto et al. 2019). This is now being tested in the treatment of lung and prostate cancer. A phase II study showed that the individuals with advanced NSCLC treated with the combination of ipilimumab and chemotherapy have enhanced progression-free survival (PFS) compared to the chemotherapy treatment (Champiat et al. 2014). A novel and intriguing instance of pseudo progression was seen in ipilimumab trials. It suggests a temporary rise in the size of the lesions followed by considerable improvement over time. As a consequence, stopping this drug after an apparent early relapse might be inappropriate (Dasanu et al. 2012).

Like ipilimumab, several other monoclonal antibodies are being made against PD-1 receptors. Several anti-PD-1 medications are currently being developed, including nivolumab and lambrolizumab (MK-3475). A completely human IgG4 monoclonal antibody called nivolumab targets the PD-1 receptor with specificity. In a study involving around 300 patients with resistant solid tumors, including 120 patients with NSCLC, nivolumab demonstrated a promising range of efficacy (Rolfo et al. 2014). Nivolumab was tested in two phase I studies for its efficacy and feasibility in patients who had advanced refractory solid tumors, including lung cancer. This drug was well accepted, and its clinical effects over all cancer types were monitored. The evaluation of these reactions is underway, and it is possible that phase II studies may be planned in the near future (Gaissmaier and Christopoulos 2021). Lambrolizumab is a monoclonal antibody used in cancer immunotherapy. It targets the PD-1 receptor and is used to treat several forms of cancer, including NSCLC. By binding to PD-1 on T-cells, lambrolizumab blocks the inhibitory signals transmitted by the PD-1 receptor, thereby enhancing the immune response against cancer cells. A trial in phase Ib examined the use of the combination of chemotherapy with lambrolizumab as the initial treatment for non-squamous NSCLC. The trials have shown that lambrolizumab is effective and safe for treating NSCLC.

16.3.4 Emerging Immune Checkpoint Inhibitors: Novel Target for the Treatment of NSCLC

(a) VISTA

VISTA (V domain-containing Ig suppressor of T-cell activation) is a type I transmembrane protein with 279 amino acids, is mostly found on helper T-cells, and is strongly found in myeloid cells (Popovic et al. 2018). It shares a great deal of homology with CD 28, PD-1, and CTLA-4. VISTA gives the function of both a receptor and a ligand, depending on the context in which it is expressed. Ligands of VISTA include VSIG 3 and PSGL-1. Phase I research on CA-170 has demonstrated its efficacy and safety (Mahoney et al. 2015).

(b) LAG-3

LAG-3 (lymphocyte activation gene 3) is a molecule that acts as a co-inhibitor and has a significant role in suppressing the immune response (Goldberg and Drake 2011). Similar to VISTA, LAG-3 is also a type I transmembrane protein expressed in tumor-infiltrating lymphocytes like NK cells, CD4+ cells, and CD8+ cells. Galectin-3 and liver sinusoidal endothelial cell lectin (LSECtin) are ligands for LAG-3 (Wang et al. 2022). LAG-3 shares structural homology to CD4. Due to this reason, this target binds to MHC-II strongly producing inhibitory signals with a higher affinity when compared to CD4. Also, it affects CD8+ activity. This LAG-3 level is elevated along with some other inhibitory receptors like PD-1, TIM-3, and so on. Previous research asserted that LAG-3 works in collaboration with PD-1 to dampen the immune response by preventing the generation of cytokines, making LAG-3 blockage less effective. Anti-LAG-3 blocking mAb BMS-986016 (relatlimab), which has undergone a phase I trial, was evaluated for its efficacy in patients with advanced illnesses when used alone or in combination with nivolumab. The outcome showed that the medication had an excellent safety profile.

(c) TIM-3

The protein TIM-3, a member of the TIM family, is abundantly expressed in myeloid cells such as dendritic cells, macrophages, and monocytes. Galectin-9 (Gal-9), high mobility group protein B1 (HMGB1), carcinoembryonic antigen cell adhesion molecule 1 (CAECAM-1), and phosphatidyl serine (PtdSer) are four TIM 3 receptor's ligands (Wang et al. 2022). Gal-9 is the first TIM-3 ligand discovered and interacts with the carbohydrate motif on TIM-3 to promote apoptosis in Th_2 cells by causing a calcium influx to their intracellular region. The removal of apoptotic bodies and the cross-presentation of antigen by dendritic cells are both mediated by interactions between PtdSer and the Ig V domain of TIM-3. The TIM-3 protein can promote T-cell activation or suppress T-cell activation and has both positive and negative effects. CEACAM-1 (carcinoembryonic antigen-related cell adhesion molecule 1) is involved in the antiviral response regulation. The connection between HMGB1 and TIM-3 is yet not completely understood. It should be emphasized that the TIM-3 inhibitor increases anti-tumor activity in a manner similar to that of other immunomodulators (Du et al. 2017).

Two patients whose samples were not subjected to anti-PD-1 antibody therapy were studied. From the moment their diseases started, both anti-PD-1-treated patients' effusions demonstrated signs of therapeutic antibody binding to CD4 and CD8 T-cells. Studies shown that other immune checkpoint molecules including TIM-3 and LAG-3 can increase CTLA-4 expression, but there was no significant increase in the expression of other markers. Additionally, it was noted that CD8 T-cells had highly elevated CTLA-4 expression (Koyama et al. 2016).

16.3.5 Integrating Chemotherapy with Immune Checkpoint Inhibitors

Conventional treatments have the power to alter immune function. The National Medical Products Administration (NMPA) has granted permission for the use of novel combination therapies that can improve the overall response rate (ORR) and PFS compared to conventional monotherapy. BLP25 is a vaccine that acts against mucin 1 that is prominent in adenocarcinomas and NSCLC. In a clinical study, patients were administered with BLP25 vaccine along with a minimal dose of cyclophosphamide, and the patients who received vaccine showed good response. In another clinical trial,

148 patients who are currently in stages III/IV received the TG4010 vaccination, which targets mucin 1, along with concurrent administration of cisplatin and gemcitabine. The group that received vaccination along with the chemotherapy had progression-free survival for 6 months. This implies that certain combinations may have synergistic effects. Combining immunosuppressive agents with chemotherapy has been proposed as a way to evaluate the possibility of long-lasting anticancer effects (Mok et al. 2019). The advantage of using ICI along with chemotherapy (ICI-chemo) compared to ICI alone (ICI-mono) in the treatment of NSCLC is currently being investigated. Another report showed that the patients who received pembrolizumab inhibitor have higher overall survival (OS) and PFS compared to those who received platinum-based chemotherapy alone. It has been demonstrated that ICI-chemo is effective against early advancement but will not influence persistent anti-cancer immunity. Patients treated with ICI-chemo exhibit CCND1 (cyclin D1) and CDKN2A (cyclin-dependent kinase inhibitor 2A) changes, which were not seen in those treated with ICI-mono. In conclusion, chemotherapy given after ICIs has greater efficacy rates, but the risks and advantages should be discussed with the patients. It may yield temporary results but it is not recommended for the long run (Hong et al. 2023). Dual immunotherapy with a limited course of chemotherapy resulted in significant improvements in OS, PFS, and ORR (Zhou et al. 2021). However, limited immunogenicity and a subpar immune response restrict the use of cancer vaccines. Patients who have a previously developed anti-tumor T-cell respond well to immune checkpoint inhibitors. For this reason, vaccination techniques have been designed specifically. After chemotherapy and pembrolizumab, addition of a neoantigen vaccine presents an opportunity to induce and expand tumor-specific immune responses (Forde et al. 2022). Injectable smart hydrogels (ISHs), which self-assemble into a network resembling a biological microenvironment, are utilized as immune modulators to localize immune cells and reprogram host cells in order to create next-generation cancer vaccines (Duong et al. 2020). The use of radiation therapy in conjunction with immune-checkpoint blockage also appears as a promising candidate.

16.3.6 Modulating T-Cell Response with Immunomodulatory Agents

Cancer immunotherapy works to enhance the immune system's inherent capacity to combat the disease by stimulating it. Dendritic cells can activate T-cells to become effector cells (either CD4+ or CD8+ cells), but in cancer patients, tolerogenic dendritic cells or TGF-β develop and curb the activity of effector cells. Many immunomodulatory agents have been used for T-cell response. In a clinical study, novel cancer vaccines containing DC transduced with the entire wild-type p53 gene were tested on 29 patients. Then the findings demonstrated that 57.1% of the patients experienced p53-specific T-cell responses after immunization. High rate of clinical responses (61.9%) was observed in patients who received chemotherapy immediately after vaccination (Antonia et al. 2006).

It was determined that the activation of an immune response to vaccination was closely related to the clinical response to subsequent treatment of chemotherapy. In another study, adherent mononuclear cells were cultured to produce autologous DCs. Then antigen-loaded DCs were administered intravenously to eight patients with late-stage NSCLC. After intranodal injection of the DC vaccine, there was no grade II/grade III toxicity; no immune response against self and moderate increase in T-cell response were observed in all patients. The result showed that five patients had advanced tumor, one had a minor tumor response, and two showed persistent tumor activity along with stronger T-cell responses (Chang et al. 2005). According to the findings, giving patients DCs pulsed with enhanced necrotic tumor cells may induce T-cell responses and may have a positive therapeutic impact in some individuals. The HDAC6 (histone deacetylase 6) inhibitor ricolinostat enhances phenotypic T-cell activation and antigen-presenting cell function. Two epigenetic modifiers working together have immunomodulatory effects that support T-cell-mediated anti-tumor immunity and have shown their therapeutic efficacy in treating NSCLC (Adeegbe et al. 2017). These changes might be used in a chemotherapy/vaccine combination to induce robust anti-tumor immunity. One research found that tumor cells administered to oxaliplatin generated larger quantities of MHC-I proteins and released cytokines that might speed up DC maturation, leading to the production of CTLs with enhanced cytotoxic capability. Additionally, TG4010 vaccine with cisplatin has been demonstrated to modify tumor cell properties toward a more immunogenic phenotype (Hodge et al. 2012).

16.3.7 Synergistic Adjuvants

Melanoma-associated antigen (MAGE)-A3 and MAGE-C2 have been identified as possible prognostic markers and appealing immunotherapy targets in a variety of cancer types. The overexpression of MAGE-A3 protein is a common occurrence in several forms of cancer, particularly in lung cancer. This overexpression contributes to the metastasis of NSCLC cells by facilitating the epithelial-mesenchymal transition (EMT). MAGE-A3 expression has been observed in 24–45% of individuals with NSCLC (Chen et al. 2017). MAGE-A3 is classified as cancer testis antigen as it is typically not found in normal adult tissues but is present in male germ cells in the testes and various cancer cell types. These antigens are produced by genes that are usually only active in the testes, but in cancer cells, they can be produced abnormally. MAGE-A3 antigens provide a true selective target for tumor-specific active immunotherapy because they are not typically found in the body, so directing treatment toward them may not harm healthy cells. The cancer immunotherapeutic agent contains recombinant MAGE-A3 protein that has been generated through genetic engineering and combined with the immunostimulant AS15 (Pujol et al. 2015). The resulting formulation consists of recombinant MAGE-A3 protein in an AS15 immunostimulant. An anti-MAGE-A3 immunotherapy clinical study in malignant melanoma indicated that immunization with a MAGE-A3 peptide can cause tumor regression. However, phase III MAGE-A3 clinical trial has been stopped in NSCLC patients since it did not achieve its objective that this adjuvant did not extend the disease-free survival rate either in the patients who did not receive chemotherapy or entire MAGE-A3-positive population (Vansteenkiste et al. 2016).

A study conducted on a stage III lung cancer patient, wherein the patient was administered with MHC class II-restricted antigen (HER 2/neu 2 peptide) along with an immunomodulatory agent (GM-CSF) as an adjuvant, showed the presence of T-cell response and antibody production against the antigen indicating a synergistic action against the cancer antigens. Dendritic cells which are the major antigen-presenting cells can directly be administered with the tumor antigen which can hasten the antigen presentation process. The autologous DC could be collected from the individuals, and the tumor antigen is readily processed after its uptake. These autologous DCs containing the processed tumor antigen can also be administered to patients as a vaccine rather than using immunomodulatory adjuvants indicating a wide range of available adjuvants that can be used according to the tumor type (Hirschowitz et al. 2006).

16.4 Conclusion

Effective treatment option and strategy in treating lung carcinoma is still an area that needs intensive exploration. Apart from existing conventional treatment strategies, immunotherapy and immunomodulatory therapeutics against lung cancer have been explored, yet the efficacy of the same is still a mixed outcome where some candidates have shown better results and some candidates have shown less or no effect on the disease end point. Immune checkpoint-modulating agents have been observed to elicit significant anti-tumor immune response, especially in tumors such as melanoma that contains high amount of neoantigens. While the existing cancer vaccines have their own set of advantages and disadvantages, combining vaccines with immunomodulatory agents could be a versatile option and treatment strategy to efficiently increase anti-tumor response and eradicate cancer progression. Existing clinical studies have compared the anti-tumor response and antibody level against specific tumor antigens in individual treatment groups (immunomodulatory agents alone and vaccines alone) and synergistic groups (immunomodulatory agents with vaccines). The outcome of these studies are in line with advantageous role of combinational treatment with immunomodulatory agents and vaccines. This chapter insists the importance, effectiveness, and the synergistic potential of antigen-specific vaccines with immunomodulatory agents which could be a potential treatment strategy to tackle lung cancer.

Acknowledgments The authors express their gratitude to the SASTRA-Deemed-to-be-University, Tamil Nadu, India, for the infrastructure and financial support. The authors also extend their appreciation for the contribution of Biopharmaceutical research lab members, SASTRA-Deemed-to-be-University.

Author Contribution Suresh Krishna Venkataramanan, Nithya Shree Raman, Karthika Rangasamy: Writing - Original Draft, Writing - Review & Editing, Collection of data; Sree Gayathri Ganapathy, Pavithra Vimala Arulrajan : Writing - Original Draft, Collection of data; Shibi Muralidar, Gayathri Gopal: Writing -Review & Editing; Senthil Visaga Ambi: Conceptualization, Visualization, Supervision, and Writing - Review & Editing

Conflict of Interest The authors declare no conflict of interest

References

Adeegbe DO, Liu Y, Lizotte PH et al (2017) Synergistic immunostimulatory effects and therapeutic benefit of combined histone deacetylase and bromodomain inhibition in non–small cell lung cancer. Cancer Discov 7:852–867. https://doi.org/10.1158/2159-8290.CD-16-1020

Aerts JG, Hegmans JP (2013) Tumor-specific cytotoxic t cells are crucial for efficacy of immunomodulatory antibodies in patients with lung cancer. Cancer Res 73:2381–2388

Altaf R, Jadoon SS, Muhammad SA et al (2022) Recent advances in immune checkpoint inhibitors for non-small lung cancer treatment. Front Oncol 12:1–10. https://doi.org/10.3389/fonc.2022.1014156

Antonia SJ, Mirza N, Fricke I et al (2006) Combination of p53 cancer vaccine with chemotherapy in patients with extensive stage small cell lung cancer. Clin Cancer Res 12:878–887. https://doi.org/10.1158/1078-0432.CCR-05-2013

Brahmer JR (2013) Harnessing the immune system for the treatment of non-small-cell lung cancer. J Clin Oncol 31:1021–1028

Butterfield LH (2015) Cancer vaccines. BMJ 350:h988

Camidge DR, Bang YJ, Kwak EL et al (2012) Activity and safety of crizotinib in patients with ALK-positive non-small-cell lung cancer: updated results from a phase 1 study. Lancet Oncol 13:1011–1019. https://doi.org/10.1016/S1470-2045(12)70344-3

Champiat S, Ileana E, Giaccone G et al (2014) Incorporating immune-checkpoint inhibitors into systemic therapy of NSCLC. J Thorac Oncol 9:144–153. https://doi.org/10.1097/JTO.0000000000000074

Chang SM, Parney IF, Huang W et al (2005) Patterns of care for adults with newly diagnosed malignant glioma. JAMA 293:557–564. https://doi.org/10.1001/jama.293.5.557

Chen X, Wang L, Liu J et al (2017) Expression and prognostic relevance of MAGE-A3 and MAGE-C2 in non-small cell lung cancer. Oncol Lett 13:1609–1618. https://doi.org/10.3892/ol.2017.5665

Chiang CLL, Benencia F, Coukos G (2010) Whole tumor antigen vaccines. Semin Immunol 22:132–143

Dasanu CA, Sethi N, Ahmed N (2012) Immune alterations and emerging immunotherapeutic approaches in lung cancer. Expert Opin Biol Ther 12:923–937

Du W, Yang M, Turner A et al (2017) Tim-3 as a target for cancer immunotherapy and mechanisms of action. Int J Mol Sci 18:1–12. https://doi.org/10.3390/ijms18030645

Duong HTT, Thambi T, Yin Y et al (2020) Degradation-regulated architecture of injectable smart hydrogels enhances humoral immune response and potentiates antitumor activity in human lung carcinoma. Biomaterials 230:119599. https://doi.org/10.1016/j.biomaterials.2019.119599

Forde PM, Spicer J, Lu S et al (2022) Neoadjuvant nivolumab plus chemotherapy in resectable lung cancer. N Engl J Med 386:1973–1985. https://doi.org/10.1056/nejmoa2202170

Gaissmaier L, Christopoulos P (2021) Immune modulation in lung cancer: current concepts and future strategies. Respiration 99:903–929

Goldberg MV, Darke CG (2011) LAG-3 in cancer immunotherapy. Curr Top Microbiol Immunol 344:269–278. https://doi.org/10.1007/82_2010_114

Hirshowitz EA, Hiestand DM, Yannelli JR (2006) State of the art: concise review, vaccines for lung cancer. J Thorac Oncol 1(1)

Hodge JW, Ardiani A, Farsaci B et al (2012) The tipping point for combination therapy: cancer vaccines with radiation, chemotherapy, or targeted small molecule inhibitors. Semin Oncol 39:323–339. https://doi.org/10.1053/j.seminoncol.2012.02.006

Hong DS, Van Tine BA, Biswas S et al (2023) Autologous T cell therapy for MAGE-A4+ solid cancers in HLA-A*02+ patients: a phase 1 trial. Nat Med 29:104–114. https://doi.org/10.1038/s41591-022-02128-z

Hu Z, Ott PA, Wu CJ (2018) Towards personalized, tumour-specific, therapeutic vaccines for cancer. Nat Rev Immunol 18:168–182

Jäger D, Jäger E, Knuth A (2001) Immune responses to tumour antigens: implications for antigen specific immunotherapy of cancer. J Clin Pathol 54(9):669–674

Koyama S, Akbay EA, Li YY et al (2016) Adaptive resistance to therapeutic PD-1 blockade is associated with upregulation of alternative immune checkpoints. Nat Commun 7:1–9. https://doi.org/10.1038/ncomms10501

Liu JKH (2014) Anti-cancer vaccines-a one-hit wonder? Yale J Biol Med 87(4):481–489

Maemondo M, Inoue A, Kobayashi K et al (2010) Gefitinib or chemotherapy for non–small-cell lung cancer with mutated EGFR. N Engl J Med 362:2380–2388. https://doi.org/10.1056/nejmoa0909530

Mahoney KM, Rennert PD, Freeman GJ (2015) Combination cancer immunotherapy and new immunomodulatory targets. Nat Rev Drug Discov 14:561–584. https://doi.org/10.1038/nrd4591

Matsushita M, Kawaguchi M (2018) Immunomodulatory effects of drugs for effective cancer immunotherapy. J Oncol 2018:8653489. https://doi.org/10.1155/2018/8653489

Mok TSK, Wu YL, Kudaba I et al (2019) Pembrolizumab versus chemotherapy for previously untreated, PD-L1-expressing, locally advanced or metastatic non-small-cell lung cancer (KEYNOTE-042): a randomised, open-label, controlled, phase 3 trial. Lancet 393:1819–1830. https://doi.org/10.1016/S0140-6736(18)32409-7

Neller MA, López JA, Schmidt CW (2008) Antigens for cancer immunotherapy. Semin Immunol 20:286–295

Offringa R, van der Burg SH, Ossendorp F, Toes RE, Melief CJ (2000) Design and evaluation of antigen-specific vaccination strategies against cancer. Curr Opin Immunol 12(5):576–582

Pardoll DM (1998) Cancer vaccine-immune tolerance. Nat Med 4.

Pinto JA, Raez LE, Oliveres H, Rolfo CC (2019) Current knowledge of Ipilimumab and its use in treating non-small cell lung cancer. Expert Opin Biol Ther 19:509–515. https://doi.org/10.1080/14712598.2019.1610380

Popovic A, Jaffee EM, Zaidi N (2018) Cancers. Emerging strategies for combination checkpoint modulators in cancer immunotherapy. J Clin Invest 128:3209–3218. https://doi.org/10.1172/JCI120775

Pujol JL, Vansteenkiste JF, De Pas TM et al (2015) Safety and immunogenicity of MAGE-A3 cancer immunotherapeutic with or without adjuvant chemotherapy in patients with resected stage IB to III MAGE-A3-positive non-small-cell lung cancer. J Thorac Oncol 10:1458–1467. https://doi.org/10.1097/JTO.0000000000000653

Rolfo C, Sortino G, Smits E et al (2014) Immunotherapy: is a minor god yet in the pantheon of treatments for lung cancer? Expert Rev Anticancer Ther 14:1173–1187

Saxena M, van der Burg SH, Melief CJM, Bhardwaj N (2021) Therapeutic cancer vaccines. Nat Rev Cancer 21:360–378. https://doi.org/10.1038/s41568-021-00346-0

Tagliamonte M, Petrizzo A, Tornesello ML et al (2014) Antigen-specific vaccines for cancer treatment. Hum Vaccin Immunother 10:3332–3346

Tomasini P, Khobta N, Greillier L, Barlesi F (2012) Ipilimumab: its potential in non-small cell lung cancer. Ther Adv Med Oncol 4:43–50. https://doi.org/10.1177/1758834011431718

Vansteenkiste JF, Cho BC, Vanakesa T et al (2016) Efficacy of the MAGE-A3 cancer immunotherapeutic as adjuvant therapy in patients with resected MAGE-A3-positive non-small-cell lung cancer (MAGRIT): a randomised, double-blind, placebo-controlled, phase 3 trial. Lancet Oncol 17:822–835. https://doi.org/10.1016/S1470-2045(16)00099-1

Wang Y, Zhang H, Liu C et al (2022) Immune checkpoint modulators in cancer immunotherapy: recent advances and emerging concepts. J Hematol Oncol 15:111

Ward S, Casey D, Labarthe MC et al (2002) Immunotherapeutic potential of whole tumour cells. Cancer Immunol Immunother 51:351–357. https://doi.org/10.1007/s00262-002-0286-2

Wu Z, Li S, Zhu X (2021) The mechanism of stimulating and mobilizing the immune system enhancing the anti-tumor immunity. Front Immunol 12:682435

Zhou J, Valentini E, Boutros M (2021) Microenvironmental innate immune signaling and cell mechanical responses promote tumor growth. Dev Cell 56:1884–1899.e5. https://doi.org/10.1016/j.devcel.2021.06.007

Important Biomarkers for Better Evaluation of Checkpoint Inhibitors and Other Immunotherapies in Lung Cancer

17

Hitesh Malhotra, Anurag Dhiman, and Rupesh K. Gautam

The most common cancer-related cause of death worldwide and in the USA is lung cancer (Siegel et al. 2021). Non-small cell lung carcinomas (NSCLC) make up the bulk of these tumours; the two most prevalent subtypes are carcinoma of squamous cells and adenocarcinoma (Antonia et al. 2018). Although responses to these medications are often moderate and the time until disease progression is quite quick, chemotherapy using platinum has historically been the primary treatment for these individuals (Reck et al. 2016). The recent developments in immunotherapy, which provide patients without an identifiable driver mutation and attractive new therapeutic option, have fundamentally changed the way advanced NSCLC is managed (Paz-Ares et al. 2018).

Utilising the immune system's potential to fight cancer is among the most promising therapeutic modalities. Because cancer cells undergo a great deal of genetic and epigenetic changes, the host immune system may recognise a variety of tumour-associated antigens, necessitating the development of unique immune resistance mechanisms in tumours. Immune resistance is greatly influenced by immunological-inhibitory pathways, sometimes referred to as immunological checkpoints, which frequently control immune tolerance and restrict collateral tissue damage. Programmed cellular death protein 1 (PD-1, also known as CD279) and cytotoxic T-lymphocyte-associated antigen 4 (also known as CD152) are the two immunological checkpoint receptors that are now being studied the most in relation to therapeutic cancer immunotherapy. They control immunological responses as inhibitory receptors in various ways and through various mechanisms. The main phase of early

H. Malhotra · A. Dhiman
Guru Gobind Singh College of Pharmacy, Yamunanagar, Haryana, India

R. K. Gautam (✉)
Department of Pharmacology, Indore Institute of Pharmacy, Indore, Madhya Pradesh, India

S. Bhatt et al. (eds.), *Immunotherapy Against Lung Cancer*,
https://doi.org/10.1007/978-981-99-7141-1_17

T-lymphocyte tolerance takes place in lymph nodes, and CTLA4 (cytotoxic T-lymphocyte-associated protein 4) is a powerful co-inhibitor implicated in this process. Activated T-cells are induced to generate the PD-1 protein during the subsequent effectors phase, which prevents them from functioning in peripheral tissues and from initiating an autoimmune reaction. Constant antigen stimulation leads to increased PD-1 expression and a "exhausted" T-cell phenotype in the absence of a successful immune response and antigen eradication. It is important to note that PD-1 is expressed more widely than CTLA-4 and that it may be triggered by other excited non-T-lymphocyte subsets, including B cells and NK (natural killer) cells, which decrease their lytic activity (Kythreotou et al. 2018). When PD-1 and its ligands, programmed mortality ligand 1 (PD-L1, also known as B7-H1) and PD-L2 (B7-DC), interact, T-lymphocyte function is decreased, including T-cell receptor signalling, cytokine production, cellular destruction, lymphocyte motility, and metabolic reprogramming (Ribas 2015).

Antigen-presenting cells (APCs), like dendritic cells (DCs), which are involved in the cancer-immunity cycle, take up antigens released by tumour cells (TC) that are perishing. The processed tumour-associated peptides are given to CD8+ T-lymphocytes together with MHC-I molecules by DCs after they have taken up the antigen in the draining lymph node. The T-cells that have been recruited go to and invade tumours, identifying and ultimately eliminating the tumour cells (Reck et al. 2016). The cancer-immunity cycle has a wide variety of potential therapeutic targets, making the creation of effective prognostic biomarkers necessary. The PD-1/PD-L1 pathway can be inhibited to treat cancer since PD-L1 is expressed at greater levels in many malignancies.

Although tumour cells have the capacity to overcome this built-in defence and tolerance can arise as a result of the overexpression of crucial immunological checkpoints, the immune system of the body is crucial in the monitoring and killing of cancer cells in a person. These checkpoints typically protect normal tissue against cytotoxic immune reactions brought by infections, but cancer cells have the ability to exploit these checkpoints to elude immune-mediated elimination. Immune resistance is supported by two checkpoints: On cancer cells, PD-L1 and, on dendritic cells or macrophages, indoleamine-2,3-dioxygenase (IDO) are present. For example, when T-cells recognise tumour antigens, interferon (INF) is released. INF may really cause the production of such checkpoints rather than just attracting more cytotoxic immune cells (IC) (Rizvi et al. 2015). Cytotoxic T-lymphocyte-associated antigen 4 (CTLA-4) is a further essential immune system suppressor that regulates early T-cell activation (Hellmann et al. 2018). The ability of the immune system to activate T-cells that are cytotoxic and effectors, which kill malignant tumour cells in the patient's body, is enhanced by immunotherapeutic medications that break these linkages between checkpoint receptors and ligands. In terms of overall survival, the three PD-1 and PD-L1 inhibitors nivolumab, pembrolizumab, and atezolizumab, which have all been approved as the second-line therapy for metastatic NSCLC, all outperformed chemotherapy (Schalper et al. 2015). Pembrolizumab, the only single-agent checkpoint inhibitor among all three medications, is only appropriate for use in first-line therapy in patients with significant PD-L1 expression (Jiang et al. 2018). A combination of two different checkpoint blockades has also been studied. Promising results have been found with the CTLA-4 inhibitor and nivolumab combination, particularly those showing improved antitumour activity and enhanced progression-free survival (PFS). Tumour mutation burden (TMB) has been discovered as a potentially important biomarker in the ipilimumab-nivolumab studies because patients with tumours that have a higher mutational load react better to dual checkpoint inhibition (Mariathasan et al. 2018). In exploratory subgroup analyses, a high blood-based TMB was associated with a longer average overall survival time for the tremelimumab-durvalumab group compared to chemotherapy alone, but the MYSTIC trial did not discover that the CTLA-4 inhibitor tremelimumab and the PD-L1 inhibitor durvalumab increased survival rates over chemotherapy in the total study population.

Testing for the expression of PD-L1 is currently the most reliable technique to assess which NSCLC patients are most likely to respond to immunotherapy. Recent lung cancer chemo-immunotherapy studies have showed promise in treating lung tumours such as adenocarcinoma and carcinoma of the squamous cells by combining checkpoint inhibitors with platinum doublet chemotherapy, even in circumstances with low expression of PD-L1 (Gide et al. 2019; Van Allen et al. 2015). The fact that the low PD-L1 expression subgroups had less favourable clinical outcomes, however, is relevant since it shows that PD-L1 is still a crucial biomarker even when utilised in combination with first-line chemo-immunotherapy. Numerous clinical studies examining single-agent checkpoint antagonists have demonstrated that certain individuals with increased levels of PD-L1 do not benefit therapeutically from these medications, revealing numerous of its limitations. Despite the importance of PD-L1 expression as a response signal, this is true. Numerous advanced NSCLC patients have benefitted greatly from immunotherapy, but many still do not react to the treatment, their condition worsens while being treated, or they experience severe immunotoxicities that are life-threatening (Thorsson et al. 2018). Practically any organ in the body may have immune-related side effects after using a checkpoint inhibitor, but endocrinopathies, colitis, pneumonitis, and dermatitis appear to be the most common. Although they are less frequent, adverse cardiovascular, renal, neurological, and haematological immunological events can also occur. Although immune-related responses tend to be mild to moderately severe in most cases, they can occasionally be severe or even deadly, especially if they are not immediately identified and treated effectively (Zhou et al. 2019). For all of these reasons, developing biomarkers that are indicative of checkpoint inhibition response is a crucial first step in maximising the potential of the new class of immunotherapy drugs. In addition to highlighting new and under research tissue and serum-based indicators, this chapter examines the presently accepted biomarkers for immunity checkpoint suppression in NSCLC.

17.1 Expression of PD-L1

The IHC (immunohistochemistry) test for expression of PD-L1 is the gold standard, as previously established, for selecting patients with advanced stage NSCLC who are more likely to respond to immunotherapy. Patients who have had conventional chemotherapy as well as those who have not been treated at all are both covered by this. According to a number of prospective studies, clinical efficacy and tissue

PD-L1 expression levels are associated. KEYNOYE-024 (16) has shown that pembrolizumab was superior to treatment in terms of overall survival in patients with high PD-L1 expression, which is defined as PD-L1 expressing on above 50% of cancer cells. This degree of expression is now required in order to be eligible for pembrolizumab therapy in patients having advanced NSCLC who have never received treatment.

Patients who received either nivolumab or atezolizumab medication, however, demonstrated the highest advantages in tumours with increased expression of PD-L1 in second-line metastatic studies (Lee et al. 2008). In the PACIFIC trial, which involved stage III patients with incurable disease who underwent final chemotherapy with radiation therapy and a year of durvalumab consolidation therapy, retrospective subgroup analysis showed no survival advantage in patients with PD-L1 1% and selectively improved survival in patients with tumours expressing 25% of PD-L1. PD-L1 is still a contentious biomarker of immunotherapy response, and a number of problems restrict its applicability, notwithstanding the compelling data from these trials connecting PD-L1 expression levels to therapeutic efficacy and response. PD-L1 expression in tumours can take many distinct forms (Newman et al. 2015), and numerous testing techniques and expression cut-points are used by different immunotherapy drugs, all of which have drawn criticism (Hastings et al. 2019).

In order to evaluate expression, each FDA-approved checkpoint inhibitor for NSCLC now in use uses a distinct PD-L1 IHC antibody, and a number of commercial testing kits are offered. In contrast to nivolumab, which uses the antibody clone, pembrolizumab and nivolumab both use the 22C3 antibody clone. Durvalumab uses the SP263 antibody, whereas atezolizumab uses the SP142 partner antibody clone. For each of these drugs, separate research employed a variety of cut-points and scoring systems to further characterise the degree of PD-L1 expression. Atezolizumab, pembrolizumab, and nivolumab all received FDA clearance for various indications as a result of the phase III studies' findings. According to FDA approvals (Yu et al. 2022), tumours with PD-L1 50% are suitable for pembrolizumab as a primary single agent; pembrolizumab, however, should only be used for cancers with PD-L1 1% if a platinum-based therapy has failed to control the tumour (Rittmeyer et al. 2017). However, nivolumab can be used in the second-line setting regardless of PD-L1 expression. PD-L1 is measured by the SP142 antibody test, which is utilised in combination with atezolizumab, as opposed to the 22C3, 28-8, and SP263 antibodies, which only evaluate PD-L1 expression on cancer cell walls. Based on how much PD-L1 is expressed by the immune system (IC) and cancerous cells (TC), atezolizumab is ranked in four distinct groups, from least to highest, according to the degree of expression. In the lowest category, denoted as TC0 and IC0, PD-L1 is present on both TC and IC to a level of 1%, whereas in the highest category, PD-L1 is present to a level of 50% on TC or 10% on IC. Atezolizumab was found to outlast docetaxel in all subgroups, including the TC0 and IC0 (PD-L11%), and is therefore approved for treatment in the second-line metastatic setting regardless of PD-L1 expression.

Studies comparing the expression across primary and metastatic locations have revealed that PD-L1 expression may also vary among tumours. Studies that specifically compared the expression of PD-L1 in brain tissue that had spread to other parts of the body with tissue from matched initial lung tumours yielded results with notable discrepancies (Newman et al. 2015; Carter et al. 2012). The histological subtype may also have an impact on PD-L1's ability to predict outcomes. Given the correlation between PD-L1 expression and that effect, checkpoint blocking may be more effective in adenocarcinoma than squamous cell. In the phase III second-line nivolumab experiment Checkmate 057 for advanced non-squamous tumours, patients with tumours that expressed more PD-L1 had better outcomes (Schalper et al. 2015). Although PD-L1 neoplasm expression was not a prognostic marker nor a predictor of response, patients with squamous cell lung cancer demonstrated superior PFS and OS over docetaxel in the Checkmate 017 trial (Campbell et al. 2016).

Despite its potential limitations as a predictor of response, testing is still the recognised standard of treatment for any recently diagnosed NSCLC. The best way for figuring out if a tumour will react to immunotherapy right now is to use IHC, which can identify the expression of PD-L1 on the outermost layer of cancer cells. Patients having elevated PD-L1 levels may not always respond well to treatment, but some do in those who have low or no PD-L1 expression, and the effects can endure for a long time. The pembrolizumab group in Keynote-024,16, which exclusively included patients whose tumours expressed PD-L1 over 50%, saw an overall response rate of 45%. This demonstrates that a sizeable proportion of individuals did not react to medication, even among a group as a whole that was differentiated by having increased levels of PD-L1 expression. The shortcomings of PD-L1 as a biomarker have led to increasing research in potential substitute response markers. The potential of TMB as a prognostic marker has attracted attention in particular.

17.2 TMB (Tumour Mutational Burden)

In certain cancer types, the percentage of tumours that react to anti-PD-1 or anti-PD-L1 treatment has been associated with cancer or tumour mutational burden (TMB), possibly significant indicators of immunotherapy response (Yarchoan et al. 2017). TMB, which includes base substitutions as well as quick insertions and deletions, measures the overall number of mutations in a cancer genome per coding region. Prior until recently, the quantity of somatic mutations was estimated using whole exome sequencing; however, the Foundation One CDx test-based next-generation sequencing techniques have now been demonstrated to significantly correlate and are currently used to assess mutational burden (Rizvi et al. 2015). Somatic mutation rates vary among various cancer types; melanoma has some of the highest rates, while gastrointestinal malignancies including pancreatic and colon cancer have some of the lowest rates (Yarchoan et al. 2017). The mutational load of NSCLC varies; smoking-related lung cancer tends to have a larger proportion of somatic mutations, whereas tumours from non-smokers have a lower burden. According to one theory, a high somatic mutation rate causes tumour cells to express more neoantigens, which in turn boosts immunogenicity and makes tumours more susceptible to immune-checkpoint therapy (Bristol-Myers Squibb 2019).

Numerous studies have demonstrated that a bigger mutational burden is clinically associated with an improved reaction to checkpoint inhibition. Pembrolizumab's effects on lung cancers with large levels of neoantigen and non-synonymous mutation were studied by Rizvi et al., and they found a correlation between these factors and a more durable clinical effect (Rizvi et al. 2015). Checkmate 227, a recent randomised experiment, looked into the usefulness of TMB in predicting how patients will react to the combined use of ipilimumab and nivolumab. This study has shown that independent of PD-L1 expression or histology, patients with high TMB who received combination immunotherapy in the initial-line metastatic situation as opposed to chemotherapy had a superior PFS. This benefit was also seen in cancers with high TMB but low PD-L1 expression. This latest research emphasises the low predictive value of PD-L1 staining for tumour immunogenicity and shows that tumour immunogenicity may be impacted by factors other than only the level of PD-L1 expression. Despite these promising early results from Checkmate 227, the significance of TMB as a biomarker identification for immunotherapy in NSCLC remains unknown because later overall survival data revealed a statistically non-significant advantage of ipilimumab with nivolumab in high TMB patients as well as a comparable surviving benefit in patients with TMB 10 mutations/megabase. This information was used to support the request for FDA clearance in the additional biologics licence application for nivolumab and ipilimumab for severe NSCLC with TMB 10 mutation per megabase (Schatton et al. 2014). TMB as a biomarker has other limitations, such as a lack of uniformity among the testing platforms used and the absence of a precise TMB threshold that would classify a tumour as having "high" TMB. Different studies have employed different TMB cutoffs, and while the latest ipilimumab plus nivolumab trials initially showed that ten mutations/megabase were clinically significant, this marker was not shown to be predictive in the abovementioned revised overall survival data.

17.3 TILs (Tumour-Infiltrating Lymphocytes)

Previous studies have shown that the degree of lymphocyte infiltration detected inside tumour tissue may have predictive importance since elevated levels of tumour-infiltrating lymphocytes (TILs) have been associated with improved survival across a number of cancer types, including NSCLC (Thomas et al. 2013; Brambilla et al. 2016). High concentrations of TILS, such as CD8+, CD3+, and CD4+, have been linked to longer survival in NSCLC, according to earlier studies. A patient's increased immune identification of tumour cells is thought to be reflected in a high TIL density, which is thought to signify an inflammatory T-cell milieu inside the tumour. Since this inflammatory neoplasm profile may be more responsive to checkpoint suppression, TIL density has also been investigated for its potential predictive utility as a biomarker for immunotherapy.

Ipilimumab checkpoint blockage in melanoma studies has been linked to both clinical response and post-treatment rise in TILs. In a study of patients with metastatic melanoma treated with pembrolizumab, a rise in intra-tumoural CD8+ T-cells was seen after therapy and was associated with a radiographic response. The level of the expression of PD-L1 on TILs and the response to atezolizumab treatment were shown to be correlated in a sample of 53 NSCLC patients, as Herbst and his colleagues reported in their study (Herbst et al. 2014). PD-L1 expression and reactivity in cancer cells were not correlated in this study, which is crucial to emphasise. The rise in immune cells that invade the tumour before and after therapy may be a good indicator of the patient's clinical and radiological response. It is necessary to do more study to corroborate this and to establish clinically significant thresholds for increasing TIL density.

17.4 Specific Genotypes for Tumours

Testing for single-gene driver mutations, such as EGFR (epidermal growth factor receptor) and ALK (anaplastic lymphoma kinase), is typical for every patient who initially comes with metastatic NSCLC. All patients will inevitably progress through therapy or quit taking it due to toxicity, even though many patients may experience good sustained responses when using an oral targeted medicine, such as an inhibitor of tyrosine kinase in cancers with EGFR exon 19 and 21 mutations. In these individuals' subsequent courses of therapy, immunotherapy has been used as a therapeutic. The second-line studies using single-agent immunotherapy did not demonstrate a survival advantage in this cohort of patients with EGFR- and ALK-positive tumours. Unfortunately, these tumours have not yet demonstrated the same responsiveness to checkpoint inhibition as cancer of other genotypes. The connection between EGFR tumour positivity and hyperprogression can be mediated by this discovery as PD-1 and PD-L1 are elevated in response to EGFR activation (Champiat et al. 2017). Additionally becoming more generally established in clinical practice is hyperprogression following immunotherapy (Kato et al. 2017). Although discontinuing TKI therapy has the potential to result in a flare-up of the illness and may help to explain the accelerated disease progression observed in certain individuals who experience checkpoint inhibition, it is not apparent if this is a true phenomenon in tumours with EGFR mutations.

PD-L1 expression has been hypothesised to be downregulated in EGFR-positive cancers, which would explain why these tumours are resistant to single-agent checkpoint inhibitors (Vokes et al. 2018), despite conflicting results that warrant more research. Although immune cells are present in the cancer microenvironment, Toki et al.'s investigation of 150 EGFR-positive NSCLC tumour samples showed that these tumours exhibited lower levels of PD-L1 expression and a larger percentage of "inactive" TILs. In this study, Granzyme B and Ki67 concentrations were assessed to assess TIL activity. Inactive TILs had lesser activity, which resulted in decreased proliferation of T-cells and cytotoxic activity. The relative absence of immunotherapy response observed in such tumours may be explained by the relatively high frequency of dormant TILs in the microenvironment of EGFR-positive tumours. According to the same study (Toki et al. 2018), KRAS-positive tumours showed greater PD-L1 expression levels and density of "active" TILs. Even though it is important to keep in mind those KRAS mutants, NSCLC is a heterogeneous category and that some subgroups react differently to checkpoint limitation; recent research has shown that KRAS mutant tumours typically have higher immunogenicity (Dong et al. 2017). Retrospective study has demonstrated that PD-L1 axis medicines are more resistant to KRAS cancers with a co-mutation in STK11/LKB1. Clinical results for STK11/LKB1 genomically altered tumours treated with checkpoint inhibitors were worse, including in PD-L1-positive tumours (Skoulidis et al. 2018).

Recent studies combining immuno-chemotherapy with VEGF inhibition show that such treatments may be able to overcome the impedance shown by EGFR- and ALK-positive cancers, even if the fundamental causes of why some tumour genotypes may not respond to checkpoint inhibition are still being understood. According to the clinical trials and retrospective subgroup analyses, patients with EGFR or ALK mutant tumours may benefit more from combining the VEGF inhibitor bevacizumab with platinum doublet chemo and the checkpoint inhibitor atezolizumab (Socinski et al. 2018). The advantages of immunotherapy may be extended to tumour genotypes that are believed to be resistant, which is a promising development. However, prospective confirmation is still required.

17.5 Biomarkers of Gene Expression

A biomarker of checkpoint blockage may one day be developed using ongoing research on gene expression profiling. Immunogenomic profiles, particularly those connected to IFN signalling and activated T-cells, have been associated with response to immunotherapy in a number of cancer types (Ayers et al. 2017), and they may be predictive. Ayers et al. showed that in cohorts of patients with melanoma, neck and head malignancies, and gastric cancer treated with pembrolizumab, the best PFS and overall reaction were predicted by an IFN-related gene profile generated from the baseline tumour tissue. The T-effector and IFN-associated gene profile was shown to be more prevalent in tumours with increased survival in the POPLAR trial, a phase II assessment of atezolizumab for the second-line therapy of advanced NSCLC. It is noteworthy to note that in IMpower150, patients with low levels of the T-effector/INF-related gene profile similarly demonstrated a PFS benefit associated with the combination of atezolizumab, platinum doublet, and bevacizumab (Socinski et al. 2018), even though those who had larger levels of this gene profile showed a more obvious advantage. By validating the expression of PD-L1, a subsequent research that looked at the NSCLC patient database from the initial Rizvi et al.'s (2015) study discovered that utilising the expression patterns of chemokines and immunosuppressive molecules improved the capacity to predict pembrolizumab response (Brogden et al. 2018). Multi-gene profiling has the potential to help identify immunogenic cancers that are more likely to react favourably to immunotherapy treatments, notwithstanding the need for more clinical research and prospective validation.

17.6 Serological Biomarkers

Peripheral blood biomarkers offer a potential alternative to tumour-based indicators due to the relative ease and lower invasiveness of blood draws, as well as the occasionally but not infrequently occurring inadequacies of tissue specimens on various cancer biopsies. It has been investigated if lab results provided during routine blood draws may be used as markers of immunotherapy response. The neutrophil-to-lymphocyte ratio (NLR), for instance, has attracted a lot of interest as a biomarker since it is simple to compute from the difference shown by a typical whole blood count. The relationship between these two components is measured by the neutrophil-to-lymphocyte ratio or NLR. It is thought that in a cancer microenvironment containing lots of neutrophil but lower lymphocyte infiltration, angiogenesis would rise, and cell death would be suppressed, boosting tumourigenesis and leading to poorer outcomes. Its effectiveness in treating several malignancies, including melanoma, breast, and other gastrointestinal cancers, has been researched (Liu et al. 2017). A poor prognosis may be indicated by rising NLR levels at baseline in NSCLC patients with advanced cancer of the lungs who are taking immunotherapy (Diem et al. 2017). Nivolumab's NLR is associated with the outcome of treatment and can be utilised as an early indicator of response, according to a retrospective research on the drug's usage in second-line therapy (Takeda et al. 2018). NLR may serve as both a prognostic and a predictive marker. Other blood count-based measurements, including absolute eosinophil count, absolute monocytes count, and platelets to lymphocyte count (PLR), are also being researched; some have shown link with response (Soyano et al. 2017). Prospective validation is required despite the limited scope and retrospective character of the research done thus far. When treating patients with checkpoint blockade, the NLR and other peripheral blood markers of a similar kind may be helpful.

Another serum-based measure under development that has generated interest is blood-based tumour mutational burden (bTMB). In their investigation, Gandara and his associates examined bTMB utilising the FoundationOne CDx test and found a positive association between tissue and blood TMB utilising a subset of the specimens obtained via second-line atezolizumab testing. This analysis also included an overview of the results from these two studies, and it was discovered that atezolizumab use was related to greater bTMB and prolonged PFS in patients with metastatic NSCLC (Gandara et al. 2018). According to their analysis, the cut-point for identifying "high" TMB may be bTMB 16 mutations/megabase, which is both clinically relevant and reliable. It was further demonstrated that bTMB may be used as a biomarker in the MYSTIC research, which looked at the immunotherapy regimen of durvalumab and tremelimumab in initial-line stage IV NSCLC.

17.7 Biomarkers in Peripheral Blood

17.7.1 NLR (Neutrophil-to-Lymphocyte Ratio)

The neutrophil-to-lymphocyte ratio (NLR) of peripheral blood cells and lymphocyte counts is directly connected to immunotherapy patients' prognoses. In NSCLC patients taking nivolumab, Diem et al. (2017) found that higher NLR was associated with poorer ORR, shorter OS, and shorter PFS. According to Ren et al. (Ho et al. 2018), compared to the group that had TMB10 mutations per Mb, patients with advanced-stage NSCLC who were undergoing immunotherapy showed a correlation between decreased NLR and prolonged OS and PFS. A low absolute lymphocyte count (ALC) was also considered to be symptomatic of a bad prognosis. Patients with reduced ALC have shown less clinical immunotherapy benefits and a shorter median PFS (Ferrucci et al. 2016). Absolute neutrophil counts (ANC) were crucial for the efficiency of anti-PD-1 therapy. In contrast to patients with lower baseline ANC and NLR levels, who had survival rates of 43% and 24%, patients with higher initial ANC levels (ANC > 7500) and larger baseline NLR levels (NLR > 3) had very poor survival rates of just 2% and 0%, respectively, at 1 and 2 years (Banna et al. 2020). When used in conjunction with other established indicators, NLR can also be utilised to forecast the prognosis for patients taking ICIs. Patients with first-line pembrolizumab monotherapy for advanced non-small cell lung cancer (aNSCLC), NLR > 5, and increased PD-L1 expression levels (>80%) showed favourable outcomes (Wang et al. 2019). NLR and PD-L1 expressions, however, were not related.

In comparison to patients with greater TMB and lower NLR (NLR > 2.5) but higher TMB and lower NLR (NLR2.5), patients with low NLR (NLR2.5) and high TMB (TMB > 10) had better OS and PFS. Additionally, lower platelet-to-lymphocyte ratio (PLR) values, which may act as a biomarker for prognosis, were associated with prolonged OS and FPS (Russo et al. 2020).

17.7.2 Lactate Dehydrogenase

Various tumours are thought to have a worse prognosis when lactate dehydrogenase (LDH) levels are high. The results of Kelderman et al. (2014) showed that the efficacy of ipilimumab therapy was limited in patients with severe melanoma having baseline blood LDH levels greater than double the upper limit of normal (ULN). A derived neutrophil/(leukocytes minus neutrophils) ratio (dNLR) of more than 3 and LDH levels above ULM are markers of suboptimal immunotherapy results, according to Mezquita et al. (2018). Clinical exams may rule out liver or muscle problems because the amount of LDH rise lacks specificity and might be brought on by any of these diseases.

17.7.3 Immunological Cells in the Peripheral Region

Immune cells in the periphery have TIL-like traits and cell divisions. Gros et al. (2016) discovered that the moving PD-1+ CD8+T-cell population contained neoantigen-specific CD8+ T-lymphocytes that were capable of recognising autologous malignancies. According to the study's findings, human peripheral blood PD-1+CD8+ T-cells as well as the success of immunotherapy may be used to predict changes in neoantigen-specific CD8+ T-lymphocytes. According to Kamphorst et al., circulating PD-1+CD8+ T-cell responses were delayed or non-existent in 70% of patients with disease progression, in contrast to individuals who saw clinical improvements after 4 weeks. The first or second treatment cycle also revealed the proliferation of circulating Ki-67+PD-1+CD8+ T-cells, suggesting a potential therapeutic effect (Kamphorst et al. 2017).

Krieg et al. found that peripheral CD14+ CD16-HLA-DRhi monocyte frequencies and peripheral T-cell counts were both associated with better ORR in patients who responded to anti-PD-1/PD-L1 treatment. The levels of CD45RO+ T memory cells were higher in responders, demonstrating the efficacy of the immunotherapy (Krieg et al. 2018).

17.7.4 ctDNA (Circulating Tumour DNA)

It is well acknowledged that the mutation burden of cancer tissues is reflected in circulating tumour DNA (ctDNA), which is simpler to obtain than TMB testing. Patients receiving pembrolizumab therapy for solid tumours showed longer overall survival (OS) in a trial by Bratman et al. (Lee et al. 2018) when their baseline ctDNA levels were lower than the median. Further predicting, the clinical advantages is enhanced by the dynamic changes in ctDNA. Thirty-three patients' ctDNA levels dropped from baseline in a cohort analysis of 73 patients, and 14 (42%) of them had objective remission. Only one (2%) of the 40 patients with higher ctDNA levels compared to baselines achieved objective remission. Following immunotherapy, lower ctDNA levels indicate that the patients' OS will be prolonged (Lee et al. 2018; Kim et al. 2018).

17.7.5 Soluble PD-L1

Similar to membrane-bound PD-L1, soluble PD-L1 (sPD-L1) promotes tumour growth and escape by obstructing T-cell proliferation and activation. Soluble PD-1 (sPD-1) was discovered to be favourably connected with favourable clinical outcomes in individuals with sophisticated pancreatic cancer. Patients with high levels of sPD-L1 (sPD-L1 > 0.012 ng/mL) have lower median overall survival times than patients with low levels of sPD-L1. Additionally, there is a substantial correlation between the levels of sPD-1 and sPD-L1. Additionally, melanoma and NSCLC patients are more likely to develop tumours if their baseline sPD-L1 levels were elevated (Zhou et al. 2017). PD-L1 levels of expression in cancer cells, however, were not correlated with sPD-L1 levels (Costantini et al. 2018). sPD-L1 concentration is simpler to quantify than tumour PD-L1 expression levels. Exosome PD-L1 levels were recently researched as an additional prognostic biomarker to sPD-L1. In the study by Theodoraki et al. (2018), there was no correlation between sPD-L1 levels and the development of squamous cell carcinoma in the head and neck. Fan et al. (2019) found that individuals with cancer of the gastric who had higher concentrations of exosome PD-L1, a separate prognostic marker, similarly had worse OS as compared to individuals who had lower concentrations of exosome PD-L1. According to Chen et al. (2018), interferon (IFN)-stimulated exosome PD-L1 synthesis increased, inhibiting CD8+ T-cell function and hastening the growth of tumours.

17.7.6 T-Cell Receptor (TCR) in Peripheral Blood

TIL counts by themselves cannot be utilised to evaluate the immune response since TILs are not necessarily tumour-recognising lymphocytes. TCR identification can represent T-cell activities of tumour cell recognition and more precisely forecast the success of immunotherapy (Reuben et al. 2020). By examining the intra-tumoural TCR repertoire of CD8+ T-lymphocytes in ovarian and colorectal cancers, Scheper et al. (2019) found that only 10% of tumour-infiltrating T-cells could differentiate autologous tumour cells. In 12 patients with metastatic melanoma, Postow et al. (2015) discovered that improved uniformity (similarities in the altered frequencies of certain V and J genes) of peripheral TCR was related to better PFS but not OS. A lower baseline level of diversity evenness in the TCR repertoire before treatment was linked to improved FPS and a favourable response to anti-PD-1 therapy, according to Hogan et al. (2019). Additionally, the early immune-related adverse events (IrAEs) related to treatment were linked to the peripheral blood TCR repertoire. Patients with significant IrAEs exhibited a lack of CD4+ and CD8+ TCR diversity.

17.7.7 Peripheral Cytokines

Peripheral cytokines might change depending on the conditions of the tumour microenvironment and the response of T-cells. Tumour evasion and immunological suppression are both attributed to TGF-. When peripheral TGF- levels are high at baseline (200 pg/mL), pembrolizumab therapy for hepatocellular carcinoma patients has a poor prognosis (Mitsuhashi and Okuma 2018). Tumour-specific T-lymphocyte distribution is more probable within the peri-tumour stroma compared to the intra-tuminal parenchyma as a result of TGF-, which is produced by peri-tumour fibroblasts (Mariathasan et al. 2018). TGF inhibitors can increase the efficacy of anti-PD-1/PD-L1 treatment in animal models of liver metastasis disorders that are advancing. This result could be a result of the powerful and durable cytotoxic T-cell reaction that TGF- inhibition incites in cancer cells (Tauriello et al. 2018).

IFN-, which is mostly produced by TILs and has the capacity to improve immune response and prevent tumour growth, may be able to modulate the levels of PD-L1 expression on cancer cells. IFN- stimulated the JAK2-STAT1 pathway, preventing the development of cancer cells (Ivashkiv 2018). IFN-, however, also stimulates the PI3K-AKT pathways, which may lead to higher levels of PD-L1 expression. The anti-tumour effects of IFN- would be enhanced by blocking the PI3K-AKT pathway. The phase II POPLAR trial found that atezolizumab-treated NSCLC patients expressed more IFN- produced by T-cell effectors. Additionally, a favourable IFN- mRNA profile suggested that anti-PD-1/PD-L1 treatment would be beneficial (Higgs et al. 2018).

IL-6 has a connection to NSCLC patients' poor prognosis. High concentrations of IL-6 are connected with an increase in Treg cells and an upregulation of PD-1 on CD4+ T-cells and CD8+ T-cells. Patients who received immunotherapy for their NSCLC had better FPS than those who received immunotherapy for those who had greater or normal levels of IL-6, in accordance with Keegan et al.'s (2020) findings. These results suggest that IL-6 levels might serve as a possible prognostic biomarker.

Even though it controls immunity, the cytokine IL-10 also encourages CD8+ T-cell expansion. Li et al.'s study (Li and Zuo 2019) found that IL-10 boosted IFN- expression while decreasing the expression of PD-1 on CD8+ T-cells in cancerous tissue and peripheral blood. IFN-/IL-10 ratios were shown to be greater in responding immunotherapy patients, according to Giunta et al. [124]. In accordance with Boutsikou et al. (2018), elevated levels of the following cytokines (TNF-, IL-1, IL-2, IL-4, and IL-8) were shown to be associated with favourable results of anti-PD-1/anti-PD-L1 treatment, and these particular cytokines were not dependent on PD-L1 expression. In addition, Sanmamed et al. (2017) reported that in individuals suffering from NSCLC and melanoma, lower levels of IL-8 were strongly associated with improved immunotherapy response and prolonged OS. The angiogenesis process, which results in tumour development and metastasis, is greatly aided by VEGF (vascular endothelial growth factor), which stands for vascular endothelial growth. VEGF has the capacity to inhibit dendritic cell (DC) development and activation and promote the recruitment of regulatory T-cells (Tregs) and myeloid-derived suppressor cells (MDSCs) (Yang et al. 2018).

Together, anti-PD-1 and anti-VEGF, as shown by Wallin et al. (2016), will encourage tumour-specific T-cell migration and increase CD8+ T-cell growth in the tumour microenvironment. According to Atkins et al. (2018), individuals with advanced carcinoma of the renal cells exhibited stronger therapeutic benefits and appeared to tolerate pembrolizumab in combination with VEGF inhibitors. Shibaki et al. (2020) found that in patients with NSCLC who were older than 75 years, increased periphery VEGF levels were associated with worse outcomes and lower immunotherapy's effectiveness.

17.8 Factors Relating to the Immune System

17.8.1 Beta-2-Microglobulin

There is beta-2-microglobulin (B2M), which is a crucial part of HLA-I (human leukocyte antigen class I) molecules. Mutations in B2M impede antigen presentation and cancer evasion. According to Sade-Feldman et al. (2017), 5 of the 17 metastatic melanoma patients receiving immunotherapy had the B2M gene showing point mutations, deletions, or a loss of heterozygosity (LOH). In comparison to respondents, non-responders had poorer OS and three times the amount of B2M LOH (30% vs. 10%). Gettinger et al. (2017) found a link between B2M deletion and reduced expression on cancer cells and PD-1 or PD-L1 therapy resistance. In lung cancer, B2M deletion-mediated class I HLA disruption causes ICIs to escape. The B2M gene knockout in immune-competent lung cancer mouse has also demonstrated resistance to ICIs. Increased PD-1+ T-cell density was linked to B2M mutations, according to Janikovits et al. (2018), suggesting that the milieu in which PD-1+ T-cells were infiltrating was where the lack of HLA-I caused by B2M mutations most frequently occurred.

According to Pereira et al. (2017), 5% of lung cancer patients had B2M mutations, the majority of which prevented the HLA-I complex from forming properly. Additional genetic alterations connected to the development of the HLA-I complex have also been found. With higher amounts of B2M and HLA-I protein, cytotoxic CD8+ lymphocyte infiltration and the expression of PD-L1 were reduced. Patients having the highest levels of heterozygosity (differing alleles at the HLA-I locus) had a greater OS with immunotherapy treatment than those who had homozygosity for at least one HLA gene, according to Chowell et al.'s (2018) findings. While MHC-II expression-positive tumour cells (>1%) indicated a positive response to anti-PD-1 therapy, MHC-I expression on tumour cells was completely lost (>50% cells) in the majority of advanced melanoma patients, indicating primary resistance towards anti-cytotoxic T-lymphocyte antigen-4 (CTLA-4) therapy.

17.8.2 B7-H4

B7-H4, an immunoglobulin from the subfamily of B7 immunoglobulins, lessens the immune response to tumours by reducing T-cell proliferation and cytokine production. Furthermore, although B7-H4 expression in normal tissues is either non-existent or extremely low, it is highly abundant in cancer tissues. B7-H4 also aids in the growth of tumours and immune evasion by suppressing T-cell activity and proliferation (Wang and Wang 2020). B7-H4 expression was associated with a reduction in PFS and OS in NSCLC patients receiving nivolumab therapy, according to Genova et al.'s research (2019). Furthermore, no association between B7-H4 expression and the outcomes of patients undergoing platinum-based chemotherapy was shown to be statistically significant. According to Shrestha et al. (2018), individuals with hepatocellular carcinoma who received immunotherapy had a poor prognosis if their B7-H4 expression levels were high. Additionally, B7-H4 expression was separately linked to a poorer prognosis.

17.8.3 TOX

The thymocyte selection gene TOX, which is linked to the expression of the high mobility group box gene, is significantly upregulated in tumour-specific T-lymphocytes and wornout T-lymphocytes following a protracted viral infection, according to Scott et al. Although the T-cell failure method is eliminated when tumour-specific T-cells lose their TOX, these non-exhausted T-cells continue to operate improperly (Scott et al. 2019). Higher TIL density and increased TOX expression were found to be positively correlated by Guo L et al. (2020), and high TOX expression was found to be an excellent predictor of prognosis for a range of tumour types, notably lung adenocarcinoma (LUAD). However, Kim et al. (2020) discovered that TOX enhanced intercellular adhesion molecules in the tumour microenvironment, which resulted in CD8+ T-cell fatigue, and that reducing TOX expression was connected to greater anti-PD-1 therapy's effectiveness. Although TOX exhibited predictive value for the efficacy of immunotherapy, routine clinical application of TOX monitoring proved difficult.

17.8.4 Biomarkers for Hyper-progressive Illness

A highly bad prognosis-related aberrant tumour development is known as hyper-progressive disease (HPD). Despite the lack of agreement on the diagnosis of HPD, it is thought that this population may include individuals whose tumour progression kinetics and/or tumour expansion rate increased at least twice while receiving medication (Saâda-Bouzid et al. 2017). According to Ferrara et al. (2018), individuals with NSCLC who underwent immunotherapy experienced HPD more frequently than those who received chemotherapy. This effect was also noted by Kim et al. (2019), who discovered that worse outcomes and greater occurrences of HPD in NSCLC patients receiving ICIs were related to reduced periphery blood levels of CD8+ T-cells, CCR7-CD45RA- T memory cells, and tired T-cells.

Ageing poses a threat to HPD. People aged 65 and older had a much higher risk of HPD (37% percent vs. 19%) than those under 65 did [154]. HPD was linked to an increase in M2 tumour-associated macrophages (TAMs), which were implicated in immunotherapy, according to Lo Russo et al.'s findings (Lo et al. 2019). Treg cells were activated and the death of the effector T-cells was sped up by increased M2 TAM infiltration in the tumour microenvironment (Wang et al. 2020). Furthermore, Chen et al. (2020) discovered that HPD was connected to elevated levels of the ctDNA and MIKI67 mutations in 22 patients with advanced NSCLC who underwent immunotherapy.

17.9 Conclusion

Immunotherapy, which has also profoundly changed how advanced sickness is handled, has ushered in an intriguing new era in the treatment of NSCLC. A number of studies have shown a relationship between expression levels and response, and IHC is now the gold standard for PD-L1 expression evaluation. Even in individuals with high expression, immunotherapy can help some patients with low or no expression, while PD-L1 testing has severe limitations. These discrepancies have motivated researchers to look for alternative response indicators. TMB originally had a lot of promise;

however, its future as a biomarker is currently questionable given the new overall survival results from Checkmate 227 revealing that ipilimumab plus nivolumab lacks predictive significance. While certain KRAS mutant tumours seem to be more susceptible to treatment, other tumour genotypes, including EGFR and ALK, tend to be less resistant to checkpoint blocking. TIL concentration, gene expression patterns, and testing for "active" TILs are a few more tissue-based indicators under research that have been linked in studies to the effectiveness of immunotherapy. Given the simplicity with which such measurements may be obtained, serum-based markers are a desirable choice, particularly when testing requires more tissue than can be sampled. Blood-based biomarkers that include the neutrophil-to-lymphocyte ratio (NLR), bTMB, and others have drawn interest despite still being researched because of their prognostic and predictive value while employing checkpoint inhibitors.

According to recent studies, the ineffectiveness of immunotherapy with a single drug in treating tumours with low PD-L1 concentrations may be addressed by using pembrolizumab in combination with a platinum doublet. The first-line treatment for advanced non-small cell lung cancer (NSCLC) currently includes this combination as the norm. Additionally, participants in this combo study were not allowed to have tumours that were positive for EGFR and ALK. The VEGF inhibitor bevacizumab is combined with the chemotherapeutic medicines carboplatin, paclitaxel, and atezolizumab in the IMpower150 regimen, which the FDA recently approved for the cure of initial-line metastatic lung adenocarcinoma. Patients with EGFR and ALK mutations were not, however, covered by this approval. Atezolizumab has also been researched and shown to improve clinical outcomes when combined with carboplatin and nab-paclitaxe or platin and pemetrexed, even though only the IMpower regimen is now authorised. While more patients will likely receive checkpoint inhibitor therapy as a result of chemotherapy and immunotherapy combinations, others may still not benefit from a response. Checkpoint blockade therapy is not without adverse effects, including potentially fatal immunotoxicities. Because of this, it is even more crucial to continue researching and creating better biomarkers that can anticipate toxicity and serve as sensitive, accurate indications of an immunotherapy's effectiveness.

References

Antonia SJ, Villegas A, Daniel D, Vicente D, Murakami S, Hui R et al (2018) Overall survival with durvalumab after chemoradiotherapy in stage III NSCLC. N Engl J Med 379(24):2342–2350

Atkins MB, Plimack ER, Puzanov I, Fishman MN, McDermott DF, Cho DC et al (2018) Axitinib in combination with pembrolizumab in patients with advanced renal cell cancer: a non-randomised, open-label, dose-finding, and dose-expansion phase 1b trial. Lancet Oncol 19:405–415

Ayers M, Lunceford J, Nebozhyn M et al (2017) IFN-γ-related mRNA profile predicts clinical response to PD-1 blockade. J Clin Invest 127(8):2930–2940

Banna GL, Signorelli D, Metro G, Galetta D, De Toma A, Cantale O et al (2020) Neutrophil-to-lymphocyte ratio in combination with PD-L1 or lactate dehydrogenase as biomarkers for high PD-L1 non-small cell lung cancer treated with first-line pembrolizumab. Transl Lung Cancer Res 9:1533–1542

Boutsikou E, Domvri K, Hardavella G, Tsiouda D, Zarogoulidis K, Kontakiotis T (2018) Tumour necrosis factor, interferon-gamma and interleukins as predictive markers of antiprogrammed cell-death protein-1 treatment in advanced non-small cell lung cancer: a pragmatic approach in clinical practice. Ther Adv Med Oncol 10:433584018

Brambilla E, Le Teuff G, Marguet S et al (2016) Prognostic effect of tumor lymphocytic infiltration in resectable non-small-cell lung cancer. J Clin Oncol 34(11):1223–1230. https://doi.org/10.1200/JCO.2015.63.0970. [PubMed: 26834066]

Bristol-Myers Squibb reports fourth quarter and full year financial results. Bristol-Myers Squibb Published 1 24, 2019

Brogden KA, Parashar D, Hallier AR et al (2018) Genomics of NSCLC patients both affirm PD-L1 expression and predict their clinical responses to anti-PD-1 immunotherapy. BMC Cancer 18(1):225. https://doi.org/10.1186/s12885-018-4134-y

Campbell JD, Alexandrov A, Kim J, Wala J, Berger AH, Pedamallu CS et al (2016) Distinct patterns of somatic genome alterations in lung adenocarcinomas and squamous cell carcinomas. Nat Genet 48(6):607–616

Carter SL, Cibulskis K, Helman E, McKenna A, Shen H, Zack T et al (2012) Absolute quantification of somatic DNA alterations in human cancer. Nat Biotechnol 30(5):413–421

Champiat S, Dercle L, Ammari S et al (2017) Hyperprogressive disease is a new pattern of progression in cancer patients treated by anti-PD-1/PD-L1. Clin Cancer Res 23(8):1920–1928. https://doi.org/10.1158/1078-0432.CCR-16-1741. [PubMed: 27827313]

Chen G, Huang AC, Zhang W, Zhang G, Wu M, Xu W et al (2018) Exosomal PD-L1 contributes to immunosuppression and is associated with anti-PD-1 response. Nature 560:382–386

Chen Y, Li X, Liu G, Chen S, Xu M, Song L et al (2020) ctDNA concentration, MIKI67 mutations and hyper-progressive disease related gene Mutatios are prognostic markers for camrelizumab and apatinib combined multiline treatment in advanced NSCLC. Front Oncol 10:1706

Chowell D, Morris L, Grigg CM, Weber JK, Samstein RM, Makarov V et al (2018) Patient HLA class I genotype influences cancer response to checkpoint blockade immunotherapy. Science 359:582–587

Costantini A, Julie C, Dumenil C, Hélias-Rodzewicz Z, Tisserand J, Dumoulin J et al (2018) Predictive role of plasmatic biomarkers in advanced non-small cell lung cancer treated by nivolumab. Oncoimmunology 7:e1452581

Diem S, Schmid S, Krapf M, Flatz L, Born D, Jochum W et al (2017) Neutrophil-to-Lymphocyte ratio (NLR) and Platelet-to-Lymphocyte ratio (PLR) as prognostic markers in patients with non-small cell lung cancer (NSCLC) treated with nivolumab. Lung Cancer 111:176–181. https://doi.org/10.1016/j.lungcan.2017.07.024. [PubMed: 28838390]

Dong ZY, Zhong WZ, Zhang XC et al (2017) Potential predictive value of TP53 and KRAS mutation status for response to PD-1 blockade immunotherapy in lung adenocarcinoma. Clin Cancer Res 23(12):3012–3024. https://doi.org/10.1158/1078-0432.CCR-16-2554. [PubMed: 28039262]

Fan Y, Che X, Qu J, Hou K, Wen T, Li Z et al (2019) Exosomal PD-L1 retains immunosuppressive activity and is associated with gastric cancer prognosis. Ann Surg Oncol 26:3745–3755

Ferrara R, Mezquita L, Texier M, Lahmar J, Audigier-Valette C, Tessonnier L et al (2018) Hyperprogressive disease in patients with advanced non-small cell lung cancer treated with PD-1/PD-L1 inhibitors or with single-agent chemotherapy. JAMA Oncol 4:1543–1552

Ferrucci PF, Ascierto PA, Pigozzo J, Del VM, Maio M, Antonini CG et al (2016) Baseline neutrophils and derived neutrophil-to-lymphocyte ratio: prognostic relevance in metastatic melanoma patients receiving ipilimumab. Ann Oncol 27:732–738

Gandara DR, Paul SM, Kowanetz M et al (2018) Blood-based tumor mutational burden as a predictor of clinical benefit in non-small-cell lung cancer patients treated with atezolizumab. Nat Med 24(9):1441–1448. https://doi.org/10.1038/s41591-018-0134-3. [PubMed: 30082870]

Genova C, Boccardo S, Mora M, Rijavec E, Biello F, Rossi G et al (2019) Correlation between B7-H4 and survival of non-small-cell lung cancer patients treated with nivolumab. J Clin Med 8:1566

Gettinger S, Choi J, Hastings K, Truini A, Datar I, Sowell R et al (2017) Impaired HLA class I antigen processing and presentation as a mechanism of acquired resistance to immune checkpoint inhibitors in lung cancer. Cancer Discov 7:1420–1435
Gide TN, Quek C, Menzies AM, Tasker AT, Shang P, Holst J et al (2019) Distinct immune cell populations define response to anti-PD-1 monotherapy and anti-PD-1/anti-CTLA-4 combined therapy. Cancer Cell 35(2):238–55.e6
Gros A, Parkhurst MR, Tran E, Pasetto A, Robbins PF, Ilyas S et al (2016) Prospective identification of neoantigen-specific lymphocytes in the peripheral blood of melanoma patients. Nat Med 22:433–438
Guo L, Li X, Liu R, Chen Y, Ren C, Du S (2020) TOX correlates with prognosis, immune infiltration, and T cells exhaustion in lung adenocarcinoma. Cancer Med 9:6694–6709
Hastings K, Yu HA, Wei W, Sanchez-Vega F, DeVeaux M, Choi J et al (2019) EGFR mutation subtypes and response to immune checkpoint blockade treatment in non-small-cell lung cancer. Ann Oncol 30(8):1311–1320
Hellmann MD, Nathanson T, Rizvi H, Creelan BC, Sanchez-Vega F, Ahuja A et al (2018) Genomic features of response to combination immunotherapy in patients with advanced non-small-cell lung cancer. Cancer Cell 33(5):843–52.e4
Herbst R, Soria J-C, Kowanetz M et al (2014) Predictive correlates of response to the anti-PD-L1 antibody MPDL3280A in cancer patients. Nature 515(7528):563–567. https://doi.org/10.1038/nature14011. [PubMed: 25428504]
Higgs BW, Morehouse CA, Streicher K, Brohawn PZ, Pilataxi F, Gupta A et al (2018) Interferon gamma messenger RNA signature in tumor biopsies predicts outcomes in patients with non-small cell lung carcinoma or urothelial cancer treated with durvalumab. Clin Cancer Res 24:3857–3866
Ho WJ, Yarchoan M, Hopkins A, Mehra R, Grossman S, Kang H (2018) Association between pretreatment lymphocyte count and response to PD1 inhibitors in head and neck squamous cell carcinomas. J Immunother Cancer 6:84
Hogan SA, Courtier A, Cheng PF, Jaberg-Bentele NF, Goldinger SM, Manuel M et al (2019) Peripheral blood TCR repertoire profiling may facilitate patient stratification for immunotherapy against melanoma. Cancer Immunol Res 7:77–85
Ivashkiv LB (2018) IFNγ: signalling, epigenetics and roles in immunity, metabolism, disease and cancer immunotherapy. Nat Rev Immunol 18:545–558
Janikovits J, Müller M, Krzykalla J, Körner S, Echterdiek F, Lahrmann B et al (2018) High numbers of PDCD1 (PD-1)-positive T cells and B2M mutations in microsatellite-unstable colorectal cancer. Oncoimmunology 7:e1390640
Jiang P, Gu S, Pan D, Fu J, Sahu A, Hu X et al (2018) Signatures of T cell dysfunction and exclusion predict cancer immunotherapy response. Nat Med 24(10):1550–1558
Kamphorst AO, Pillai RN, Yang S, Nasti TH, Akondy RS, Wieland A et al (2017) Proliferation of PD-1+ CD8 T cells in peripheral blood after PD-1-targeted therapy in lung cancer patients. Proc Natl Acad Sci U S A 114:4993–4998
Kato S, Goodman A, Walavalkar V, Barkauskas DA, Sharabi A, Kurzrock R (2017) Hyperprogressors after immunotherapy: analysis of genomic alterations associated with accelerated growth rate. Clin Cancer Res 23(15):4242–4250. https://doi.org/10.1158/1078-0432.CCR-16-3133. [PubMed: 28351930]
Keegan A, Ricciuti B, Garden P, Cohen L, Nishihara R, Adeni A et al (2020) Plasma IL-6 changes correlate to PD-1 inhibitor responses in NSCLC. J Immunother Cancer 8:e000678
Kelderman S, Heemskerk B, van Tinteren H, van den Brom RR, Hospers GA, van den Eertwegh AJ et al (2014) Lactate dehydrogenase as a selection criterion for ipilimumab treatment in metastatic melanoma. Cancer Immunol Immunother 63:449–458
Kim ST, Cristescu R, Bass AJ, Kim KM, Odegaard JI, Kim K et al (2018) Comprehensive molecular characterization of clinical responses to PD-1 inhibition in metastatic gastric cancer. Nat Med 24:1449–1458
Kim CG, Kim KH, Pyo KH, Xin CF, Hong MH, Ahn BC et al (2019) Hyperprogressive disease during PD-1/PD-L1 blockade in patients with non-small-cell lung cancer. Ann Oncol 30:1104–1113

Kim K, Park S, Park SY, Kim G, Park SM, Cho JW et al (2020) Single-cell transcriptome analysis reveals TOX as a promoting factor for T cell exhaustion and a predictor for anti-PD-1 responses in human cancer. Genome Med 12:22

Krieg C, Nowicka M, Guglietta S, Schindler S, Hartmann FJ, Weber LM et al (2018) High-dimensional single-cell analysis predicts response to anti-PD-1 immunotherapy. Nat Med 24:144–153

Kythreotou A, Siddique A, Mauri FA, Bower M, Pinato DJ (2018) PD-L1. J Clin Pathol 71:189–194

Lee E, Chuang HY, Kim JW, Ideker T, Lee D (2008) Inferring pathway activity toward precise disease classification. PLoS Comput Biol 4(11):e1000217

Lee JH, Long GV, Menzies AM, Lo S, Guminski A, Whitbourne K et al (2018) Association between circulating tumor DNA and pseudoprogression in patients with metastatic melanoma treated with anti-programmed cell death 1 antibodies. JAMA Oncol 4:717–721

Li C, Zuo W (2019) IL-10 *in vitro* could enhance IFNγ expression and suppress PD-1 expression in CD8 T cells from esophageal cancer patients. Exp Cell Res 379:159–165

Liu X, Qu JK, Zhang J et al (2017) Prognostic role of pretreatment neutrophil to lymphocyte ratio in breast cancer patients. Medicine (United States) 96(45):e8101

Lo RG, Moro M, Sommariva M, Cancila V, Boeri M, Centonze G et al (2019) Antibody-Fc/FcR interaction on macrophages as a mechanism for hyperprogressive disease in non-small cell lung cancer subsequent to PD-1/PD-L1 blockade. Clin Cancer Res 25:989–999

Mariathasan S, Turley SJ, Nickles D, Castiglioni A, Yuen K, Wang Y et al (2018) TGFbeta attenuates tumour response to PD-L1 blockade by contributing to exclusion of T cells. Nature 554(7693):544–548

Mezquita L, Auclin E, Ferrara R, Charrier M, Remon J, Planchard D et al (2018) Association of the lung immune prognostic index with immune checkpoint inhibitor outcomes in patients with advanced non-small cell lung cancer. JAMA Oncol 4:351–357

Mitsuhashi A, Okuma Y (2018) Perspective on immune oncology with liquid biopsy, peripheral blood mononuclear cells, and microbiome with non-invasive biomarkers in cancer patients. Clin Transl Oncol 20:966–974

Newman AM, Liu CL, Green MR, Gentles AJ, Feng W, Xu Y et al (2015) Robust enumeration of cell subsets from tissue expression profiles. Nat Methods 12(5):453–457. https://doi.org/10.1038/nmeth.3337

Paz-Ares L, Luft A, Vicente D, Tafreshi A, Gumus M, Mazieres J et al (2018) Pembrolizumab plus chemotherapy for squamous non-small-cell lung cancer. N Engl J Med 379(21):2040–2051

Pereira C, Gimenez-Xavier P, Pros E, Pajares MJ, Moro M, Gomez A et al (2017) Genomic profiling of patient-derived xenografts for lung cancer identifies B2M inactivation impairing immunorecognition. Clin Cancer Res 23:3203–3213

Postow MA, Manuel M, Wong P, Yuan J, Dong Z, Liu C et al (2015) Peripheral T cell receptor diversity is associated with clinical outcomes following ipilimumab treatment in metastatic melanoma. J Immunother Cancer 3:23

Reck M, Rodriguez-Abreu D, Robinson AG, Hui R, Csoszi T, Fulop A et al (2016) Pembrolizumab versus chemotherapy for PD-L1-positive non-small-cell lung cancer. N Engl J Med 375(19):1823–1833

Reuben A, Zhang J, Chiou SH, Gittelman RM, Li J, Lee WC et al (2020) Comprehensive T cell repertoire characterization of non-small cell lung cancer. Nat Commun 11:603

Ribas A (2015) Adaptive immune resistance: how cancer protects from immune attack. Cancer Discov 5:915–919

Rittmeyer A, Barlesi F, Waterkamp D, Park K, Ciardiello F, von Pawel J et al (2017) Atezolizumab versus docetaxel in patients with previously treated non-small-cell lung cancer (OAK): a phase 3, open-label, multicentre randomised controlled trial. Lancet 389(10066):255–265

Rizvi NA, Hellmann MD, Snyder A, Kvistborg P, Makarov V, Havel JJ et al (2015) Cancer immunology. Mutational landscape determines sensitivity to PD-1 blockade in non-small cell lung cancer. Science 348(6230):124–128. https://doi.org/10.1126/science.aaa1348

Russo A, Russano M, Franchina T, Migliorino MR, Aprile G, Mansueto G et al (2020) Neutrophil-to-Lymphocyte Ratio (NLR), Platelet-to-Lymphocyte Ratio (PLR), and outcomes with

nivolumab in pretreated non-small cell lung cancer (NSCLC): a large retrospective multicenter study. Adv Ther 37:1145–1155
Saâda-Bouzid E, Defaucheux C, Karabajakian A, Coloma VP, Servois V, Paoletti X et al (2017) Hyperprogression during anti-PD-1/PD-L1 therapy in patients with recurrent and/or metastatic head and neck squamous cell carcinoma. Ann Oncol 28:1605–1611
Sade-Feldman M, Jiao YJ, Chen JH, Rooney MS, Barzily-Rokni M, Eliane JP et al (2017) Resistance to checkpoint blockade therapy through inactivation of antigen presentation. Nat Commun 8:1136
Sanmamed MF, Perez-Gracia JL, Schalper KA, Fusco JP, Gonzalez A, Rodriguez-Ruiz ME et al (2017) Changes in serum interleukin-8 (IL-8) levels reflect and predict response to anti-PD-1 treatment in melanoma and non-small-cell lung cancer patients. Ann Oncol 28:1988–1995
Schalper KA, Brown J, Carvajal-Hausdorf D, McLaughlin J, Velcheti V, Syrigos KN et al (2015) Objective measurement and clinical significance of TILs in non-small cell lung cancer. J Natl Cancer Inst 107(3):dju435
Schatton T, Scolyer RA, Thompson JF, Mihm MC (2014) Tumor-infiltrating lymphocytes and their significance in melanoma prognosis. Methods Mol Biol 1102:287–324. https://doi.org/10.1007/978-1-62703-727-3_16. [PubMed: 24258985]
Scheper W, Kelderman S, Fanchi LF, Linnemann C, Bendle G, de Rooij M et al (2019) Low and variable tumor reactivity of the intratumoral TCR repertoire in human cancers. Nat Med 25:89–94
Scott AC, Dündar F, Zumbo P, Chandran SS, Klebanoff CA, Shakiba M et al (2019) TOX is a critical regulator of tumour-specific T cell differentiation. Nature 571:270–274
Shibaki R, Murakami S, Shinno Y, Matsumoto Y, Yoshida T, Goto Y et al (2020) Predictive value of serum VEGF levels for elderly patients or for patients with poor performance status receiving anti-PD-1 antibody therapy for advanced non-small-cell lung cancer. Cancer Immunol Immunother 69:1229–1236
Shrestha R, Prithviraj P, Anaka M, Bridle KR, Crawford D, Dhungel B et al (2018) Monitoring immune checkpoint regulators as predictive biomarkers in hepatocellular carcinoma. Front Oncol 8:269
Siegel RL, Miller KD, Fuchs HE, Jemal A (2021) Cancer statistics, 2021. CA Cancer J Clin 71(1):7–33. https://doi.org/10.3322/caac.21654
Skoulidis F, Goldberg ME, Greenawalt DM et al (2018) STK11/LKB1 mutations and PD-1 inhibitor resistance in KRAS-mutant lung adenocarcinoma. Cancer Discov 8(7):822–835
Socinski MA, Jotte RM, Cappuzzo F et al (2018) Atezolizumab for first-line treatment of metastatic nonsquamous NSCLC. N Engl J Med 378(24):2288–2301
Soyano A, Dholaria B, Marin J et al (2017) Blood biomarkers correlate with outcome in advanced non-small cell lung cancer patients treated with anti PD-1 antibodies. J Thorac Oncol 12(11):S2011–S2011
Takeda T, Takeuchi M, Saitoh M, Takeda S (2018) Neutrophil-to-lymphocyte ratio after four weeks of nivolumab administration as a predictive marker in patients with pretreated non-small-cell lung cancer. Thorac Cancer 9(10):1291–1299. https://doi.org/10.1111/1759-7714.12838. [PubMed: 30126063]
Tauriello D, Palomo-Ponce S, Stork D, Berenguer-Llergo A, Badia-Ramentol J, Iglesias M et al (2018) TGFβ drives immune evasion in genetically reconstituted colon cancer metastasis. Nature 554:538–543
Theodoraki MN, Yerneni SS, Hoffmann TK, Gooding WE, Whiteside TL (2018) Clinical significance of PD-L1(+) exosomes in plasma of head and neck cancer patients. Clin Cancer Res 24:896–905
Thomas NE, Busam KJ, From L et al (2013) Tumor-infiltrating lymphocyte grade in primary melanomas is independently associated with melanoma-specific survival in the population-based genes, environment and melanoma study. J Clin Oncol 31(33):4252–4259. https://doi.org/10.1200/JCO.2013.51.3002. [PubMed: 24127443]
Thorsson V, Gibbs DL, Brown SD, Wolf D, Bortone DS, Ou Yang TH et al (2018) The immune landscape of cancer. Immunity 48(4):812–30 e14

Toki MI, Mani N, Smithy JW et al (2018) Immune marker profiling and programmed death ligand 1 expression across NSCLC mutations. J Thorac Oncol 13(12):1884–1896. https://doi.org/10.1016/j.jtho.2018.09.012. [PubMed: 30267840]

Van Allen EM, Miao D, Schilling B, Shukla SA, Blank C, Zimmer L et al (2015) Genomic correlates of response to CTLA-4 blockade in metastatic melanoma. Science 350(6257):207–211

Vokes N, Jimenez Alguilar E, Adeni A, Al E (2018) Efficacy and genomic correlates of response to anti-PD1/PD-L1 blockade in non-small cell lung cancers harboring targetable oncogenes. In: 2018 IASLC world conference on lung cancer

Wallin JJ, Bendell JC, Funke R, Sznol M, Korski K, Jones S et al (2016) Atezolizumab in combination with bevacizumab enhances antigen-specific T-cell migration in metastatic renal cell carcinoma. Nat Commun 7:12624

Wang JY, Wang WP (2020) B7-H4, a promising target for immunotherapy. Cell Immunol 347:104008

Wang X, Cao L, Li S, Wang F, Huang D, Jiang R (2019) Combination of PD-L1 expression and NLR as prognostic marker in patients with surgically resected non-small cell lung cancer. J Cancer 10:6703–6710

Wang X, Wang F, Zhong M, Yarden Y, Fu L (2020) The biomarkers of hyperprogressive disease in PD-1/PD-L1 blockage therapy. Mol Cancer 19:81

Yang J, Yan J, Liu B (2018) Targeting VEGF/VEGFR to modulate antitumor immunity. Front Immunol 9:978

Yarchoan M, Hopkins A, Jaffee EM (2017) Tumor mutational burden and response rate to PD-1 inhibition. N Engl J Med 377(25):2500–2501

Yu C, Luo D, Yu J, Zhang M, Zheng X, Xu G et al (2022) Genome-wide CRISPRCas9 knockout screening identifies GRB7 as a driver for MEK inhibitor resistance in KRAS mutant colon cancer. Oncogene 41(2):191–203

Zhou J, Mahoney KM, Giobbie-Hurder A, Zhao F, Lee S, Liao X et al (2017) Soluble PD-L1 as a biomarker in malignant melanoma treated with checkpoint blockade. Cancer Immunol Res 5:480–492

Zhou Y, Zhou B, Pache L, Chang M, Khodabakhshi AH, Tanaseichuk O et al (2019) Metascape provides a biologist-oriented resource for the analysis of systems-level datasets. Nat Commun 10(1):1523

Insight on the Clinical Trials of Immunotherapy for the Treatment of Lung Cancer

18

Dhruv Sanjay Gupta, Vaishnavi Gadi, and Saritha Shetty

18.1 Introduction

In the United States, lung cancer is the second most common cancer diagnosed and the leading cause of cancer-associated death (Hoy et al. 2019). Adenocarcinoma, squamous carcinoma, big cell carcinoma (also known as non-small cell lung cancer) and small cell lung cancer are some of the different histologic subtypes of lung cancer (Ruiz-Cordero and Devine 2020). There are several risk factors that have been considered to be directly linked to the aetiology of lung cancer, even though tobacco smoking is the primary risk factor responsible for 80–90% of all lung cancer diagnoses (Nooreldeen and Bach 2021). Public health concerns about lung cancer have increased. Along with global industrialization, urbanization and environmental pollution, the aetiology of lung cancer has become more composite. The tertiary prevention techniques of lung cancer as well as the investigation of novel diagnostic and therapeutic approaches have advanced based on data obtained from the studies on the epidemiologic features of lung cancer and its relative risk factors (Mao et al. 2016).

Over the past few decades, lung cancer survival has only slightly increased, but the development of screening techniques, early identification by low-dose CT, breakthroughs in targeted therapy and immunotherapy will potentially lower mortality rates and enhance patient survival (Schabath and Cote 2019). For diagnosis and staging, numerous techniques are being developed. The subtype and stage of the cancer determine the course of treatment; there are now a number of personalized therapies being implemented (Nasim et al. 2019).

D. S. Gupta · V. Gadi · S. Shetty (✉)
NMIMSDepartment of Pharmaceutics, Shobhaben Pratapbhai Patel School of Pharmacy & Technology Management, SVKM's Narsee Monjee Institute of Management Studies (NMIMS) Deemed-to-University, Mumbai, India

S. Bhatt et al. (eds.), *Immunotherapy Against Lung Cancer*,
https://doi.org/10.1007/978-981-99-7141-1_18

Recent studies have established significant treatment advancements for patients with metastatic non-small cell lung cancer (mNSCLC), prompting much higher survival rates. A portion of patients with mNSCLC have experienced unusually extended survival due to the development of specific antibodies that target the programmed death (PD-1) receptor, programmed death-ligand 1 (PD-L1) and the cytotoxic T-lymphocyte-associated protein 4 receptor (Reck et al. 2022).

The key component of the amelioration of advanced-stage NSCLC has been systemic cytotoxic chemotherapy, but its efficacy has plateaued. New therapeutic modalities are also needed. Despite a greater understanding of the role of driver mutations in NSCLC and strategies to target these mutations in the management of NSCLC, for instance, epidermal growth factor receptor (EGFR) mutation and anaplastic lymphoma kinase (ALK) fusion oncogene, success is still only partially achieved. Immunotherapy is unquestionably the most effective new treatment for lung cancer (Lee et al. 2013).

Through this chapter, the authors aim to provide a holistic overview of the various immunotherapeutic strategies being explored, along with their present clinical status. Immune checkpoint inhibitors, immunostimulatory molecules, vaccines, cellular immunotherapy and immune cell engineering, among others, have been described with respect to their clinical success and interrogation.

18.1.1 Lung Cancer

Lung cancer is a complex health condition with a range of clinicopathological characteristics (Travis et al. 2015). Whether it has to do with the patient's vulnerability to lung cancer or responsiveness to biologic therapy, there is an underlying genetic basis influencing the pathogenesis of lung cancer. Thus, testing for driver mutations in particular genes in lung tumours has fundamentally altered the ways in which the disease is treated clinically as well as how it advances (Fois et al. 2021). The most frequently seen oncogene in non-small cell lung cancer (NSCLC) is KRAS, which has historically been ineffective in targeted therapy methods such as farnesyl transferase inhibition, MEK (mitogen-activated protein kinase kinase) inhibition and synthetic lethality screens (Adderley et al. 2019). Compared to non-smokers, lifelong smokers have a 20–40 times increased risk of developing lung cancer (Ozlü and Bülbül 2005).

The nature of the tumour and the degree of the metastases may govern the signs and symptoms. Patients suspected to suffer from lung cancer undergo a tissue diagnosis, a thorough staging procedure and an operational patient evaluation as part of the diagnostic process (Collins et al. 2007). Surgical removal of the tumour is most commonly adopted as a treatment strategy for the pharmacological management of non-small cell carcinoma stages I through IIIA. A multimodal strategy is used to treat advanced non-small cell carcinoma and may involve radiation, chemotherapy and hospice treatment (Temel et al. 2022).

A considerable number of patients have tumours displaying mutations that can be managed with molecularly targeted treatment (MTT), according to a recent study. These targeted treatments are utilized with considerable effectiveness in elderly lung cancer patients because they have a significantly better tolerable adverse effect profile. Immune checkpoint inhibitors, a novel class of medications, have recently entered the market and are showing promising outcomes in the second-line treatment of lung cancer with a manageable side effect profile (Kanesvaran et al. 2016). Histology-based therapy for advanced lung cancer is built on the foundation of chemotherapy. But during the past few decades, the findings on predictive biomarkers have presented novel treatment approaches for lung cancer, by way of immunotherapy and targeted therapy (Thai et al. 2021).

The degree of benefit of non-small cell lung cancer treatment is judged on the basis of the patient's responsiveness, morphological diagnosis and clinical stage. Surgery is often recommended for individuals in the early stages. Adjuvant treatment is recommended in specific circumstances. Chemotherapy, biological treatment and most recently immunotherapy have been recommended at locally advanced and metastatic stages (Skřičková et al. 2018). The treatment of advanced non-small cell lung cancer (NSCLC) has seen a massive shift, with the introduction of immune checkpoint inhibition. Significant interest in using these drugs in early stages of disease has been prompted by impressive results in the metastatic context (Broderick 2020).

18.1.2 Immunotherapy and Lung Cancer

Lung cancer remains the most common cancer-related cause of mortality and its treatment is complex. Despite having previously failed to treat lung cancer, immunotherapy has recently become a very successful new treatment, and interest in it is developing on a global scale (Woodard et al. 2016). It is crucial to understand the processes involved in immune identification and cancer cell elimination (Steven et al. 2016).

There are seven steps involved in the immunotherapy-based treatment of tumours by tumour-specific cluster of differentiation 8 T (CD8 T) cells. Each of these processes is vital, and each one can be regulated to increase or decrease responses and prevent collateral damage to healthy cells. A tumour must include cancer neoantigens, and these antigens must load professional APCs, like dendritic cells (DCs), so that the immune cells in the draining lymph node can be exposed to the antigen. Prior to becoming activated and proliferating, tumour-specific T-cells must first recognize these antigens via T-cell receptor (TCR) identification of the MHC: peptide complex receives the proper co-stimulatory signals and then receive further support (such as CD40 ligation). Then, activated tumour-specific T-lymphocytes circulate outside the dLN before arriving at the tumour site. These T-cells must overcome several local immune-suppressive mechanisms once they enter the tumour, and they are likely to be re-stimulated by the APCs there. Finally, after completing these six processes, these activated T-cells must attack the tumour. This entails recognizing the antigen produced by the tumour and releasing powerful chemicals like perforin and granzymes that kill the tumour cell. This mechanism can also produce memory cells, which may be crucial in the management of developing micrometastases (Steven et al. 2016).

The CLTA-4 pathway is of key importance in immunotherapy. The immune system possesses counterregulatory systems such as CTLA-4, LAG-3, PD-1/PD-2 and TIM-3 that prevent the immune response from amplifying in ways that could be detrimental. The expression of CTLA-4 is constitutive in Tregs but only increases in conventional T-cells following activation. Anti-CTLA-4 antibodies function as an intermediary and stop CTLA-4 from interacting with its receptor, maintaining the antitumour immune response (Topalian et al. 2015; Pardoll 2012). CLTA-4 inhibitors currently under study include ipilimumab (Weber 2007) and tremelimumab (Zatloukal et al. 2009).

The PD-1/PD-L1 pathway is also targeted by immunotherapy. The primary purpose of the PD-1 receptor (programmed cell death-1) is to regulate T-cell activity in peripheral tissues. It is expressed on T-/B-cells, NK cells and MDSCs. Two PD-1 ligands are expressed as a result of IFN-y, which lowers T-cell activation. Blocking PD-1 signalling can improve antitumour immunity, improve CD8+ T-cell activities and restore their capacity for cytotoxicity (Postow et al. 2015; Nguyen and Ohashi 2015). Anti-PD-1 drugs currently under study include nivolumab (Wang et al. 2014) and pembrolizumab (Hui et al. 2017).

Additionally, monoclonal antibodies that block PD-L1 reduce inflammation and maintain lung tissue (Philips and Atkins 2015). Anti-PD-L1 drugs can lessen immune-related toxicity while also suppressing a different harmful T-cell control (Haile et al. 2013). The anti-PD-L1 drugs under research include durvalumab (MEDI4736) (Antonia et al. 2016), atezolizumab (MPDL3280A) (Fehrenbacher et al. 2016), avelumab (Collins and Gulley 2019) and BMS-936559 (Philips and Atkins 2015).

18.1.3 Approved Therapeutics for Lung Cancer

The Food and Drug Administration (FDA) has approved various anti-cancer drugs for lung cancer. Both generic and brand names are included in Table 18.1. The information has been summarized based on the latest data available on the National Cancer Institute's webpage.

Despite their widespread use, drug combinations typically do not have the FDA approval.

Table 18.1 FDA-approved and emerging immunotherapeutic agents for lung cancer management (encompassing generic and brand names)

Category	Name of drugs	Reference
Drugs for non-small cell lung cancer (approved)	• Abraxane (paclitaxel albumin-stabilized nanoparticle formulation) • Adagrasib • Afatinib dimaleate • Afinitor (everolimus) • Afinitor Disperz (everolimus) • Alymsys (bevacizumab) • Amivantamab-vmjw • Atezolizumab • Avastin (bevacizumab) • Bevacizumab • Brigatinib • Capmatinib hydrochloride • Cemiplimab-rwlc • Ceritinib • Crizotinib • Cyramza (ramucirumab) • Docetaxel • Doxorubicin hydrochloride • Everolimus • Fam-trastuzumab deruxtecan-nxki • Gefitinib • Gilotrif (afatinib dimaleate) • Imfinzi (durvalumab) • Iressa (gefitinib) • Keytruda (pembrolizumab) • Lorlatinib • Mobocertinib succinate • Necitumumab • Nivolumab • Opdivo (nivolumab) • Osimertinib mesylate • Paclitaxel • Retevmo (selpercatinib) • Rozlytrek (entrectinib) • Rybrevant (amivantamab-vmjw) • Selpercatinib • Sotorasib • Hydrochloride • Trametinib dimethyl sulfoxide • Tremelimumab-actl • Yervoy (ipilimumab) • Zirabev (bevacizumab) • Zykadia (ceritinib)	National Cancer Institute (2016)

(continued)

Table 18.1 (continued)

Category	Name of drugs	Reference
Drug combinations for non-small cell lung cancer (combinations not FDA approved)	• Carboplatin-taxol • Gemcitabine-cisplatin	National Cancer Institute (2016)
Drugs for small cell lung cancer (approved)	• Afinitor (everolimus) • Atezolizumab • Doxorubicin hydrochloride • Durvalumab • Etoposide • Everolimus • Imfinzi (durvalumab) • Methotrexate sodium • Nivolumab • Opdivo (nivolumab) • Tecentriq (atezolizumab) • Trexall (methotrexate sodium) • Zepzelca (lurbinectedin)	National Cancer Institute (2016)

18.2 Emerging Targets for Immunotherapeutics

While PD-1 has gained foremost attention and continues to be one of the most widely explored targets, there are several other immunotherapeutic targets that have gained clinical attention. This section offers an overview of their origin and brief mechanism of action based on pre-clinical studies, in addition to notable clinical advancements.

18.2.1 CTLA-4

The cytotoxic T-lymphocyte antigen 4 (CTLA-4), belonging to the immunoglobulin family, is primarily expressed on the surface of T-cells. It undergoes binding on antigen-presenting cells (APCs), as is chiefly responsible for inhibiting the activation and migration of T-cells, by induction of a negative feedback mechanism (Shiravand et al. 2022).

T-cells, more specifically regulatory T-cells, mediate an immunosuppressive effect through the upregulation of indoleamine 2,3-dioxygenase (IDO), following interaction with APCs. It has been established through research that cancer cells do not express CD80 or CD86 (the cluster of differentiation 80 and 86, respectively), and anti-CTLA4 antibodies exert their therapeutic effects through the priming of T-cells, even at a microenvironmental level (Patel and Weiss 2020). Given its mechanism of action, it has gained interest as an alternative treatment strategy to overcome resistance arising from monotherapy. This may be attributed to its mechanism of action being different from targeting the PD-1/PD-L1 pathway. In a meta-analysis conducted over a 12-year period (2008–2020), the polymorphism of CTLA-4 was not observed to be an independent risk factor in lung cancer pathogenesis; however, it was observed to be a risk factor specifically in NSCLC (Wei et al. 2021).

Ipilimumab, an IgG-1 monoclonal antibody, has demonstrated promising therapeutic efficacy in melanoma management, in combination with other agents such as nivolumab. This has warranted further exploration in the management of various cancers, such as lung cancer. CheckMate-012, a phase I clinical trial, yielded results of a satisfactory safety profile of the combination of the aforementioned agents (Negrao et al. 2019).

CheckMate-568, a phase II clinical trial exploring the outcome of delivery of the same agents, assessed the dosage in a ratio of 3:1 (nivolumab: ipilimumab) for a period of 6 weeks. A higher rate of progression-free survival was observed in patients, with the occurrence of mild adverse events. The promising findings obtained from the first two phases prompted the exploration of these agents in a phase III trial, exploring dosing independently, and in combination with chemotherapy. In subjects showing a PD-L1 expression greater than or equal to 1%, a survival rate of 40% was observed over a 2-year period (Ready et al. 2019).

To sum it up, immunotherapeutic agents such as PD-1 and PD-L1 have received widespread attention; however, newer targets such as CTLA-4 are slowly but steadily changing the therapeutic landscape, with chief applications in the management of multiple malignancies (Zhang et al. 2021). The Akeso Inc. is engaged in developing Cadonilimab (®), a PD-1/CTLA-4-bispecific antibody for the amelioration of solid tumours, including lung cancer. Its usage has been approved in China since June 2022 for cervical cancer management, and it is expected to gain popularity in other countries with time (Keam 2022).

A phase Ib clinical trial has explored the usage of tremelimumab, a CTLA-4, IgG2 monoclonal antibody, in combination with durvalumab, for the management of advanced-stage NSCLC. At a dosage of 1 mg/kg, it showed a satisfactory toxicity profile, with a grade 4 adverse events observed in a small percentage of the population (Antonia et al. 2016).

18.2.2 TIM-3

Recent research reveals that the two T-cell inhibitory receptors PD-1 and TIM-3 govern T-cell fatigue and immunotherapy effectiveness, although the molecular mechanism is still unknown. These receptors are expressed during T-cell exhaustion, and PD-1 has been observed to bind to TIM-3 ligand galectin-9 (Gal-9), thereby reducing the propensity for cell death. Anti-Gal-9 plus an agonistic anti-GITR (glucocorticoid-induced tumour necrosis factor receptor-related protein) antibody combination has been observed to deplete T-regulatory cells, resulting in a synergistic anti-cancer action. Interferons increase Gal-9 expression and secretion, and high Gal-9 expression is associated with a poor prognosis in a variety of cancers, thereby making it an interesting therapeutic target (Yang et al. 2021).

A study by Datar et al. showed up to 25% TIM-3 levels in tumour-infiltrating lymphocytes, in patients with NSCLC. In addition to other biomarkers such as PD-1 and LAG-3, it was observed to play a prominent role in lung cancer prognosis, more so in patients receiving immunotherapy (Datar et al. 2019).

This has sparked further research into the domain of checkpoint receptors. A variety of immune cells, including leukemic stem cells, express T-cell immunoglobulin and mucin domain 3 (Tim-3). In preclinical models, concurrent blockade of Tim-3 and PD-1 can suppress tumour growth and enhance antitumour T-cell responses in cancer patients (Acharya et al. 2020).

A study by Yasinska et al. revealed that localized galectin-9 and TIM-3 overexpression was observed in breast cancer tumours, accompanied by translocation. The presence of these biomarkers was seen to protect cells from cellular death, thereby reducing clinical efficacy of therapeutic agents and preventing the exertion of an antitumour activity (Yasinska et al. 2019).

Sabatolimab is a monoclonal antibody that has been observed to bind to TIM-3. A phase I/phase II study evaluated its effects in the management of solid tumours, in combination with other agents such as spartalizumab. It was observed to be well tolerated by the subjects, with the exertion of an antitumour activity (Curigliano et al. 2021). Recent research has demonstrated the significance of TIM-3 in T-cell exhaustion and its relationship to the effectiveness of anti-PD-1 treatment (He et al. 2018).

In addition to this, the efficacy of the agents in this category has been evaluated alongside oncolytic vaccinia viruses (oVV), for lung cancer management. Although systemic administration of oVV kills tumour cells directly and attracts and activates T-cells for indirect tumour killing, combination with PD-1 and TIM-3 blockers has shown promising results in the management of refractory lung cancer (Lahiri et al. 2023).

A clinical study undertaken on NSCLS patients in Zhoushan Hospital, China, over a 3-year period, indicated an improved survival time on controlling TIM-3 expression. This fortifies its position as a robust biomarker and as an independent governor of the prognosis of patients, chiefly in cases of adenocarcinomas and NSCLC (Zhang et al. 2023).

18.2.3 LAG-3

An immunological inhibitory receptor known as the lymphocyte activation gene-3 (LAG3; CD223), which is chiefly expressed on activated T-cells, binds the class II major histocompatibility complex (MHC). The inhibition of Th1-cell proliferation and the decrease in inflammatory biomarkers such as IL-2 and TNF are a few of its primary roles (Pockley et al. 2020).

LAG-3 has also been observed to bind to adhesion molecules in the liver. According to research on melanoma cells, the expression of this biomarker has been observed to encourage cancer cells to evade the immune system while reducing the ability of T-cells to control tumours (Beumer-Chuwonpad et al. 2021).

Cytotoxic T-cells that express LAG-3 have lower proliferation rates and reduced cytokine production, but suppressive T-cells that express LAG3 have a proven heightened activity despite the lack of a fully understood mechanism of action. As a result, the immune response becomes worn out as a result of LAG3's constant overexpression. LAG-3 has been gaining clinical importance as an immunotherapeutic target, more so in combination with other immune checkpoint inhibitors (Huang et al. 2004).

Ieramilimab, a novel anti-LAG3 agent, is currently being evaluated in two clinical trials, as independently and in combination with anti-PD-1 agents. In a phase I/ phase II trial, a promising safety profile of these agents was observed, chiefly with respect to solid lung carcinomas (Schöffski et al. 2022).

The same combination of agents was further evaluated in a phase I/phase II trial, focused on patients with advanced-stage SCLC and lymphomas. A satisfactory therapeutic outcome was observed; however, there is a need to undertake a greater number of clinical studies to assess its efficacy in the management of NSCLC (NCT03365791).

18.3 Immunostimulatory Molecules on T-Cells

18.3.1 OX40

OX40 is responsible for the delivery of co-stimulatory signals, in the late phase of survival and activation of T-cells. It belongs to the TNFR family and is primarily expressed in the form of its ligand in APCs and macrophages. The activation of this molecule has been linked with the enhancement of Th-1 and Th-2 immune responses, thereby regulating subsequent differentiation and expression of pro-inflammatory molecules, such as Th-9 (De Giglio et al. 2021).

In addition to this, OX40 fulfils the role of maintenance of the function of helper T-cells, controls proliferation and improves coordination between signalling molecules, such as CD4+ and CD8 (Fu et al. 2020). Initial work undertaken in models of sarcoma and breast cancer yielded positive results. However, a major drawback is that clinically significant outcomes have been observed only in strongly immunogenic tumours, necessitating the usage of combinations with different immunotherapeutic agents, such as interleukins, synthetic chemotherapeutic agents and radiotherapy. Various OX40 antagonists have been clinically assessed, with most studies being undertaken in advanced-stage models (Halim et al. 2018).

MOXR0916, an OX40 agonist monoclonal antibody, is being evaluated in combination with atezolizumab, for the management of solid malignancies. As we wait for an overall official outcome of the trial, preliminary dose escalation has not led to any adverse effects, and good therapeutic adherence has been observed (Kim et al. 2022). In addition to this, OX40 antagonists have been studied in combination with PD-L1 inhibitors, such as sintilimab and tislelizumab (Alves Costa Silva et al. 2020).

The triple regimen of OX40 agonists, PD-1 inhibitors and CTLA-4 inhibitors is being tested in a number of trials. OX40 agonist MEDI0562 is being tested in a dose escalation phase I trial either alone or together with the anti-CTLA-4 tremelimumab and the anti-PD-1 durvalumab (Goldman et al. 2022). Preliminary results showed that the novel agent was generally well tolerated, with a small percentage of volunteers experiencing grade 3 adverse effects and no reporting of grade 4 adverse effects (Glisson et al. 2020).

18.3.2 ICOS

It is vital to develop mechanisms for response monitoring and prediction to enhance clinical management of cancer immunotherapy. Inducible T-cell co-stimulator (ICOS) has been identified to be a mediator of immune response across various cancer models. Its monitoring has been analysed as a strategy for monitoring and evaluating responses to immunotherapy and has gained attention owing to its nature as a non-invasive technique (Xiao et al. 2020).

In a study undertaken by Rochigneux et al., ICOS levels, along with the expression of natural killer (NK) cells, were associated with an improvement in overall survival rates. It is crucial to understand the interplay of these biomarkers in pathogenesis, as they determine the efficacy of immunotherapeutic agents (Rochigneux et al. 2022).

ICOS undergoes binding with its ligand (ICOSL) and triggers adaptive immunity, which in turn facilitates an antineoplastic response, paving the way for emerging potentials for clinical translation. Various advancements in delivery, including the usage of a soluble form (ICOS-Fc), have been observed to arrest the migration of tumour cells, thereby arresting metastasis of lung cancer cells. A study by Clemente et al. assessed the loading of the soluble form of ICOS onto biodegradable nanoparticles, in an attempt to improve bioavailability. Nanosponges and cyclodextrin nanoparticles have been harnessed as nanotherapeutic strategies, and results from in vivo studies in mice models have indicated a suppression of the proliferation of solid tumours, by controlling angiogenesis and downregulating key inflammatory markers, such as interleukins (Clemente et al. 2020).

Declining levels of ICOS have been linked with lowered lung functioning, independent of demographic factors and the medical history of patients. Patients with higher expression had a prolonged survival time, owing to the onset of T-cell-mediated immunity (Bonham et al. 2019).

In phase I clinical study undertaken by Yap et al., the effects of dose escalation of vopratelimab, independently and in combination with nivolumab, were evaluated. The study was further escalated and focused on ICOS-positive tumours, and a promising safety and efficacy profile was obtained. There was an overall improvement in survival time; however, further clinical testing is required to enable the identification of a greater number of biomarkers influencing therapeutic outcomes (Yap et al. 2022).

18.3.3 Other Immunostimulatory Molecules

In addition to cultivating an understanding of widely explored immunostimulatory molecules, it is essential to explore a number of other agents. These include CD27, NKG2A and 4-IBB. In cancer cells, a concurrent expression of CD70 and CD27 has been directly linked with proliferation and survival time of malignancies (Flieswasser et al. 2022). CD27 agonistic antibodies have been explored in combination with immune checkpoint inhibitors and have yielded positive results in the management of solid malignancies (Starzer and Berghoff 2019). As for the immune checkpoint NKG2A, monalizumab was initially explored for the management of melanomas but is now being employed for a variety of cancers. It is chiefly associated with natural killer (NK) cells and has demonstrated positive results with respect to checking tumour growth in mouse models (Van Hall et al. 2019). 4-IBB is a co-stimulatory molecule and has been observed to play a vital role in the regulation of immune responses. Its mechanism of action may chiefly be attributed to the inactivation of cytotoxic T-lymphocytes, mediating the expression of interferons, making it a viable immunotherapeutic target (Vinay and Kwon 2014). Table 18.2 offers an overview of the clinical trials undertaken to assess the involvement of immunostimulatory molecules in lung cancer pathogenesis, as well as agents used for effective targeting.

Table 18.2 Clinical studies on immunostimulatory molecules for lung cancer management

Therapeutic strategy	Target	Clinical trial reference number	Number of volunteers	Study design	Outcome	Reference
Durvalumab, as monotherapy or in combination with oleclumab or monalizumab (anti-NKG2A monoclonal antibody)	NKG2A	NCT03822351	189 patients with stage III lung cancer	Phase II clinical trial	Improved progression-free survival and response rate on adopting combination therapy, reduction in tumour burden and satisfactory safety profile	Herbst et al. (2022)
Ivuxolimab, in combination with utomilumab	OX40 and 4-1BB	NCT02315066	57 patients with a variety of cancers, including advanced NSCLC	Multicentre, phase I, dose escalation trial	Exertion of preliminary antitumour activity, promising safety profile and relatively high rate of disease control	Hamid et al. (2022)
MOXR0916, anti-OX40 monoclonal antibody	OX40	NCT02219724	Patients with solid tumours	First-in-human, phase I study	No observation of dose-related toxicity, low-grade adverse effects, satisfactory pharmacokinetic profile and potentials for synergism on combination with other immunotherapeutic agents	Kim et al. (2022)
BMS-986178 (OX40 agonist), independently or in combination with nivolumab and/or ipilimumab	OX40	NCT02737475	165 patients with a variety of solid tumours, including NSCLC	Phase I/ phase IIa clinical study	Satisfactory safety and toxicity profile and need for further assessment of synergistic potentials	Gutierrez et al. (2021)
Durvalumab and tremelimumab, independently or in combination with radiotherapy	ICOS	NCT02701400	18 patients with relapsed SCLC	Randomized, phase II clinical trial	Achievement of stability of disease progression, improved progression-free survival time, low-grade adverse effects and improved activation of ICOS+ T-cells	Pakkala et al. (2020)

18.4 Tumour Vaccines

Oncolytic immunotherapy and cancer vaccines are promising therapeutic modalities that have the potential to benefit patients with advanced-stage cancer. Recombinant vaccinia viruses (VV), in particular, show significant promise as therapeutic agents.

Combinatorial methods, especially those that employ immune checkpoint inhibition, have yielded promising preclinical outcomes that call for the design of novel clinical investigations. For instance, dendritic cell (DC) vaccines based on neoantigens exhibit interesting benefits in the treatment of various malignant tumours.

A clinical trial by Ding et al. explored the potentials of a personalized, neoantigen peptide-pulsed autologous DC vaccine, in patients with metastatic lung cancer. Mild, grade 1–2 adverse effects were observed, with the spread of the disease being controlled up to 75%, in addition to an overall survival period of nearly 8 months. This study prompts the need for further exploration of the potentials of neoantigen vaccines and designing newer therapeutic strategies for lung cancer management (Ding et al. 2021). Figure 18.1 offers a complete overview of the topics discussed in this chapter.

Despite promising findings from translational research conducted on animal models, human trials using VV vectors independently as cancer vaccines have typically produced negative outcomes. However, notwithstanding negative findings with respect to monotherapy, better clinical efficacy has been achieved when regular treatments and VV vaccinations were combined. Researchers are also engaged in the exploration of novel vaccine approaches, such as the stimulation of antitumour immunity via stimulator of interferon genes (STING) activation in Batf3-dependent dendritic cells (DCs), primarily through the applications of VV vectors attenuated via replication. Table 18.3 offers an insight into the clinical trials conducted on vaccines, for the amelioration of lung cancer.

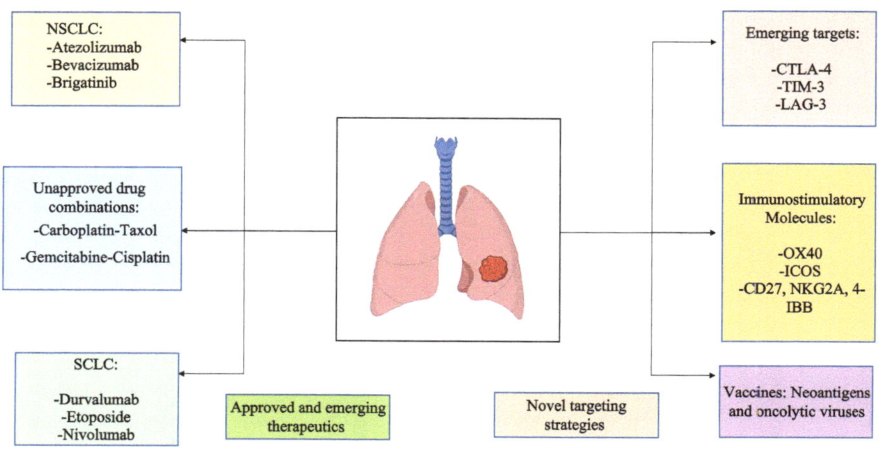

Fig. 18.1 Overview of approved and emerging therapeutics as well as novel targets for lung cancer management

Table 18.3 Clinical trials conducted on vaccines for the amelioration of lung cancer

Therapeutic strategy	Clinical trial reference number	Number of volunteers	Study design	Outcome	Reference
Neoantigen-based vaccine (NEO-PV-01)+ PD-1 blockade	NCT02897765	82 patients with a variety of cancers, including NSCLC	Phase Ib, open-label clinical trial	Promising safety profile and efficacy, no observation of adverse effects, localization of tumour cells and exertion of cytotoxic effects	Ott et al. (2020)
Neoantigen-based vaccine (NEO-PV-01)+ PD-1 blockade + chemotherapy	NCT03380871	38 patients with advanced, non-squamous NSCLC	Phase Ib, open-label clinical trial	Exertion of cytotoxic effects, reduced tumour cell infiltration and satisfactory safety profile in advanced-stage disease management	Awad et al. (2022)
Dendritic cell (DC) vaccines + low-dosage of cyclophosphamide and PD-1 blocking antibody	NCT02808416	10 patients with advanced-stage lung cancer	Clinical trial	No observation of adverse effects, improved progression-free survival time and potentials for combination with immunotherapeutic agents in the management of solid tumours	Wang et al. (2020)
Vx-001 vaccine, targeting telomerase reverse transcriptase (TERT)	NCT01935154	221 patients with TERT-positive NSCLC, having received chemotherapy	Randomized, double-blind, phase IIb clinical trial	Low toxicity reporting, initiation of an immune response and arrested disease progression over a 6-month period	Gridelli et al. (2020)
DCVAC/LuCa (dendritic cell vaccines), in combination with conventional chemotherapeutic agents	NCT02669719	61 chemotherapy-naïve patients with advanced stage IV lung cancer	Prospective, open-label, phase II clinical trial	Over 50% rate of a 2-year survival, low-grade adverse effects and progression-free survival period of 8 months achieved. Potentials for further exploration in a phase III trial	Zhong et al. (2022)

18.5 Conclusion

Immunotherapy for the management of malignancies is a rapidly evolving, dynamic domain. As a large number of therapies continue to gain FDA approval, there is a need to develop a better understanding of their mechanisms of action and potentials in cancer management. This chapter started out with the aim to establish a foundation by offering a basic understanding of the role of immunotherapy in cancer management and then narrowing the scope to lung cancer. Readers are offered an overview of the evolution of the concept of immunotherapy in the context of lung cancer, as well as a comprehensive list of FDA-approved molecules. This was followed by a discussion of the various emerging targets that have gained considerable clinical attention, backed by a discussion of recent clinical advancements. Our discussion would remain incomplete without a holistic understanding of other paradigms and aspects, such as the role of immunostimulatory molecules, novel strategies such as nanotechnological interventions to improve therapeutic outcomes and vaccines for disease management. However, a key observation that must be highlighted is the need for a greater number of clinical trials, in more diverse populations. This must also include the exploration of a combination of various immunotherapeutic agents, in an attempt to unravel synergistic potentials and any potential adverse effects that may emerge. As we move forward, scaling up of these technologies and ensuring access for improvement of quality of life of patients must be addressed.

References

Acharya N, Sabatos-Peyton C, Anderson AC (2020) Tim-3 finds its place in the cancer immunotherapy landscape. J Immunother Cancer 8(1):e000911. https://doi.org/10.1136/jitc-2020-000911

Adderley H, Blackhall FH, Lindsay CR (2019) KRAS-mutant non-small cell lung cancer: converging small molecules and immune checkpoint inhibition. EBioMedicine 41:711–716. https://doi.org/10.1016/j.ebiom.2019.02.049

Alves Costa Silva C, Facchinetti F, Routy B, Derosa L (2020) New pathways in immune stimulation: targeting OX40. ESMO Open 5(1):e000573. https://doi.org/10.1136/esmoopen-2019-000573

Antonia S, Goldberg SB, Balmanoukian A, Chaft JE, Sanborn RE, Gupta A, Narwal R, Steele K, Gu Y, Karakunnel JJ, Rizvi NA (2016) Safety and antitumour activity of durvalumab plus tremelimumab in non-small cell lung cancer: a multicentre, phase 1b study. Lancet Oncol 17(3):299–308. https://doi.org/10.1016/S1470-2045(15)00544-6

Awad MM, Govindan R, Balogh KN, Spigel DR, Garon EB, Bushway ME, Poran A, Sheen JH, Kohler V, Esaulova E, Srouji J, Ramesh S, Vyasamneni R, Karki B, Sciuto TE, Sethi H, Dong JZ, Moles MA, Manson K et al (2022) Personalized neoantigen vaccine NEO-PV-01 with chemotherapy and anti-PD-1 as first-line treatment for non-squamous non-small cell lung cancer. Cancer Cell 40(9):1010–1026.e11. https://doi.org/10.1016/j.ccell.2022.08.003

Beumer-Chuwonpad A, Taggenbrock RLRE, Ngo TA, Van Gisbergen KPJM (2021) The potential of tissue-resident memory T cells for adoptive immunotherapy against cancer. Cells 10(9):2234. https://doi.org/10.3390/cells10092234

Bonham CA, Hrusch CL, Blaine KM, Manns ST, Vij R, Oldham JM, Churpek MM, Strek ME, Noth I, Sperling AI (2019) T cell Co-Stimulatory molecules ICOS and CD28 stratify idiopathic pulmonary fibrosis survival. Respir Med X 1:100002. https://doi.org/10.1016/j.yrmex.2019.100002

Broderick SR (2020) Adjuvant and neoadjuvant immunotherapy in non-small cell lung cancer. Thorac Surg Clin 30(2):215–220. https://doi.org/10.1016/j.thorsurg.2020.01.001

Clemente N, Boggio E, Gigliotti LC, Raineri D, Ferrara B, Miglio G, Argenziano M, Chiocchetti A, Cappellano G, Trotta F, Caldera F, Capucchio MT, Yagi J, Rojo MJ, Renò F, Cavalli R, Dianzani C, Dianzani U (2020) Immunotherapy of experimental melanoma with ICOS-Fc loaded in biocompatible and biodegradable nanoparticles. J Control Release 320:112–124. https://doi.org/10.1016/j.jconrel.2020.01.030

Collins JM, Gulley JL (2019) Product review: avelumab, an anti-PD-L1 antibody. Hum Vaccin Immunother 15(4):891–908. https://doi.org/10.1080/21645515.2018.1551671

Collins LG, Haines C, Perkel R, Enck RE (2007) Lung cancer: diagnosis and management. Am Fam Physician 75(1):56–63

Curigliano G, Gelderblom H, Mach N, Doi T, Tai D, Forde PM, Sarantopoulos J, Bedard PL, Lin C-C, Hodi FS, Wilgenhof S, Santoro A, Sabatos-Peyton CA, Longmire TA, Xyrafas A, Sun H, Gutzwiller S, Manenti L, Naing A (2021) Phase I/Ib clinical trial of sabatolimab, an anti–TIM-3 antibody, alone and in combination with spartalizumab, an anti–PD-1 antibody, in advanced solid tumors. Clin Cancer Res 27(13):3620–3629. https://doi.org/10.1158/1078-0432.CCR-20-4746

Datar I, Sanmamed MF, Wang J, Henick BS, Choi J, Badri T, Dong W, Mani N, Toki M, Mejías LD, Lozano MD, Perez-Gracia JL, Velcheti V, Hellmann MD, Gainor JF, McEachern K, Jenkins D, Syrigos K, Politi K et al (2019) Expression analysis and significance of PD-1, LAG-3, and TIM-3 in human non–small cell lung cancer using spatially resolved and multiparametric single-cell analysis. Clin Cancer Res 25(15):4663–4673. https://doi.org/10.1158/1078-0432.CCR-18-4142

De Giglio A, Di Federico A, Nuvola G, Deiana C, Gelsomino F (2021) The landscape of immunotherapy in advanced NSCLC: driving beyond PD-1/PD-L1 inhibitors (CTLA-4, LAG3, IDO, OX40, TIGIT, vaccines). Curr Oncol Rep 23(11):126. https://doi.org/10.1007/s11912-021-01124-9

Ding Z, Li Q, Zhang R, Xie L, Shu Y, Gao S, Wang P, Su X, Qin Y, Wang Y, Fang J, Zhu Z, Xia X, Wei G, Wang H, Qian H, Guo X, Gao Z, Wang Y et al (2021) Personalized neoantigen pulsed dendritic cell vaccine for advanced lung cancer. Signal Transduct Target Ther 6(1):26. https://doi.org/10.1038/s41392-020-00448-5

Fehrenbacher L, Spira A, Ballinger M, Kowanetz M, Vansteenkiste J, Mazieres J, Park K, Smith D, Artal-Cortes A, Lewanski C, Braiteh F, Waterkamp D, He P, Zou W, Chen DS, Yi J, Sandler A, Rittmeyer A (2016) Atezolizumab versus docetaxel for patients with previously treated non-small-cell lung cancer (POPLAR): a multicentre, open-label, phase 2 randomised controlled trial. Lancet (London, England) 387(10030):1837–1846. https://doi.org/10.1016/S0140-6736(16)00587-0

Flieswasser T, Van Den Eynde A, Van Audenaerde J, De Waele J, Lardon F, Riether C, De Haard H, Smits E, Pauwels P, Jacobs J (2022) The CD70-CD27 axis in oncology: the new kids on the block. J Exp Clin Cancer Res 41(1):12. https://doi.org/10.1186/s13046-021-02215-y

Fois SS, Paliogiannis P, Zinellu A, Fois AG, Cossu A, Palmieri G (2021) Molecular epidemiology of the main druggable genetic alterations in non-small cell lung cancer. Int J Mol Sci 22(2):612. https://doi.org/10.3390/ijms22020612

Fu Y, Lin Q, Zhang Z, Zhang L (2020) Therapeutic strategies for the costimulatory molecule OX40 in T-cell-mediated immunity. Acta Pharm Sin B 10(3):414–433. https://doi.org/10.1016/j.apsb.2019.08.010

Glisson BS, Leidner RS, Ferris RL, Powderly J, Rizvi NA, Keam B, Schneider R, Goel S, Ohr JP, Burton J, Zheng Y, Eck S, Gribbin M, Streicher K, Townsley DM, Patel SP (2020) Safety and clinical activity of MEDI0562, a humanized OX40 agonist monoclonal antibody, in adult patients with advanced solid tumors. Clin Cancer Res 26(20):5358–5367. https://doi.org/10.1158/1078-0432.CCR-19-3070

Goldman JW, Piha-Paul SA, Curti B, Pedersen KS, Bauer TM, Groenland SL, Carvajal RD, Chhaya V, Kirby G, McGlinchey K, Hammond SA, Streicher K, Townsley DM, Chae YK, Voortman J, Marabelle A, Powderly J (2022) Safety and tolerability of MEDI0562, an OX40 agonist mAb, in combination with durvalumab or tremelimumab in adult patients with advanced solid tumors. Clin Cancer Res 28(17):3709–3719. https://doi.org/10.1158/1078-0432.CCR-21-3016

Gridelli C, Ciuleanu T, Domine M, Szczesna A, Bover I, Cobo M, Kentepozidis N, Zarogoulidis K, Kalofonos C, Kazarnowisz A, Korozan M, de Las Penas R, Majem M, Chella A, Griesinger F, Bournakis E, Sadjadian P, Kotsakis A, Chinet T et al (2020) Clinical activity of a htert (vx-001) cancer vaccine as post-chemotherapy maintenance immunotherapy in patients with stage IV non-small cell lung cancer: final results of a randomised phase 2 clinical trial. Br J Cancer 122(10):1461–1466. https://doi.org/10.1038/s41416-020-0785-y

Gutierrez M, Moreno V, Heinhuis KM, Olszanski AJ, Spreafico A, Ong M, Chu Q, Carvajal RD, Trigo J, Ochoa De Olza M, Provencio M, De Vos FY, De Braud F, Leong S, Lathers D, Wang R, Ravindran P, Feng Y, Aanur P, Melero I (2021) OX40 agonist BMS-986178 alone or in combination with nivolumab and/or ipilimumab in patients with advanced solid tumors. Clin Cancer Res 27(2):460–472. https://doi.org/10.1158/1078-0432.CCR-20-1830

Haile ST, Dalal SP, Clements V, Tamada K, Ostrand-Rosenberg S (2013) Soluble CD80 restores T cell activation and overcomes tumor cell programmed death ligand 1-mediated immune suppression. J Immunol (Baltimore, Md.: 1950) 191(5):2829–2836. https://doi.org/10.4049/jimmunol.1202777

Halim TYF, Rana BMJ, Walker JA, Kerscher B, Knolle MD, Jolin HE, Serrao EM, Haim-Vilmovsky L, Teichmann SA, Rodewald H-R, Botto M, Vyse TJ, Fallon PG, Li Z, Withers DR, McKenzie ANJ (2018) Tissue-restricted adaptive type 2 immunity is orchestrated by expression of the costimulatory molecule OX40L on group 2 innate lymphoid cells. Immunity 48(6):1195–1207.e6. https://doi.org/10.1016/j.immuni.2018.05.003

Hamid O, Chiappori AA, Thompson JA, Doi T, Hu-Lieskovan S, Eskens FALM, Ros W, Diab A, Spano J-P, Rizvi NA, Wasser JS, Angevin E, Ott PA, Forgie A, Yang W, Guo C, Chou J, El-Khoueiry AB (2022) First-in-human study of an OX40 (ivuxolimab) and 4-1BB (utomilumab) agonistic antibody combination in patients with advanced solid tumors. J Immunother Cancer 10(10):e005471. https://doi.org/10.1136/jitc-2022-005471

He Y, Cao J, Zhao C, Li X, Zhou C, Hirsch F (2018) TIM-3, a promising target for cancer immunotherapy. Onco Targets Ther 11:7005–7009. https://doi.org/10.2147/OTT.S170385

Herbst RS, Majem M, Barlesi F, Carcereny E, Chu Q, Monnet I, Sanchez-Hernandez A, Dakhil S, Camidge DR, Winzer L, Soo-Hoo Y, Cooper ZA, Kumar R, Bothos J, Aggarwal C, Martinez-Marti A (2022) COAST: an open-label, phase II, multidrug platform study of durvalumab alone or in combination with oleclumab or monalizumab in patients with unresectable, stage III non–small-cell lung cancer. J Clin Oncol 40(29):3383–3393. https://doi.org/10.1200/JCO.22.00227

Hoy H, Lynch T, Beck M (2019) Surgical treatment of lung cancer. Crit Care Nurs Clin North Am 31(3):303–313. https://doi.org/10.1016/j.cnc.2019.05.002

Huang C-T, Workman CJ, Flies D, Pan X, Marson AL, Zhou G, Hipkiss EL, Ravi S, Kowalski J, Levitsky HI, Powell JD, Pardoll DM, Drake CG, Vignali DAA (2004) Role of LAG-3 in regulatory T cells. Immunity 21(4):503–513. https://doi.org/10.1016/j.immuni.2004.08.010

Hui R, Garon EB, Goldman JW, Leighl NB, Hellmann MD, Patnaik A, Gandhi L, Eder JP, Ahn M-J, Horn L, Felip E, Carcereny E, Rangwala R, Lubiniecki GM, Zhang J, Emancipator K, Roach C, Rizvi NA (2017) Pembrolizumab as first-line therapy for patients with PD-L1-positive advanced non-small cell lung cancer: a phase 1 trial. Ann Oncol 28(4):874–881. https://doi.org/10.1093/annonc/mdx008

Kanesvaran R, Roy Chowdhury A, Krishna L (2016) Practice pearls in the management of lung cancer in the elderly. J Geriatr Oncol 7(5):362–367. https://doi.org/10.1016/j.jgo.2016.05.004

Keam SJ (2022) Cadonilimab: first approval. Drugs 82(12):1333–1339. https://doi.org/10.1007/s40265-022-01761-9

Kim TW, Burris HA, De Miguel Luken MJ, Pishvaian MJ, Bang Y-J, Gordon M, Awada A, Camidge DR, Hodi FS, McArthur GA, Miller WH, Cervantes A, Chow LQ, Lesokhin AM, Rutten A, Sznol M, Rishipathak D, Chen S-C, Stefanich E et al (2022) First-in-human phase I study of the OX40 agonist MOXR0916 in patients with advanced solid tumors. Clin Cancer Res 28(16):3452–3463. https://doi.org/10.1158/1078-0432.CCR-21-4020

Lahiri A, Maji A, Potdar PD, Singh N, Parikh P, Bisht B, Mukherjee A, Paul MK (2023) Lung cancer immunotherapy: progress, pitfalls, and promises. Mol Cancer 22(1):40. https://doi.org/10.1186/s12943-023-01740-y

Lee CK, Brown C, Gralla RJ, Hirsh V, Thongprasert S, Tsai C-M, Tan EH, Ho JC-M, Chu DT, Zaatar A, Osorio Sanchez JA, Van Vu V, Au JSK, Inoue A, Lee SM, Gebski V, Yang JC-H (2013) Impact of EGFR inhibitor in non-small cell lung cancer on progression-free and overall survival: a meta-analysis. J Natl Cancer Inst 105(9):595–605. https://doi.org/10.1093/jnci/djt072

Mao Y, Yang D, He J, Krasna MJ (2016) Epidemiology of lung cancer. Surg Oncol Clin N Am 25(3):439–445. https://doi.org/10.1016/j.soc.2016.02.001

Nasim F, Sabath BF, Eapen GA (2019) Lung cancer. Med Clin North Am 103(3):463–473. https://doi.org/10.1016/j.mcna.2018.12.006

National Cancer Institute (2016) Drugs approved for lung cancer. National Cancer Institute

Negrao MV, Lam VK, Reuben A, Rubin ML, Landry LL, Roarty EB, Rinsurongkawong W, Lewis J, Roth JA, Swisher SG, Gibbons DL, Wistuba II, Papadimitrakopoulou V, Glisson BS, Blumenschein GR, Lee JJ, Heymach JV, Zhang J (2019) PD-L1 expression, tumor mutational burden, and cancer gene mutations are stronger predictors of benefit from immune checkpoint blockade than HLA class I genotype in non–small cell lung cancer. J Thorac Oncol 14(6):1021–1031. https://doi.org/10.1016/j.jtho.2019.02.008

Nguyen LT, Ohashi PS (2015) Clinical blockade of PD1 and LAG3—potential mechanisms of action. Nat Rev Immunol 15(1):45–56. https://doi.org/10.1038/nri3790

Nooreldeen R, Bach H (2021) Current and future development in lung cancer diagnosis. Int J Mol Sci 22(16):8661. https://doi.org/10.3390/ijms22168661

Ott PA, Hu-Lieskovan S, Chmielowski B, Govindan R, Naing A, Bhardwaj N, Margolin K, Awad MM, Hellmann MD, Lin JJ, Friedlander T, Bushway ME, Balogh KN, Sciuto TE, Kohler V, Turnbull SJ, Besada R, Curran RR, Trapp B et al (2020) A phase Ib trial of personalized neoantigen therapy plus anti-PD-1 in patients with advanced melanoma, non-small cell lung cancer, or bladder cancer. Cell 183(2):347–362.e24. https://doi.org/10.1016/j.cell.2020.08.053

Ozlü T, Bülbül Y (2005) Smoking and lung cancer. Tuberk Toraks 53(2):200–209

Pakkala S, Higgins K, Chen Z, Sica G, Steuer C, Zhang C, Zhang G, Wang S, Hossain MS, Nazha B, Beardslee T, Khuri FR, Curran W, Lonial S, Waller EK, Ramalingam S, Owonikoko TK (2020) Durvalumab and tremelimumab with or without stereotactic body radiation therapy in relapsed small cell lung cancer: a randomized phase II study. J Immunother Cancer 8(2):e001302. https://doi.org/10.1136/jitc-2020-001302

Pardoll DM (2012) The blockade of immune checkpoints in cancer immunotherapy. Nat Rev Cancer 12(4):252–264. https://doi.org/10.1038/nrc3239

Patel SA, Weiss J (2020) Advances in the treatment of non–small cell lung cancer. Clin Chest Med 41(2):237–247. https://doi.org/10.1016/j.ccm.2020.02.010

Philips GK, Atkins M (2015) Therapeutic uses of anti-PD-1 and anti-PD-L1 antibodies. Int Immunol 27(1):39–46. https://doi.org/10.1093/intimm/dxu095

Pockley AG, Vaupel P, Multhoff G (2020) NK cell-based therapeutics for lung cancer. Expert Opin Biol Ther 20(1):23–33. https://doi.org/10.1080/14712598.2020.1688298

Postow MA, Callahan MK, Wolchok JD (2015) Immune checkpoint blockade in cancer therapy. J Clin Oncol 33(17):1974–1982. https://doi.org/10.1200/JCO.2014.59.4358

Ready N, Hellmann MD, Awad MM, Otterson GA, Gutierrez M, Gainor JF, Borghaei H, Jolivet J, Horn L, Mates M, Brahmer J, Rabinowitz I, Reddy PS, Chesney J, Orcutt J, Spigel DR, Reck M, O'Byrne KJ, Paz-Ares L et al (2019) First-line nivolumab plus ipilimumab in advanced non–small-cell lung cancer (CheckMate 568): outcomes by programmed death ligand 1 and tumor mutational burden as biomarkers. J Clin Oncol 37(12):992–1000. https://doi.org/10.1200/JCO.18.01042

Reck M, Remon J, Hellmann MD (2022) First-line immunotherapy for non-small-cell lung cancer. J Clin Oncol 40(6):586–597. https://doi.org/10.1200/JCO.21.01497

Rochigneux P, Lisberg A, Garcia A, Granjeaud S, Madroszyk A, Fattori S, Gonçalves A, Devillier R, Maby P, Salem N, Gorvel L, Chanez B, Gukasyan J, Carroll J, Goldman J, Chretien AS, Olive D, Garon EB (2022) Mass cytometry reveals classical monocytes, NK cells, and ICOS+

CD4+ T cells associated with pembrolizumab efficacy in patients with lung cancer. Clin Cancer Res 28(23):5136–5148. https://doi.org/10.1158/1078-0432.CCR-22-1386

Ruiz-Cordero R, Devine WP (2020) Targeted therapy and checkpoint immunotherapy in lung cancer. Surg Pathol Clin 13(1):17–33. https://doi.org/10.1016/j.path.2019.11.002

Schabath MB, Cote ML (2019) Cancer progress and priorities: lung cancer. Cancer Epidemiol Biomarkers Prev 28(10):1563–1579. https://doi.org/10.1158/1055-9965.EPI-19-0221

Schöffski P, Tan DSW, Martín M, Ochoa-de-Olza M, Sarantopoulos J, Carvajal RD, Kyi C, Esaki T, Prawira A, Akerley W, De Braud F, Hui R, Zhang T, Soo RA, Maur M, Weickhardt A, Krauss J, Deschler-Baier B, Lau A et al (2022) Phase I/II study of the LAG-3 inhibitor ieramilimab (LAG525) ± anti-PD-1 spartalizumab (PDR001) in patients with advanced malignancies. J Immunother Cancer 10(2):e003776. https://doi.org/10.1136/jitc-2021-003776

Shiravand Y, Khodadadi F, Kashani SMA, Hosseini-Fard SR, Hosseini S, Sadeghirad H, Ladwa R, O'Byrne K, Kulasinghe A (2022) Immune checkpoint inhibitors in cancer therapy. Curr Oncol 29(5):3044–3060. https://doi.org/10.3390/curroncol29050247

Skřičková J, Kadlec B, Venclíček O, Merta Z (2018) Lung cancer. Casopis Lekaru Ceskych 157(5):226–236

Starzer AM, Berghoff AS (2019) New emerging targets in cancer immunotherapy: CD27 (TNFRSF7). ESMO Open 4:e000629. https://doi.org/10.1136/esmoopen-2019-000629

Steven A, Fisher SA, Robinson BW (2016) Immunotherapy for lung cancer. Respirology 21(5):821–833. https://doi.org/10.1111/resp.12789

Temel JS, Petrillo LA, Greer JA (2022) Patient-centered palliative care for patients with advanced lung cancer. J Clin Oncol 40(6):626–634. https://doi.org/10.1200/JCO.21.01710

Thai AA, Solomon BJ, Sequist LV, Gainor JF, Heist RS (2021) Lung cancer. Lancet 398(10299):535–554. https://doi.org/10.1016/S0140-6736(21)00312-3

Topalian SL, Drake CG, Pardoll DM (2015) Immune checkpoint blockade: a common denominator approach to cancer therapy. Cancer Cell 27(4):450–461. https://doi.org/10.1016/j.ccell.2015.03.001

Travis WD, Brambilla E, Nicholson AG, Yatabe Y, Austin JHM, Beasley MB, Chirieac LR, Dacic S, Duhig E, Flieder DB, Geisinger K, Hirsch FR, Ishikawa Y, Kerr KM, Noguchi M, Pelosi G, Powell CA, Tsao MS, Wistuba I (2015) The 2015 World Health Organization classification of lung tumors: impact of genetic, clinical and radiologic advances since the 2004 classification. J Thorac Oncol 10(9):1243–1260. https://doi.org/10.1097/JTO.0000000000000630

Van Hall T, André P, Horowitz A, Ruan DF, Borst L, Zerbib R, Narni-Mancinelli E, Van Der Burg SH, Vivier E (2019) Monalizumab: inhibiting the novel immune checkpoint NKG2A. J Immunother Cancer 7(1):263. https://doi.org/10.1186/s40425-019-0761-3

Vinay DS, Kwon BS (2014) 4-1BB (CD137), an inducible costimulatory receptor, as a specific target for cancer therapy. BMB Rep 47(3):122–129. https://doi.org/10.5483/BMBRep.2014.47.3.283

Wang C, Thudium KB, Han M, Wang X-T, Huang H, Feingersh D, Garcia C, Wu Y, Kuhne M, Srinivasan M, Singh S, Wong S, Garner N, Leblanc H, Bunch RT, Blanset D, Selby MJ, Korman AJ (2014) In vitro characterization of the anti-PD-1 antibody nivolumab, BMS-936558, and in vivo toxicology in non-human primates. Cancer Immunol Res 2(9):846–856. https://doi.org/10.1158/2326-6066.CIR-14-0040

Wang Q-T, Nie Y, Sun S-N, Lin T, Han R-J, Jiang J, Li Z, Li J-Q, Xiao Y-P, Fan Y-Y, Yuan X-H, Zhang H, Zhao B-B, Zeng M, Li S-Y, Liao H-X, Zhang J, He Y-W (2020) Tumor-associated antigen-based personalized dendritic cell vaccine in solid tumor patients. Cancer Immunol Immunother 69(7):1375–1387. https://doi.org/10.1007/s00262-020-02496-w

Weber J (2007) Review: anti-CTLA-4 antibody ipilimumab: case studies of clinical response and immune-related adverse events. Oncologist 12(7):864–872. https://doi.org/10.1634/theoncologist.12-7-864

Wei Z, Zhang S, Hu J (2021) CTLA-4 +49 A/G polymorphism and the risk of lung cancer: a meta-analysis. Zhongguo Fei Ai Za Zhi 24(3):173–181. https://doi.org/10.3779/j.issn.1009-3419.2021.102.09

Woodard GA, Jones KD, Jablons DM (2016) Lung cancer staging and prognosis. Cancer Treat Res 170:47–75. https://doi.org/10.1007/978-3-319-40389-2_3

Xiao Z, Mayer AT, Nobashi TW, Gambhir SS (2020) ICOS is an indicator of T-cell–mediated response to cancer immunotherapy. Cancer Res 80(14):3023–3032. https://doi.org/10.1158/0008-5472.CAN-19-3265

Yang R, Sun L, Li C-F, Wang Y-H, Yao J, Li H, Yan M, Chang W-C, Hsu J-M, Cha J-H, Hsu JL, Chou C-W, Sun X, Deng Y, Chou C-K, Yu D, Hung M-C (2021) Galectin-9 interacts with PD-1 and TIM-3 to regulate T cell death and is a target for cancer immunotherapy. Nat Commun 12(1):832. https://doi.org/10.1038/s41467-021-21099-2

Yap TA, Gainor JF, Callahan MK, Falchook GS, Pachynski RK, LoRusso P, Kummar S, Gibney GT, Burris HA, Tykodi SS, Rahma OE, Seiwert TY, Papadopoulos KP, Blum Murphy M, Park H, Hanson A, Hashambhoy-Ramsay Y, McGrath L, Hooper E et al (2022) First-in-human phase I/II ICONIC trial of the ICOS agonist vopratelimab alone and with nivolumab: ICOS-high CD4 T-cell populations and predictors of response. Clin Cancer Res 28(17):3695–3708. https://doi.org/10.1158/1078-0432.CCR-21-4256

Yasinska IM, Sakhnevych SS, Pavlova L, Teo Hansen Selnø A, Teuscher Abeleira AM, Benlaouer O, Gonçalves Silva I, Mosimann M, Varani L, Bardelli M, Hussain R, Siligardi G, Cholewa D, Berger SM, Gibbs BF, Ushkaryov YA, Fasler-Kan E, Klenova E, Sumbayev VV (2019) The Tim-3-Galectin-9 pathway and its regulatory mechanisms in human breast cancer. Front Immunol 10:1594. https://doi.org/10.3389/fimmu.2019.01594

Zatloukal P, Heo DS, Park K, Kang J, Butts C, Bradford D, Graziano S, Huang B, Healey D (2009) Randomized phase II clinical trial comparing tremelimumab (CP-675,206) with best supportive care (BSC) following first-line platinum-based therapy in patients (pts) with advanced non-small cell lung cancer (NSCLC). J Clin Oncol 27(15_suppl):8071. https://doi.org/10.1200/jco.2009.27.15_suppl.8071

Zhang Q, Tang L, Zhou Y, He W, Li W (2021) Immune checkpoint inhibitor-associated pneumonitis in non-small cell lung cancer: current understanding in characteristics, diagnosis, and management. Front Immunol 12:663986. https://doi.org/10.3389/fimmu.2021.663986

Zhang C, Xu L, Ma Y, Huang Y, Zhou L, Le H, Chen Z (2023) Increased TIM-3 expression in tumor-associated macrophages predicts a poorer prognosis in non-small cell lung cancer: a retrospective cohort study. J Thorac Dis 15(3):1433–1444. https://doi.org/10.21037/jtd-23-227

Zhong R, Ling X, Cao S, Xu J, Zhang B, Zhang X, Wang H, Han B, Zhong H (2022) Safety and efficacy of dendritic cell-based immunotherapy (DCVAC/LuCa) combined with carboplatin/pemetrexed for patients with advanced non-squamous non-small-cell lung cancer without oncogenic drivers. ESMO Open 7(1):100334. https://doi.org/10.1016/j.esmoop.2021.100334

Future Perspectives of Cancer Immunotherapy for the Treatment of Lung Cancer

19

Dhruv Sanjay Gupta and Saritha R. Shetty

Abbreviations

AI	Artificial intelligence
CAR-T	Chimeric antigen receptor T
DSTYK	Dual serine/threonine and tyrosine non-receptor protein kinase
EZH2	Enhancer of zeste homolog 2
FOXM1	Forkhead box protein M1
ICIs	Immune checkpoint inhibitors
MDSCs	Myeloid-derived suppressor cells
NSCLC	Non-small cell lung cancer
OTUD6B	Ovarian tumour domain-containing 6B
PD-L1	Programmed death ligand-1
PR C2	Polycomb repressive complex 2
PRKDC	DNA-PK inhibitor
TME	Tumour microenvironment

19.1 Brief Discussion of Evolution of Immunotherapy

Over the last few decades, there has been a massive shift in the conversation for cancer management, from chemotherapy to immunotherapy. It originated as a line of treatment relying on the induction of infections, in order to enhance tumour

D. S. Gupta · S. R. Shetty (✉)
Department of Pharmaceutics, Shobhaben Pratapbhai Patel School of Pharmacy & Technology Management, SVKM's Narsee Monjee Institute of Management Studies (NMIMS) Deemed-to-University, Mumbai, India
e-mail: saritha.shetty@nmims.edu

S. Bhatt et al. (eds.), *Immunotherapy Against Lung Cancer*,
https://doi.org/10.1007/978-981-99-7141-1_19

responses. Immunotherapy may be dated back to the late nineteenth century, with the discovery of the role played by streptococcal infections in patients with osteosarcoma (Říhová and Šťastný 2015). This was a prime example of how an infection caused by a xenobiotic could trigger an immune response and aid cancer management. While the domain of oncolytic virus therapy has been evaluated for its benefits and clinical applications over decades, its efficacy has been observed to decline over time (Kaufman et al. 2015).

With time, there has been a growing interest in the field of cancer immunotherapy. In the 1980, researchers demonstrated the efficacy of interleukins, which are chief inflammatory biomarkers, and natural killer cells in arresting tumorigenesis (Rosenberg 2014). This was the first major advancement in the field, and while several side effects such as toxicity have now been identified, it was a crucial step in leading us to where we stand now.

Coming to the twenty-first century, a prime area of interest has been the blockade of programmed cell death, mediated by programmed death ligand-1 (PD-L1) and several other checkpoints, which have yielded very promising clinical results (Gou et al. 2020). A hallmark in this century, with respect to immunotherapy, has been immune checkpoint blockade, with the first FDA-approved therapy (ipilimumab) being utilised for the management of advanced melanoma (Youssef and Dietrich 2020).

Moving forward, chimeric antigen receptor T (CAR-T) cell therapy has steadily gained attention and originated as a strategy for leukaemia management (Haslauer et al. 2021). Immunotherapy has garnered attention across the world, with several breakthroughs fortifying its importance in clinical settings. With a special focus on lung cancer, the FDA approved two key anti-PD-L1 antibodies, Keytruda (pembrolizumab) (Marcus et al. 2021) and Opdivo (nivolumab), for lung cancer management (Leal and Ramalingam 2022). This paved the way for further research and development, bringing to us pembrolizumab, approved by the FDA in 2016 for the management of non-small cell lung cancer (NSCLC) patients showcasing PD-L1 expression (Forde et al. 2022). Over the years, other monoclonal antibodies such as nivolumab have been approved, owing to their satisfactory safety and efficacy profiles, based on results gathered from clinical trials.

Over the course of the last decade, immunotherapy has gathered attention owing to its usage in conjunction with other treatment strategies. This includes the combination of chemotherapeutic and immunotherapeutic agents, which have demonstrated lowered disease progression and an overall improvement in the quality of life of patients (Yu et al. 2019). This has helped immunotherapy establish its position as a first-line treatment, in combination with chemotherapy, chiefly in the treatment of NSCLC (Mamdani et al. 2022).

As research continues to flourish, there is a need to develop several predictor models for the detection of biomarkers, which may provide an indication of the efficacy and safety of these treatments (Kong et al. 2022). There is a need to conduct a greater number of focused clinical trials, in order to develop a complete understanding of the involvement of different biomarkers. In addition to this, as interest around the tumour microenvironment (TME) and a genomic underlying continues to grow, a greater number of studies would help in the effective utilisation of resources and improve outcomes.

The authors aim to offer an understanding of the future perspectives of immunotherapy, with a focus on recently discovered targets and their scope for clinical translation. In addition to this, the emergence of resistance to immunotherapy and novel measures to tackle the same have been discussed. Any discussion with respect to the future of medical science would be incomplete without delving into the influence of artificial intelligence (AI), which has been explored at length through this chapter. Finally, an understanding of the influence of the microbiome in pathogenesis and combinatorial therapeutic approaches has been presented.

19.2 Discovery of New Checkpoints for Exploration as Targets

In recent years, programmed death ligand-1 (PD-L1) has captured interest as a prominent immunotherapeutic target. However, this target has been found to work best with the management of smaller tumours and has been linked with a variety of adverse effects in various organ systems. This has prompted the need to explore novel targets, some of which are detailed in this section.

The need for exploring newer targets is also boosted by the fact that most NSCLCs have achieved resistance to treatment regimens currently in place. The studies being undertaken recently direct a greater focus on the genomic basis for disease progression, enabling more specific and personalised strategies for lung cancer management. There is a pressing need to explore newer target moieties and identify key biomarkers, which may be used for predictive analysis in clinical settings (Wang et al. 2021b).

A relatively new target, forkhead box protein M1 (FOXM1) bears an association with PD-L1 and has been observed to reduce its expression. In addition to this, studies in animal models have demonstrated its efficacy in arresting cellular proliferation and exerting protective effects on healthy cells. Combined administration with antibiotics and antibodies has been seen to exert synergistic effects, offering a greater number of benefits as opposed to monotherapy, for the management of lung cancer (Madhi et al. 2022).

A study by Valencia et al. aided the identification of DSTYK (dual serine/threonine and tyrosine kinase), which plays an integral role as a dual serine/threonine and tyrosine non-receptor protein kinase. Its increased expression has been linked with a higher rate of morbidity and mortality, creating a need for exploring strategies to effectively target it. Various studies have indicated an improved level of therapeutic sensitivity of lung cancer cells, following the inhibition of this target (Valencia et al. 2022).

Another emerging area of therapeutics is the targeting of chimeric antigen receptor (CAR)-T cells, which effectively modify immune responses and greatly reduce the effects of antigens in furthering cancer spread (Qu et al. 2021). However, there are certain challenges associated with this line of therapy, including problems with penetration, a complex microenvironment and potentials for toxicity (Chen et al. 2022b). There is a need to undertake a greater degree of assessment and develop an optimised therapeutic regimen with fewer side effects.

Researchers have also identified DNA-PK inhibitor (PRKDC) as a potential target, which has been observed to enhance the biological effects of monoclonal antibodies in animal models, with a chief focus on PD-L1. It has been recently explored for its benefits as a biomarker for ICI activity and may be targeted to improve patient outcomes and prolong survival time (Tan et al. 2020).

Folate receptors play a crucial yet overlooked role in cancer management. By becoming binding sites for chemotherapeutic drugs, over time, a vast number of immunotherapeutic agents are useful in the management of cancers showing folate receptor overexpression. In addition to this, they play a vital role in imaging and detecting biomarkers, which when coupled with deep learning technologies and may be used to yield better post-operative management and a lowered tumour burden (Scaranti et al. 2020).

Ovarian tumour domain-containing 6B (OTUD6B) is another new target that is gaining research attention. Interestingly, increased OTUD6B has been seen in a variety of cancers, including lung adenocarcinomas. Designing of therapeutic regimens to bring about its knockdown may be beneficial in limiting the spread of lung cancer and may be used to trigger cellular apoptosis. This is chiefly due to its strong linkage with a variety of genes responsible for catalysing inflammatory responses and immune suppression (Zhao et al. 2022).

An arena that cannot be overlooked is the involvement of myeloid-derived suppressor cells (MDSCs) in the pathogenesis of lung cancer. They have been found to play a role in immune suppression, directly impacting the proliferation and growth of tumours. In addition to this, their overactivity has been linked with an increased propensity for resistance to treatment. Hence, there is a need to effectively target these cells (Yang et al. 2020). By effectively controlling their expression, it is possible to achieve a lowered rate of cellular infiltration, angiogenesis and genetic mutations. However, certain challenges must be overcome in order to maximise the targeting potential, including the largely heterogeneous nature of these cells and a need for greater clinical characterisation (De Cicco et al. 2020). Figure 19.1 encapsulates a few novel targets, for immunotherapeutic agents.

19.3 Discussion of Immunotherapy Resistance and Novel Approaches for Its Management

As previously discussed, PD-L1 has established its clinical significance, with time. While patients have been observed to have benefits in the long run, the onset of resistance complicates treatment, causing them to show signs of disease progression over the course of the treatment or post completion of a treatment cycle (Rolfo et al. 2021). The onset of immunotherapy resistance is complicated by a number of genetic features and lifestyle factors and may be chiefly classified as primary and acquired resistance (Zugazagoitia et al. 2016).

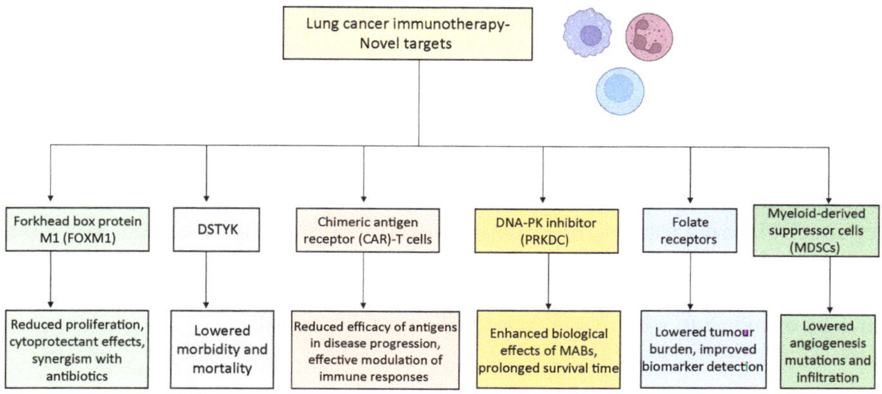

Fig. 19.1 Overview of novel targets for lung cancer immunotherapy

19.3.1 Primary Resistance

Primary resistance chiefly encompasses tumour-related mechanisms, relying on the blockade to the entry of immune cells, into the TME. This causes an initial non-response to therapy, owing to impaired recognition by the T-cells. Primary resistance has been seen to account for up to 27% and 44% resistance cases in the usage of immune checkpoint inhibitors (ICIs) as first- and second-line treatment options (Boyero et al. 2020).

The major mechanisms involved in primary resistance include epigenetic modulation, miRNA dysregulation, disruption in chemokine levels, post-transcription changes and stromal cells (Passaro et al. 2022). One of the most widely observed mechanisms of resistance is epigenetic modulations, which are seen to occur due to reversible genomic changes, which do not involve the disruption of nucleic acid sequences. These changes result in abnormal genetic expression, which in turn accelerates disease progression. These alterations have resulted in impediments to immunotherapy, in malignant cells as well as the body's immune cells. Changes such as methylation may affect the migration of T-cells as well as presentation of antigens to the immune system. Additionally, epigenetic changes may affect the expression of genes responsible for triggering apoptosis (Lahiri et al. 2023).

19.3.2 Secondary Resistance

Acquired resistance, also referred to as secondary resistance, dabbles in factors extrinsic to the tumour. It is chiefly characterised by a successful period of initial response to treatment, followed by the development of resistance, chiefly due to immune evasion of the cells (Chen et al. 2022a). As in the case of PD-L1 blockade, acquired resistance is commonly observed following initial rounds of treatment. However, there is a lack of a clear clinical definition for acquired resistance to immunotherapy. Several scientists and clinicians have undertaken efforts to lay down a clear clinical picture, focusing on exposure of patients to PD-L1 blockade treatment, initial stability and response to therapy, followed by disease progression post discontinuing the therapy (Schoenfeld et al. 2021).

Another explored area of acquired resistance is the resistance to tyrosine kinase inhibitors, especially in the case of patients diagnosed with EGFR (epidermal growth factor receptor) mutant neoplasms. Instances of resistance have been reported following usage as both first- and second-line treatments, indicated by histopathological studies. The most commonly adopted approach to overcoming this type of resistance is the combination of third-generation immunotherapeutic agents such as osimertinib with chemotherapy (Wu and Shih 2018).

19.3.3 Novel Approaches for the Management of Resistance

The discussion of resistance to lung cancer immunotherapy would be incomplete without discussing novel strategies to overcome it. A widely explored strategy has been the usage of nanoparticles, in order to effectively target the tumour microenvironment. Researchers have explored the benefits of loading agents such as cisplatin, gold, siRNA, doxorubicin and immunomodulatory agents, in order to improve the efficacy of immunotherapy (Zhang et al. 2023). Another recommended approach to tackle PD-L1 resistance is the targeting of enhancer of zeste homolog 2 (EZH2), a sub-unit of the polycomb repressive complex 2 (PRC2), through the delivery of oral inhibitory agents. This may be an interesting approach for the management of resistance in tumours at an advanced stage (Shin et al. 2022). The usage of combinatorial strategies has emerged as a promising strategy, with immunotherapeutic agents being combined with angiogenesis inhibitors and metabolic enzyme-targeting agents (Horvath et al. 2020). Keeping with the theme of combined treatment, marked benefits have been reported following the combination of radiotherapy with immunotherapy, chiefly in the improvement of survival and quality of life of patients (Shang et al. 2021). However, there is a need for a greater number of clinical trials to demonstrate the efficacy of these strategies and to permit scaling up and usage at a wider level. The following section discusses the advent of radiomics and deep learning, which may be harnessed in the monitoring of treatment efficacy and potentials for the onset of resistance, as well as suitable strategies for the management of the same.

19.4 Usage of Radiomics and Deep Learning

Radiomics and deep learning have emerged as interesting avenues in furthering our understanding of malignancies. Radiomics has been applied to conventional imaging, in order to provide clinically significant data. This encompasses a thorough description of the nature of tumours, the stage of malignancy and underlying genetic factors (Avanzo et al. 2020).

In a study undertaken by Trebeschi et al., radiomics was employed in order to quantify responses of patients to immunotherapy, chiefly for non-small cell lung cancer (NSCLC). Non-invasive techniques have been developed for biomarker analysis. In the present study, radiomics was used to elucidate the linkage between the cell cycle of cancerous cells and administration of immunotherapeutic agents, based on the lesions assessed (Trebeschi et al. 2019). Tong et al. explored the immune implications of the tumour microenvironment in determining the efficacy of immunotherapy. Following a genomic screening and obtaining results from imaging procedures, a model was developed. This model was observed to yield more robust data than imaging studies alone and gave a clearer picture of the immune modulation brought about by immunotherapeutic interventions (Tong et al. 2022).

Carrying out an analysis of the mutations furthering cellular proliferation may be harnessed in order to obtain a clinical picture of the pharmacological effects of ICIs (immune checkpoint inhibitors). On distinguishing the degree of mutation, He et al. evaluated the survival time to draw a predictive inference with respect to the treatment administered (He et al. 2020). This goes on to show that once certain key factors like the degree of mutation and nature of the lesion are known, deep learning tools may be effectively utilised to make predictive analyses with respect to treatment efficacy. Table 19.1 highlights the recently developed radiomic models for lung cancer, chiefly for predictive analysis. It also encapsulates their clinical implications in disease management.

19.5 Other Potentials for Harnessing AI for Prediction of Clinical Outcomes

Over time, the limitations of administering ICI agents independently have been identified. In an attempt to design more powerful treatment regimens, researchers have tapped into artificial intelligence (AI) tools, for enhancement of treatment outcomes. One major area of application is the identification of specific biomarkers, a process that has been expedited by automation of sample analysis. AI tools may be employed to develop histopathological interpretations and map out complex cellular interactions (Chen et al. 2022c). Neural networks, mimicking the neuronal layout in the brain, have been steadily gaining attention. Li et al. evaluated the overall survival and progression-free survival in patients with squamous cell carcinoma. Using the neural network model developed, the benefits of combinatorial immunotherapeutic approaches were studied (Li et al. 2022a).

Specific biomarkers like programmed cell death ligand-1 (PD-L1), chiefly responsible for inhibition of inflammatory biomarkers and triggering apoptosis, have been assessed using AI models. Cheng et al. used multiple models for biomarker detection and were able to achieve highly accurate results, bearing a significant correlation with those obtained from conventional techniques (Cheng et al. 2022b). This was a key indicative of the robustness of the models developed and potentials for scaling up and clinical translation.

Table 19.1 Overview of recently developed radiomic models and their clinical implications in lung cancer management

Patients/ volunteers	Data assessed	Clinical outcome	Reference
Patients with NSCLC ($n = 139$)	Analysis of CT scans following multiple cycles of ICI administration	On evaluation of the changes in the radiomic texture obtained from the scans, inferences may be drawn with respect to treatment efficiency at initial stages	Khorrami et al. (2020)
Patients with NSCLC ($n = 33$)	Analysis of CT scans of lesions, following ICI therapy	The difference between the initial size of lesions and reduction following therapy may be used to distinguish between various factors influencing disease progression and may aid in identification of critical factors	Barabino et al. (2022)
Patients with NSCLC ($n = 255$)	Assessment of scans obtained pre- and post-treatment	PD-L1 expression was correlated with tumour shrinkage, and a variety of individual related factors such as age and lifestyle factors were evaluated. The development of such a model may be useful in highlighting underlying characteristics contributing to disease progression	Li et al. (2021)
Stage III/stage IV NSCLC patients	CT scans of large tumour obtained before and after three cycles of immunotherapy	A shrinkage in tumour size was correlated with patient survival and was a strong indicator of immunotherapy efficiency (on the basis of the rate of disease progression). The development of such a model could assist individualisation of treatment	Xie et al. (2022)
Patients with NSCLC ($n = 126$)	CT scans of lung tissue	The development of this predictive model aided the distinguishing of pneumonitis caused by chemotherapy and immunotherapy, thereby providing a grounding to clinicians for a sound prognosis	Qiu et al. (2022)
Patients with NSCLC and pneumonitis	CT scans and medical history of patients	This model may assist in narrowing in on the cause of pneumonitis in patients and attributing it to either chemotherapy or immunotherapy, helping to further validate clinical decision-making	Cheng et al. (2022a)

Another noteworthy advancement has been the usage of AI tools in lung cancer management, in the backdrop of the COVID-19 pandemic. They key area of application discussed is the usage of AI technologies to distinguish between the histopathological effects of the virus and those produced by immunotherapy. In addition to this, the advent of AI has facilitated improved recruitment for clinical trials, has paved the way for improved diagnosis and offers higher specificity over traditional detection and imaging methods (Boddu et al. 2022). Mu et al. undertook a non-invasive, AI-assisted analysis of immunotherapeutic efficacy. The analysis was centred around PD-L1 expression, and a measurement of survival time was obtained. Machine learning-based analysis helped in distinguishing between patients showing expression of this biomarker and those who did not, poising it as an alternative to traditionally used biochemical analysis techniques. However, there is a need for a greater number of focused clinical trials to determine the efficiency of these methods and to develop a complete understanding of the extent to which they may be useful (Mu et al. 2021).

While human intervention has been instrumental in diagnosis and designing the most optimum treatment strategies, there is a distinct margin for error. This may primarily be attributed to a large number of samples to be analysed. AI tools have gained acceptance owing to their ease of analysing voluminous data, as well as providing useful insights with respect to the usage of immunotherapeutic agents (Li et al. 2022b). Significant lowering of cost and other resources may be achieved by more effective screening of patients, to deem their fitness for immunotherapy, and this may be achieved by bringing in AI-based screening technologies (Yan et al. 2022).

19.6 Role of Lung Microbiome

Recent advancements have paved the way for broadening our understanding of the role played by the microbiome in cancer progression and management. While the intestinal microbiota has gained precedence owing to its involvement in a large number of metabolic disorders and chronic ailments, there is a need to direct our focus to local microbiomes as well. In the case of lung cancer, there is a significant underlying influence of the mucosal cells, the secretions of which are rich in microbes. These bear specificity and uniqueness to the type of tumour they are present in and respond differently to different treatment measures (Wong-Rolle et al. 2021).

The microbes making up the lung microbiota have been observed to gain entry into the body chiefly through airways and play a mediating role in the release of key biomarkers. Various in vivo studies have pointed to dysbiosis resulting from tumour growth, which may be essential in diagnosis and exploring newer targets for therapy (Dong et al. 2021). In a study undertaken by Tsay et al., dysregulation of the microbial composition in the lower airways upregulates inflammatory biomarkers, such as interleukins. In addition to this, a modulation in the microbial load was seen to accelerate tumorigenesis (Tsay et al. 2021). A major reason why it is important to understand the role played by the lung microbiome in cancer progression is that these microbes regulate immune responses, which in turn influence the trajectory of immunotherapy (Ramírez-Labrada et al. 2020). In terms of their pharmacological effects, the microbes in the respiratory system modulate inflammatory responses and angiogenesis and also play a vital role in controlling migration and further proliferation of cancerous cells. They have also been linked with suppressing the side effects resulting from the administration of antibiotics and immunotherapeutic agents (Wang et al. 2021a).

Oster et al. assessed the impact of helicobacter pylori infestation on immunotherapy outcomes in a mouse model as well as human subjects. It was observed that microbial infection inhibited tumour shrinkage and reduced the overall survival time due to the onset of resistance (Oster et al. 2022). This study was a hallmark in establishing the interplay between tumour growth and microbiota from different parts of the body. Additionally, Tomita et al. established the interplay between the usage of proton pump inhibitors and reduced effects of ICIs. This was effectively tackled using *Clostridium* sp. bacteria, which when administered may improve survival rates and minimise the side effects of other agents administered (Tomita et al. 2022).

19.7 Discussion of Gut Microbiome and Implications with Respect to Lung Cancer Management

A major reason for the growing interest around the gut microbiota, with a special reference co cancer, is the influence of microbial populations on immune system functioning. Various species have been linked with immune memory and maturation of cells, all of which may be crucial in modulating anti-neoplasm responses (Carbone et al. 2019). Liu et al. explored a model centred around important microbial metabolic processes and their role in tumour progression. It was observed that these processes played a significant role in the blockade of various immune checkpoints, necessitating more focused investigation (Liu et al. 2022). However, it is crucial to understand that this relationship is quite intricate and complex, owing to a number of factors. Studies have indicated that some types of bacteria improve clinical responses to the administration of ICIs, indicating potentials for boosting their intestinal population through the administration of probiotics and prebiotics. However, certain types of microbes have shown a negative relation with respect to arresting cancer magnification (Grenda et al. 2022).

It is also essential to develop an overview of the various agents that could influence microbial growth and viability. Certain antibiotics, chemotherapeutic drugs and immunotherapeutic agents influence the sustenance of these microbes. In certain cases, an upregulation is required while populations need to be controlled in certain scenarios. Hence, it is essential to cultivate a thorough understanding of multiple clinical angles, to maximise the benefits offered by these commensals and to minimise any potential harmful effects (Guo et al. 2022).

A study undertaken by Chau et al. made use of predictive analysis to distinguish between the microbial compositions of healthy volunteers and patients with lung cancer. In addition to this, the response to immunotherapeutic drugs was monitored in each case, and a strong interplay of microbial populations in different body sites was found. However, a common recommendation in several such studies undertaken is the need for a greater number of clinical studies, with larger more diverse populations, as well as preliminary testing in animal models (Chau et al. 2021).

Cancer researchers across the globe are dedicated to studying the effects of toxicity of immunotherapeutic agents, as well as potentials for the onset of resistance in chronic therapy, which may be key determinants of progression-free survival and in improving the overall quality of life of patients (Bredin and Naidoo 2022). Owing to the differences in individual genetic makeup and the need for personalised medicine, especially for immunotherapy, has prompted the need to closely monitor the effects of the microbiome on inflammatory responses and immune functioning (Zhou et al. 2019). The usage of ICIs has revolutionised immunotherapy and specialised cancer medicine. However, to ensure that the greatest possible extent of clinical benefits is obtained, there is a need to direct a focus on microbial populations, which are robust predictors of the specificity and sensitivity of treatments administered (Shaikh et al. 2019).

19.8 Discussion of Current Pitfalls and Future Scope

Moving forward, there is a need to direct a greater focus on combinatorial treatment strategies, to reduce the possibility of resistance and improve clinical outcomes. Immunotherapy has been explored in combination with radiotherapy, chiefly in early stages of the disease, to arrest tumour growth (Wirsdörfer et al. 2018). Radiotherapy adds the benefit of providing treatment to patients with inoperable tumours or in the case of local disease advancements. In addition to providing local benefits, it offers systemic benefits as well. The results from a number of studies have elucidated its influence on the tumour microenvironment, with synergism recorded in combination with immunotherapeutic agents, to enhance treatment outcomes (Ko et al. 2018). Radiotherapy has been combined with a number of FDA-approved immunotherapeutic agents, such as pembrolizumab and nivolumab, to control cellular proliferation. However, there is a need to validate these results through a greater number of clinical trials, chiefly phase III clinical trials in diverse populations (Theelen et al. 2021). Following promising results from studies and the demonstration of a satisfactory safety profile (Geng et al. 2021), a greater number of approved agents have been integrated into regimens, including durvalumab as maintenance therapy, and atezolizumab, supported by promising results of combinatorial administration (Agrawal et al. 2021). However, a key strategy to improving outcomes is the personalisation of immunotherapy. Its functioning is intrinsically complicated by a number of factors, as previously discussed, and the personalisation of medicine through machine learning and deep learning technologies is certainly the way forward (Bogart et al. 2022).

Another interesting avenue of research has been the applications of nanomedicine, in overcoming resistance and challenges to delivery. It has enabled researchers to effectively modulate microenvironmental conditions and use them for therapeutic benefits (Ovais et al. 2020). Nanoparticles have steadily gained attention owing to the protective effects offered to the agents to be delivered and have enabled specification of targeting (Chiang et al. 2018). Various nanotechnological platforms, such as vaccines (Butts et al. 2011) and liposomes, have been explored for their benefits (Doroudian et al. 2023). However, the scalability of these delivery systems remains a major challenge and must be addressed to maximise potentials.

It is important to understand, however, that immunotherapy is still in its nascent stages of development, and its standardisation is a major challenge, owing to different requirements of patients. As a result, a greater number of studies are required to monitor the pharmacokinetic and pharmacodynamic profiles of these agents (Sanmamed et al. 2016). With the advent of AI, there is a scope for personalisation of therapy, and this may be harnessed to keep up with the dynamism of the tumour microenvironment (Lapuente-Santana et al. 2021). Each therapeutic regimen comes with the risk of adverse effects, and it is important to understand those pertinent to immunotherapy. Reports from clinical trials have indicated rashes, oedema, overactivity of the immune system and pain as a few side effects (Haanen et al. 2017), and these must be duly looked into, in order to bring about a minimisation in their occurrence. The results obtained from research and experimentation so far have yielded promising results for the future of immunotherapy, and it is poised to grow exponentially in the years to come.

References

Agrawal V, Benjamin KT, Ko EC (2021) Radiotherapy and immunotherapy combinations for lung cancer. Curr Oncol Rep 23(1):4. https://doi.org/10.1007/s11912-020-00993-w

Avanzo M, Stancanello J, Pirrone G, Sartor G (2020) Radiomics and deep learning in lung cancer. Strahlenther Onkol 196(10):879–887. https://doi.org/10.1007/s00066-020-01625-9

Barabino E, Rossi G, Pamparino S, Fiannacca M, Caprioli S, Fedeli A, Zullo L, Vagge S, Cittadini G, Genova C (2022) Exploring response to immunotherapy in non-small cell lung cancer using Delta-radiomics. Cancers 14(2):350. https://doi.org/10.3390/cancers14020350

Boddu RSK, Karmakar P, Bhaumik A, Nassa VK, Vandana, Bhattacharya S (2022) Analyzing the impact of machine learning and artificial intelligence and its effect on management of lung cancer detection in covid-19 pandemic. Mater Today Proc 56:2213–2216. https://doi.org/10.1016/j.matpr.2021.11.549

Bogart JA, Waqar SN, Mix MD (2022) Radiation and systemic therapy for limited-stage small-cell lung cancer. J Clin Oncol 40(6):661–670. https://doi.org/10.1200/JCO.21.01639

Boyero L, Sánchez-Gastaldo A, Alonso M, Noguera-Uclés JF, Molina-Pinelo S, Bernabé-Caro R (2020) Primary and acquired resistance to immunotherapy in lung cancer: unveiling the mechanisms underlying of immune checkpoint blockade therapy. Cancers 12(12):3729. https://doi.org/10.3390/cancers12123729

Bredin P, Naidoo J (2022) The gut microbiome, immune check point inhibition and immune-related adverse events in non-small cell lung cancer. Cancer Metastasis Rev 41(2):347–366. https://doi.org/10.1007/s10555-022-10039-1

Butts C, Maksymiuk A, Goss G, Soulières D, Marshall E, Cormier Y, Ellis PM, Price A, Sawhney R, Beier F, Falk M, Murray N (2011) Updated survival analysis in patients with stage IIIB or IV non-small-cell lung cancer receiving BLP25 liposome vaccine (L-BLP25): phase IIB randomized, multicenter, open-label trial. J Cancer Res Clin Oncol 137(9):1337–1342. https://doi.org/10.1007/s00432-011-1003-3

Carbone C, Piro G, Di Noia V, D'Argento E, Vita E, Ferrara MG, Pilotto S, Milella M, Cammarota G, Gasbarrini A, Tortora G, Bria E (2019) Lung and gut microbiota as potential hidden driver of immunotherapy efficacy in lung cancer. Mediat Inflamm 2019:1–10. https://doi.org/10.1155/2019/7652014

Chau J, Yadav M, Liu B, Furqan M, Dai Q, Shahi S, Gupta A, Mercer KN, Eastman E, Hejleh TA, Chan C, Weiner GJ, Cherwin C, Lee STM, Zhong C, Mangalam A, Zhang J (2021) Prospective correlation between the patient microbiome with response to and development of immune-mediated adverse effects to immunotherapy in lung cancer. BMC Cancer 21(1):808. https://doi.org/10.1186/s12885-021-08530-z

Chen Y, Chen Z, Chen R, Fang C, Zhang C, Ji M, Yang X (2022a) Immunotherapy-based combination strategies for treatment of EGFR-TKI-resistant non-small-cell lung cancer. Future Oncol 18(14):1757–1775. https://doi.org/10.2217/fon-2021-0862

Chen L, Chen F, Li J, Pu Y, Yang C, Wang Y, Lei Y, Huang Y (2022b) CAR-T cell therapy for lung cancer: potential and perspective. Thorac Cancer 13(7):889–899. https://doi.org/10.1111/1759-7714.14375

Chen P, Zhang J, Wu J (2022c) Artificial intelligence in digital pathology to advance cancer immunotherapy. 21 Century Pathol 2(3):120

Cheng J, Pan Y, Huang W, Huang K, Cui Y, Hong W, Wang L, Ni D, Tan P (2022a) Differentiation between immune checkpoint inhibitor-related and radiation pneumonitis in lung cancer by CT radiomics and machine learning. Med Phys 49(3):1547–1558. https://doi.org/10.1002/mp.15451

Cheng G, Zhang F, Xing Y, Hu X, Zhang H, Chen S, Li M, Peng C, Ding G, Zhang D, Chen P, Xia Q, Wu M (2022b) Artificial intelligence-assisted score analysis for predicting the expression of the immunotherapy biomarker PD-L1 in lung cancer. Front Immunol 13:893198. https://doi.org/10.3389/fimmu.2022.893198

Chiang C-S, Lin Y-J, Lee R, Lai Y-H, Cheng H-W, Hsieh C-H, Shyu W-C, Chen S-Y (2018) Combination of fucoidan-based magnetic nanoparticles and immunomodulators enhances tumour-localized immunotherapy. Nat Nanotechnol 13(8):746–754. https://doi.org/10.1038/s41565-018-0146-7

De Cicco P, Ercolano G, Ianaro A (2020) The new era of cancer immunotherapy: targeting myeloid-derived suppressor cells to overcome immune evasion. Front Immunol 11:1680. https://doi.org/10.3389/fimmu.2020.01680

Dong Q, Chen ES, Zhao C, Jin C (2021) Host-microbiome interaction in lung cancer. Front Immunol 12:679829. https://doi.org/10.3389/fimmu.2021.679829

Doroudian M, Zanganeh S, Abbasgholinejad E, Donnelly SC (2023) Nanomedicine in lung cancer immunotherapy. Front Bioeng Biotechnol 11:1144653. https://doi.org/10.3389/fbioe.2023.1144653

Forde PM, Spicer J, Lu S, Provencio M, Mitsudomi T, Awad MM, Felip E, Broderick SR, Brahmer JR, Swanson SJ, Kerr K, Wang C, Ciuleanu T-E, Saylors GB, Tanaka F, Ito H, Chen K-N, Liberman M, Vokes EE et al (2022) Neoadjuvant nivolumab plus chemotherapy in resectable lung cancer. N Engl J Med 386(21):1973–1985. https://doi.org/10.1056/NEJMoa2202170

Geng Y, Zhang Q, Feng S, Li C, Wang L, Zhao X, Yang Z, Li Z, Luo H, Liu R, Lu B, Wang X (2021) Safety and efficacy of PD-1/PD-L1 inhibitors combined with radiotherapy in patients with non-small-cell lung cancer: a systematic review and meta-analysis. Cancer Med 10(4):1222–1239. https://doi.org/10.1002/cam4.3718

Gou Q, Dong C, Xu H, Khan B, Jin J, Liu Q, Shi J, Hou Y (2020) PD-L1 degradation pathway and immunotherapy for cancer. Cell Death Dis 11(11):955. https://doi.org/10.1038/s41419-020-03140-2

Grenda A, Iwan E, Chmielewska I, Krawczyk P, Giza A, Bomba A, Frąk M, Rolska A, Szczyrek M, Kieszko R, Kucharczyk T, Jarosz B, Wasyl D, Milanowski J (2022) Presence of Akkermansiaceae in gut microbiome and immunotherapy effectiveness in patients with advanced non-small cell lung cancer. AMB Express 12(1):86. https://doi.org/10.1186/s13568-022-01428-4

Guo H, Zhao L, Zhu J, Chen P, Wang H, Jiang M, Liu X, Sun H, Zhao W, Zheng Z, Li W, Chen B, Fang Q, Yang M, He Y, Yang Y (2022) Microbes in lung cancer initiation, treatment, and outcome: boon or bane? Semin Cancer Biol 86:1190–1206. https://doi.org/10.1016/j.semcancer.2021.05.025

Haanen JBAG, Carbonnel F, Robert C, Kerr KM, Peters S, Larkin J, Jordan K (2017) Management of toxicities from immunotherapy: ESMO Clinical Practice Guidelines for diagnosis, treatment and follow-up. Ann Oncol 28:iv119–iv142. https://doi.org/10.1093/annonc/mdx225

Haslauer T, Greil R, Zaborsky N, Geisberger R (2021) CAR T-cell therapy in hematological malignancies. Int J Mol Sci 22(16):8996. https://doi.org/10.3390/ijms22168996

He B, Dong D, She Y, Zhou C, Fang M, Zhu Y, Zhang H, Huang Z, Jiang T, Tian J, Chen C (2020) Predicting response to immunotherapy in advanced non-small-cell lung cancer using tumor mutational burden radiomic biomarker. J Immunother Cancer 8(2):e000550. https://doi.org/10.1136/jitc-2020-000550

Horvath L, Thienpont B, Zhao L, Wolf D, Pircher A (2020) Overcoming immunotherapy resistance in non-small cell lung cancer (NSCLC)—novel approaches and future outlook. Mol Cancer 19(1):141. https://doi.org/10.1186/s12943-020-01260-z

Kaufman HL, Kohlhapp FJ, Zloza A (2015) Oncolytic viruses: a new class of immunotherapy drugs. Nat Rev Drug Discov 14(9):642–662. https://doi.org/10.1038/nrd4663

Khorrami M, Prasanna P, Gupta A, Patil P, Velu PD, Thawani R, Corredor G, Alilou M, Bera K, Fu P, Feldman M, Velcheti V, Madabhushi A (2020) Changes in CT radiomic features associated with lymphocyte distribution predict overall survival and response to immunotherapy in non–small cell lung cancer. Cancer Immunol Res 8(1):108–119. https://doi.org/10.1158/2326-6066.CIR-19-0476

Ko EC, Raben D, Formenti SC (2018) The integration of radiotherapy with immunotherapy for the treatment of non–small cell lung cancer. Clin Cancer Res 24(23):5792–5806. https://doi.org/10.1158/1078-0432.CCR-17-3620

Kong J, Ha D, Lee J, Kim I, Park M, Im S-H, Shin K, Kim S (2022) Network-based machine learning approach to predict immunotherapy response in cancer patients. Nat Commun 13(1):3703. https://doi.org/10.1038/s41467-022-31535-6

Lahiri A, Maji A, Potdar PD, Singh N, Parikh P, Bisht B, Mukherjee A, Paul MK (2023) Lung cancer immunotherapy: progress, pitfalls, and promises. Mol Cancer 22(1):40. https://doi.org/10.1186/s12943-023-01740-y

Lapuente-Santana Ó, Van Genderen M, Hilbers PAJ, Finotello F, Eduati F (2021) Interpretable systems biomarkers predict response to immune-checkpoint inhibitors. Patterns 2(8):100293. https://doi.org/10.1016/j.patter.2021.100293

Leal TA, Ramalingam SS (2022) Neoadjuvant therapy gains FDA approval in non-small cell lung cancer. Cell Rep Med 3(7):100691. https://doi.org/10.1016/j.xcrm.2022.100691

Li J, Ge S, Sang S, Hu C, Deng S (2021) Evaluation of PD-L1 expression level in patients with non-small cell lung cancer by 18F-FDG PET/CT radiomics and clinicopathological characteristics. Front Oncol 11:789014. https://doi.org/10.3389/fonc.2021.789014

Li S, Li W, Ma T, Fu S, Gao X, Qin N, Wu Y, Zhang X, Wang J, Pan Y, Liu Z (2022a) Assessing the efficacy of immunotherapy in lung squamous carcinoma using artificial intelligence neural network. Front Immunol 13:1024707. https://doi.org/10.3389/fimmu.2022.1024707

Li Y, Wu X, Yang P, Jiang G, Luo Y (2022b) Machine learning for lung cancer diagnosis, treatment, and prognosis. Genomics Proteomics Bioinformatics 20(5):850–866. https://doi.org/10.1016/j.gpb.2022.11.003

Liu B, Chau J, Dai Q, Zhong C, Zhang J (2022) Exploring gut microbiome in predicting the efficacy of immunotherapy in non-small cell lung cancer. Cancers 14(21):5401. https://doi.org/10.3390/cancers14215401

Madhi H, Lee J, Choi YE, Li Y, Kim MH, Choi Y, Goh S (2022) FOXM1 inhibition enhances the therapeutic outcome of lung cancer immunotherapy by modulating PD-L1 expression and cell proliferation. Adv Sci 9(29):2202702. https://doi.org/10.1002/advs.202202702

Mamdani H, Matosevic S, Khalid AB, Durm G, Jalal SI (2022) Immunotherapy in lung cancer: current landscape and future directions. Front Immunol 13:823618. https://doi.org/10.3389/fimmu.2022.823618

Marcus L, Fashoyin-Aje LA, Donoghue M, Yuan M, Rodriguez L, Gallagher PS, Philip R, Ghosh S, Theoret MR, Beaver JA, Pazdur R, Lemery SJ (2021) FDA approval summary: pembrolizumab for the treatment of tumor mutational burden–high solid tumors. Clin Cancer Res 27(17):4685–4689. https://doi.org/10.1158/1078-0432.CCR-21-0327

Mu W, Jiang L, Shi Y, Tunali I, Gray JE, Katsoulakis E, Tian J, Gillies RJ, Schabath MB (2021) Non-invasive measurement of PD-L1 status and prediction of immunotherapy response using deep learning of PET/CT images. J Immunother Cancer 9(6):e002118. https://doi.org/10.1136/jitc-2020-002118

Oster P, Vaillant L, Riva E, McMillan B, Begka C, Truntzer C, Richard C, Leblond MM, Messaoudene M, Machremi E, Limagne E, Ghiringhelli F, Routy B, Verdeil G, Velin D (2022) *Helicobacter pylori* infection has a detrimental impact on the efficacy of cancer immunotherapies. Gut 71(3):457–466. https://doi.org/10.1136/gutjnl-2020-323392

Ovais M, Mukherjee S, Pramanik A, Das D, Mukherjee A, Raza A, Chen C (2020) Designing stimuli-responsive upconversion nanoparticles that exploit the tumor microenvironment. Adv Mater 32(22):2000055. https://doi.org/10.1002/adma.202000055

Passaro A, Brahmer J, Antonia S, Mok T, Peters S (2022) Managing resistance to immune checkpoint inhibitors in lung cancer: treatment and novel strategies. J Clin Oncol 40(6):598–610. https://doi.org/10.1200/JCO.21.01845

Qiu Q, Xing L, Wang Y, Feng A, Wen Q (2022) Development and validation of a radiomics nomogram using computed tomography for differentiating immune checkpoint inhibitor-related pneumonitis from radiation pneumonitis for patients with non-small cell lung cancer. Front Immunol 13:870842. https://doi.org/10.3389/fimmu.2022.870842

Qu J, Mei Q, Chen L, Zhou J (2021) Chimeric antigen receptor (CAR)-T-cell therapy in non-small-cell lung cancer (NSCLC): current status and future perspectives. Cancer Immunol Immunother 70(3):619–631. https://doi.org/10.1007/s00262-020-02735-0

Ramírez-Labrada AG, Isla D, Artal A, Arias M, Rezusta A, Pardo J, Gálvez EM (2020) The influence of lung microbiota on lung carcinogenesis, immunity, and immunotherapy. Trends Cancer 6(2):86–97. https://doi.org/10.1016/j.trecan.2019.12.007

Říhová B, Šťastný M (2015) [History of immuno-therapy—from coley toxins to check-points of the immune reaction]. Klin Onkol 28(Suppl. 4):4S8–4S14

Rolfo C, Ordóñez-Reyes C, Cardona AF (2021) Immunotherapy resistance in non-small cell lung cancer: a Rubik's cube to assemble. J Immunother Precis Oncol 4(4):185–188. https://doi.org/10.36401/JIPO-21-7

Rosenberg SA (2014) IL-2: the first effective immunotherapy for human cancer. J Immunol 192(12):5451–5458. https://doi.org/10.4049/jimmunol.1490019

Sanmamed MF, Chester C, Melero I, Kohrt H (2016) Defining the optimal murine models to investigate immune checkpoint blockers and their combination with other immunotherapies. Ann Oncol 27(7):1190–1198. https://doi.org/10.1093/annonc/mdw041

Scaranti M, Cojocaru E, Banerjee S, Banerji U (2020) Exploiting the folate receptor α in oncology. Nat Rev Clin Oncol 17(6):349–359. https://doi.org/10.1038/s41571-020-0339-5

Schoenfeld AJ, Antonia SJ, Awad MM, Felip E, Gainor J, Gettinger SN, Hodi FS, Johnson ML, Leighl NB, Lovly CM, Mok T, Perol M, Reck M, Solomon B, Soria J-C, Tan DSW, Peters S, Hellmann MD (2021) Clinical definition of acquired resistance to immunotherapy in patients with metastatic non-small-cell lung cancer. Ann Oncol 32(12):1597–1607. https://doi.org/10.1016/j.annonc.2021.08.2151

Shaikh FY, Gills JJ, Sears CL (2019) Impact of the microbiome on checkpoint inhibitor treatment in patients with non-small cell lung cancer and melanoma. EBioMedicine 48:642–647. https://doi.org/10.1016/j.ebiom.2019.08.076

Shang S, Liu J, Verma V, Wu M, Welsh J, Yu J, Chen D (2021) Combined treatment of non-small cell lung cancer using radiotherapy and immunotherapy: challenges and updates. Cancer Commun 41(11):1086–1099. https://doi.org/10.1002/cac2.12226

Shin DS, Park K, Garon E, Dubinett S (2022) Targeting EZH2 to overcome the resistance to immunotherapy in lung cancer. Semin Oncol 49(3–4):306–318. https://doi.org/10.1053/j.seminoncol.2022.06.005

Tan KT, Yeh C-N, Chang Y-C, Cheng J-H, Fang W-L, Yeh Y-C, Wang Y-C, Hsu DS-S, Wu C-E, Lai J-I, Chang PM-H, Chen M-H, Lu M-L, Chen S-J, Chao Y, Hsiao M, Chen M-H (2020) *PRKDC*: new biomarker and drug target for checkpoint blockade immunotherapy. J Immunother Cancer 8(1):e000485. https://doi.org/10.1136/jitc-2019-000485

Theelen WSME, Chen D, Verma V, Hobbs BP, Peulen HMU, Aerts JGJV, Bahce I, Niemeijer ALN, Chang JY, de Groot PM, Nguyen Q-N, Comeaux NI, Simon GR, Skoulidis F, Lin SH, He K, Patel R, Heymach J, Baas P, Welsh JW (2021) Pembrolizumab with or without radiotherapy

for metastatic non-small-cell lung cancer: a pooled analysis of two randomised trials. Lancet Respir Med 9(5):467–475. https://doi.org/10.1016/S2213-2600(20)30391-X
Tomita Y, Goto Y, Sakata S, Imamura K, Minemura A, Oka K, Hayashi A, Jodai T, Akaike K, Anai M, Hamada S, Iyama S, Saruwatari K, Saeki S, Takahashi M, Ikeda T, Sakagami T (2022) *Clostridium butyricum* therapy restores the decreased efficacy of immune checkpoint blockade in lung cancer patients receiving proton pump inhibitors. OncoImmunology 11(1):2081010. https://doi.org/10.1080/2162402X.2022.2081010
Tong H, Sun J, Fang J, Zhang M, Liu H, Xia R, Zhou W, Liu K, Chen X (2022) A machine learning model based on PET/CT radiomics and clinical characteristics predicts tumor immune profiles in non-small cell lung cancer: a retrospective multicohort study. Front Immunol 13:859323. https://doi.org/10.3389/fimmu.2022.859323
Trebeschi S, Drago SG, Birkbak NJ, Kurilova I, Călin AM, Delli Pizzi A, Lalezari F, Lambregts DMJ, Rohaan MW, Parmar C, Rozeman EA, Hartemink KJ, Swanton C, Haanen JBAG, Blank CU, Smit EF, Beets-Tan RGH, Aerts HJWL (2019) Predicting response to cancer immunotherapy using noninvasive radiomic biomarkers. Ann Oncol 30(6):998–1004. https://doi.org/10.1093/annonc/mdz108
Tsay J-CJ, Wu BG, Sulaiman I, Gershner K, Schluger R, Li Y, Yie T-A, Meyn P, Olsen E, Perez L, Franca B, Carpenito J, Iizumi T, El-Ashmawy M, Badri M, Morton JT, Shen N, He L, Michaud G et al (2021) Lower airway dysbiosis affects lung cancer progression. Cancer Discov 11(2):293–307. https://doi.org/10.1158/2159-8290.CD-20-0263
Valencia K, Echepare M, Teijeira Á, Pasquier A, Bértolo C, Sainz C, Tamayo I, Picabea B, Bosco G, Thomas R, Agorreta J, López-Picazo JM, Frigola J, Amat R, Calvo A, Felip E, Melero I, Montuenga LM (2022) DSTYK inhibition increases the sensitivity of lung cancer cells to T cell–mediated cytotoxicity. J Exp Med 219(12):e20220726. https://doi.org/10.1084/jem.20220726
Wang D, Cheng J, Zhang J, Zhou F, He X, Shi Y, Tao Y (2021a) The role of respiratory microbiota in lung cancer. Int J Biol Sci 17(13):3646–3658. https://doi.org/10.7150/ijbs.51376
Wang M, Herbst RS, Boshoff C (2021b) Toward personalized treatment approaches for non-small-cell lung cancer. Nat Med 27(8):1345–1356. https://doi.org/10.1038/s41591-021-01450-2
Wirsdörfer F, De Leve S, Jendrossek V (2018) Combining radiotherapy and immunotherapy in lung cancer: can we expect limitations due to altered Normal tissue toxicity? Int J Mol Sci 20(1):24. https://doi.org/10.3390/ijms20010024
Wong-Rolle A, Wei HK, Zhao C, Jin C (2021) Unexpected guests in the tumor microenvironment: microbiome in cancer. Protein Cell 12(5):426–435. https://doi.org/10.1007/s13238-020-00813-8
Wu S-G, Shih J-Y (2018) Management of acquired resistance to EGFR TKI–targeted therapy in advanced non-small cell lung cancer. Mol Cancer 17(1):38. https://doi.org/10.1186/s12943-018-0777-1
Xie D, Xu F, Zhu W, Pu C, Huang S, Lou K, Wu Y, Huang D, He C, Hu H (2022) Delta radiomics model for the prediction of progression-free survival time in advanced non-small-cell lung cancer patients after immunotherapy. Front Oncol 12:990608. https://doi.org/10.3389/fonc.2022.990608
Yan W, Tang X, Wang L, He C, Cui X, Yuan S, Zhang H (2022) Applicability analysis of immunotherapy for lung cancer patients based on deep learning. Methods 205:149–156. https://doi.org/10.1016/j.ymeth.2022.07.004
Yang Z, Guo J, Weng L, Tang W, Jin S, Ma W (2020) Myeloid-derived suppressor cells—new and exciting players in lung cancer. J Hematol Oncol 13(1):10. https://doi.org/10.1186/s13045-020-0843-1
Youssef G, Dietrich J (2020) Ipilimumab: an investigational immunotherapy for glioblastoma. Expert Opin Investig Drugs 29(11):1187–1193. https://doi.org/10.1080/13543784.2020.1826436
Yu W-D, Sun G, Li J, Xu J, Wang X (2019) Mechanisms and therapeutic potentials of cancer immunotherapy in combination with radiotherapy and/or chemotherapy. Cancer Lett 452:66–70. https://doi.org/10.1016/j.canlet.2019.02.048

Zhang X, Wang X, Hou L, Xu Z, Liu Y, Wang X (2023) Nanoparticles overcome adaptive immune resistance and enhance immunotherapy via targeting tumor microenvironment in lung cancer. Front Pharmacol 14:1130937. https://doi.org/10.3389/fphar.2023.1130937
Zhao G, Song D, Wu J, Yang S, Shi S, Cui X, Ren H, Zhang B (2022) Identification of OTUD6B as a new biomarker for prognosis and immunotherapy by pan-cancer analysis. Front Immunol 13:955091. https://doi.org/10.3389/fimmu.2022.955091
Zhou H, Suo J, Zhu J (2019) [Therapeutic relevance of human microbiota and lung cancer]. Zhongguo Fei Ai Za Zhi 22(7):464–469. https://doi.org/10.3779/j.issn.1009-3419.2019.07.09
Zugazagoitia J, Guedes C, Ponce S, Ferrer I, Molina-Pinelo S, Paz-Ares L (2016) Current challenges in cancer treatment. Clin Ther 38(7):1551–1566. https://doi.org/10.1016/j.clinthera.2016.03.026

MIX
Papier aus verantwortungsvollen Quellen
Paper from responsible sources
FSC® C105338

If you have any concerns about our products,
you can contact us on
ProductSafety@springernature.com

In case Publisher is established outside the EU,
the EU authorized representative is:
Springer Nature Customer Service Center GmbH
Europaplatz 3, 69115 Heidelberg, Germany

Printed by Libri Plureos GmbH
in Hamburg, Germany